OLYMPIC WEIGHTLIFTING
A Complete Guide for Athletes & Coaches

Third Edition

GREG EVERETT

Catalyst Athletics

APOD
2018 Revised Edition

ISBN 978-0-9907985-4-5

Catalyst Athletics, Inc
www.catalystathletics.com

Anatomical illustrations by Glen Oomen

Publisher's Cataloging-in-Publication
(Provided by Quality Books, Inc.)

    Everett, Greg, author.
       Olympic weightlifting : a complete guide for athletes
    & coaches / Greg Everett. -- Third edition.
       pages cm
       Includes bibliographical references and index.
       ISBN 978-0-9907985-4-5

       1. Weight lifting. 2. Weight lifting--Coaching.
    3. Olympics.   I. Title.

    GV546.3.E84 2015   796.41
                    QBI15-600186

Contents

The Jerk

Error Correction

Program Design & Training

Acknowledgments

I feel compelled to first recognize the achievements and contributions to weightlifting of the coaches and athletes who have come before me. My respect for these individuals is limitless, whether or not we agree on any given topic, because of their passion, commitment, and their work in and out of the gym that has propelled the development of training and coaching methodology. Without these individuals, I would not have had the opportunities that have allowed me to reach this point.

Coach Mike Burgener has been particularly important to my education as my first weightlifting coach and mentor. Without him and his generosity, it's likely this book wouldn't exist. I would also like to thank coaches Bob Morris, John Thrush, Jim Schmitz and Bob Takano in particular for the things I've learned from them and their support in various capacities of both me and this book since its original publication, although many other coaches have been helpful and supportive along the way. I hope you know who you are.

Of course, thank you to all of my weightlifters, on whom I get to experiment and through the coaching of whom I'm able to continue to learn, as well as for allowing me to use photographs of you throughout this book.

My wife Aimee deserves a great deal of gratitude for her support of my absurd choice to try to make a living on the creation of educational material for an obscure and impoverished sport, and for helping me in too many ways to enumerate to accomplish what I have. I also want to thank my daughter Jade for enduring numerous weightlifting competitions and many hours in the gym, and for understanding my often long work hours.

Finally, thank you to Robb Wolf and Nicki Violetti of NorCal Strength & Conditioning for bringing me into their gym years ago and convincing me I could in fact earn a living doing what I love.

Introduction to the Third Edition

It's been eight years since I originally released *Olympic Weightlifting: A Complete Guide for Athletes & Coaches*. In this time, it has become and remained the most successful book on the topic in the world. However, as a coach, I am continually learning through my work with my weightlifters and interactions with other successful coaches, and as a consequence, my approaches to various elements of lifting or coaching, my thoughts on certain elements of program design and training, and my opinions regarding the management of lifters of all types are somewhat fluid. Additionally, in these years I've been able to learn how well information in the previous edition was conveyed to readers, where confusion was common, and what new popular information and practices need to be addressed, and have made appropriate changes to improve clarity in these instances.

This newest edition reflects these alterations, none of which are particularly dramatic and certainly not contradictory to anything in previous versions. Additionally, I have taken advantage of the opportunity to improve the way the information is organized and presented to maximize its utility and accessibility. I have added significantly more information, with new chapters as well as expansion of existing material, and components to improve the book's use as a reference, such as an index, a glossary, more tables and additional section headings. Finally, photographs and illustrations have been improved to ensure the best possible communication of the concepts in the text.

I'm incredibly grateful to all of the readers of this book who have supported me and Catalyst Athletics through the years and allowed us to grow into such a dominant source of information and education for the sport of weightlifting. I hope that my continued efforts to provide more and better information, like this new edition of the book, will be adequate expressions of my gratitude.

—Greg Everett, January 2016

How to Use This Book

The size of this book may be daunting to some readers, but I have gone to considerable lengths to present the material in an organized, rational fashion, as well as include helpful summaries and simplifications along the way, to make it as accessible and useful as possible to readers of all levels of experience. The book has changed significantly since its original release in 2008 to continue improving upon this intention.

The book as a whole is a single continuous progression, beginning with a foundation of fundamentals and building to the finer details of execution and principles. As much as possible, I have tried to avoid redundancy by presenting universal principles at a single point and then expanding upon them in ways specific to a given lift later, and later sections often build on information presented in preceding sections. It's consequently recommended that the book be read start to finish initially, and then specific sections returned to as desired or needed.

I have provided summaries throughout the book as a way of concisely presenting the most important points in each section for two basic reasons: First, to help reinforce what has been read, and second, to provide a simplified system for the less experienced lifter or coach to focus on practical information that can be implemented immediately. This progression of summaries can be found in its own section at the end of the book for quick reference.

If you're a beginner, either as a lifter or a coach, you can rely primarily or exclusively on the summaries of each step in the progression to get simple and clear instructions on what exactly to do and how to do it—these summaries are numbered sequentially from start to finish. Later, you can return and delve deeper into the details as your increasing experience improves your ability to understand and apply more of the information in a useful manner.

The table of contents and index can be used to locate specific sections or topics in the book, and a glossary is also provided in the back of the book for quickly looking up terminology.

Very often the book addresses the coach specifically despite being intended for both coaches and athletes. If you are an athlete training without a coach, don't make the mistake of thinking you're being neglected—you are your own coach.

Please note that while photographs are included to help illustrate and clarify certain points throughout the book that it's extremely difficult, if not impossible, to capture intended movements and moments perfectly. Additionally I have used photographs of actual lifts in training as much as possible, and of many different athletes, to best represent reality. Please rely on written descriptions as the final word in cases in which photographs may appear to not perfectly represent the associated explanation.

Understanding the Lifts

Throughout the learning process, a continually improving understanding of the principles and mechanics of the Olympic lifts will remain an important component of technique development and coaching. The fundamental principles of the snatch, clean and jerk are universal, although expressed in distinctive manners. Described in the simplest possible terms, all three lifts employ the generation of force against the ground to first elevate and accelerate the barbell upward, then use force against the inertia of the elevated barbell to accelerate the athlete downward and into position to receive the bar. Despite the segmented description, the lifts are performed with remarkable fluidity in their ideal execution.

Phases of the Lifts

The snatch, clean and jerk can all be considered as being comprised of two basic phases. In the first phase, the lifter elevates the barbell with the lower body; in the second phase, the lifter moves his or her body down underneath the elevated barbell with the upper body (Figure 1.1).

More specifically, the snatch and clean will be considered primarily in terms of three different phases in order to aid analysis—the first pull, second pull, and third pull. In addition to these phases, there will be the preparatory position, starting position, receiving position, and recovery. The three-pull method is both simple and logical and consequently effective in communication among athletes and coaches.

Preparatory Position: This is the position the lifter assumes once at the barbell, prior to actively setting the starting position. This is a relaxed or semi-relaxed position the lifter habitually holds at least momentar-

ily while focusing and finalizing any pre-lift mental rituals. Often this is gripping the bar lightly and either leaning over it or sitting in a squat position behind it.

Starting Position: This is the position from which the lifter actually begins the lift; that is, it's the last position of the lifter prior to any elevation of the barbell off the floor. Depending on the lifter's style, this may be a static position that can be easily seen and distinguished, or it may be a position the lifter passes through when using a dynamic start.

First Pull: The first pull is the phase of the lift in which the barbell is lifted from the floor to the point at which the final upward explosion is initiated—when the barbell reaches approximately mid-thigh level.

Second Pull: The second pull is the final upward explosion effort and brings the athlete into the fully

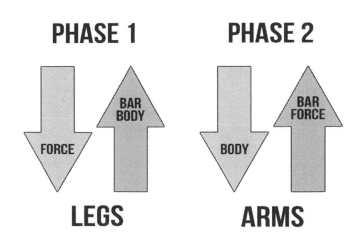

FIGURE 1.1 The snatch, clean and jerk can all be thought of in two phases, delineated by the change in the direction of force, the direction of movement of the barbell and body, and the parts of the body primarily responsible for creating the force and movement.

extended position of the lift. This includes the *transition*, *scoop* or *double knee bend*, and begins at the point at which the barbell is at approximately mid-thigh and finishes at the point at which the lifter has finished extending the knees and hips maximally.

Third Pull: The third pull is the athlete's transition from the extended position into the receiving position under the barbell—that is, it is the active relocation of the lifter under the barbell.

Receiving Position: The receiving position is the position of the lifter when the barbell has reached its final position relative to the body—overhead in the snatch and on the shoulders in the clean.

Recovery: The recovery is the movement of the lifter from the receiving position into the final standing position to complete the lift. In the snatch, this means standing up from the bottom of an overhead squat, and in the clean, standing from the bottom of a front squat.

Russian literature commonly breaks the lifts into three periods and six phases, which can also be used to analyze the lifts and teach specific elements (Medvedyev 1986/1989). It's helpful for coaches to be familiar with these phases, but the three-pull system will be used exclusively throughout this book when discussing the snatch and clean.

Period 1 (The Pull)

Phase 1: This phase is simply the lifter's first application of force to the barbell. It begins with that application of force and ends when the bar separates from the floor. This phase can be compared to the starting position.

Phase 2: The second phase consists of the pull between the separation of the bar from the floor and the beginning of the double knee bend. This phase is equivalent to the first pull.

Period 2 (The Explosion)

Phase 3: Phase three is essentially the double knee bend or scoop—it is the movement of the knees forward and their slight rebending as the torso moves into a vertical orientation. This phase is the first part of the second pull.

Phase 4: This phase is the final upward extension of the body and acceleration of the bar—it begins from the point of greatest knee flexion in the double knee bend and ends with the complete extension of the body. This phase is the final part of the second pull.

Period 3 (The Squat Under)

Phase 5: Phase 5 consists of the lifter's initial movement under the bar. It begins at the lifter's complete extension in phase 4 and ends when the barbell reaches its maximum height (the barbell continues to move upward under the momentum created in the explosion and in reaction to the lifter pulling against it to move down).

Phase 6: The final phase lasts from the point of the barbell's maximum height to the point at which the lifter receives the barbell in the squat position.

The jerk can similarly be broken into pieces for ease of discussion. While these segments don't perfectly align with those of the snatch and clean, they are similar enough that a pattern should be recognizable.

Preparatory Position: This is the position the lifter assumes prior to initiating the jerk. It may or may not be the same position used in the jerk itself.

Starting Position: This is the position from which the lifter actually begins the lift; that is, it's the last position of the lifter prior to the initiation of the dip.

Dip: The dip is the bending of the knees to elastically load the muscles and barbell, and position the body to allow the legs to drive the barbell upward.

Drive: The drive is the aggressive push against the ground with the legs to accelerate and elevate the barbell maximally.

Push Under: This is akin to the third pull of the snatch and clean; it is the lifter's intentional push against the bar with the arms to preserve as much of the bar's upward momentum and relocate the body under the bar.

Receiving Position: This is the position in which the lifter secures the jerk overhead. Typically this will be the split position, although it may also be a partial or full squat.

Recovery: The recovery is the movement of the lifter from the receiving position into the final standing position to complete the lift. In the jerk, this means standing from the split, partial squat or squat into a full standing position with the barbell locked out overhead.

Russian literature also breaks the jerk into three periods and five phases, which can be used alternatively to analyze the lifts and teach specific elements (Medvedyev 1986/1989). Again, while these may not be as practically useful for many coaches, it's helpful to be familiar with them.

Period 1 (The Half Squat)

Phase 1: This is the dip of the jerk: the bending of the knees from the initial standing position into the bottom of the dip position.

Period 2 (The Thrust)

Phase 2: This is the braking of the dip to stop the downward movement of the lifter and barbell.

Phase 3: This is the drive of the legs out of the dip to accelerate and elevate the barbell.

Period 3 (The Squat Under)

Phase 4: This is the movement of the legs into the receiving position, typically the split, and the movement of the rest of the body into the proper position under the bar.

Phase 5: The final phase is the securing of the barbell in the overhead position and establishing stability.

Laws of Motion in Weightlifting

The principles dictating the results of the lifter's movements are described by the constant interaction of Newton's Laws of Motion:

Law of Inertia: *Every body perseveres in its state of being at rest or of moving uniformly straight forward, except insofar as it is compelled to change its state by force impressed.* In other words, an object will maintain its present motion or lack thereof unless and until acted upon by an external force. A barbell will remain on the platform until a lifter moves it; likewise, a moving barbell will continue traveling upward due to the lifter's force as long as that applied force and/or the resulting momentum remains greater than the force of gravity acting on the barbell in the opposite direction. Additionally, the barbell will travel in whatever direction the lifter applies force to it (this becomes important when considering the contact of the barbell and the hips or upper thighs during the final extension of the snatch or clean, for example).

Law of Acceleration: *The rate of change of momentum of a body is proportional to the resultant force acting on the body and is in the same direction.* An object's acceleration is proportional to the applied force, but inversely proportional to its mass. That is, more force will create greater acceleration on a given object, but the greater an object's mass, the less acceleration will be created by a given magnitude of force. To increase the acceleration of a given barbell, more force must be applied, and the same amount of force will produce less acceleration as the weight on the barbell increases.

Law of Reciprocal Actions: *All forces occur in pairs, and these two forces are equal in magnitude and opposite in direction.* This law is most commonly paraphrased as, *For every action, there is an equal and opposite reaction.* When a lifter drives against the ground to lift the barbell, the ground delivers the same magnitude of force in return. The earth's far greater mass than the lifter/barbell system results in all noticeable movement being undertaken by the lifter and the bar when driving against the ground. This law will also come into play as the lifter applies force against the barbell's mass in an elevated position to relocate his or her body underneath it.

In the initial stage of the snatch or clean, the athlete generates muscular force with the legs and hips against the platform, lifting and accelerating the barbell upward. When the athlete reaches the peak of productive body extension and can consequently no longer drive against the platform to further elevate and accelerate the bar, the barbell will now possess upward momentum, and it will continue its upward travel temporarily even with the removal of any further force application by the athlete; how much higher the bar will travel under its own momentum will depend on both the weight on the barbell and the amount of force that's been applied by the lifter.

If performing the lift correctly, the lifter will not cease applying force to the barbell at this point, however. The effort to pull against the barbell will continue aggressively with the arms, but the lifter will cease applying force against the ground through the feet. As predicted by the law of reciprocal actions, this application of force to the bar without pressure against the platform will result in both the barbell continuing its upward travel and the lifter beginning and continuing his or her downward travel in reaction. The degree to which each object travels relative to each other will depend on their relative masses and the magnitude of momentum of the barbell; that is, the heavier the barbell relative to the athlete and the more slowly it's moving, the less it will travel upward and the more the lifter will travel downward (Of course, we have to also consider the influence of gravity on this interaction, which will assist the downward movement of the athlete and limit the upward travel of the barbell).

In short, during the first phase of the lift (the first and second pulls), the lifter is applying force against the ground with the lower body to elevate the barbell; in the second phase (the third pull), the lifter is apply force against the barbell and its inertia with the upper body to move his or her body down.

What distinguishes a power snatch or power clean from a snatch or clean is the interplay of force application, barbell mass and athlete mass. If a lifter applies maximal force to the barbell, the depth at which it must be received will be dictated entirely by the mass of the barbell and the mass of the athlete. That is, a light barbell will accelerate more and travel higher, whereas the heavier barbell will accelerate less and not travel as high.

The force application can of course be controlled by the lifter, however. A light barbell can be received in the full squat position by reducing the force applied to elevate the barbell. The lifter's effort to pull under the bar when not applying force against the platform will continue the barbell's upward motion to a greater degree the lighter the barbell is, requiring even less initial acceleration to receive the bar at full depth.

The previous applies equally to the jerk—the difference is merely that instead of pulling against the barbell, the lifter pushes against it.

The entirety of these principles can be distilled into some simple rules for the execution of the lifts, which will be discussed in detail throughout the book. During the first and second pulls, the lifter must maintain contact with the platform until maximal productive body extension is achieved in order to impart maximal acceleration to the barbell; in order to move into position under the barbell to receive it, the lifter must actively and aggressively continue pulling against the barbell with the pressure of the feet against the platform eliminated or reduced; and the transition between these phases of the lift must be as rapid as possible—in fact, the final explosion of the bar up and the transition of the lifter under it will, with a proficient athlete, become in essence a single continuous action.

Center of Mass, Center of Pressure & Line of Gravity

One of the most fundamental elements involved in weightlifting is the constant balancing of the lifter-barbell system over the base of support as the positions of the body and weight change both dramatically and quickly relative to the ground and each other.

Center of Mass The center of mass is the point around which the total mass of an object is equally distributed. In other words, it's the center of the object in terms of balance—supporting the object directly under the center of mass will keep the object balanced over the base of support. In weightlifting, the concern primarily is with the combined center of mass of the athlete and the barbell. This point will move continuously as the athlete performs the lift, but must always remain essentially balanced over the feet for a successful lift.

Line of Gravity The athlete's line of gravity is an imaginary vertical line that passes through the athlete's center of mass and runs through the point at the base (feet) over which the athlete is balanced. In other words, the athlete-barbell system is balanced over the point of the foot where the line of gravity passes. Different sources place the line of gravity of a naturally standing, unloaded individual to be anywhere between approximately the front edge of the heel and the center of the distance between the balls of the foot and the heel.

In reality, a person will be able to stand without falling on any point from the balls of the foot to the back of the heel, as can be demonstrated easily by anyone with decent balance. However, it's important to distinguish between possible and ideal, particularly when introducing the elements of a weighted external object and movement. Throughout a lift, the combined mass of the barbell and the athlete need to remain balanced over their base of support (the feet); otherwise, there will be movement forward or backward at some point in the lift, making it more difficult, or impossible, for the lifter and barbell to remain stable. With the additional weight of the barbell, which is also not fixed in a constant relative position to the lifter, shifts in balance can very quickly

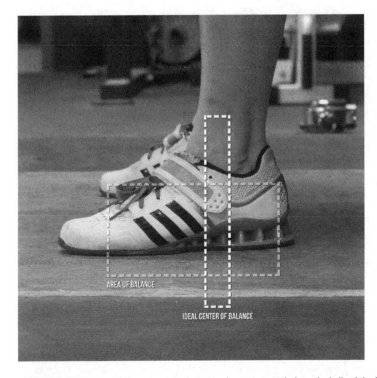

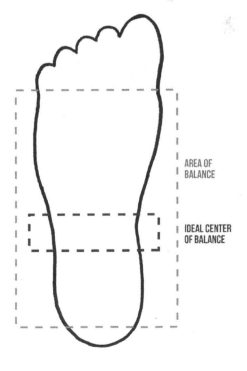

FIGURE 1.2 The area of balance over the foot extends approximately from the balls of the foot to the back edge of the heel. The ideal center of balance—the point at which the athlete's line of gravity should pass—is approximately the area at the front edge of the heel, slightly behind the middle of the possible area of balance.

be magnified to degrees beyond control.

Standing still, this ideal balance can be felt simply by the slightly greater pressure on the heel relative to the balls of the feet. During the snatch and clean, the athlete will be attempting to maintain the line of gravity of the bar-body system through this same point of balance irrespective of where the center of pressure is at any given moment, which will change throughout a lift. For our purposes, this point will be called the front edge of the heel because generally speaking, it will benefit us to maintain balance slightly farther back within the above-described range (Figure 1.2).

In any case, the balance of the athlete should be slightly behind the middle of the foot, i.e. closer to the heel than the toes. The front edge of the heel is a convenient landmark to use, and this will give us the proper sense of balancing over the foot slightly behind the center of the actual area of balance of the foot (balls of the feet to the back of the heel; essentially the middle of the foot without the toes).

Center of Pressure The center of pressure represents the point of the foot at which the downward force of the barbell-body system is focused. For example, if an athlete stood still on his or her toes, the center of pressure would be at the balls of the foot; if the athlete rocked back onto the heels by lifting the toes off the floor, the center of pressure would be at the heel. Normally, the line of gravity will pass essentially through the center of pressure—this is true for any still object in order for it to remain balanced.

However, it's important to understand that the line of gravity and the center of pressure do not necessarily align in a moving athlete. During movement of sufficient speed, it's entirely possible to maintain a line of gravity over a point other than that on which the pressure on the foot is maximal, such as during the ankle extension of the second pull of the snatch and clean or finish of the drive of the jerk—at this moment, all pressure is on the balls of the feet, but the line of gravity is still over the front edge of the heel.

As a simple demonstration of this concept, imagine an athlete performing a vertical jump in which he or she lands in the same place from which the jump originated—that is, there is no movement forward or backward. For this to happen, the center of mass

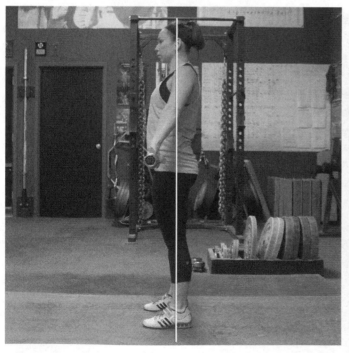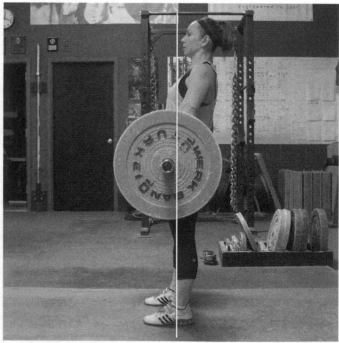

FIGURE 1.3 Maintaining the same line of gravity in a standing position with the addition of a weighted barbell at arms' length will require a degree of backward inclination (of the trunk or body as a whole) proportional to the relative masses of the barbell and body. The heavier the barbell is relative to the body, the closer it will need to be to the desired line of gravity in order to balance the combined center of mass over that point. Pictured with no additional weight (left) and 135% of bodyweight (right).

and line of gravity must remain in the same place throughout the movement; however, the center of pressure will shift forward to the balls of the feet as the jump is completed with the natural plantar flexion of the ankle. This demonstrates a divergence of center of pressure and the line of gravity. We can exaggerate this divergence with an athlete jumping backward rather than directly vertically. The center of pressure will still shift forward as the jump is completed with plantar flexion, but the center of mass and line of gravity will move backward—in the opposite direction.

This divergence is what occurs during the Olympic lifts, and is an important concept to understand— an athlete rising up onto the balls of the foot during a lift does not necessarily indicate a forward shift of the athlete's center of mass or a change of balance in any direction.

Athletes and coaches are most likely not working with tools that allow the monitoring or measuring of weight distribution over the foot with any kind of genuine precision—certainly not in real-time or in any way that would allow immediate adjustments during a lift. Athletes can simply keep slightly more pressure on the heel than on the balls of the feet while the full foot is in contact with the floor and attempt to maintain that same balance as the heels rise. This maintenance of balance (or the failure thereof) will be observable by the final position of the lifter, e.g., if a lifter jumps forward in a snatch, that athlete is clearly allowing his or her center of mass to shift forward at some point during the lift.

Strength Versus Technique

There is ongoing discussion and confusion regarding the roles of strength and technique in the sport of weightlifting, although largely carried on outside the competitive weightlifting community, presumably attributable to the sport's relative obscurity and consequent lack of understanding. At the extreme ends of the discussion are the ideas that the sport is wholly dependent on technique, or that that technique is es-

sentially irrelevant with enough strength.

The fact is that neither strength nor technique will adequately compensate for a significant lack of the other. No amount of technical proficiency will allow a lifter to magically defy the laws of physics—200 kilograms will not suddenly jump from the floor to over a lifter's head without the application of a great magnitude of muscular force. Likewise, even enormous amounts of strength cannot be applied effectively to the snatch or clean & jerk without reasonable technical proficiency.

Technique is the medium through which strength is expressed—the lifts are limited, then, by the weakest part of the equation. Neither strength nor technique can be neglected for the sake of developing the other. Program design and training must always take into account each lifter's strengths and weaknesses— maximal success will be achieved through strengthening the weaknesses and exploiting the strengths.

Legs Versus Hips

Another common argument, or at least point of confusion, is regarding the relative contributions to the lifts of knee extension and hip extension. In short, both knee and hip extension are critical for optimal pulling in the snatch and clean. While it's not perfectly accurate or complete, it's helpful conceptually to consider knee extension (or leg drive against the floor) to be responsible primarily for elevation of the barbell, and hip extension to be responsible for the speed of the barbell. In other words, the lifter requires maximal hip and knee extension to create maximal elevation and acceleration of the barbell, rather than relying on one significantly more than the other, although variations in lift technique among individuals will typically emphasize one over the other to some degree, depending on the lifter's natural strengths and structure. With respect to the jerk, any contribution from hip extension is largely eliminated by the necessary positioning of the dip and drive, forcing the movement to rely nearly entirely on knee extension.

Learning & Teaching the Lifts

There is no single perfect learning progression for the snatch and clean & jerk. Different approaches are rooted in technical style variation, tradition, available time and resources, and the needs of individual athletes, including circumstances such as age. Consideration of the broad spectrum of coaching methods in relation to the large number of successful weightlifters worldwide suggests this is not necessarily a problem. That said, it's also apparent that the breadth of successful coaching invariably relies on the same sound technical principles.

Just as there is with instruction, there is variation of lifting technique among athletes and coaches. Setting aside differences as symptoms of what could be considered universally to be poor technique, there exist iterations of correct technique. Some of these are products of given lifters' anatomical peculiarities or particular natural strengths, and some are products of environment and coaching. For nearly any detail of lifting technique presented in this book, at least one successful lifter who violates it can be found.

This book is written with the assumption that the reader intends to learn or teach the lifts in accordance with the technical style presented. There will be occasional discussion of different technical styles when appropriate and helpful, or for the sake of comparison, but this will make up a relatively small portion of the content of the book. It is correct to infer by this that the technical style presented in the book is my preferred style; if it were not, it would not be taught in the book.

However, part of my coaching philosophy is that I will use anything that works; what works best varies among athletes as mentioned previously. When reading this book, bear in mind that very little is set in stone and adjustments should always be made when appropriate to maximize each lifter's potential based on their natural strengths and weaknesses. In short,

there is truly no right or wrong in weightlifting: there is effective or ineffective, and these things are not universal among athletes.

All athletes should be taught textbook lifting technique initially and spend the early period of their development practicing and improving their proficiency and consistency with this conventional technique. Over time, lifters can be allowed to naturally gravitate toward more idiosyncratic technique that best exploits their unique strengths as long as it does not violate basic principles and create problems. This process will better ensure that divergence from textbook technique is beneficial and not simply the product of a failure to properly address a weakness or invest adequate time into developing baseline technical proficiency.

Over-Coaching Over-coaching is an easy mistake to make in consideration of the volumes of detailed information existing regarding the lifts. The coach must remain disciplined and provide the athlete what is needed, resisting the urge to delve into details for which the athlete is not ready and consequently cannot use productively. This kind of over-coaching can be a product of the coach's desire to impress with his or her knowledge, but at least as often, it's simply the result of the coach's eagerness to achieve progress with the athlete. Unfortunately, overwhelming the athlete with information he or she doesn't yet have the experience to apply is often counterproductive.

With this in mind, the information in this book needs to be used by both the coach and athlete discriminately. For the novice lifter, much of the detail can be overlooked and the attention focused on only the most fundamental points. I have placed summaries and lists in each section of the learning progression: these are enough to get a new athlete started learning the lifts without superfluous detail.

As the athlete progresses, more of the information contained in the book will begin to make sense and be successfully applicable in training. That is, the athlete can progress to conceptual understanding from a starting point of simple execution.

Progression I have made an effort to deliver a learning progression encompassing the snatch and clean & jerk that is simultaneously exhaustive and flexible. While the strategy must be complete, it must also be easily adaptable to individual athletes and circumstances. In a sense, then, it's as much a framework for teaching the lifts as it is a specific progression. This framework provides much opportunity for addition, omission and alteration by each coach and athlete as deemed appropriate. Steps may be omitted in some cases; in others they may be added or modified. And of course, the process can be executed exactly as written, as it should likely be for those just starting out in coaching.

The flexibility of the progression extends beyond the movements themselves. Each component can be considered merely a physical drill for the body, or an opportunity for education regarding the principles on which it's based. This accommodates athletes of all levels of experience, as well as the spectrum of coaching and learning styles. Inexperienced athletes can quickly learn the lifts with little or no explanation of principle simply through the repetition of drills, while more advanced athletes will be able to improve their technical performances by learning and better understanding the underlying principles easily underscored with each segment of the progression. Likewise, coaches who prefer the minimalist approach to instruction will be successful with the drills alone, while more cerebral coaches will be able to easily inject detailed but digestible lessons with each one.

The drills that comprise the learning progressions will also in many cases serve as remedial exercises for lifters who have already learned the lifts and need to improve technical proficiency.

Repetition Learning movement patterns is ultimately and unavoidably a matter of quality repetition, feedback, and effort. No advanced teaching technique or science will change this to any considerable degree—there will never be a substitute for time, focus and hard work, and eliminating these things would strip much of the potential for satisfaction from the process.

With respect to repetition, the emphasis needs to be on quality. Not only is poor execution of a movement ineffective for developing technique, it's counterproductive in the sense that it demands time and energy that could be put to better use, as well as creating similar but incorrect motor patterns with which the correct patterns must compete. Of course movements will not be perfect in the early stages of learning, and there will be few if any demonstrating true perfection throughout an entire lifting career. This doesn't mean learning technique is a futile endeavor—it simply means that conscious effort must be made to execute each repetition as precisely as possible for the given stage of development. In other words, sloppiness, laziness, inattentiveness and impatience need to be avoided as much as possible. This is a responsibility shared by the coach and athlete.

Feedback Tied in closely with repetition quality is the quality and quantity of feedback. Feedback will exist in forms of varying utility and accessibility. Easily the most productive will be the guidance and instruction of a qualified coach based on observation and analysis of the athlete. The primary concern in this case is the ability of the coach and athlete to effectively communicate with each other—no amount of accurate technique analysis by the coach will have any effect if the athlete doesn't understand the coach's feedback. Similarly, the athlete must be able to relay to the coach his or her experience with each lift. This kind of clear communication takes time to develop as the coach and athlete become better acquainted, but from the beginning, effort should be made continually to establish and improve the kind of rapport necessary to support the athlete's technical progress.

It's unnecessary for coaches to have been elite weightlifters in order to be successful with their athletes. It is, however, necessary for coaches to have legitimate experience with weightlifting training and competition. Being familiar with the feel of the lifts, responses to programming, and the process of competing will allow the coach to produce more effective programming and communicate far more successfully with his or her weightlifters. There is also a unique culture of the sport that can only be learned through immersion, along with many details of training and competition etiquette. The most important experience any future coach can have is that of training as a dedicated competitive weightlifter under the guidance of an experienced weightlifting coach in a gym full of other competitive weightlifters. This kind of experience cannot be replaced with books, seminars or even internships.

Each coach will develop over time his or her own style of instruction and interaction with the athlete. The intention of this book is not to prescribe any particular style, but instead to provide a collection of both reliable principles and recommended strategies to be used as a solid foundation on which each coach can construct his or her own unique approach.

One that warrants mention here is the notion of positive and negative cues. Commonly the coach will instruct an athlete to *not* do something, or to act in a way inconsistent with the nature of the movement. As an example of the former, the coach may tell the lifter to not lift the hips too quickly when lifting the bar from the floor; a more effective cue would be to instruct the athlete to lift the chest with the hips. As an example of the latter, the coach may tell the lifter to keep the hips down; a more effective cue may be to instruct the lifter to instead keep the chest or shoulders up. Whereas the first instruction causes the lifter to think *down* when needing to move *up*, the second keeps the instruction consistent with the nature of the movement. In short, athletes are more likely to respond as desired when told explicitly what to do instead of being told what not to do and left to figure out corrections on their own. Much of the time, an athlete is aware of a technical error, in which case telling them not to do it is unnecessary and unhelpful; what they're lacking is the knowledge of what specific actions to perform in order to correct it.

Video review can be an excellent means of feedback for athletes without access to a coach, or as an additional means for those who are receiving coaching. The effectiveness of video review is of course predicated on not only knowing what to look for but how to respond—in other words, it's not helpful for an athlete to watch video of a lift if he or she is unable to recognize faults and their causes, and then to develop strategies to correct them. This is simply a matter of combined education and experience. The better athletes understand the principles of the lifts,

the better they will understand the rationale of positioning and movement mechanics, allowing them to recognize the roots of technique errors and to create drills or cues to correct them.

Video can be used in a number of ways. Most effective is access to immediate review following a single lift. This can be accomplished these days with the use of video cameras on the cell phones nearly every athlete carries. There are also now several applications for phones and tablets that provide simple tools to aid in video analysis, such as slow-motion playback, frame-by-frame progression, drawing tools and bar path tracing.

It should be noted here that this recent explosion in availability of analysis tools has delivered an attendant increase in over-analysis. That is, many new lifters and coaches are dissecting lifts to such an extent that it actually becomes counterproductive. As a coach, it's imperative to be able to recognize errors in a lift in real time, and in fact, many technical problems can truly only be diagnosed in real time, as they pertain to speed and rhythm, and diagnosis can also be aided in many cases by sound. As a lifter, it's equally imperative to learn to feel a lift, and use the additional live feedback of sound. Excessive reliance on analysis tools can limit the development of these abilities in terms of both speed and ultimate degree.

The least effective method of video review is to record entire training sessions and watch the video well after the completion of the session—this allows neither immediate feedback when the feeling of the movement is still fresh, nor the opportunity to immediately attempt chosen corrections. The inherent problems of this kind of lag time notwithstanding, this type of video review is much better than none at all. In addition, these videos can serve in an archive as means by which to measure progress and evaluate training productivity over the long term. They of course can also be shared with coaches or other lifters in remote locations for feedback.

The most basic feedback available is simply the athlete's own collective senses. The greater the athlete's understanding of the guiding principles of the movement's technique, the better a framework he or she will have within which to make sense of what he or she feels. For example, it does no good for an athlete to recognize his or her weight is on the balls of the feet if he or she doesn't know the weight shouldn't be there at that particular moment. Again, this awareness of the sensations involved in lifting is part of the language used between the coach and athlete to most effectively produce improvements.

Simple Versus Complex The Olympic lifts are complex movements demanding great precision and focus. Patience and discipline will carry both athletes and coaches a long way, and attempts to circumvent or artificially accelerate the process will invariably result in failure to achieve mastery. Coaches disagree about how comprehensive the process for teaching the lifts should be. Some are extreme minimalists, preferring to show athletes what the lift should look like and allowing them over time to learn how to make it happen on their own. Others have very basic progressions that get athletes started but still require they essentially teach themselves through the observation of other lifters and feedback from what turns out to be experimentation in training. Still others use extensive and detailed teaching progressions that teach the mechanics of every segment of each lift.

The minimalist approach generally works well for very naturally talented athletes and very young athletes, as these are the type of individuals who are able to mimic observed actions well and who have a natural feel for athletic movement. Even with such athletes, however, this approach can leave holes in technical performance or understanding that come back to haunt the athlete much later in his or her lifting career. Further, this approach often falls very short when teaching adults, who not only do not pick up motor skills as quickly and easily as their young counterparts, but who also tend to be interested in the conceptual element of learning.

This book unquestionably takes a very comprehensive and detailed approach for two basic reasons. First, such an approach will work for any individual, from the athletically talented to the completely unathletic. Any coach who works with anyone other than those destined for weightlifting greatness will need to be prepared to work with lifters who will need a great deal more guidance. And second, a detailed approach can always be simplified when appropriate. As a coach, it's always better to have more tools than you need than to need more tools than you have.

The Progression Process

The process of teaching or learning the snatch and clean & jerk will vary considerably in duration. The progression presented in this book is not intended to be undertaken in any specific period of time; it will need to be implemented appropriately for each athlete. This can range from teaching the foundational elements, snatch, clean and jerk each over the course of a few training sessions, to spending several weeks, and possibly longer, building to the complete lifts. It is presented, however, with the steps in the recommended order, from foundational elements through the completion of each lift.

Further, what occurs after the lifter has learned to perform the snatch and clean & jerk reasonably well will vary. For example, an athlete of an appropriate age who learns very quickly may move in short order into a training cycle with significant loading in the competition lifts; on the other end of the spectrum, a lifter may spend a long period of time performing the lifts or segments of the lifts with an empty barbell or very light loading while the training program focuses on developing elements like strength, mobility, stability and work capacity. The former will be more typical of an individual with an extensive athletic background who comes to weightlifting with a solid foundation of strength, mobility and motor skill; the latter will be more typical of children being first introduced to the sport or adults arriving at the sport without an athletic background or in need of considerable remediation.

The various approaches will be addressed in more detail in the Program Design section of the book.

Implementing the Progression Drills

The teaching progression drills for the snatch, clean and jerk are presented in following sections of the book. When and how these drills are introduced and practiced by various athletes can vary considerably. In most situations of athletes in the late teens to adult age with existing training experience, the drills for a given lift will all be learned and practiced together in a single training session or in a handful of consecutive sessions, and most athletes will be able to transition to using at least a training bar from the hang in this time, if not actually transitioning to performing the full lift from the floor.

In other cases, the coach may choose to introduce only certain drills in a given session, and expose the athlete to the complete progression in smaller individual doses over a longer period of time. A more gradual progression is usually a better choice for young athletes beginning to specialize in weightlifting in combination with instruction and practice of general and specific strength exercises. For example, these athletes may train the snatch or power snatch from the hang only and perform snatch pulls and overhead squats for a period of time, and then later learn the full snatch once a solid foundation has been built. How exactly this is done must be left to the coach, as what works best can vary considerably based on the circumstances and athlete.

The effectiveness of these drills can be significantly diminished through poor execution. It needs to be understood very clearly that there is a simple order of priorities throughout the learning process: Position, movement, speed, load. Performing a correct movement from an incorrect position is impossible, because it is, by definition, a different movement, and the introduction of excessive speed or weight before the development of sound movement is counterproductive, because again, the lifter simply practicing an incorrect movement. These points are critical to keep in mind at this earliest stage of learning. If the coach or athlete fails to ensure correct positioning, or insists on speed over accuracy, the execution of the drills is far less likely to be correct and consequently will create poor motor patterns that will have to be overwritten later—this process is much more difficult than simply ingraining the correct patterns from the beginning.

Athletes are often in a hurry to complete these drills, and will attempt to perform a series in immediate succession at high speed and without even the briefest pause in the starting position. This needs to be stopped immediately, and the reps controlled by the coach to allow him or her to ensure correct positioning and better guide the athlete through the movements.

This hierarchy should become clear as the learning progressions first establish positions, then introduce movement from and to these positions, and finally increase these movements to full speed. Increases in loading are introduced only after a foundation of proper positions, movement and speed is established. It applies equally at all scales—that is, from the learning process as a whole to each individual component thereof. With these learning drills, practically this means each section must begin with correct positioning, and may be performed initially as slowly as necessary for the athlete to repeatedly execute the movement correctly. Certain sections cannot be performed slowly, but these fall at a point at which a solid enough foundation for that particular movement should already exist to prevent any considerable trouble.

In some cases, additional drills may need to be created to help the athlete through the following progression. With a legitimate understanding of the principles of the lifts, this should present no problem. In short, we first isolate the problem as much as possible, determine a method of improving it, practice that corrective method, and gradually reintegrate the corrected component into its parent movement. This basic method is precisely what will often be used later for effective fault correction.

With these progression drills, generally the attempt is to mimic the actual movements toward which the athlete is working as well as possible; in some instances, however, drills that deviate from what will actually occur in the lift are used in order to more effectively teach a given component of the whole skill (an example being a muscle snatch or muscle clean). As long as these deviations are recognized as such by the athlete and coach, they will present no problems.

Certain movements and positions will change very slightly with the addition of a loaded barbell. This load shifts the athlete-barbell system's center of mass and consequently changes the necessary positioning of the body at any given phase of the movement. These changes are minor and, if understood, will not prevent successful learning. Ultimately, every lift, irrespective of the weight on the bar or lack thereof, must be performed according to the present center of mass of the athlete-barbell system. The principles guiding the positions and movements do not change—if they are observed correctly, the resulting movements will be correct at any weight.

These learning drills should be performed in sets of 3-5 repetitions. Even while the weight is very light, or essentially non-existent, more than five consecutive repetitions will usually result in a degradation of accuracy.

Coaching

Coaching is an art form encompassing multiple disciplines and fields of knowledge that must be blended in such a way that the lines of delineation among them are blurred if not erased. It's the knowledge and understanding of relevant scientific principles, the experience of implementation of training methodologies, the accurate assessment of disparate athletes and their varying needs, the prediction of responses to training, the proper and productive social interaction with a wide array of individuals, the psychological support and guidance of athletes of many different backgrounds and needs, the institution of reasoned discipline, and the qualities of respected leadership.

Many of the qualities of the successful coach are inherent within an individual, although needing to be intentionally cultivated, and no amount of technical knowledge will make up for their absence. The most perfectly constructed training program will fail miserably if the lifter isn't sufficiency motivated and disciplined, and doesn't possess absolute certainty that the coach is dedicated to his or her success.

The coach needs to be committed fully to the preparation and success of his or her weightlifters, not only to create the optimal programming prescriptions, but to provide the lifter reassurance that his or her dedication to training is warranted and will result in progress. For any coach, the success of the athletes must be the top priority by a significant margin—any interest on the coach's part in public recognition, appreciation or fame is misplaced energy and focus that diminishes his or her ability to manage the lifter. Coaches who consistently produces exemplary weightlifters will receive their due credit and recognition eventually without actively seeking it.

All athletes are individuals with varying sensibilities, experiences, needs and understanding. Coaches must adapt to each athlete to some extent to maximize the effectiveness of their work, providing them the ideal nature and degree of support, motivation

and accountability. However, this is not an instruction for coaches to coddle their athletes. Part of the coach's responsibility is to create and enforce high standards and provide all athletes with clear expectations regarding behavior, effort and performance. If the coach fails in this regard, the standards and expectations of the team or gym will rapidly deteriorate to match the level of the least ambitious athlete in the group.

Lineage & Legacy All great craftsmen learn from those who have come before them—the best learn from experience working directly under the masters. It's in this way that knowledge is passed among the coaching generations. A new coach can learn from books, video, magazines and articles, but this kind of learning is incomplete and lacking the intangible quality that is truly the key to solving the puzzle.

Lineage in coaching is an idea that's overlooked to a stunning extent in weightlifting in this confusing new era of the internet. And most troubling, it seems evident that giving credit and paying respect to lineage is often not overlooked, but actually intentionally avoided. Presumably the individuals posing as spontaneously materializing coaches are doing so because they believe it bolsters their image—geniuses who needed no teaching or assistance to get to where they are (which is often not where they claim). Unfortunately, it seems this image is too frequently believed, but all great coaches have roots they celebrate and to which they pay their respects.

One of the characteristics of great coaches is the understanding that giving credit to their mentors is not the same thing as surrendering the credit due for their own original ideas or work. There is not only a willingness to give this credit, but an eagerness. There is pride in the pedigree. Trying to hide your lineage (or lack thereof) and pretending to be someone you're not is the behavior of amateurs and frauds.

It's easy to be a technician—to learn protocols and algorithms and repeat what has been said or written, particularly these days when so much information is so readily available. Technicians can help a lot of people become better lifters, and introduce a lot of people to the sport. But being a technician is very different from being a coach, which is a teacher in all the best senses of the word, and one who understands the whys and hows in a way that allows them to truly coach—not just run people through the motions.

Lineage doesn't mean you can't be original. It's a foundation.

Weightlifting Experience In order to become a great weightlifting coach, an individual arguably has to be a weightlifter for a period of time—genuinely BE a weightlifter. Not practice the lifts, not enjoy the lifts, not do the lifts as part of another sport or activity, but live the life—live a life that is constructed around the demands of being a competitive weightlifter, train under an established coach, in a true weightlifting gym, and ideally in a team environment.

If one hasn't had this experience, its importance can't ever truly be appreciated—but it's glaringly ob-vious when coaches have not. This doesn't mean coaches have to have been world-class weightlifters by any means. It's the experience of the life and the culture that matters, not the competitive results. There are too many subtleties and intangibles that can only be learned through this experience that build the foundation for the understanding and communication required of a successful coach.

Understand that this doesn't mean that without such experience as a lifter and apprenticeship as a new coach an individual can't possibly teach people how to lift, help people enter the sport, or any number of other things. But without the experience, the individual will probably never become a truly great weightlifting coach.

Individual Variation

One of the great difficulties in both presenting and learning information regarding weightlifting is the great natural variation among athletes and the consequent differences in numerous aspects, such as actual body positions in various phases of a lift, the relative ability of a given lifter in different exercises, the ultimate technical style each lifter develops over time, and the response to training.

However, while a superficial survey of these disparities may seem to contradict basic recommendations, this variation remains within the scope of the most fundamental principles of weightlifting. Following are some of the most significant areas of variations that can be expected.

Body Proportions & Effects

The unique structure of each lifter's body, such as the relative lengths of the limbs and the trunk, the width and shape of the pelvis, the shape of the skeletal components of the shoulder complex, and the precise alignment of various joints, will dictate the actual positions each lifter will be able to achieve. This is, of course, one of the primary elements of successful recruiting for the sport—some athletes are simply better suited physically by virtue of their anatomy, and this is a significant component of the natural selection of the sport; that is, those athletes best suited for the sport continue to thrive and improve to the highest levels, while those not possessed of ideal physical characteristics fall away as the level of competition increases due to the inability to overcome significant physical disadvantages.

Body Types

The human body exists in infinite variations in terms of proportions. Each variation provides advantages and disadvantages for certain physical tasks. Individuals with given proportions will excel in the sports in which such proportions provide an advantage, and will eventually fail in sports in which they are disadvantageous. Obvious examples include basketball, in which height is a clear advantage, and gymnastics, in which a shorter stature is an advantage. While there are occasional exceptions to the rule, they are extremely rare, and virtually never (if ever) prove more successful than more advantageously proportioned athletes. Weightlifting is no different. Despite a wide range of weight categories and therefore possible

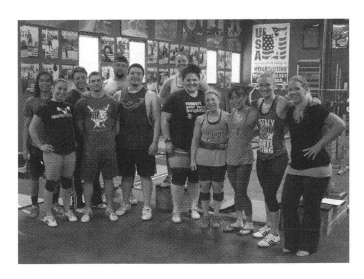

FIGURE 3.1 Between two genders and twenty weight classes, there is an enormous variety in the physical characteristics of weightlifters at all levels of performance.

overall height and mass differences, there are certain proportions that invariably confer an advantage.

There are three basic body types with regard to proportions: brachiomorph, mesomorph, and dolicomorph.

Brachiomorphic: The brachiomorphic body type describes individuals with relatively long torsos and short legs and arms. These proportions tend to be advantageous for squatting and the clean & jerk, as the shorter legs reduce mechanical disadvantage at the knee and hip. These individuals are typically successful in weightlifting unless the disproportionality is extreme.

Mesomorphic: The mesomorphic body type describes individuals with what would be considered balanced proportions. These athletes have no specific significant advantage or disadvantage, although they will tend to be successful in weightlifting as long as their bodyweights are proper for their heights.

Dolichomorphic: The dolichomorphic body type describes individuals with short torsos and long legs and arms. These athletes are at a considerable disadvantage in the sport of weightlifting for numerous reasons, including poor mechanics for leg strength and non-optimal positioning with regard to the barbell's interaction with the body during the pulls of the snatch and clean.

Positions

The most obvious and visible differences among lifters are displayed in the most basic positions of weightlifting: the starting and receiving positions of the snatch, clean and jerk. The actual joint angles and limb and trunk positions and orientations can vary significantly, making precise measurements essentially useless, and often making the identification of proper positions by inexperienced athletes and coaches difficult. It's important to note that anatomical structure and mobility are distinct characteristics—the former is permanent while the latter can be modified (and must be modified if not optimal for successful lifting). Following are explanations of what the body structure will affect in each position, and examples of multiple athletes who all meet criteria for correct positions despite varied appearance.

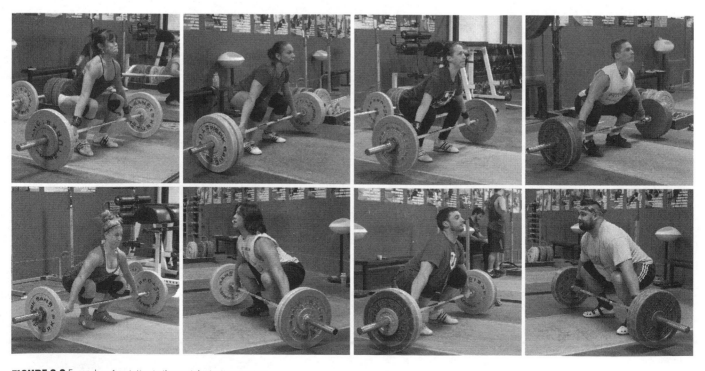

FIGURE 3.2 Examples of variation in the snatch starting position

Starting Position In the starting position of the snatch and clean, body structure will affect the joint angles of the ankle, knee and hip, the height of the hip relative to the knee, the angle of the back relative to the floor, the angle and width of the feet, and to a small degree, the placement of the barbell relative to the foot and the distance of the shoulders in front of the barbell. Nearly all athletes will be capable of meeting the criteria provided in this book for a proper starting position if possessed of adequate mobility, with the exception of the extremely tall. (Figure 3.2)

Clean Receiving Position In the receiving position of the clean—the front squat—body structure will affect the depth of the squat, the angles of the ankle, knee and hip, the angle of the torso relative to the floor, the angle and width of the feet, the width of the grip on the bar, the position of the hands on the bar, and the position of the elbows in the rack position. The most significant variation will be in the rack position—some lifters, for example, will be able to maintain a full grip around the bar while others will have only a few fingertips under the bar; some will be capable of elevating the elbows until the upper arm

is horizontal, while others will not be able to elevate the elbows significantly. (Figure 3.3)

Snatch Receiving Position In the receiving position of the snatch—the overhead squat—body structure will affect the depth of the squat, the angles of the ankle, knee and hip, the angle of the torso relative to the floor, the angle and width of the feet, the width of the grip on the bar, the hand and wrist positions, the rotation of the arms at the shoulders, the degree of elbow extension, and the relative positions of the barbell and head. (Figure 3.4)

Jerk Rack Position In the jerk rack position, body structure will affect the width of the grip on the bar, the position of the hands on the bar and the angle of the elbows. This may be the position in which there is the largest degree of variation among lifters; an excellent jerk rack position requires the right arm segment proportions and optimal mobility. Ideally lifters will be capable of keeping the palms under the bar and the elbows relatively low; many lifters will have to rely on a jerk rack position with higher elbows and the hands in a less than optimal position on the bar. (Figure 3.5)

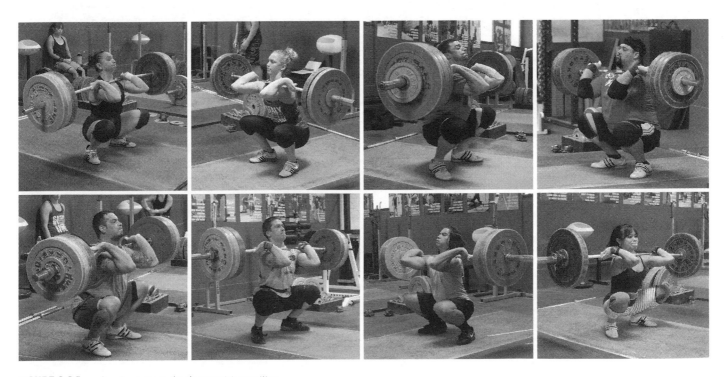

FIGURE 3.3 Examples of variation in the clean receiving position

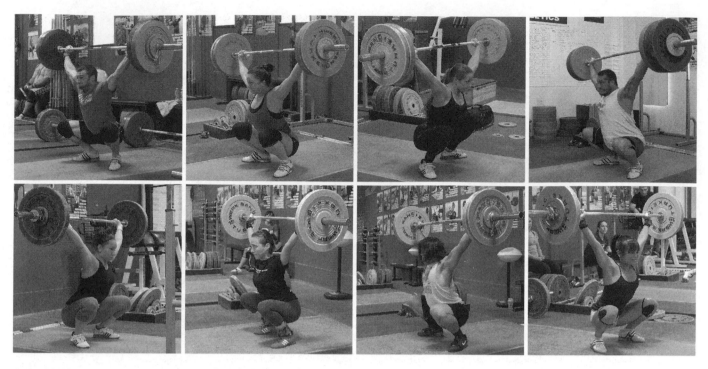

FIGURE 3.4 Examples of variation in the snatch receiving position

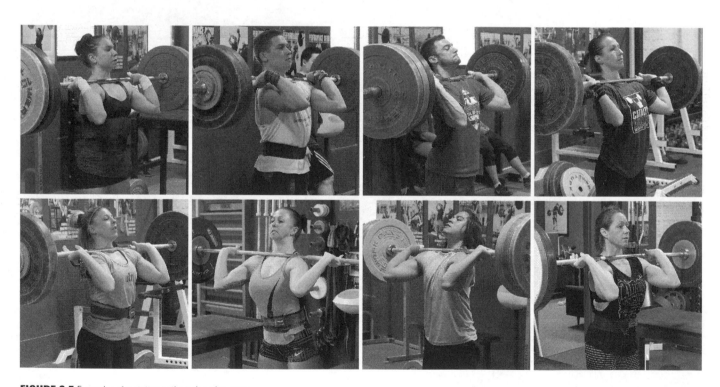

FIGURE 3.5 Examples of variation in the jerk rack position

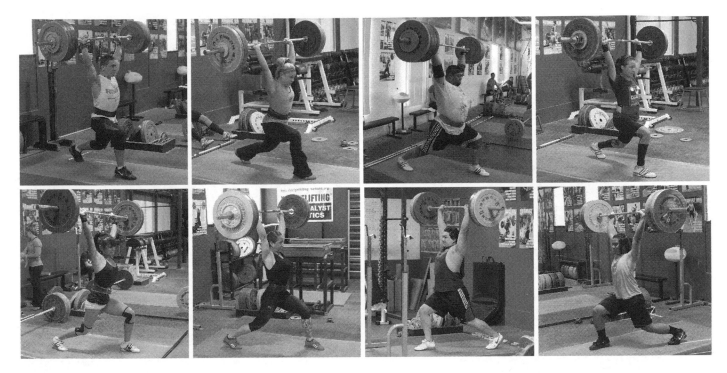

FIGURE 3.6 Examples of variation in the jerk split position

Jerk Split Position In the jerk split position, body structure will affect the length and width of the split, the angle of the trunk, the angle of the back leg segments and degree of knee flexion, the angle of the front thigh, the width of the grip on the bar, the hand and wrist positions, the rotation of the arms at the shoulders, the degree of elbow extension, and the relative positions of the barbell and head. (Figure 3.6)

Leverage

There is a general ability of athletes in lighter weight classes to be capable of lifting more weight relative to bodyweight than their heavier weight class counterparts. This is a simple issue of leverage, although of course many other factors are involved in each athlete to produce the ultimate level of ability; that is, we cannot always state with certainty that all short lifters are stronger than all tall lifters relative to bodyweight. However, shorter limbs do confer a basic advantage for lifting weight in terms of leverage.

Lever mechanics are at play in the movement of any joint by muscular effort. Muscles contract to move the limb onto which they attach across the joint in question; the length of that limb and the distance to the attachment point of the muscle that moves it decide the actual resistance with a given weight; the longer the lever arm, the greater the difficulty of moving the weight. To conceptualize this simply, imagine holding a pole with a 5kg weight at one end in one hand and trying to lift the weighted end—the closer to the weight you grip the pole, the easier it will be to lift. This is a simple demonstration of leverage—the weight at the end of the pole didn't change, but the amount of resistance, and your ability to lift it, did.

If we consider the leg of a weightlifter performing a squat, we have the knee as the fulcrum, the thigh as the lever arm, the distance between the point around which the knee pivots and the point where the force is applied by the quadriceps muscle group via the patellar tendon as the force lever arm (Figure 3.7). This is of course a simplified description of the system, as we also have the hip joint and musculature participating in a squat, and even the ankle joint and musculature to some degree, as well as the fact that the knee is a complex joint with the patella creating changing leverage throughout the range of motion, but will serve this explanation satisfactorily.

The lifter's body is attached to the upper legs at their proximal ends (the hip joints), and this, along with whatever additional weight the lifter is holding (on the back, on the shoulders, or overhead), is the resistance in the system. The longer the femur (i.e. taller and/or longer-legged the athlete), the greater the distance between the load and the fulcrum, and consequently, the more difficult it is to move any given amount of weight. Of course, larger individual's anatomy will also mean that the force arm is longer as well (the distance between the point around which the joint pivots at the knee and where the force is applied), but to a smaller degree than the resistance arm, meaning the two will not balance each other out, and the mechanical disadvantage increases as the total length of the leg increases.

Contributing to the disadvantage is that an athlete's muscular cross-sectional area does not increase proportionally with height or limb length indefinitely. A comparison between a longer and shorter legged lifter will not necessarily have a proportional increase in the size of the muscles of the leg. In other words, one of the major sources of potential force generation becomes proportionally smaller as the leverage disadvantage increases.

In short, this means that a lifter with shorter femurs will have better mechanics for squatting than a lifter with longer femurs. For example, if we compare two lifters of the same height and bodyweight with similar training experience, the lifter with shorter legs will nearly always out-squat the lifter with longer legs unless there is a combined advantage from several other factors. Similarly, if we compare two lifters of the same level of performance in their respective weight classes, the lifter from the lighter weight class will more than likely squat a larger percentage of his or her bodyweight than the lifter from the heavier weight class.

Of course, this mechanical difference really only dictates potential ability; there are many other factors that contribute to a lifter's ultimate level of performance that can mitigate the limitations of relatively poor leverage (such as a higher fast-twitch to slow-twitch fiber composition of the involved

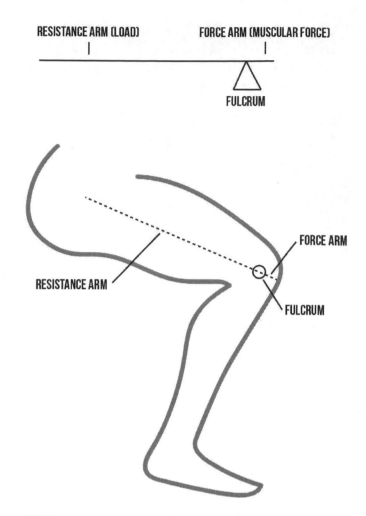

FIGURE 3.7 Longer limbs create greater mechanical disadvantage for the muscles responsible for moving that limb around a joint. This means that shorter limbs confer a basic advantage for lifting weight, and provide lifters in lighter weight classes the general ability to lift more relative to their bodyweight than lifters from heavier weight classes.

musculature, greater neurological efficiency, muscle cross-sectional area, etc.) or that can limit the advantage conferred by relatively good leverage (such as a lower fast-twitch to slow-twitch fiber ratio, relatively low neurological efficiency, etc.).

Additionally, this kind of anatomical variation will affect the technique of the snatch, clean and jerk to some extent as well. An athlete with shorter legs and a longer torso, for example, will tend to pull the snatch and clean with a more upright posture that is more reliant on leg strength than hip strength. In other words, the exact technical execution and positions of the lift will eventually reflect the natural strengths of the athlete to some extent.

Greg Everett

Competition Lift Ratios

Generally lifters demonstrate a fairly consistent ratio between the snatch and clean & jerk. However, this ratio can vary considerably in some cases. This may be an indication of a problem, such as a mobility limitation, technical issue, or improper bodyweight, or it may be the manifestation of a given lifter's natural strengths and weaknesses or anatomy that will not be changed to any considerable degree through training.

Possible reasons for a high snatch relative to clean & jerk include:

- Tall or long-limbed athlete
- Bodyweight too low for height
- Athlete is more explosive than strong

Possible reasons for a low snatch relative to clean & jerk include:

- Short or short-limbed athlete
- Limited mobility
- Limited technical proficiency
- Athlete is less explosive than strong

As was discussed earlier, taller and longer-limbed athletes are at a disadvantage with regard to moving weight in a basic sense; this means that they tend to clean & jerk less in relative terms than their shorter and shorter-limbed counterparts, as the clean & jerk is more dependent on strength generally and squatting strength specifically. However, taller lifters tend to have at least a small advantage in the snatch, as they will naturally have a greater distance between the height of the bar at their fully-extended positions and their receiving positions (assuming adequate mobility in the bottom position) than their shorter counterparts.

Physical Traits

In addition to the basic structure of the body, other innate physical characteristics will dictate the abilities of each lifter to some extent. These are traits that individuals possess by virtue of birth, not due to any intentional intervention. Of course, these elements can be improved to varying degrees with proper training, but an individual naturally endowed with an exceptional degree of these traits (if a reasonable level of training is undertaken) will always remain ahead of an individual who is not. This is not to say that less advantaged lifters with an extremely high level of dedication and hard work cannot be competitive with such athletes, but they will certainly never be capable of surpassing a more advantaged lifter with equal work ethic and commitment.

Speed and explosiveness are arguably the most dramatically naturally-influenced traits with relevance to weightlifting. This is determined by many factors, including the natural ratio of fast twitch to slow twitch muscle fibers, hormone levels, skeletal structure and neurological factors that influence motor unit recruitment, rate coding, synchronization, and intra- and intermuscular coordination. All athletes can increase their speed to some degree through training (in weightlifting, the most dramatic improvements will be the result of technical proficiency and timing), but a naturally slow athlete will never achieve the levels of actual movement speed of a naturally fast athlete.

Natural levels of strength and flexibility also vary considerably. Some of the most flexible athletes in the world have invested little to no time in their entire lives to stretching; likewise, there are many individuals possessed of impressive strength who have never engaged in strength training (or even particularly physically demanding work). These two traits can be influenced to a greater extent through training than speed, although their rate of progress and ultimate levels are still largely genetically predetermined.

The athlete's capacity for motor skill learning is also largely innate, just like intellectual learning. Some athletes are able to pick up skills with relative ease and reach mastery in a very short period, while others will struggle over long periods of time to learn the same skills, and often never reach the same ultimate level of proficiency. This can also be influenced in the earliest year's of an athlete's life (such as through participation in an array of athletic activity), but is essentially unchangeable by the time an older athlete reaches a coach.

Joint ranges of motion and end positions are

also determined genetically—mobility and flexibility work can improve an athlete's access to the available range of motion allowed anatomically, but it cannot change the basic shape and structure of a joint. The joint in which this element has the greatest influence on weightlifting performance is the elbow. While some lifters will be capable of achieving slight hyperextension of the elbow and consequently a very secure, stable lockout position for holding weight overhead in the snatch and jerk that relies largely on bone structure, other lifters will be unable to even achieve a perfectly straight arm with maximal elbow extension effort, leaving them to rely more on muscular strength and effort to maintain the overhead position and struggling to support heavier weights (Figure 3.8).

Of course, with proper program design, instruction and enough hard work and long term commitment, natural disadvantages in these areas can largely be overcome or at least mitigated. A less naturally advantaged lifter who consistently works hard for a long time can usually beat a naturally talented lifter who does not; however, the elite of any sport will always be those who are both the most naturally gifted and the hardest working, most committed athletes. That is simply a combination that cannot be beat.

Program design and training must take into account each lifter's natural physical traits and seek to exploit his or her strengths and mitigate the negative effects of his or her weaknesses.

Training Response & Recovery

No two athletes will respond in an identical manner to any given set of training stimuli. This is the very basis for the complexity and difficulty of effective weightlifting program design. If all athletes responded identically to the same training program, the job would be very simple.

Aside from the fact that each athlete will require somewhat different training programs in terms of exercise selection, rep ranges, intensity, volume and

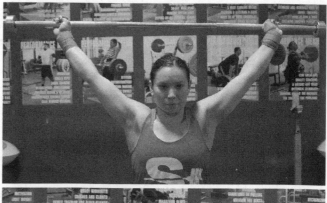

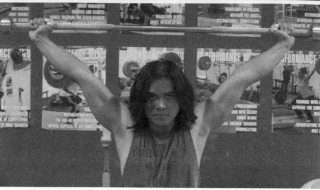

FIGURE 3.8 The natural structure of the athlete's joints will dictate their ultimate possible ranges of motion and end positions. The elbows are the joint with the most influence on weightlifting performance; the ability to completely lock the joint will confer a significant advantage.

similar parameters, athletes possess innate characteristics that govern their ability to recover effectively from training, meaning one athlete can tolerate more and progress more quickly and to a greater magnitude than another, even if all other factors are equal.

This is primarily an issue of natural hormonal status, but also involves factors like an athlete's quality of sleep and basic constitution with regard to elements like managing stress. These are things that are largely innate and cannot be altered significantly through training or other means (with the exception of PED use on hormonal levels).

Although we can make many useful generalizations to guide the program design process, ultimately program design must be individualized to account for all of the peculiarities of each athlete if maximal progress is to be obtained.

Individualized Competition Lift Technique

A quick survey of weightlifters at the highest level of competition will make it clear that there is considerable variation in the details of technical execution of the snatch and clean & jerk. For any generally accepted rule of lifting technique, one can find exceptions among even world class lifters. However, this is not evidence that these common rules are incorrect or of no use; it is evidence that in order to reach the highest levels of performance, technique over time will need to adapt to some degree to each athlete's physical peculiarities.

I.P. Zhekov (1976/1992) wrote that "the weightlifter-barbell system is a self-organizing, self-tuning system. It continually adjusts itself, searching for the right movement variation which helps it to best execute the motor task." This is an enlightening statement in that it reminds us that the human body is incredibly adept when it comes to motor skills. However, it does not mean that the athlete will naturally develop and establish optimal weightlifting technique without instruction and feedback. It simply means that, along with such instruction and guidance, within the established parameters of effective lift technique, each athlete will naturally develop idiosyncratic variations that maximize his or her abilities by exploiting strengths and mitigating weaknesses.

All lifters should begin the process by learning the fundamentals and training the lifts with textbook technique. This develops a solid base that acts as a framework for later modification. Additionally, without this base early in a lifter's career, there is no true way to accurately evaluate divergence from it; it will never be clear if the individual style is genuinely optimal for that athlete, or if it's the product of never having properly developed a certain aspect of the lift and is actually harming the lifter's performance.

When to begin allowing a lifter to diverge from this base of standard technique is not a simple answer, as it will always be a decision based largely on subjective criteria. In any case, it will be important for the coach and athlete to communicate clearly about what the athlete is feeling during the process of development—this will often reveal elements that are holding the athlete back. It's also important to recognize that mistakes may be made, and that reverting to the previous method of execution should always be considered an option.

Training Progress

All weightlifters will progress at different rates and be capable of reaching different ultimate levels. Each of these things is influenced significantly by factors such as starting age, the details of the training program, and general circumstances related to training, recovery, motivation and the like, but there are additional factors specific to each individual beyond control or manipulation that will dictate the nature and extent of progress.

Lifters of the lighter weight classes typically progress more quickly than their larger weight class counterparts, while lifters in the heavier classes tend to be capable of sustaining progress for a longer period of time (Medvedyev 1986/1989).

Athletes who naturally possess a greater number of individual muscle fibers per muscle, and those with a high percentage of fast twitch fibers, have greater potential for ultimate levels of strength and explosiveness, and will improve at greater rates (Zatsiorsky 1995).

Complex factors like the ability to achieve quality sleep regularly, the management of stress with relatively little physiological effect, and hormonal balance will all contribute to an athlete's potential and rate of progress.

Facility & Equipment

Weightlifting is a unique sport and mode of training, and as such makes very specific demands on the training facility and equipment. With the exception of a barbell and plates, none of the following items are absolutely necessary in the most fundamental sense, but many, such as weightlifting shoes, are required for legitimate training. As with any sport, the higher the level of performance is intended, the higher the quality and greater the amount of equipment will be necessary.

It should be noted that all weightlifting competition is conducted with metric weights. Regardless of national convention outside of the sport, all weightlifters and weightlifting coaches need to be familiar with recognizing and communicating weights in kilograms. While not absolutely necessary to be successful, training with metric equipment is the most sensible approach unless legitimately impossible.

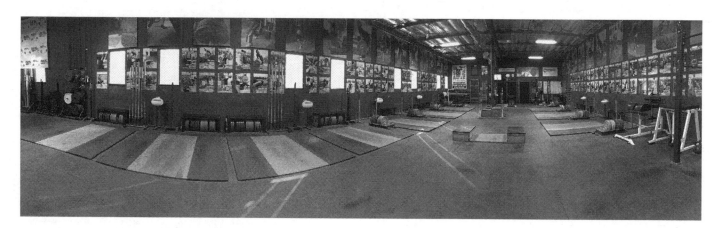

FIGURE 4.1 The Catalyst Athletics training facility in Sunnyvale, California.

Barbells

The principal requirement for the Olympic lifts is an Olympic barbell (Figure 4.2). These bars are remarkably strong yet provide flexibility without permanent deformity—that is, they are intentionally built to be very elastic. This elasticity provides what is called "whip" to the bar, and every barbell brand and type will have a somewhat different feel in this regard, although the best bars will be quiet similar.

The sleeves rotate smoothly on the shaft using a series of needle bearings to allow the bar to be rotated by the lifter during the turnover of the snatch and clean without having to overcome the rotational inertia of the plates. A bar that doesn't spin well results in more difficult lifts at best and injuries at worst. The needle bearings better distribute the force to prevent pitting of the barbell shaft and maintain smooth and consistent spin.

Competition regulation men's bars are 20kg

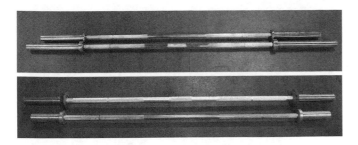

FIGURE 4.2 Regulation men's and women's bars (top)
FIGURE 4.3 Light training bars for technique instruction (bottom)

(44lbs), with a shaft diameter of 28mm and a length of 2200mm. Women's bars are 15kg (33lbs), with a shaft diameter of 25mm and a length of 2010 mm. Both bars are the same length between the sleeves—1310mm—and have the same markings in the knurling (the position of the 0.5cm knurling breaks among men's and women's bars may differ extremely slightly in position in non-competition-certified barbells). Women's barbells often do not have knurling in the center, while men's bars more often do. Competition barbells must also have color markings on their end caps corresponding to the international color-coding system: blue for 20kg barbells and yellow for 15kg barbells. This color-coding is only occasionally used on training barbells.

For women in an athletic training setting, women's bars may not be absolutely necessary, but for many women, grip security on a men's bar will be a problem. Competitive female weightlifters should always train on women's barbells because they will always be used in competition. (One exception in training is for back squats, for which women will often prefer using a men's barbell; this is also preferred because heavy squatting can be tough on the thinner barbell itself.)

Spending more money on a barbell will prevent a lot of frustration and likely save money in the long run—the barbell should be considered a long-term investment. Less expensive bars will spin poorly, have poor elasticity, oxidize more, bend permanently more easily, fit plates either too tightly or too loosely, and will have to be replaced more often than more expensive bars. The application will help determine the choice of bar—if lifting will be performed for competition, consider spending more money as the bar will be used more frequently and loaded with more weight, and movement precision will be a pri-

ority; if lifting will be performed simply for athletic training, less expensive bars may suffice, but will not be as durable as higher quality bars. In any case, the barbell should be the primary concern; its quality will have a more significant effect on training than any other piece of equipment aside from shoes.

There are two basic categories of Olympic bars: training and competition. The most noticeable differences—aside from price—are the deeper and sharper knurling and certification by the IWF of the competition bars. Certification and the extreme precision it indicates is unnecessary for training applications and even the local level of competition. More importantly, the deeper and sharper knurling of competition bars will typically prove too severe for daily use and destroy lifters' hands in short order.

In the early stages of learning or teaching the lifts, technique bars are important (Figure 4.3). These bars are ideally of regulation diameter and may be as light as 5kg. This allows a more gradual loading progression for athletes while keeping the feel of the bar correct. Prior to this, 5-ft lengths of ¾" PVC pipe can be used for introducing the movements and will be the tool of choice for the initial snatch progression drills in this book.

Bumper Plates & Change

Bumper plates allow the barbell to be dropped after lifts or in cases of missed attempts with less damage to the bar, plates and flooring. Bumper plates are 450mm in diameter with a center hole diameter of 50mm. The thickness of the plate varies with the brand and model depending on the construction and characteristics of the rubber compound used.

Color	Bumper	Change
Red	25kg	2.5kg
Blue	20kg	2kg
Yellow	15kg	1.5kg
Green	10kg	1kg
White		5kg / 0.5kg

TABLE 4.1 Weight Color Chart

There is a wide range of quality in the realm of bumper plates. Just as with barbells, bumpers can be of competition quality and consequently extremely expensive. Their training counterparts are more than adequate for the highest level lifters in training. Very inexpensive bumpers, often composed of recycled rubber, are also available and are appropriate for many athletic training situations. It's common that the metal hubs used in many of these plates will become loose over time, but this is generally not problematic aside from being annoying. If the bumpers will be used frequently by a large number of athletes, such as in a college or high school athletic training facility, more expensive training bumpers will be a wise investment to withstand the abuse.

Bumper plates come in weights of 10kg, 15kg, 20kg and 25kg. Change plates come in weights of 0.5kg, 1kg, 1.5kg, 2kg, 2.5kg and 5kg. Weights are color-coded for recognition with the following international convention: 25kg is red; 20kg is blue; 15kg is yellow; 10kg is green. Training change plates are usually a single color (such as gray or black), but officially and in competition, these plates are also color-coded in a manner that corresponds to the bumper plates: 2.5kg are red; 2kg are blue; 1.5kg are yellow; 1kg are green; and 0.5 and 5kg are white (Table 4.1). Gyms often do not have 1.5kg plates, as they are a relatively new item and generally not worth the expense (the combination of a 1kg and 0.5kg plate on the bar is easy and costs nothing additional). In recent years, friction plates have become common in competition—these are change plates with a rubber coating that prevents their easy sliding off the bar. This means that weights smaller than 2.5kg can be loaded outside of the collar, which reduces weight change times in competition.

Less expensive bumper plates may be all black. A common practice is to run a line of properly colored tape around the diameter of such bumpers to help with weight recognition.

Technique plates are helpful in the early stages of learning and teaching the lifts. These plates are the standard diameter of bumpers, allowing the athlete to pull the bar from the normal position on the floor, but are as light as 2.5kg and even less in some homemade instances.

Collars

Weightlifting collars are comprised of two threaded components—a screw that tightens the collar against the sleeve of the barbell, and a screw around the circumference of the collar that then extends against the plates to tighten the assembly and prevent shifting of the plates (Figure 4.6). This creates a simple system for securing the plates snugly on the ends of the barbell. These collars are a standard weight of 2.5kg and are, for the obvious reason, included in the account of the total weight on the bar.

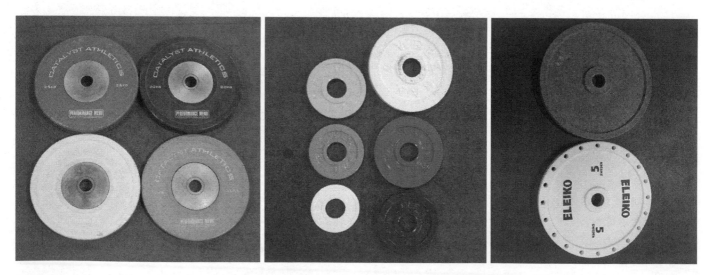

FIGURE 4.4 Bumper plates: 10kg, 15kg, 20kg and 25kg (left). Change plates: 0.5kg, 1kg, 1.5kg, 2kg, 2.5kg and 5kg (center).
FIGURE 4.5 Technique plates allow athletes to pull from the correct height off the floor while weighing only fractions of the lightest bumper plate. (right)

Greg Everett

It's fairly uncommon for collars to be used regularly in a weightlifting gym, largely because of the additional time and effort required and the frequent weight changes, but also because they tend to be in comparatively short supply due to their expense. This is not a safety concern with experienced lifters training with high quality barbells and plates because the tight manufacturing tolerances mean plates don't slide on the barbell's sleeves too easily to slide off during the expected jostling of a lift, and because experienced lifters rarely if ever put a barbell in an orientation in which plates will slide significantly. With less expensive equipment, or inexperienced lifters who are more likely to tilt the bar and allow plates to slide, collars are a good idea.

Competitive lifters are encouraged to use collars periodically, particularly in the weeks prior to a competition, to get accustomed to the different feeling of the bar. Without collars, both the sleeves of the barbell and the plates on the sleeves are free to spin; with tightly applied collars, as will be seen in competition, the plates are unable to spin on the sleeves, and rotation is confined to the actual bearings of the barbell. While quality bars will still spin very well, there is a definite and noticeable difference between a collared and un-collared bar, even in the sound it makes during a lift. It can be surprising and disrupting to lift on a collared bar in a meet without prior experience of the feeling.

Spring collars or similar simpler and less expensive collars can also be used in the gym if securing the plates is desired (Figure 4.6). These are lightweight enough to not need to be considered in the total weight of the bar.

Lifting Platform

A weightlifting platform is the ideal lifting surface and should be considered necessary for competitive weightlifters (Figure 4.7). Quality platforms can be built easily and inexpensively, or can be purchased very expensively and unnecessarily. A wooden lifting surface can also be sunk into rubber flooring for a simple and unobtrusive platform.

However the platform is built, a wooden lifting surface will provide a stable, smooth and incompressible lifting platform, and rubberized landing pads will reduce the beating the bar and bumpers take and extend their useful lives, as well as reduce the abuse to the underlying flooring and limit noise somewhat.

To build an inexpensive platform, start with two 4'x8' sheets of inexpensive ½" or ¾" plywood alongside each other to create an 8'x8' footprint. Place two more sheets perpendicularly on top of these and screw them together tightly over the entire surface to prevent any lifting of the second layer. These sheets can also be glued together, but this will prevent their disassembly for moving or replacement of individual sheets in the future.

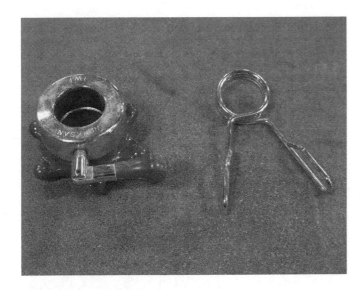

FIGURE 4.6 Barbell collars

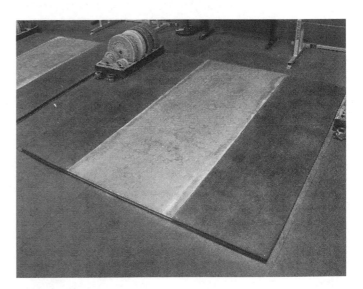

FIGURE 4.7 Lifting platform

Center a 4'x8' sheet of smooth ½" or ¾" high-quality plywood or MDF on top of this base, again perpendicular to the top sheets of plywood and screw down. Cover the remaining 2'x8' sections with rubber of the same thickness as the center sheet—horse stall matting is relatively inexpensive and does the job well, or rolled rubber sheeting can be purchased.

If time, tools and ambition are available, it's recommended that the top sheet be cut narrower. The bumpers on a bar will sit just barely outside the width of a 4'-wide top sheet, meaning more accidental dropping on the wood. Cutting the top sheet to 3'6" and the rubber sides to 27" wide will provide more than enough lifting surface and more landing area for the bumpers. (These are the dimensions pictured in Figure 4.7.)

To place a platform in existing rubber flooring, simply cut a sheet of plywood or MDF of the same thickness of the rubber flooring to the desired dimensions and lay it over the flooring where it will be placed. Trace the sheet on the rubber, remove the wood, and cut the rubber. Be sure to place the cuts inside the drawn lines to ensure a tight fit. The wood can be secured to the floor with construction adhesive to prevent warping or shifting.

Squat Rack

Squat racks will allow the athlete to perform heavier squats, jerks, presses and a number of other possible exercises without having to first lift the weight from the floor, which ranges from unnecessarily difficult and taxing to impossible (Figure 4.8). For the weightlifter, the squat rack is not optional.

Racks can either be a single unit, or two individual uprights. Individual uprights are helpful in terms of storage space and ease of relocation, but single-unit racks are more stable and generally easier to work with. The width of all quality single-unit racks is adjustable, so this is not a reason for individual uprights.

In any case, like a barbell and bumper plates, more money spent on a rack will mean one that functions better, lasts longer and supports more weight. The last thing that needs to go through an athlete's mind when finishing an extremely heavy squat is whether or not the rack will support the bar.

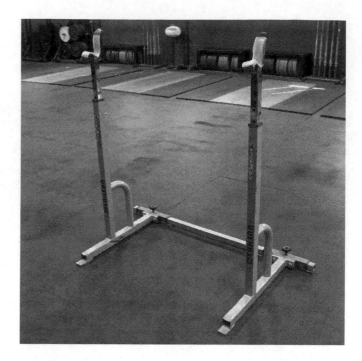

FIGURE 4.8 Squat rack

A couple basic elements to consider are possible heights, the mechanism of height and width adjustment, and the shape of the cradle. For athletes who want to use the squat rack for bench pressing, or for those who are particularly short, greater low-end height adjustability will be necessary. It's rare to find a rack that won't adjust high enough for any athlete, but it's fairly common for racks to not go low enough for bench pressing.

Some racks have awkward mechanisms for height and width adjustment, and sometimes those of questionable reliability. Find a rack that adjusts easily and securely.

Finally, racks can have different shapes for the bar cradle. Typically these are flat-bottomed with a high vertical back and a lower, forward-slanting front. Occasionally the front is vertical as well, making replacement of the bar far more difficult. Other racks' cradles are curved at the bottom, meaning that the bar settles into a single position rather than being able to roll back and forth somewhat. Ideally the cradle has a Teflon or similar surface on which the bar rests to help protect the knurling from being worn down over time, although protection can be added to most racks if desired.

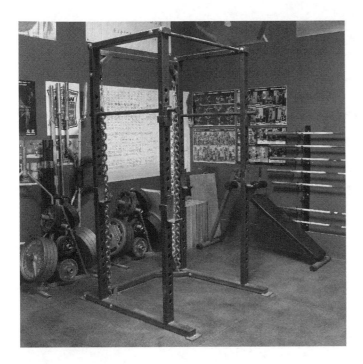

FIGURE 4.9 Power rack

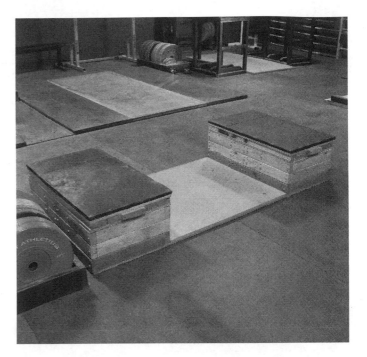

FIGURE 4.10 Pulling blocks

Power Rack

Power racks can also be used instead of squat racks, or in addition to squat racks (Figure 4.9). The drawback of using a power rack instead of a squat rack is the amount of space it takes up—placing a full-size rack on a standard-size platform will take up far too much space for non-rack lifting, and moving such racks is not an easy task. Power racks do offer options for more exercises or exercise variations, however, so if space and money allow, they're a nice addition to any facility.

Power racks can be used for exercises such as rack supports, jerk supports and jerk recoveries, heavy partial squats or jumping squat variations in which the bar needs to be lifted from an elevated height or there is a need for safety reasons to prevent the bar from dropping to the floor. Half-racks take up less space but need to be bolted to a wall, and full racks are self-supporting but have a large footprint.

Pulling Blocks

Pulling blocks are small elevated platforms that can be used to snatch or clean from by starting the barbell

at a level higher than the floor (Figure 4.10). These can be constructed relatively inexpensively in a number of different ways and made adjustable in height for maximal utility—ideally a set of blocks can adjust from a level at which the bar is around mid-shin all the way up to mid-thigh. Metal pulling stands are also manufactured by a few different companies, but tend to be very expensive and not very adjustable.

A variation of pulling blocks are pulling stands, but these are usually very small and not very stable—bars can't be dropped on them after lifts—so their real use is limited to partial pulls and deadlifts or very light snatches and cleans.

Stair Blocks

Stair blocks are an unusual and unnecessary piece of equipment that can also be built easily (Figure 4.11). This is a single block with multiple heights in a stair-step configuration. Unlike pulling blocks, which support the barbell with the bumper plates on each end, stair blocks support the barbell directly at its center and the lifter straddles the block. This allows partial

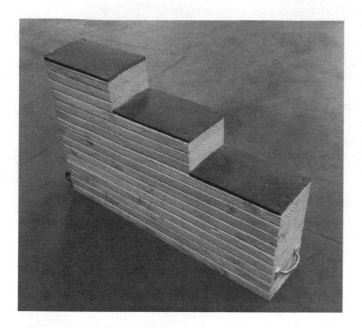

FIGURE 4.11 Staircase blocks

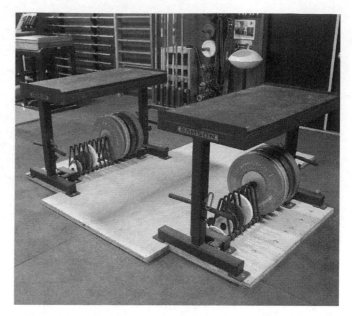

FIGURE 4.12 Jerk tables

snatch and clean pulls to be done with an elastic rebound of the bar to increase its speed at the start of the pull. Such use is not particularly good for the barbell, so less expensive bars should be used.

Jerk Tables / Blocks

Jerk blocks have become much more common in recent years, but are still somewhat of a luxury, in part because of cost, but also because of their large space requirement (Figure 4.12). They can be built, or they can be purchased now from a few different manufacturers.

The purpose of jerk blocks is to simply provide an elevated surface for the plates on the bar, just like pulling blocks, but higher. The athlete can lift the bar from this elevated position much as he or she would from a squat rack, but more importantly, following a jerk, the athlete can drop the bar back to this elevated platform rather than dropping it to the floor or lowering it back to the shoulders. In this way, jerk blocks allow the athlete to perform multiple successive reps in the jerk with much heavier loads than could be lowered back to the shoulders safely by the athlete. Depending on how they're constructed, jerk blocks can sometimes be lowered enough to be used as pulling blocks for snatches and cleans.

Risers

A riser is a simple piece of equipment that can generally be made with leftover wood (Figure 4.13). This small platform on which the athlete stands elevates the athlete without changing the barbell's starting height; in other words, it increases the range of the pull from the floor. Pulls and deadlifts from the riser can be effective for increasing a lifter's pulling strength and speed from the floor. Most important when building a riser is ensuring a smooth, flat top surface for the lifter to stand on without any risk of tripping or catching a shoe on an edge, and a flat bottom surface that keeps the riser flat and stable on the platform.

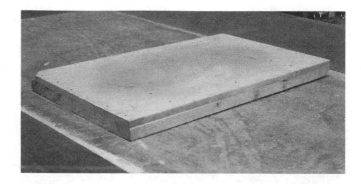

FIGURE 4.13 Riser

Plyo Boxes

Plyo boxes can be purchased or built fairly inexpensively (Figure 4.14). A few boxes of various heights will allow an enormous number of options for jump training, step-ups and various stretches and odd uses.

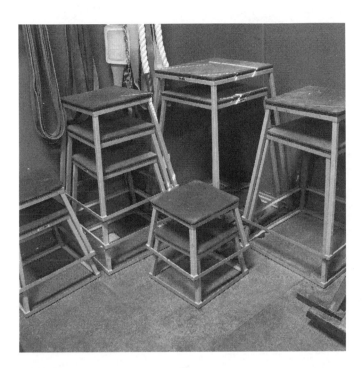

FIGURE 4.14 Plyo boxes

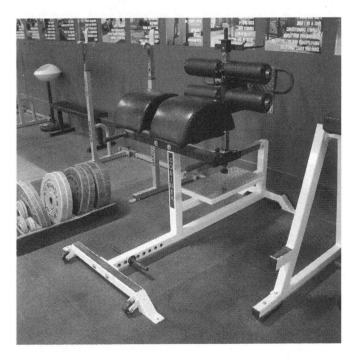

FIGURE 4.15 Glute-ham bench

Glute-Ham Bench

A glute-ham bench is a large and expensive piece of equipment that is certainly not necessary, but valuable if space and finances allow its purchase (Figure

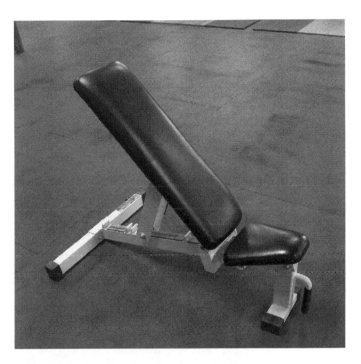

FIGURE 4.16 Adjustable bench

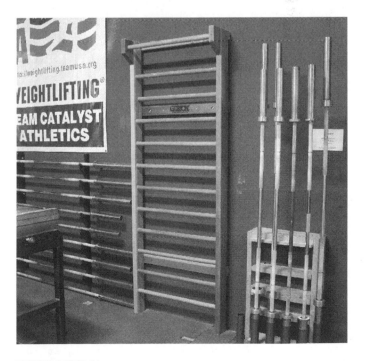

FIGURE 4.17 Stall bars

4.15). It can be used for a number of supplemental back, hip and core exercises such as back and hip extensions, glute-ham raises, roman chair/GHB sit-ups, and reverse hyperextensions.

Adjustable Bench

Although much less common since the elimination of the press in competition, it is not unheard of for weightlifters to bench press at certain times (Figure 4.16). If budget and space allow, a quality adjustable bench is worth having in the facility to allow both flat and incline bench pressing. Incline bench pressing will be more commonly used because of the more vertical top position and because when used to build mass for a lifter, will help put that mass more in the shoulders and upper chest where it's more helpful for the jerk rack position in particular. Benches can also be useful for various ab and shoulder prehab exercises.

Stall Bars

Stall bars, while by no means a necessary piece of equipment, are useful if available (Figure 4.17). Primarily their use is for stretching and ab training, but they're also useful to provide a selection of attachment points for elastic bands used for shoulder prehab exercises.

Shoes

Weightlifting shoes (Figure 4.18) are an absolute must for all lifters for two primary reasons. First, the hard soles don't compress under loads, eliminating the instability found in soft-soled shoes as well as ensuring that generated force is transmitted more completely from the platform to the bar. Second, the lifted heels effectively increase the ankles' range of motion, allowing the lifter to keep the hips forward and torso upright as needed in the squat (Figure 4.19).

It's important to find a pair of shoes that support the arches well. Orthotics should be used by any athletes with collapsing arches to ensure proper foot and ankle position, which will in turn ensure the lifter

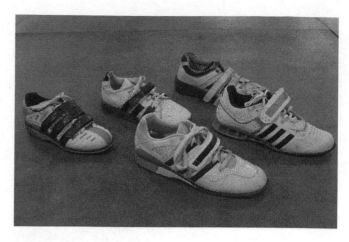

FIGURE 4.18 Weightlifting shoes

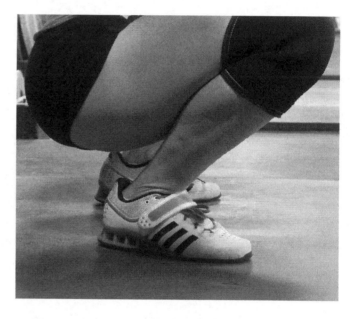

FIGURE 4.19 The lifted heels of weightlifting shoes increase the ankles' range of motion and allow better positioning in the bottom of the squat.

is able to recognize his or her full strength potential and better avoid injury to the ankles, knees, hips and back.

Weightlifting shoes are fairly expensive, but should be considered an investment in both performance and longevity. Typically the shoes' uppers will hold up well over time, so with occasional repairs and resoling, a single pair of shoes will often last many years. It's important to retire shoes when the uppers are no longer supportive, however; this can lead to foot and ankle instability and cause injuries up the chain from the knees to the hips to the back and even the shoulders, elbows and wrists.

Chalk

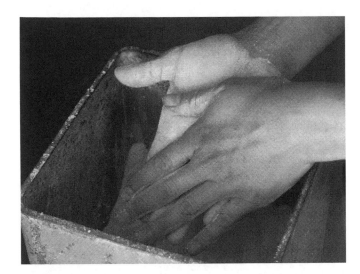

FIGURE 4.20 Chalk

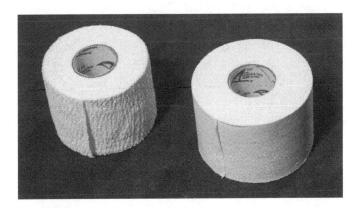

FIGURE 4.21 Elastic and non-elastic athletic tape

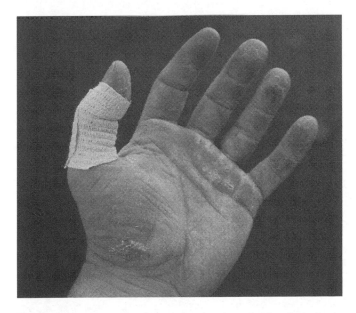

FIGURE 4.22 Taping the thumbs can help reduce discomfort from the hook grip and increase grip integrity for some lifters.

Chalk will improve the grip on the bar by keeping the hands dry as well as provide some protection from bar friction (Figure 4.20). It's usually best purchased from gymnastics equipment suppliers as broken blocks. The broken pieces are less expensive and are already partway to the state in which they'll end up anyway. Purchasing chalk from rock climbing or fitness equipment stores will prove unnecessarily expensive.

Chalk belongs in four primary places: the lifter's hands, the bar, clothing from bar and hand contact, and in the container it came from. Spreading chalk all over the facility because of an unwillingness to take the extra five seconds to rub it into the hands over the bucket is disrespectful to the owner of the facility and a hassle for those who are responsible for cleaning it up; more importantly, loose chalk on lifting surfaces can result in potentially serious injuries from slipping feet. Remember—chalk trails on the floor lead to amateurs.

Along with chalk, hand-drying products such as Tite-Grip can be used to keep hands dry during training. Such products are extremely helpful for allowing tape to continue to adhere.

Tape

Tape may be used for a number of reasons (Figure 4.21). For the hands, it can serve as a means of prevention of injuries or protection of existing injuries. Taping parts of the hands that receive the most friction can reduce the potential for callus tears and sometimes improve grip. Taping the thumb can reduce the discomfort of the hook grip, and for some lifters, improve the security of the grip (Figure 4.22). It's important in cases of taping over any joints in the hands to use elastic tape—non-elastic tape will prevent normal joint movement and often result in spraining of adjacent joints. In competition, tape may not extend past the end of the thumb—keep the end of the thumb visible to avoid problems.

Tape is also commonly used on the wrists for support in the overhead positions of the snatch and jerk. In cases of existing injuries, it can provide some added support to reduce movement outside the comfortable range of motion. It's sometimes used as well in a preventative fashion to limit the extension of the wrists and reduce translation of the distal heads of the ulna and radius under heavy overhead loads. Such use should be avoided as much as possible unless and until necessary to allow the joints to develop along with the rest of the body; taping unnecessarily in the earlier stages of a lifting career will limit the strength and conditioning of the wrists and create more potential problems in the future.

Wrist Wraps

Wrist wraps are an alternative to tape for support of the wrists (Figure 4.23). Their tension can be easily adjusted to avoid dramatic movement limitation and they can be used loosely to keep the joints warm; additionally, they will prevent the spending of large sums of money on tape. Wrist wraps come in a number of styles. Like knee sleeves, wrist wraps should not be used unnecessarily—the longer a lifter can train without them, the stronger and more conditioned the wrists will become as they develop in pace with the rest of the body, and the less likely he or she will experience problems later due to limitations in the wrists' ability to keep up with the rest of the body.

Caution should also be exercised to ensure wrist wraps are not over-tightened—this can too greatly

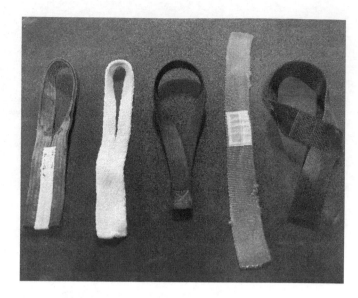

FIGURE 4.24 There are several styles of lifting straps.

limit the mobility of the wrist and hand, preventing the correct overhead position and increasing the risk of elbow and shoulder injury. Wraps should support the proper hand and wrist position, not prevent it.

Straps

The use of straps is generally limited to pulls and variations, multiple rep, block or hang work in the snatch, or in times when the hands are too beat-up to grip the bar (Figure 4.24). Of course, using straps will by no means remove the need for grip strength

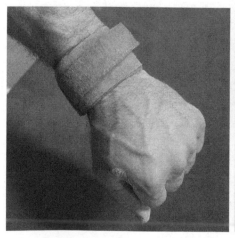
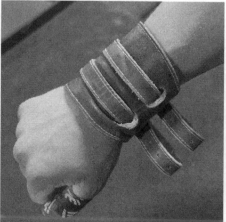
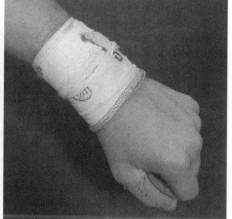

FIGURE 4.23 Wrist wraps can be used to provide additional support for the wrists in the overhead positions of the snatch and jerk.

Greg Everett

entirely and may not have a particularly dramatic effect for some athletes—it's simply a matter of judicious use to prevent excessive reliance on them and the feeling of security they provide. Ultimately, if an athlete can't hold onto it, he or she can't lift it, so it's important to not allow overall body strength development to outpace grip strength development to a significant enough degree that an athlete is missing lifts due to grip failure. However, for athletes who are on heavy classic lift emphasis cycles, using straps for the snatch in some workouts is often necessary to prevent undue stress to the hands.

Generally it's advisable to limit the use of straps as an athlete approaches a competition, with the exception of cases in which strap use will prevent possible damage to the hands. For athletes with exceptional grip strength and no history of the hands slipping during lifts, straps can be used as much as desired.

Simple straps can be purchased or made inexpen-

sively with nylon webbing. Smoother nylon will feel better on the hands, but it will take a period of use to roughen up enough to stick well to the bar. Wider straps will also feel better on the hands, but often they will interfere with the necessary mobility of the hand and wrist.

Straps can be wrapped somewhat differently depending on the exercise. For exercises like pulls and deadlifts, during which the bar will simply remain hanging from the hands rather than in or above them, a tighter wrap is acceptable. Some lifters may even wrap the straps twice around the bar to limit slipping and friction on the hands during extremely heavy, high-rep pulls or shrugs.

For the snatch, the manner of wrapping is more important. Because the hand and wrist must turnover as the bar is received overhead, the straps cannot limit mobility. Wrapping them too tightly or placing the straps over the wrists rather than the hands

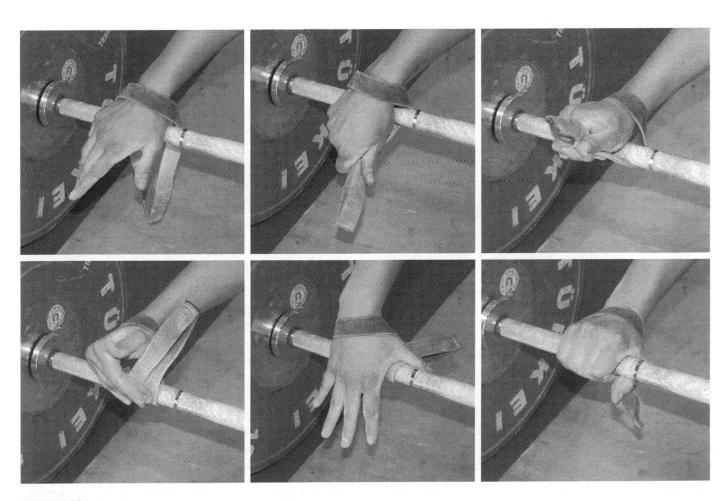

FIGURE 4.25 Placing straps

will prevent this turnover and correct hand position. Straps during these exercises can be left seemingly loose and still function as needed. An easy way to check a proper wrap is, before beginning the lift, to simply extend the wrist and flatten the hand against the bar as if holding it overhead. If this isn't possible, the straps are too tight or too high. Also, if the wrist cannot remain neutral when pulling—that is, it's in a partially extended position—the straps are too tight.

The use of straps for cleans is not recommended. Because the clean rack position for most lifters involves the bar moving nearer to the ends of the fingers from its starting point deeper in the hands, straps will prevent the athlete from racking the bar correctly, placing a great deal of strain on the wrists, elbows and shoulders. Even for athletes who are able to still rack the bar well with straps on, there is a concern about missing lifts. In the snatch, no matter which direction the bar is lost, the straps will quickly and easily unwrap and present no problems. When missing a clean, because of the hand position, the bar is not able to roll out of the straps easily, and will more likely remain in the hands, forcing the elbows down and creating opportunity to strain the wrists, elbows and shoulders, and possibly causing the elbows to strike the thighs, opening the athlete up for serious wrist and lower arm injury. In the case of

falling backward under a clean, an already precarious situation is made much worse by the lifter's ability to release the bar being limited. This has in more than one instance sprained and broken lifters' wrists when their elbows hit the floor at their sides with the bar still stuck in their hands.

To place the straps (Figure 4.25), slide the hand through the loop with the palm down and the length of the strap hanging. The surface of the strap should lie flat against the hand—if it doesn't, the strap needs to be flipped around the other way or moved to the other hand. In sewn-loop straps, the inner length should be on top of the outer length as pictured.

Place the hand on the bar with the strap hanging down behind it. With the fingers, pull the strap under and around the bar to wrap it, and close the hand around it. To adjust the position or tension of the straps, rotate the bar and hands, or slide in and out. The hook grip is not necessary (or possible for most) when using straps.

Knee Sleeves & Wraps

Neoprene or woven elastic knee sleeves are common pieces of gear among lifters. These sleeves are tight enough to provide joint support, but not as tight

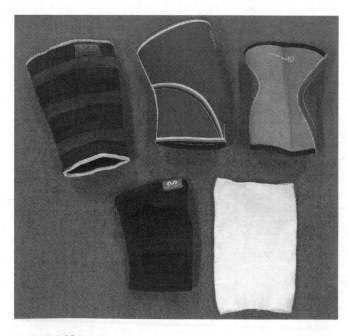

FIGURE 4.26 Knee sleeves come in different materials and thicknesses to provide varying feels, performance and levels of support.

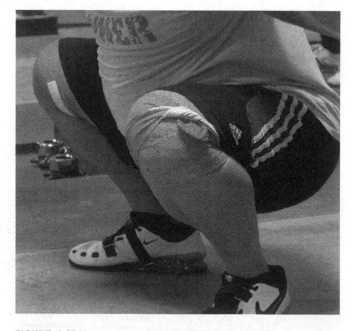

FIGURE 4.27 Knee wraps can be made tighter around the joint to create more rebound than knee sleeves.

Greg Everett

as wraps, which must be loosened in between sets. They keep the knees warm during training and consequently may reduce injury risk and improve function in addition to reducing achiness. They will also provide a degree of assistance in the bottom of the squat and in the dip of the jerk, but little enough that they remain legal in competition.

When joint warmth is not a concern, knees sleeves should be considered much like belts in that their use should be limited to heavier training. Many athletes choose, also like belts, to wear them only for the clean & jerk and not for the snatch. In training, their use may be restricted to heavy squatting and cleaning. Some athletes will find they provide some beneficial support when jerking as well by improving the elasticity in the dip and drive.

In some cases, athletes will find that knee sleeves actually cause knee pain by opening the joint excessively when the material behind the knee bunches up in the bottom of the squat. Clearly in such cases, sleeves should not be used, or the athlete should experiment with thinner sleeves.

For older or particularly beat-up lifters, knee sleeves may be a necessity during all training. At this point, this is really not a concern and their use is encouraged to allow continued training. For younger and newer lifters, the longer sleeve use can be postponed, both in terms of a career and a given training session, the better off the athlete will be.

Thin knee sleeves that don't provide any real support can also be used to simply keep the joints warm during training, especially in colder weather.

Knee wraps are an alternative to knee sleeves (Figure 4.27). The primary benefit is that their greater stiffness assists in the rebound out of the bottom of the squat or jerk dip to a greater degree than knee sleeves. However, if wrapped tightly enough for this effect, they will usually need to be unwrapped in between sets. Many weightlifters consequently find wraps to be more of a hassle than they're worth.

Like with wrist wraps and tape, knee sleeves and wraps should only be used as an athlete advances to higher stages of training and competition and determines them necessary. New lifters should avoid their use to ensure more complete development of a foundation that will allow more productive training over the long term.

Belts

Opinions regarding the use of belts (Figure 4.28) vary widely among coaches and athletes. At the root of many of the arguments is the consideration of them as safety devices. The debate can be quickly ended (or at least attenuated) by agreeing that belts should be used for a single purpose: performance enhancement.

The spine is protected during heavy structural loading by the combination of internal thoracic and abdominal pressure and both deep and superficial muscular effort. Belts allow the athlete to increase the pressure in the torso by limiting the possible expansion of the abdominal cavity. In other words, they primarily reinforce the musculature around the circumference of the trunk to better maintain stabilizing pressure, rather than support the spine directly. The consequence of this increased pressure is increased rigidity of the torso, allowing it to function as both a more effective transmitter of force from the legs and hips to the bar as well as a more stable foundation for compressive loads. Additionally, increased intraabdominal pressure reduces pressure on the intervertebral discs significantly.

The notion that belts should not be considered safety devices is not at all intended to imply their correct use will not increase the safety of heavy structur-

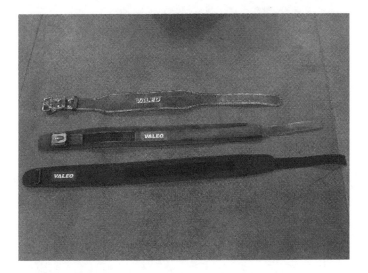

FIGURE 4.28 Belts increase the rigidity of the trunk under load, improving performance and safety, but should be used judiciously.

al lifts. It's simply a perspective that helps discourage improper and excessive use.

In the case of competitive weightlifters, belts can generally be reserved for the heaviest squats, cleans and jerks, or for higher-rep sets in which the core musculature is likely to fatigue significantly and increase the risk of postural instability. With weights lighter than this, refraining from the use of a belt will demand more effort from the musculature necessary to stabilize the torso as well as the athlete's conscious and unconscious control of body positions and muscular activation, consequently improving the development of both. This is not to say, of course, that belts eliminate the need for great effort or the development of trunk strength—only that athletes can achieve better trunk strength and stability development by limiting their use, particularly early in their development, and then adding them as a final performance boost.

A variety of belts are available. Four-inch belts are wholly adequate and don't limit mobility in the deep squat or starting position of the pulls like 6-inch belts can. If the athlete intends to compete, note that belt width is limited to 120 mm—about 4.7 inches—so 6-inch belts are not legal anyway.

As long as it's reliable, the closure type is not important and the choice can be made based on personal preference. However, a traditional belt buckle's adjustability is limited, so for some lifters, the belt will always be either too tight or too loose. Cam devices avoid this problem by being adjustable to any position.

Belts should not be tightened excessively—their role is to reinforce the muscular wall, not to force abnormal compression of the abdomen. In other words, the belt should be tight enough to support the abdominal bracing position, not to prevent it and force the athlete into a hollow position. The lifter should place the belt in position, fill the stomach with air, brace, and tighten the belt down enough to pull the abs just inside their braced position—this will ensure the abs when braced will be both pressurizing the torso as well as pushing out against the belt for reinforcement.

The use of belts should be postponed by new lifters as long as possible. Some world class lifters, in fact, never use a belt in their entire careers because they've developed adequate strength, stability and control. All new lifters should strive to train as much and as long as possible without belts.

Warming Up

Warming up properly before training is critical not only for reducing the chance of injury through the preparation of joints and muscles, but also for optimizing performance through the improvement of nerve transmission and communication between the CNS and motor units (Bompa 1999). This stage of training is neglected by a surprising number of athletes and coaches simply out of impatience or unfamiliarity with protocols. Any athlete who is unwilling to spend ten minutes warming up is not serious about training.

If the facility is particularly cold or the athlete unusually stiff, some light monostructural activity such as rowing, jumping rope, cycling or jogging can be performed for 2-5 minutes. The idea is to get the body moving in a way that increases its temperature, blood flow through the muscles, and synovial fluid release in the joints without taxing it metabolically or introducing any excessive demands on range of motion, speed of movement, or force production.

Following this, the athlete can spend a few minutes foam-rolling lightly to generate some body heat and prepare the muscles for smoother action. The athlete can then progress to a series of dynamic range of motion exercises (DROMs) and a select few static stretches to begin preparing the joints and muscles for greater degrees of movement.

Another consideration with regard to warming up is the basic time requirement for the body to get up to speed. Even when lifters perform an entire warm-up protocol, they may find that they don't begin feeling "warm" until partway through a training session. A simple way to add more time to allow the body to adjust and prepare without actually adding more time to a training session is to perform the initial steps of the warm-up, such as any monostructural or foam rolling work, and even some initial DROMs, then take

a break to perform the several common preparatory tasks: taping, preparing a pre-workout drink, making notes in the training journal, etc. This places the warm-up, or at least part of it, further from the time the athlete actually begins lifting without extending the total time of the training session, and for most athletes, this additional time will make the warm-up feel more effective sooner into the workout.

Additionally, some simple warm-up-type activity, such as a quick series of light DROMs, performed first thing in the morning will help the athlete warm up more quickly later in the day and feel looser and more prepared generally. This is especially helpful for lifters who train relatively early in the morning—this even earlier initiation of the warm-up process will help the lifter prepare far more effectively and feel considerably better at the time of the actual training session.

Static Stretching

Static stretching, with exceptions such as the wrists, ankles, shoulder girdle and hip flexors, generally is not ideal for warming-up. It will be less effective for improving flexibility than when done after training, is not an effective way to increase body temperature, and does a relatively poor job of preparing an athlete for movement. There is also evidence that static stretching can temporarily reduce explosiveness and proprioception, which makes it undesirable prior to training or competition for high-level athletes.

Exceptions to this are specific areas of muscle tightness that prevent an athlete from correctly assuming a given position. For example, a very tight new lifter may need to use a bout of static stretching prior to lifting and even in between sets to help maintain his or her lumbar curve in the squat or starting position of the pulls. This static stretching should be placed closer to the end of the warm-up to ensure the muscles are warm and adequately pliable to maximize effectiveness. If an athlete is inflexible to such a degree, there should be no concern about the possible negative effects of pre-training static stretching—such an athlete is not performing at a high enough level for such extremely minor effects to even warrant consideration.

Mobility training is discussed at greater length in its own section at the end of this book.

Warm-up Protocol

The following is a complete warm-up protocol that involves foam-rolling, dynamic range of motion exercises, and a selection of static stretches in the suggested order of execution. Athletes can modify this series to address specific needs. More flexible athletes will likely be able to omit most or all of the static stretches. This sequence should be done at a relatively quick pace for the sake of efficiency and a better warming effect.

Foam Rolling Sequence

For the pre-training foam rolling series, the intention is to simply loosen the muscles up and improve fluidity in their movement. We are not attempting to do deep, aggressive work on problem areas. This is better reserved for the post-workout window. Each area should be rolled for 10-15 easy passes.

Thoracic Spine Lie on the roller with it oriented perpendicularly to the spine. Start with your arms crossed loosely over your chest and roll the length of your thoracic spine, gradually relaxing more over the roller. After several passes, you can lift your arms overhead for further rolling. You will likely feel and hear some popping. After rolling, you may also want to lie still on the roller and allow your back to bend over it, further loosening the thoracic spine, moving

a few inches after each hold to cover the area immediately above the thoracolumbar junction in particular. (Figure 5.1)

Underarm Lie on your side with the roller at the area where your underarm meets your trunk with your arm extended overhead. Roll this attachment area and rotate your body to hit a range of aspects. You'll find areas that are more sensitive than others on which you'll want to focus. (Figure 5.2)

Glutes Sit on the roller with one leg crossed over the other knee and lean onto the glute of the crossed leg. Shift as you roll to find the areas of sensitivity on which to focus. (Figure 5.3)

Adductors & Hamstrings Sit with the roller under one leg and shift pressure to the inside of the roller leg, rotating that leg inward somewhat. Focus on the origin area of the adductors and hamstrings. (Figure 5.4)

Quads & Hip Flexors Start lying face down with both quads on the roller and make passes straight along the front of the quads. If more pressure is needed, move one leg off the roller. After your passes here, roll to the side of one leg and focus on the lateral quad, making sure to reach all the way around to the edge where it folds into the IT band (without rolling directly on the IT band), from just above the knee all the way to the hip. Staying on the side of one leg, move up to the hip flexor area, hitting the lateral aspect and then shifting toward the front. (Figure 5.5)

VMOs & Adductors Lie face down on the quads with the legs spread to the ends of the roller. Rotate the legs and shift your weight to one leg at a time to hit the VMO and adductors on each leg. (Figure 5.6)

Calves You can wrap up the foam rolling series with some quick passes on the calves, focusing primarily on the lower area, by resting the calves with straight legs on the roller and holding yourself up with the hands on the floor by your hips. (Figure 5.7)

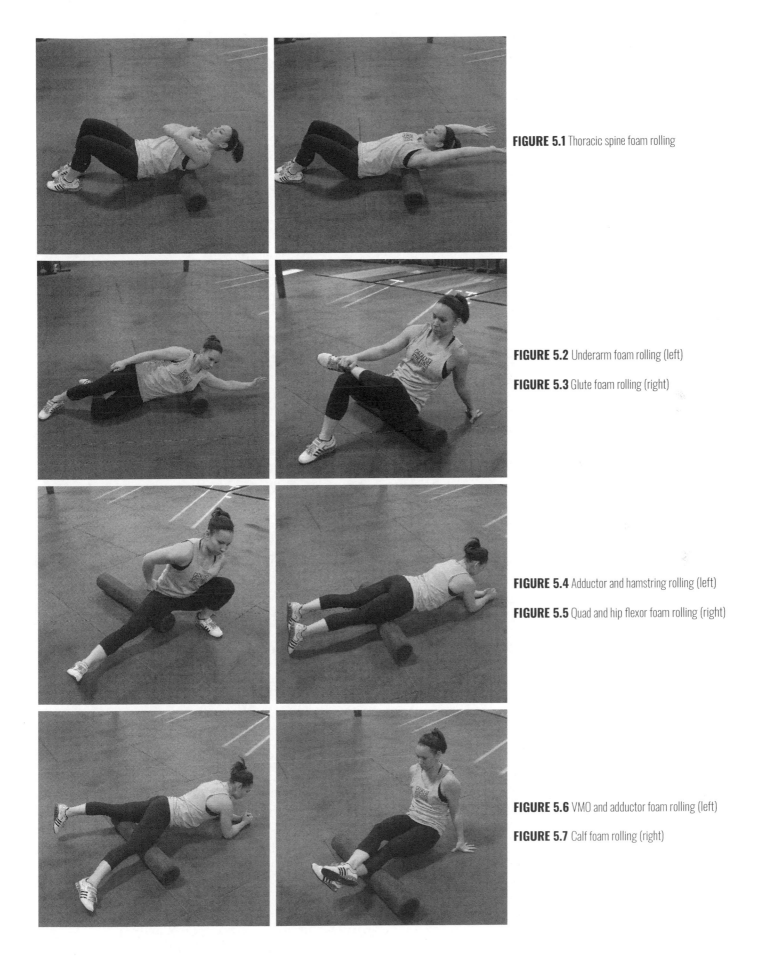

FIGURE 5.1 Thoracic spine foam rolling

FIGURE 5.2 Underarm foam rolling (left)

FIGURE 5.3 Glute foam rolling (right)

FIGURE 5.4 Adductor and hamstring rolling (left)

FIGURE 5.5 Quad and hip flexor foam rolling (right)

FIGURE 5.6 VMO and adductor foam rolling (left)

FIGURE 5.7 Calf foam rolling (right)

Dynamic & Static Stretch Sequence

Dynamic range of motion exercises should be performed with 10-15 reps (in each direction or per side where applicable). Static stretches should be held for 20-30 seconds, or if preferred, 10-15 repetitions of 2-second holds. Keeping a quick pace and not resting while working through this series will improve the warming effects and reduce the time demand.

Wrist Circles Wrist circles in both directions will warm and loosen up the joints to prepare them to support weight at extreme ranges of motion. Keep the hands and forearms close together to ensure maximal range of motion. (Figure 5.8)

Elbow Circles Elbow circles in both directions will help prepare the elbows for the stress of receiving and supporting heavy loads. The hands should be rotated along with the wrists to get more complete movement of the radius and ulna. (Figure 5.9)

Freestyle Bounce Start with one arm up and one arm down, the elbows bent slightly. Simultaneously pull the up arm and push the down arm backward, bouncing 2-3 times before switching arms and repeating until reaching the rep count. (Figure 5.10)

Over & Back Over & backs will further loosen up the shoulders, triceps, biceps and lats. Keep your abs tight and lower ribs down as you swing back overhead to ensure the shoulder is opened fully. (Figure 5.11)

Arm Circles Bilateral arm circles will help open up the chest and shoulders. This should involve maximal movement of the shoulder blades in all directions, not just of the arms. Perform a series of swings forward, and then a series backward. (Figure 5.12)

Shoulder Girdle Stretch With the elbow bent and above the shoulder, place the forearm against a doorjamb, upright of a power rack or similar structure, and lean the chest forward to stretch the pec and delt. (Figure 5.13)

Underarm Stretch Bend your elbow and lift it above your head so you can place the underside of your upper arm near the elbow against the upright of a power rack or similar. Hold the wrist of this arm with your other hand to push it outward slightly as you lean forward to push the elbow back, keeping your abs tight. (Figure 5.14)

Back Squat Lean-Through Grip a barbell in a squat rack with your hands a little outside shoulder width. Position yourself under the bar as if you're going to lift it from the rack for a back squat and push your chest forward away from the bar, keeping the elbows down. (Figure 5.15)

Leaning Bar Hang Hold a pull-up bar with a jerk-width grip and place your feet on the floor or box as needed a couple feet in front of the bar. Hang while leaning your chest forward through your arms, keeping the toes attached to the floor to allow this forward leaning angle along with the hang. (Figure 5.16)

Apley Push This is a simple internal rotation stretch that is more accessible to larger, less-flexible athletes. Place the back of one hand against the lower back with the elbow bent at about a 90-degree angle (similar to the Apley scratch test position). Rather than reaching across the body to grab the opposite elbow, press the back of the elbow against a power rack, door frame or wall to push it forward and toward the opposite side of the body. (Figure 5.17)

Trunk Rotations With a slightly wider than squat stance, rotate the trunk from side to side, using the generated momentum to push the range of motion. Allow the back foot to pivot on the toes to reduce twisting on the knee. Perform the series as a continuous motion. (Figure 5.18)

Bow & Bend With the knees unlocked slightly, reach to the floor by bending at the hips and back, return to standing with your hands on your hips, push the hips forward, and lean the torso back without allowing the knees to bend. Tightening the glutes while leaning back will help prevent hyperextension of the lower back and improve the stretch of the hip flexors. Perform the series as a continuous motion. (Figure 5.19)

Leg Swings Leg swings to the front will loosen up the hamstrings and to the back will loosen up the quads and hip flexors. Keep the trunk tight and pelvis in a constant neutral position during the swings to improve the stretch at the hips rather than allowing the lower back to absorb some of the movement. Perform the series as a continuous motion. (Figure 5.20)

Knee Circles In a narrow stance, bend the knees slightly and rest your hands on your thighs just above the knee. Perform a series of circles with both knees at the same time, first clockwise and then counter-clockwise. You can also circle both knees toward the outside and then the inside. (Figure 5.21)

Spiderman Lunge + Hip Flexor Stretch With your hands on the floor on either side of your lead leg, reach the front foot into a long lunge position, with the lead shin approximately vertical, and push the hips and torso down as low as possible inside the lead leg. Hold this position for a few seconds, then bring the trunk upright, squeeze the glute of the back leg, and push the hips forward to stretch the hip flexor of the back leg and hold a few seconds. Perform a series of this combination, alternating legs. (Figure 5.22)

Russian Baby Maker With your feet slightly wider than your normal squat stance, squat and bend down to place your hands on top of your feet and wedge your elbows as deep in toward your groin as possible. Partially rest your legs on your elbows as you push out against the insides of your thighs. The key is to attempt to spread the thighs apart where they meet the hips, rather than at the knees. You will not be in a full-depth squat—your thighs will be around horizontal and your trunk leaned forward. (Figure 5.23)

Squatting or Lunging Ankle Stretch Sit into the bottom of a squat, place both forearms on the top of one knee, and lean your weight onto it to close that ankle as much as possible, keeping the foot flat against the floor. If your calves or hips are too tight for you to sit in this position comfortably, modify the squat into a lunge and stretch the calf of the lead leg. (Figure 5.24)

Wrist Stretches If the forearms are particularly tight, the athlete may also need to add flexion, extension and hook grip stretching to help prepare the wrists to manage heavy loading in awkward positions. Before flexion and extension stretches, the wrist should be decompressed by pulling it straight out from the arm. This will help allow the small carpal bones to move more freely and correctly. (Figure 5.25)

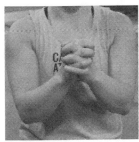 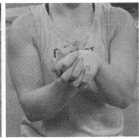 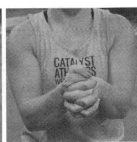 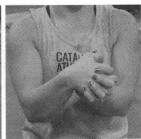 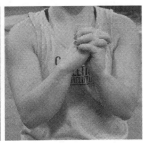

FIGURE 5.8 Wrist circles

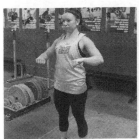 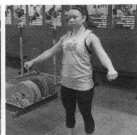 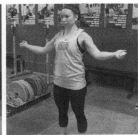 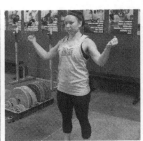 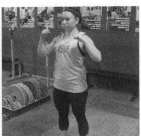

FIGURE 5.9 Elbow circles

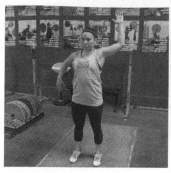 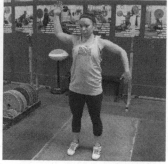 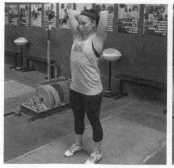 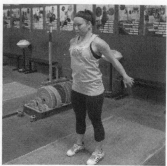

FIGURE 5.10 Freestyle bounce

FIGURE 5.11 Over & back

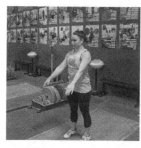 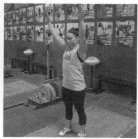 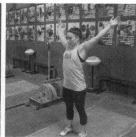 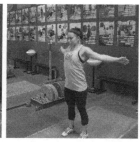 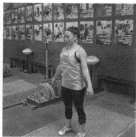

FIGURE 5.12 Arm circles

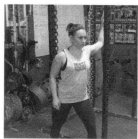 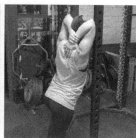 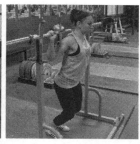 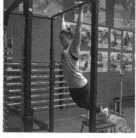 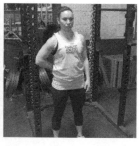

Left to Right: **FIGURE 5.13** Doorjamb shoulder girdle stretch; **FIGURE 5.14** Underarm stretch; **FIGURE 5.15** Back squat lean-through; **FIGURE 5.16** Leaning bar hang; **FIGURE 5.17** Apley push.

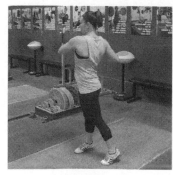 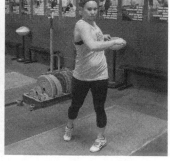 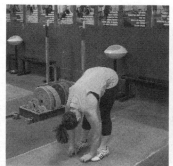 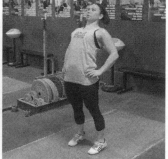

FIGURE 5.18 Trunk rotations

FIGURE 5.19 Bow & bend

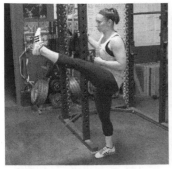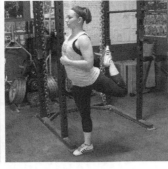

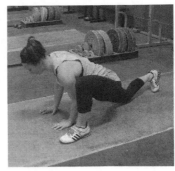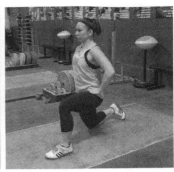

FIGURE 5.20 Leg swings

FIGURE 5.22 Spiderman lunge + hip flexor stretch

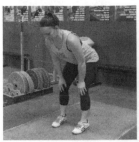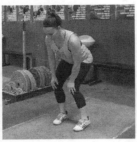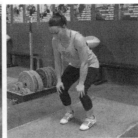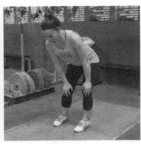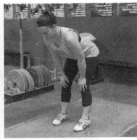

FIGURE 5.21 Knee circles

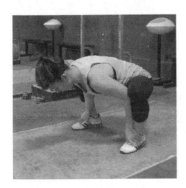

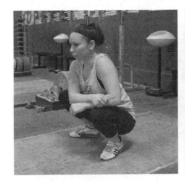

FIGURE 5.23 Russian baby maker

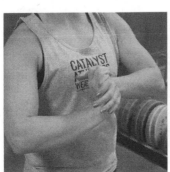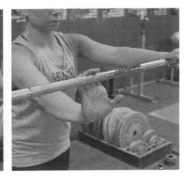

FIGURE 5.24 Squatting (left) and lunging (right) ankle stretch

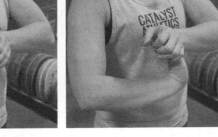

FIGURE 5.25 Wrist stretches

Barbell Warm-ups

Following the warm-up described above, the athlete will begin working with a barbell in preparation for the session's training. This will provide a specific warm-up for the training to follow, and accordingly, this barbell work will vary depending on the content of the training session as well as the needs of each athlete.

Athletes will generally perform a series of movements with the empty bar initially such as press, squat and pull variations. This initial work is a very basic warm-up that largely bridges the gap between the completely general warm-up and the more specific work to come. These movements are chosen by each athlete according to his or her needs or comfort. Examples for a snatch workout are snatch presses and push presses, overhead squats, back squat + snatch push press, snatch balances, press in snatch, and muscle snatch variations. An athlete may rotate among a few of these each session. For example, 5 snatch presses, 5 snatch back squat + snatch push press, 5 mid-hang muscle snatches + overhead squats. Following this series, the athlete will move on to the first exercise of the session, for which he or she will likely start with an empty barbell.

The basic notion of progressive loading of course applies here—that is, the specific warm-up will use gradually increasing weights to bring the athlete up to the working weight of the exercise. There are a number of approaches to this among athletes and coaches, and even among different training sessions for a single athlete. The fundamental principle of any warm-up is to encourage the body to perform optimally—that means preparing the muscles and joints for the necessary ranges of motion and movements and preparing the nervous system for force production and motor skill execution without incurring unnecessary fatigue.

The athlete will increase the load on the bar in progressively smaller increments as it makes its way to the working weight. That is, near the lighter end of the range, larger jumps in weight will be possible and desirable. In addition to this, the more technically demanding the exercise, the smaller the increments will be as the working weight is approached. For example, warm-up weight increases for the snatch will typically be smaller than for the clean & jerk, and much smaller than for squats or pulls.

Most athletes will perform better by spending more time with the lighter weights and subsequently taking larger jumps than by taking a greater number of warm-up weights. The former will allow adequate motor pattern practice and joint and muscle preparation with less muscular fatigue than the latter. For example, an athlete might spend some time with the empty bar, then snatch 50kg for 2-4 sets of doubles or triples, then jump to 70kg for a double, then 90 for a single, then 100, then 110, then 115. When compared to snatching 50 x 2, 60 x 2, 70 x 2, 80 x 1, 90 x 1, 100 x 1, 110 x 1, 115 x 1, the larger jumps with the longer light-weight warm-up will nearly always be preferred by athletes. However, this method is something that the athlete will need to practice regularly to become accustomed to it—it may be difficult and uncomfortable initially if a more extensive and even progression has been the protocol used previously. Athletes who are not yet technically consistent will tend to perform better with more warm-up lifts using smaller jumps. Athletes should experiment with both types of warm-ups to find which approach suits them better.

Specific warm-ups are also an opportunity for small amounts of technique training. Athletes can take advantage of the need to prepare the body for performance to practice corrective or helpful training drills. The *technique primer* is an exercise used to prepare for a training exercise that follows immediately by practicing specific technique elements. An example would be performing a few sets of tall snatches prior to the session's snatches for an athlete who needs to focus on pulling under the snatch more aggressively or accurately.

Another option is using a *warm-up couplet*—this is a complex of a technique-oriented exercise with the primary exercise to be trained. Common examples are power snatch + snatch for an athlete who may have trouble extending fully or aggressively at the top, or turning the bar over quickly enough; snatch + overhead squat for an athlete who is unstable in the bottom position; and muscle snatch + snatch for an athlete who has trouble turning over the bar aggressively or precisely enough. Of course, more than one exercise can be added, in which case we might be performing a *warm-up triplet*; more than this is arguably excessive and counterproductive.

Warm-up couplets can be used as the athlete works his or her way up the weight increments, and then the technique exercise dropped at the point at which it becomes too demanding to be considered a warm-up anymore. For example, using our previous snatch increments, the athlete may power snatch + snatch 50kg for 2-3 sets, then 70kg for 1-2 sets, then drop the complex and begin snatching only at 90kg.

If the training session is more of a technique focus than load focus, or if the movements in the chosen complex indicate it, smaller increments may be used. An example might be a muscle snatch + snatch complex—because the muscle snatch loading is considerably lower than the snatch and will consequently be dropped relatively quickly, smaller increases may be desirable to ensure an adequate volume of work. In this case, the athlete may muscle snatch + snatch 50kg for a double, 60kg for a double, 70kg for a single, 75kg for a single, and then only snatch at 90kg.

An additional consideration is developing the athlete's ability to manage unfamiliar conditions. Athletes will naturally use identical warm-up weights for long periods of time and become very accustomed to these weights. This can occasionally make it difficult mentally for the athlete to lift weights other than these, and may cause problems in a competition situation when circumstances require an unexpected change in attempt weights and according adjustment to the warm-up. While it's important for the athlete to be extremely comfortable with a given warm-up protocol for competition in order to minimize variables and fortify confidence, occasionally changing warm-up weights in training can help prepare the athlete for uncomfortable situations and improve mental toughness and resilience.

A final consideration is that the initial barbell warm-ups may not feel strong or quick. It's advisable to focus more on the movement and use a slower speed initially until the body feels looser and warmer after a set or two. Often all it takes is one or two initial sets with the bar with a minute or two rest in between to suddenly feel a significant improvement. Ideally the lifter will not begin adding weight until this threshold is crossed.

Breathing & Trunk Rigidity

Breath control is critical for increasing and maintaining the structural integrity of the trunk while under heavy loads. The supporting musculature is alone inadequate—in order to adequately stabilize the spine, the abdominal and thoracic cavities must be pressurized. Intraabdominal pressure can also reduce pressure on intervertebral discs by 20% on average and as much 40% (Zatsiorsky 1995). Additionally, we need to create a broad base with the torso—the rationale for this should be obvious if one considers the structural integrity of a pyramid versus an upside-down pyramid. Drawing in the abs may look nice on the beach, but it will diminish the ability of the body to support the kind of forces we intend to introduce.

The torso has only a single supporting structure along its height—the spine—on one side, and this structure articulates in all directions, requiring additional support to maintain rigidity. The weak point is the circumference below the ribcage in which there is no rigid structure tying the torso into the pelvis—this creates a compressible area into which the torso can collapse forward and to the sides.

This area is filled with organs, the tissues of which are relatively incompressible, but the space inside of which we cannot directly make more resistant to compression. Above this, separated by the diaphragm, are the lungs. This provides us a convenient way to reduce the compressibility of the contents of the torso. By filling the lungs, we increase the rigidity of the thoracic cavity, and we also force the diaphragm down, which compresses the organs of the abdominal cavity somewhat.

To improve further on this compression, we can tighten the musculature surrounding the trunk, which prevents unwanted expansion of the container walls and reduces the potential for the torso to collapse. This includes both the muscles surrounding the trunk circumferentially, as well as the diaphragm and pelvic floor at the top and bottom, respectively.

In addition to improving the rigidity of the trunk, this action increases muscular excitability; muscular force is increased with exhalation relative to inhalation, and with the Valsalva maneuver relative to exhalation (Zatsiorsky 1995). In other words, pressurizing the trunk and holding the breath during a lifting effort actually increases the muscles' ability to generate force. However, breath-holding must be used judiciously and combined typically with properly-timed and controlled exhalation as discussed later in this chapter.

The athlete will need to draw in as much air as possible, allowing the abdomen to expand and the diaphragm to contract, ensuring the lungs are able to fill completely; filling the lungs partially by only allowing the chest to lift and expand is not adequate. Inhaling through the nose, or at least initiating the breath through the nose and then completing it through the

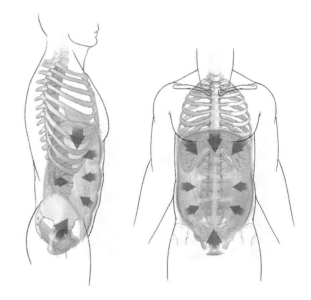

FIGURE 6.1 Trunk rigidity is created through the pressurization of the trunk with air and the activation of the musculature surrounding the trunk in all directions.

mouth, can encourage improved diaphragm activation and achieve a deeper breath. The athlete can also think of breathing from the bottom of the lungs first—that is, filling the bottom of the torso first and then filling upward toward the chest (this is the rationale behind the cue "stomach breath"). In any case, the abs will need to be relaxed to allow expansion of the abdomen—a full breath cannot be taken with the abdomen already tight, as the diaphragm cannot contract and move downward if the organs below it have nowhere to move.

Once this breath is taken, the lifter will tighten down the abdominal and back musculature around the circumference of the trunk and the pelvic floor to increase the internal pressure and reduce the potential for flexion or extension of the torso. This effort to tighten down around the pressurized torso will push air out of the lungs and up the trachea—the athlete will need to close the glottis in order to keep the air in (this should happen naturally with the effort to hold the breath).

It's important that the athlete not "hollow", or draw in the abdominals as many have been taught to do or believe is correct. If the abdominals are drawn in, the base of support is reduced in circumference, reducing stability. We want the muscles activated tightly while keeping the torso as wide and deep as possible, allowing us a broad foundation to support the load. It may help athletes having difficulty with this activation to think of pushing the abs down. (This does not mean that the transversus abdominis is not active; it simply means that it should not be the sole focus of the stabilization effort and should not be cinched in to a degree that limits the ability to fill the trunk adequately with air.)

Pressurization should be maintained throughout as much of the movement as possible. There will be times, however, such as during the recovery of a clean, that the lifter will feel dizzy and even near unconsciousness. This can be because the athlete is not properly racking the barbell and the pressure is compressing the carotid arteries and reducing blood flow to the brain (this will be addressed in later chapters), but it can also be from actually holding the breath and bearing down simultaneously; these actions, especially when combined, result in vagus nerve stimulation and reduce heart rate and blood pressure (this can be easily demonstrated by feeling your pulse while breathing normally, then holding your breath—you will typically feel an almost immediate reduction in heart rate). In some cases, this can cause unconsciousness, but this can be avoided by paying attention and reacting appropriately. Additionally, increased intrathoracic pressure can reduce cardiac output, also potentially causing dizziness or unconsciousness (Zatsiorsky 1995).

If dizziness or light-headedness occurs during lifts, the athlete should release a small amount of air during the highest-pressure moment of the lift by making some noise. This will release some air and prevent dizziness while maintaining trunk stability. Some athletes will be more comfortable, and even feel stronger, making a habit of always releasing air with noise during the recovery of the squat, as long as the release is controlled and minimal. In fact, this aggressive release of air can actually help improve the rigidity of the trunk if performed properly. If dizziness is considerable, the athlete should drop the bar immediately and sit down safely to recover.

During the explosive second pulls of the snatch and clean, and even sometimes during the drive of the jerk, some lifters will make noise with an expulsion of a small amount of air. This is not problematic and is usually helpful in increasing the athlete's aggressiveness. Again, however, this release must be of only a fraction of the air in the lungs.

The effect of torso pressurization can be demonstrated easily with unweighted squats. The athlete can pressurize the torso and perform a few squats with a bounce. Following this, the athlete will expel as much air as possible, and squat again with the bounce. Invariably the difference is dramatic enough to elicit some kind of exclamation from the athlete.

The Squat

The squat is foundational to the Olympic lifts as a position, a movement and a strength exercise. Without a well-developed and consistent squat, neither pulling technique nor pulling power will produce entirely successful Olympic weightlifting. The great natural physical variation among athletes dictates that there will never be a universally perfect prescription for body positioning, but irrespective of this variation, the fundamental principles remain consistent. Continued reliance on them will ensure that modifications from the strict prescription are rational and sound instead of haphazard and likely improper.

Be cautious of defying the underlying principles with the excuse of individual variation—often this is inappropriately cited when the actual cause of an athlete's inability to adhere to these prescriptions is entirely correctable over time, such as mobility-related limitations or simply stubborn habits. It's necessary to critically evaluate each athlete individually to make accurate determinations—coaches should avoid allowing an athlete to continue poor habits due simply to laziness or frustration with slow progress and, more importantly, increase the risk of injury.

The Squat Position

As the base from which all movement and positioning originates, the placement of the feet will dramatically influence the squat. The width of the stance and degree of external rotation will affect the

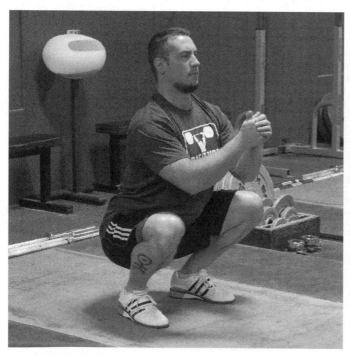
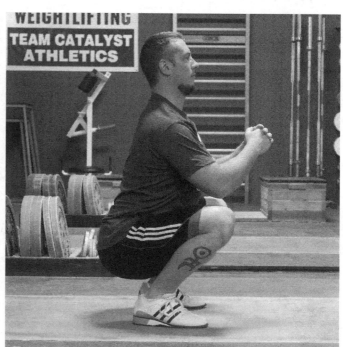

FIGURE 7.1 The basic squat position

movement and position of the hips and back, and will often be the deciding factor in whether a squat is successful or failed, mechanically sound or injurious. Individual variation notwithstanding, the feet must be positioned in a manner that allows and encourages proper biomechanics of the legs, hips and back, while allowing the greatest possible range of motion and supporting the unique positional and movement characteristics of the Olympic lifts.

Anthropometrics—in particular relative leg segment lengths—and hip anatomy will dictate appropriate width and rotation of the feet. Mobility limitations and similar impediments may prevent an athlete from immediately achieving this ultimately proper positioning, but again, these are temporary obstacles that should be corrected over time.

The starting foot placement will be slightly outside hip-width at the heels with the toes turned out comfortably—generally between approximately 20-30 degrees from center. With the athlete sitting at the bottom of the squat in this basic position, adjustments can be quickly made according to leg segment and trunk lengths, hip anatomy, and ankle and knee alignment to place him or her in the proper position.

From this relaxed, starting bottom position, there are two basic criteria with which to be concerned:

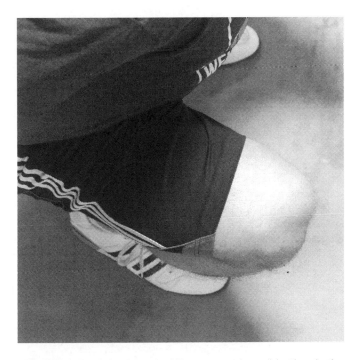

FIGURE 7.2 The thigh and foot should be approximately parallel with each other when viewed from directly above.

When viewed from directly above, the foot and thigh are approximately parallel with each other (Figure 7.2); when viewed from the front of the toe, the foot is approximately underneath the knee. The hips should sit in between the heels somewhat; in other words, the heel will not be directly under the thigh, but slightly outside of its centerline. This positioning will keep the knees and ankles aligned well, but will also allow for slightly improved depth, and, more importantly, a more absorptive bottom position—that is, the final position will be structurally sound without having an abrupt and jarring stop from a perfectly vertical stacking of the bones.

With these relationships established—assuming the hips are at full possible depth—the remaining positional relationships will be unavoidably correct. This allows for a wide range of potential external rotation—athletes will in general naturally find what is most comfortable for them. That said, some athletes will need to be told explicitly to spread the knees farther than they wish; occasionally athletes will prefer a stance that prevents the hips from reaching adequate depth between the thighs due to the structures of the upper thighs being pushed into the forward edges of the pelvis. If the athlete is unable to achieve adequate depth and back extension, particularly if he or she is also feeling pressure near the front of the hips, a more externally rotated stance is more than likely needed.

Turning the toes out to an extreme degree is also problematic, in part because the lifter's base of support is reduced in depth and consequently balance will become more difficult, and because this can place the muscles acting on the hips and legs in positions from which optimal force cannot be generated. Additionally, it will likely force the thighs to move through a plane that restricts hip mobility as the squat deepens.

What proper squat positioning achieves is simple but important—biomechanically sound alignment of the involved joints and muscles, optimizing performance and reducing the risk of injury.

These relationships of the feet and leg segments should be maintained for the duration of the movement—in other words, the knees should follow the line described by the angle of the feet as the athlete descends and recovers. For some athletes, this will, at least initially, require they consciously make an effort to push the knees out to the sides as the tendency will be for the knees to collapse inward. However, these cases should not be misinterpreted to mean that all athletes should be actively pushing the knees out during the squat—this is strictly an action and cue for lifters whose knees are moving inside the feet during the squat. There is no shortage of speculation regarding valgus knee movement in the squat and its potential to cause injury, but this relationship is apparently contradicted by the practical evidence—that of many weightlifters over many years lifting with such valgus movement without knee injury. However, it's recommended that lifters and coaches work to minimize valgus knee movement in the squat to limit injury potential.

From this basic position, there will be a degree of adjustment possible without considerable violation of these relationships. That is, once in this position, the athlete will find he or she can move the feet in and out and turn the toes in and out slightly and continue to meet the criteria fairly well. This small range will allow some latitude, and the lifter is encouraged to experiment within this range until the most comfortable position is found.

The effect of hip width on foot placement should be self-explanatory—this is the origin of the legs and consequently the starting point for the stance (this is easier to picture if you consider an athlete in a standing position). Relative leg segment length affects how far back the foot travels relative to the thigh as the knee flexes. The longer the lower leg is relative to the upper leg, the farther toward the hip the foot will be when the knee is closed—this means that the longer the lower leg is relative to the upper leg, the closer the feet will be in a sound squat position. In other words, the overall length of the legs is not the only factor that determines squat stance—how that length is created contributes as well. (Figure 7.3)

The foot position should be identical for all squat variations—back squat, front squat, overhead squat—and all receiving positions except the split in the jerk—snatch, clean, power snatch, power clean, power jerk, squat jerk. Many athletes will assume different foot positions for each type of squat—this is an indicator that the athlete has not learned and developed a correct squat position, and is likely working around mobility restriction.

Depth

The depth of an Olympic squat should not even be a topic of discussion, but because there has been and continues to be discussion among coaches and athletes in sports outside of weightlifting, it warrants at least clarification: proper depth is full depth; full depth means full depth. Full depth is not parallel, nor is it breaking parallel—it is squatting to the lowest position possible without surgical alteration of body parts while maintaining correct posture. To clarify, the goal is to close the knee joint as much as possi-

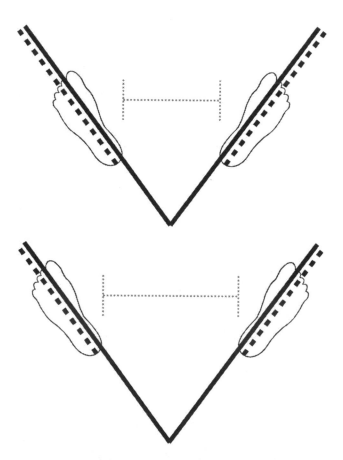

FIGURE 7.3 The width of the feet in the correct squat stance is not only a product of total leg length or total height, but also of relative leg segment length. This diagram represents two athletes with identical upper leg and foot lengths, but different lower leg lengths. If hip anatomy and external rotation is the same, the athlete with the longer lower leg (and therefore longer total leg length, and likely even greater total height) actually has a narrower foot placement. Athletes and coaches cannot simply assume that taller athletes will need wider stances than shorter athletes—each athlete's foot placement needs to be determined individually according to the criteria described.

ble while maintaining a correctly arched back and the proper balance over the foot.

Depth is measured by the position of the hips, and the depth of the hips is governed by the position of the knees, the degree of dorsiflexion of the ankles, the absolute and relative lengths of the upper and lower leg, the horizontal position of the hips relative to the feet, the width and degree of external rotation of the feet, and the mass of the upper and lower legs. These factors are largely interdependent, and a change in one will typically effect change in others.

If the knees are prevented from moving forward over the feet, as is believed by many individuals to be safer for the knees (incorrectly), the hips must travel farther back behind the feet. With the hips behind the athlete's base, the torso must be inclined forward to a greater degree in order for the athlete's center of mass to remain balanced over the feet. If the hips are lowered from this position, flexibility will restrict the spine's ability to remain correctly arched, forcing the athlete to curl forward, again to remain balanced. For what should be fairly obvious reasons, neither of these positions will allow the safe and effective support of a barbell in the positions it must be received in the snatch and clean. (Note that shorter athletes may be able to achieve a proper squat depth and po-

sition without the knees passing forward of the toes dramatically, and very flexible athletes or certain proportions may be able to sit in between the feet in a manner that keeps the shins relatively upright.)

Inadequate ankle mobility will also result in the knees remaining too far back—if the ankles are unable to dorsiflex to a great enough degree, the lower leg cannot reach an angle sufficient to bring the knees into a position that allows the hips to reach their intended placement. This is the reason for the lifted heel of weightlifting shoes—elevation of the heel effectively increases the ankles' range of motion and allows the hips to move in more under the shoulders.

Femur length will affect the depth of each athlete's squat simply by dictating how far away from the knees the hips will be. Athletes with great hip flexibility and long femurs will typically be capable of extraordinarily deep squat positions, while their shorter-femured counterparts will appear higher even when at their maximal depth. For some athletes, femur length will exceed what can be compensated for through ankle flexibility in the basic squat position, and adjustments will need to be made to allow a better bottom position.

For individuals with largely muscled legs and who are capable of very upright torso positions in the

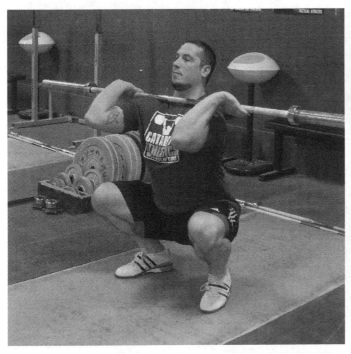 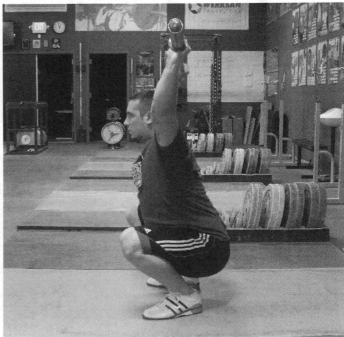

FIGURE 7.4 The placement of the barbell in the clean and snatch demands the torso remain extremely upright.

bottom of the squat, the hips may not be particularly low relative to the knees even when the knees are closed completely. These individuals' lowest position may be very near horizontal thigh orientation.

The Hips

The positional priority of the Olympic squat is maintaining essentially as upright a torso as possible (As will be discussed later, in the overhead squat, the torso should not be completely vertical because of the demands of correct shoulder positioning). In the clean, the barbell is supported directly by the torso on the shoulders, and for this to be possible, the torso must be erect. In the snatch, the barbell is supported overhead with locked elbows. This position is strong and stable within only a very small range of torso positions—excessive forward lean of the torso not only makes unreasonable demands on shoulder mobility, but undermines the structural integrity of the system. (Figure 7.4)

This requirement of an erect torso position dictates all remaining body positions. In order to maintain an upright torso, the hips must remain as near to under the shoulders as possible. Because the athlete must of course remain balanced over his or her base, this in turn requires the knees travel forward (to a degree dependent on leg segment lengths and the stance being used) to allow the hips to move in closer to the feet.

For athletes accustomed to more traditional squat mechanics, this quad-dominant movement will feel weak and unnatural. While rising from the squat, these lifters will have a tendency to elevate the hips prematurely in order to give the quads better leverage on the knee and to engage the hamstrings more, which, initially, will allow a stronger movement for them. This hip elevation, however, will result in a problematic forward inclination of the torso. Aside from creating difficulty in supporting the barbell, this habit will limit the development of the quads and consequently become self-preserving. Eventually the athlete will reach a point at which he or she is handling loads that are literally impossible to support with such a posture and progress will cease completely. This can be avoided by forcing correct positioning and movement from the outset despite any temporary reductions in loading that may occur as a consequence.

When squatting, the hips must unavoidably travel in a slight arc backward, which will momentarily force the trunk to lean forward slightly more to maintain balance of the system. This movement of the hips and trunk will be minimal and not problematic as long as the athlete focuses on standing straight up by moving the hips and knees simultaneously rather than leading with one or the other, working to preserve the same upright posture, and trains to strength this movement properly (Figure 7.5).

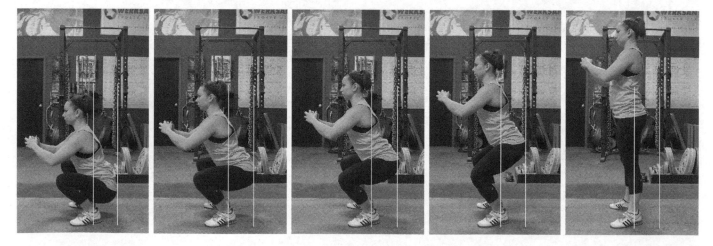

FIGURE 7.5 The hips will have to move backward slightly as the lifter rises from the bottom of the squat. However, this shifting can and should be minimized by focusing on maintaining an upright posture, moving the knees and hips simultaneously, and keeping the "hips in"—as near to under the shoulders as is possible. The lines in these photos remain at the same distance from each other as a reference to illustrate the minimal backward movement of the hips through the middle of the squat.

Greg Everett

The Back

The spine in its neutral position curves through lordosis in the lumbar region and kyphosis in the thoracic region. Because of their accordingly angled surfaces, it is in this position that pressure is evenly distributed over the vertebrae and intervertebral disks and the back is structurally soundest when the body is standing vertically under a compressive load. However, in the squat, as in the pull from the floor, the athlete is dealing only partly with compressive forces—torque on the spine and hip must also be considered.

The first priority in the squat is the maintenance of the lumbar spine's lordotic arch. The joints of the lumbar vertebra and the joint of the fifth lumbar vertebra with the sacrum are the most susceptible to injury, and consequently warrant the greatest attention. This is due in large part simply to the fact that these joints are farthest from the application of force with a load on the shoulders or overhead and are therefore the natural fulcrums of the torque.

Contributing to this unavoidable structural characteristic are the correctable factors of thoracic spine immobility and hip immobility and the resulting hypermobility of the lumbar spine. It's extremely common for the natural kyphotic curvature of the upper spine to be exaggerated through years of poor postural habits and musculature weakness and inactivation, and for the mobility of the thoracic vertebrae to be reduced significantly over time from the lack of movement. The lumbar spine must compensate for the inability of the thoracic spine and hips to move properly, and in doing so, must move through a range of motion greater than intended, creating laxity in the connective tissue and allowing continued exacerbation of both the source and symptoms of the problem.

While hyperextension is of course potentially injurious, the potential is essentially limited to instances of compressive force in nearly vertical positions. The erect posture of the front and overhead squats allows opportunity for such compression, but the more common force acting on the spine and hip is forward torque, and consequently the greater concern in regard to the safety of the lumbar spine is flexion under load. This places immense strain on the posterior connective tissue and undue pressure on the anterior aspects of the vertebrae and intervertebral discs. Because the torso will be inclined forward to a small degree—the consequent line of force along with the tension of the hip extensors will encourage flexion of the spine and make hyperextension more difficult within the confines of correct body and bar positioning. Further, the hip extensors and adductors pull the pelvis when under tension (such as in the bottom of a squat) in the direction of posterior rotation, which causes lumbar flexion.

Because of this, we want to actually exaggerate the lumbar spine's lordotic arch somewhat in most cases. This slight exaggeration acts as a hedge against flexion during the movement in a few ways: By increasing the degree of curvature, the length of the moment arm is reduced and therefore the ability to resist the applied force is improved; greater extension improves the leverage of the spinal extensors and consequently their ability to maintain extension; and a greater degree of curvature means a larger margin of error—it will take more unintended movement to bring the spine into a compromised flexed position.

This exaggeration of the lumbar curve should obviously be most pronounced at the point of greatest forward torso inclination and reduced as the torso nears vertical to reflect the changing torque and compression on the joints—in other words, the exaggeration should be greatest at the point at which the tendency for spinal flexion is greatest, and curvature should be closer to neutral as the spine nears a fully erect position with greater compressive forces.

In the back and overhead squats, the torso will never reach a perfectly vertical orientation even when the athlete is standing fully because the placement of the bar dictates slight forward inclination in order to maintain balance over the base—the lumbar spine will therefore never quite return to completely neutral, although it will be close. In the front squat, the torso can reach vertical in the standing position because of the placement of the bar in front of the hips. Neutral lumbar curvature can be achieved, and vigilance to maintain it will remain necessary, as there is now a possibility of hyperextension. Protection against hyperextension of the lumbar spine during any lifting movement will primarily be the responsibility of the abdominal musculature.

While simple in theory, this spinal curvature is often difficult to achieve and maintain in practice due to flexibility limitations. Inflexible hip extensors and adductors will prevent the pelvis from rotating anteriorly to maintain its positional relationship with the spine as the hip is flexed to move into the bottom of the squat. This inability of the pelvis to rotate adequately results in the lumbar spine taking up the slack in the system, at best limiting the maintenance of the lordotic exaggeration and at worst resulting in considerable lumbar flexion.

A very slight degree of flexion is acceptable in the earliest stages of training—at this point, the loads being handled by the athlete will rarely be great enough to create significant injury risk, and the speed of movements is typically low. In reality, it's rare for adult athletes to possess entirely adequate mobility initially, so this is somewhat beyond control. This must, however, be corrected as soon as possible, and certainly before the athlete is allowed to lift legitimately heavy weights. Mobility training is discussed in detail in a later section of the book. More advanced athletes will typically experience a slight reduction in lumbar spine extension at the bottommost position of the squat; this is not problematic if the resulting degree

of extension is still equal to or greater than neutral. However, the goal for all athletes is to maintain an essentially static spine position throughout a lift.

The thoracic spine curvature will need to be manipulated as well. Its natural kyphosis reduces the structural integrity of the system when resisting forward torque, as in the clean, or overhead, as in the snatch. The forward curvature places the load farther forward in relation to the base of the spine, increasing the moment on the joints and consequently the tendency for the spine to flex and the torso to drop forward. This can be effectively countered in the same manner lumbar flexion is prevented. In the case of the lumbar spine, the existing curve is simply exaggerated; in the case of the thoracic spine, the curve needs to be reduced as much as possible. Except in rare cases of hypermobility, the thoracic spine will not actually be extended into lordosis—its curvature will simply be reduced. This flattening of the thoracic spine effectively creates a single arch through the entire spine, or what will be referred to throughout the book as complete extension.

By creating this complete extension, effectively a

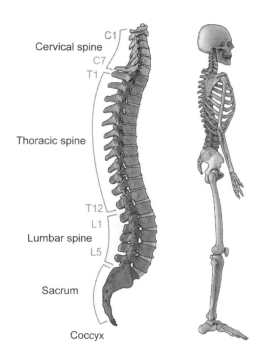

FIGURE 7.6 Neutral spinal curvature

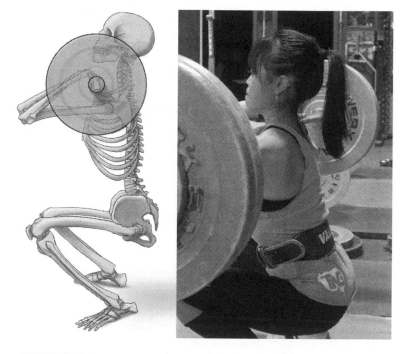

FIGURE 7.7 For both improved performance and safety, the athlete should create complete extension of the back—essentially a continuous arch over the full length of the spine.

Greg Everett

continuous arch from the sacrum to the base of the skull, the lever arm of the back is shortened slightly, reducing the mechanical disadvantage of the muscles extending it and the hip, the leverage of those muscles is improved, and consequently the strength and stability of the system is increased. This of course improves performance and further protects the spine from flexion injuries. As with the lumbar curve, this thoracic positioning should be adjusted according to the inclination of the torso—most pronounced at the point of greatest forward inclination, and returning closer to neutral as the torso nears vertical.

The Head

The head should remain upright and the face directed forward throughout the movement of the squat. Commonly lifters will tilt the head back, occasionally to an extreme degree, and redirect their focus upward to help drive through the sticking point of a squat. While cervical extension does reinforce and actually strengthen thoracolumbar extension, cervical extension should not be allowed to become extreme to avoid straining the neck.

The eyes should remain directed approximately straight ahead or slightly above and focused on a fixed point. It's important the focal point be distant enough from the lifter to not noticeably change its relative position and cause the lifter's head or eyes to move significantly during the squat. Lowering the head or even merely the gaze will commonly cause the lifter to drop the chest and shift the weight forward during the ascent because of the tendency for the body to follow the eyes and head, potentially resulting in a failed lift. If a lifter demonstrates that an upwardly-directed gaze improves his or her squatting, it's perfectly acceptable as long as it does not create any other problems.

Weight Distribution

Throughout the squat, the lifter's weight should balanced just slightly behind the middle of the foot—that is, slightly closer to the heel than the balls of the foot. A simple landmark to conceptualize this is the front edge of the heel—this is approximately the point through which the lifter's line of gravity should pass.

Inadequate mobility of the hips and ankles will commonly force the heels to rise and the weight to shift to the balls of the feet as the lifter descends. This imbalance becomes particularly problematic when attempting to stabilize a system that includes a barbell weighing sometimes dramatically more than the athlete. In the bottom position of a proper squat, the pressure may shift slightly farther forward over the feet; this is not necessarily problematic, and the weight simply needs to be shifted back as soon as possible as the lifter recovers from the bottom position.

If the root of the problem is inadequate mobility, a stretching prescription will be necessary. The lifter's squat stance should also be evaluated to ensure it's not preventing proper positioning and balance. Otherwise, practice and coaching cues for the lifter to remain flatfooted and keep slightly more pressure on the heels than on the balls of the feet should be sufficient.

Occasionally the outside edges of the athlete's feet will rise at the bottom of the squat, and the feet even rotate outward. This is typically the result of inadequate ankle mobility and the body's attempt to continue moving the knees into the necessary position after maximal ankle dorsiflexion has occurred. Ankle mobility work is a must.

This may also be the result of an excessively wide foot placement. If the feet are positioned such that the knees must track inside them, the feet may be pulled along with them. This improper foot positioning may be due to nothing more than ignorance, but it can also be an unconscious attempt to compensate for inadequate ankle mobility. This can be easily tested by placing the athlete into the correct position and observing the result.

Variation & Modification

Modifications to the basic squat position may be necessary or desirable in certain cases. Most commonly, the position is modified inappropriately due to mobility restrictions, and consequently increases the risk of injury and limits the lifter's progress in the lifts.

Occasionally athletes will find their ankle and

knee joints are not in perfect alignment with each other when standing upright—in these cases, the angle of the feet should be adjusted accordingly, giving priority to the maintenance of proper knee mechanics. In other words, the proper alignment of the lower leg with the upper leg takes precedence over the alignment of the foot with the upper leg. This kind of misalignment is invariably minor and should have little if any effect on the squat. Athletes are typically able to feel this when in the squat position as a twisting sensation in the knee—the position should be adjusted until such pressure is eliminated.

Long-legged lifters may find it simply impossible to meet perfectly the alignment criteria while achieving a full-depth squat with correct spinal curvature. In these cases, the foot placement may be widened and externally rotated slightly more. This will allow the hips to remain closer to the feet as they travel down and in their bottom position, which will reduce the demand on hip extensor flexibility for the maintenance of spinal curvature. Such adjustments should be made incrementally and tested with caution—hip and spine position improvements should not force compromise of knee alignment to a degree that increases injury risk. Note that this will still require an improvement of hip and ankle mobility.

In short, variation in the appearance of the squat position is not necessarily problematic and in need

of correction—if this variation is a product of permanent anatomical factors (e.g. skeletal structure) rather than correctible factors (e.g. immobility) and the fundamental criteria are met, the position is perfectly acceptable. If these criteria are not met due to uncorrectable factors, the safety of the positions and movement will need to be evaluated on an individual basis.

Defying the Basics

There are successful weightlifters who defy—sometimes dramatically—the positional relationships described here. In some cases, this defiance is simply the product of ignorance, unchallenged habit or improper instruction; in other cases, it's entirely intentional and serves to achieve specific objectives. The most common example of this is widening of the foot placement in order to allow the hips to drop farther in between the feet and achieve greater depth. This places enormous stress on the connective tissue of the knees by introducing torque on the joints not experienced in their natural alignment (Figure 7.9).

Whether this positioning will result in chronic pain, a career-ending injury, or no apparent problems is impossible to predict, and consequently these kinds of fundamental positional violations are strongly dis-

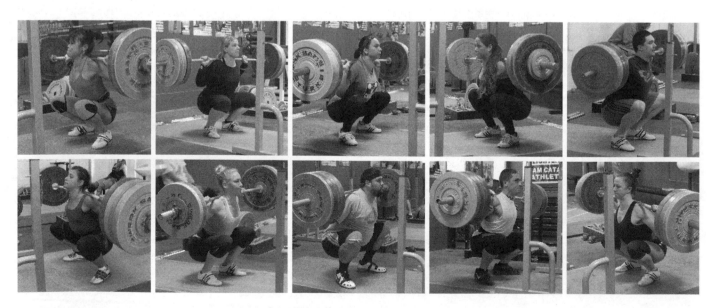

FIGURE 7.8 Lifters' body types will determine what their ultimate positions in the squat will be. This individual variation can produce dramatic differences in appearance of the squat position while still meeting the criteria of a correct, full-depth squat. Note that these individual peculiarities are independent of temporary mobility limitations.

Greg Everett

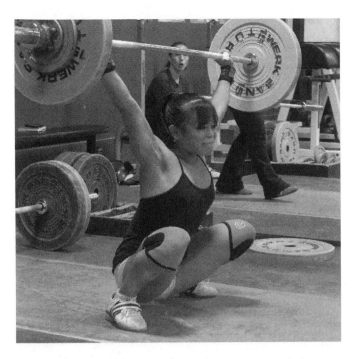

FIGURE 7.9 An excessively wide stance and the resulting torque on the knees.

couraged for anyone but the highest caliber athletes, who have not only proven to be extremely well-suited for the sport and able to tolerate a great deal of abuse, but whose careers depend on making lifts, and for whom the risk is consequently worth the potential benefit.

That said, it should be noted that athletes will occasionally find themselves in such positions unintentionally during particularly heavy lifts. This is infrequent enough to not be a concern if the athlete is possessed of appropriate mobility, which provides a margin of error beyond the minimal degree necessary to achieve the perfect positions.

The Bounce

In most squatting, particularly during the recovery of the clean, lifters will "bounce" out of the bottom of the squat. This potentiates the concentric contraction of the muscles and increases the speed of the recovery, allowing the athlete to pass more quickly and easily through the sticking point of the squat at which mechanical disadvantage is greatest, which in turn reduces the fatigue of the legs, leaving

them fresher for the subsequent jerk after a clean or the next repetition in a set of squats. For lifters who rely more on explosiveness and elasticity than a large strength reserve, a proper bounce in a clean or front squat can be the deciding factor in the success or failure of the recovery.

The bounce is actually the summation of three distinct but interrelated elements: the muscles' stretch reflex, the collision of the upper and lower legs, and the whip of the barbell.

When stretched at a great enough rate, muscles will respond with an immediate and powerful involuntary contraction. This stretch reflex—or myotatic reflex—is the same phenomenon at play in plyometric training. By performing the squat with adequate speed and tension, this reflex can be harnessed to increase the total force production of the concentric movement and generate greater momentum during the recovery of the squat to carry the lifter through the most difficult point.

This movement can be easily misinterpreted as relaxing under the bar, and is occasionally practiced as such by athletes who have learned it solely through observation and possess no understanding of its principles. This is a critical mistake for two reasons. First, anything even resembling relaxation under heavy loads is an opportunity for injury. Second, any relaxation will reduce the stability of the relative position of the hips and spine, meaning that downward force at the bottom of the squat will cause changes in these positions that will absorb some of that force; consequently, less of that force can be stored as elastic energy to then contribute to the recovery from the bottom.

This is a blow to performance and safety that can't be afforded when handling significant loads. The athlete must remain tight and structurally sound throughout the movement, bracing for the abrupt arrest of downward movement and the subsequent rapid change of direction. This being said, the athlete must also allow the weight to push his or her body down rapidly as he or she nears the bottom.

The second component of the bounce is simply the collision of the upper and lower legs with each other. This is no different than bouncing a ball—after colliding with the lower legs, the remainder of the lifter's body rebounds away from the feet. The larger the athlete's legs, the more pronounced this rebound effect will be. It's important to note here too that if an athlete is not mobile enough to close the knee joint to such a degree, the ability for that athlete to catch a legitimate bounce in the bottom of a squat is greatly reduced—this structural arrest of the downward movement allows greater speed into the bottom position than can be managed under muscular force alone.

Olympic barbells are intentionally manufactured to possess a high degree of elasticity. In other words, the bars are capable of bending to great degrees without permanent deformity. This characteristic creates the opportunity for the final component of the bounce. If the lifter reaches the bottom of the squat with any reasonable speed, the plates on the barbell will have a considerable amount of downward momentum. The bar's elasticity in concert with the narrow area of support at its center leaves the weighted ends free to move somewhat independently, allowing the weights to continue traveling downward after the lifter's downward motion has ceased. This generates elastic energy in the bar, like loading a spring, and at the limits of the bar's elasticity, the weights will rebound back up. This whip of the bar reduces the downward force of the bar temporarily—an immediate transition out of the bottom of the squat will allow the lifter to take advantage of this temporarily reduced load to accelerate rapidly and pass through the sticking point of the squat with more speed and therefore less work. The degree of bar whip is of course related directly to the load on the bar (more weight means more bending, and also means more plates, moving more of the total weight toward the ends of the bar, further increasing its bending), making this component of the bounce the most variable among lifters and lifts.

The bounce is of particular importance to athletes in possession of comparatively weak legs, who will be cleaning loads much nearer to their greatest squat efforts than their stronger-legged counterparts. Likewise, athletes whose jerks are weak in comparison to their cleans will need to conserve as much leg strength for the jerk as possible. Often a correct bounce will be the difference between success and failure for these lifters.

In cases of missed timing in which the lifter finds him- or herself stuck in the bottom position of the squat, the effects of the bounce can still be created to a lesser degree to assist in the recovery attempt. The athlete can initiate a small upward movement and drop again to create a small bounce, and repeat this cycle, in which each subsequent bounce will be incrementally greater, in an attempt to generate a final summative bounce great enough to power through the sticking point. While this can work, it will never be as effective as a correct single bounce.

Generally the bounce should be used when training front squats to improve technique, timing and the neurological adaptations of the stretch reflex for the clean. The back squat more often should be performed with a more controlled speed through the bottom range of motion to ensure strength development in the lowest possible position, which is the weakest range of motion, although some degree of stretch reflex will always exist unless the lifter comes to a complete stop and holds the bottom position for approximately three seconds or more.

If an athlete is already squatting heavy loads but has not had experience with bouncing out of the bottom, bouncing should be introduced gradually to allow time for the connective tissue to adapt to the new stress.

A common mistake is diving from the top of a squat in the attempt to catch the bounce. So much distance at such a speed increases the downward force of the weight to a point that makes supporting it and changing its direction far more difficult. Athletes will find more success using a natural downward speed until nearing approximately horizontal with the thighs, and then increasing the speed into the bottom while remaining tight. This will create the speed to the bottom necessary for the bounce, but keep the total downward force with the realm of control. Because cleans will be received at levels considerably lower than standing, this also more accurately mimics the shorter distance of downward acceleration that will be experienced in the clean.

Breathing

Breath control during the squat is no different than what was described in the previous chapter for all structural lifting. Pressurization of the torso will improve the structural integrity of the spine during the movement, improving both performance and safety, and increases muscular activation. The more rigid the trunk remains during the squat, the more completely the force generated by the legs will be transferred to the bar. Movement within the trunk will absorb force of the legs and hips and result in the need for the legs to work harder than necessary to move the barbell. This is particularly true when bouncing out of the bottom of the squat. This rigidity will also minimize extraneous movement and improve the stability and balance of the athlete.

Some athletes will only begin to draw in air as they initiate their descent. This can work if the breath is taken in quickly enough, but it can prevent the best possible pressurization of the torso, and can also shift the athlete's balance enough to be problematic with heavier lifts. More effective, and more predictable, is drawing in air and settling into the pressurization before any movement begins. This ensures ideal pressurization and adds only a couple seconds at most to each rep's execution time—nothing too unreasonable considering the benefits.

Often under heavy squats—particularly front squats—athletes may find it difficult to take in as much air as they'd like. In these cases, an initial breath can be taken and held, and then the bar popped up slightly by the legs in order to momentarily lighten the load, during which time a final top-off of air can be taken in before beginning the descent into the squat.

The maintenance of this trunk pressurization is most critical through the transition at the bottom of the squat during which the forces threatening the body's structure are the most intense. The breath as a whole should be maintained throughout the lift; however, some of the air can be released by making some noise during the recovery if the athlete finds it helpful, and such a release may also actually increase the rigidity of the trunk. Such a release will also help prevent dizziness without significantly reducing the integrity of the trunk.

Learning & Teaching the Squat

With the previous information in hand, learning and teaching the squat is fairly simple. That said, it can for certain athletes be difficult, primarily due to limitations of mobility, and occasionally due to limitations in an individual's body awareness and muscle recruitment abilities. These situations will require additional steps, but are all completely resolvable with a little patience and creativity. The importance of a well-developed squat, no matter how difficult attaining it may prove to be, cannot be overstated.

Foot Placement

The first step is to find the correct foot position—because this will be the base, there is no use in considering other positions until the placement of the feet is sound. The athlete will simply place the heels just outside the width of the hips and turn the toes out comfortably, approximately 20-30 degrees from the midline.

With this stance established, he or she will squat down and relax as much as possible in the bottom-

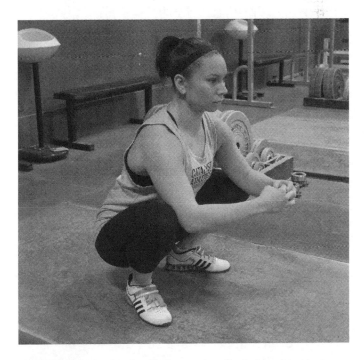

FIGURE 7.10 Sitting in a relaxed bottom squat position to determine stance

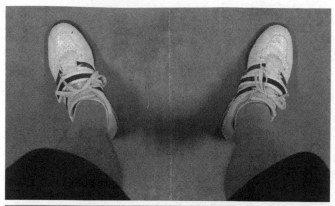

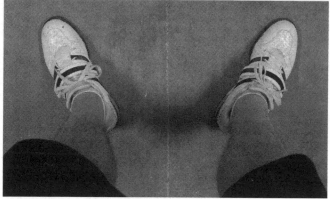

FIGURE 7.11 The range of foot positions is between approximately 20 and 30 degrees relative to the centerline.

most position—literally attempt to sit on the heels with no concern for posture. From this bottom position, the athlete will adjust the feet and thighs until they achieve the relationship discussed previously. The width of the feet will likely need to be adjusted slightly as well to ensure the thigh is approximately parallel with the foot and the knee is approximately above the toe when viewed from the front of the foot. The degree of external rotation of the legs can be experimented with as well until a comfortable position is established. Once this position has been established, the athlete will return to standing without moving the feet.

In this standing position, the athlete should view the feet and attempt to commit the stance to memory for quicker future positioning. For practice, the foot position can be first changed, and then the above process repeated until the athlete can find his or her correct stance reasonably well in the standing position.

Back & Posture

With the stance now established, we need to place the athlete into the bottom of the squat with the proper posture and trunk stabilization. This is the stage in which mobility limitations and muscle recruitment problems will become most evident.

For the sake of not complicating things unnecessarily, the athlete should first be simply instructed to draw in and hold a complete breath, set the back in complete extension, and lower him- or herself into the bottom position of the squat while maintaining back extension. He or she will not be able to reach the same depth possible with the back relaxed, but it will be similar if the athlete is adequately mobile.

If the athlete is unable to reach the bottom of the squat with the back set properly in extension, there are a number of possible problems. Most common are inadequate mobility, an inability to activate the spinal extensors sufficiently, or a combination of these (this is assuming, of course, that the foot placement is already correct).

Inflexible hip musculature will rotate the pelvis posteriorly as the athlete squats, preventing the maintenance of lumbar extension. No amount of spinal erector activation will be great enough to completely counteract the pull of these muscles. Limited ankle mobility will also prevent an athlete from achieving the proper bottom position. This will usually be obvious from the shins being too upright rather than inclined forward, and the appearance of the athlete nearly falling backward. Increasing mobility is the only option in these cases.

Occasionally an athlete will be possessed of obviously adequate mobility, but unable to establish the proper bottom position as would be expected. In these cases, the problem most often lies in that athlete's inability to activate the spinal extensors and/or stabilize the trunk as a whole. This can be a difficult problem to fix and will typically require a good deal of patience from both the coach and athlete.

To combat the inability of the athlete to maintain the proper alignment of the spine and pelvis in the squat—assuming the problem isn't mobility—activation of the spinal extensors will need to be improved (This activation will actually counteract some degree of limited mobility).

Spinal Extensor Activation

There are numerous possible ways in which to teach an athlete to better activate the spinal extensors, and the method should be selected based on its effectiveness for the athlete in question. In essence the goal is to place the athlete into a position in which he or she is able to forcefully extend the back without necessarily knowing how to do so conceptually, and without the interference of antagonist inflexibility.

Back Extension Hold Ideally the athlete has access to a glute-ham bench in which he or she can do back extension holds. With the footpads placed at about the same level as the fulcrum, and the fulcrum positioned under the hips, the athlete will lift the head and chest up as high as possible. The athlete should feel a forceful contraction of the spinal extensors from the upper to lower back. This position should be held for a few seconds before the athlete relaxes.

It may help for the athlete to place the hands behind the head. Additionally, hand contact by the coach on the athlete's erectors during this drill can sometimes further encourage activation and help the athlete feel exactly what they're attempting to contract. Pressure with a finger or two on either side of the spine, particularly in the lumbar region, should be adequate. (Figure 7.12)

Superman If a glute-ham bench is not available, the athlete can alternatively perform a superman hold. Lying prone (face down) on the floor with the hands behind the head, he or she will lift the chest and legs as high as possible and hold this arched position for a few seconds. This will produce the same basic result as the back extension hold—the sensation of forceful extensor contraction along the entire length of the back. (Figure 7.13)

The Back Squat

The most basic weighted squat variation is the back squat, which is a staple for all strength training, including Olympic weightlifting. Only a few details need to be addressed with regard to its performance as all the previous information on the squat in this chapter applies. (The front squat and overhead squat will be addressed in detail in the Clean and Snatch sections of the book, respectively.)

First is the placement of the barbell on the back. For most athletes, the correct positioning of the bar will be very natural. In cases in which this is not true, the coach can provide some simple instruction to ensure correct bar placement.

The athlete will first retract the shoulder blades completely and elevate them slightly. This will create somewhat of a muscular shelf with the traps and shoulder blades on which the bar can sit very securely. The bar will sit between the top of the traps and the top of the shoulders and be in contact with muscle—it should not be in contact with the bony protrusions (spinous processes) of the cervical or thoracic spine.

The athlete should grip the bar with the hands

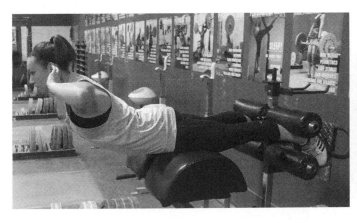

FIGURE 7.12 Back extension hold

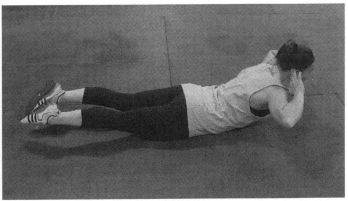

FIGURE 7.13 Superman

fairly close to the shoulders—a width that will place the forearms approximately vertical or just outside vertical when viewed from the front or back of the athlete. This close hand placement will help reinforce the retraction of the shoulder blades and the extension of the upper back. The elbows should be kept under the bar or only slightly behind it. Allowing the elbows to rotate too far behind the bar will encourage forward rounding of the upper back and forward leaning of the torso during the recovery from the bottom of the squat.

The thumbs should be wrapped around the bar along with the rest of the fingers, and the grip moderately tight. Because of the security of the barbell's placement on the back, a tight grip is not necessary to maintain its position; however, many lifters find that tightly squeezing the bar helps them recover from the squat more easily.

The squat is performed identically to the descriptions provided throughout this chapter. The athlete will draw in a breath and stabilize the trunk, control the speed of the descent, transition quickly in the bottom position, and drive through the recovery as quickly as possible (with the exception of intentionally slow squats).

Back squats will of course be taken out of squat racks. The athlete will position him- or herself under the bar with the correct bar placement by bending the legs partially. Once the bar is settled into position, the athlete will extend the legs and hips to lift the bar from the rack. With heavy squats, this lift from the racks should be aggressive to inspire confi-

dence in the lifter—a slower, less aggressive lift from the rack will make the weight feel much heavier, and no athlete will feel confident squatting a weight that feels heavy right out of the rack. The athlete will take a couple small steps back away from the rack and set the squat position with the feet. A new breath should generally be taken for each rep in a set unless the weight is light and multiple reps are being performed in quick succession.

Following completion of the set, the athlete will step forward between the squat rack uprights and squat the bar down into the cradles in the same manner he or she lifted it initially. The athlete should not simply get close to the rack and lean forward to dump the bar into it. This practice is risky for a number of reasons, and is unnecessarily abusive of the equipment.

Spotting & Missing

There will unfortunately be times when an athlete is unable to complete a back squat. As with all lifts used by the weightlifter, with the exception of the rare bench press, the athlete should be able to bail out of the lift safely without a need for spotters. This is done simply by leaning back to dump the bar backward and jumping forward out of the way. This is best done from the bottom of the squat because there will be no movement to contend with. Because most misses will occur above the bottom, the athlete can simply allow the weight to push him or her back down to the bottom (under control of course) and then dump the weight from there. In cases in which failure is due to forward leaning of the torso, this is even more important—this return to the bottom is an opportunity to bring the torso more upright and get the weight balanced across the feet again to allow a dump of the bar behind the lifter.

Occasionally it will be desirable to spot an athlete during a back squat set in which a miss is possible. This can be done for two basic reasons—one, to save the athlete the trouble of having to bail out, strip the bar down, and lift it back up to the rack; and two, to force the athlete to complete the rep with as much of the weight as possible (as a forced rep).

This spotting can be done by a single individual standing behind the lifter. In most cases of failed

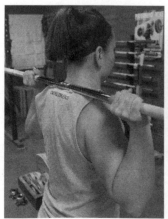 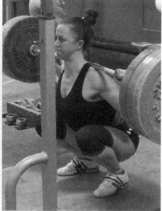

FIGURE 7.14 Correct placement of the barbell for the back squat

squats, the athlete will be incapable of completing the lift by only a fraction of the total weight—they will not suddenly cease to be capable of lifting anything at all. For this reason, a single spotter is usually able to provide enough assistance to unload that fraction of the weight momentarily to allow the athlete to drive through the sticking point and complete the lift.

Standing behind the lifter far enough to allow space for the hips as they travel back slightly during the squat, the spotter will simply keep his or her hands in close proximity to the bar as the athlete performs the squat. This can be done with the hands under or over the bar, and outside the athlete's hands unless the athlete uses a wide grip. In any case, it's important any assistance the spotter gives is directed upward and not either forward or backward, unless the bar is unintentionally moving in one of those directions (in many cases it will be drifting forward slightly because the athlete's chest is dropping, in which case the spotter can pull it back into position).

If the athlete requires more assistance than the spotter can provide, it will be obvious, and the spotter should instruct the athlete to bail out. The athlete will dump the bar as normal, while the spotter helps guide it back and gets out of the way. It's important that the lifter and spotter communicate clearly before and during the lift so that both are working together in the case of a miss and know what the other intends to do.

Spotting the back squat in particular, but also the front squat to a lesser extent, can encourage better squat performance by increasing a lifter's confidence. A lifter who isn't confident in squatting a certain weight will not fully commit to doing so in a unconscious effort to make sure he or she ends up in a position from which he or she can easily bail out, i.e. sitting in a solid, balanced position in the bottom of the squat rather than struggling to stand halfway up and potentially tipping forward. A coach standing behind the lifter to provide help if needed will make the lifter less concerned about missing and allow them to focus on the lift itself rather than what they're planning to do in case of failure. No contact with the bar by the coach even needs to be made—his or her mere presence is all that's required for this effect. However, the coach should always be ready to intervene in case help is required.

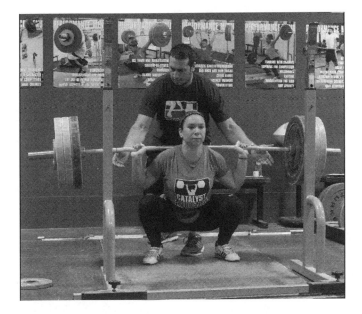

FIGURE 7.15 If desired, the back squat can be spotted. The hands can be placed either under or over the barbell.

2 Progression Summary

The Squat

Place the heels slightly outside hip-width with toes turned out comfortably.

Sit the hips down and relax in the bottom position, adjusting the foot position until the thighs are parallel with the feet and the hips comfortable.

Stand, arch the entire back and pressurize the trunk, and squat slowly to maximal depth with the back remaining arched and the torso upright.

Keep the feet flat and the weight balanced over the front edge of the heels.

Foot Positions & Transition

With the exception of the split position used in the split jerk (or the rare split snatch and split clean) there will be only two foot positions—*pulling* (or *drive* in the context of the jerk) and *receiving*.

The receiving position has already been established—it is the same stance used for the squat. This will be the foot position used to receive the snatch, clean, power snatch, power clean, and power jerk, and will be the stance used in all squat variations. Again, consistency in the fundamentals is imperative for developing consistency in the lift as a whole. The more consistent the receiving position of the feet, the more predictable the required positioning of the remainder of the body, and the fewer adjustments and corrections the athlete will need to make in a very brief window to produce a successful lift.

The pulling position will be predicated on three basic criteria—allowing maximal power production during the pull of the snatch and clean, allowing a sound starting position, and allowing the athlete to work with any structural peculiarities that may make a divergence from a conventional pulling position necessary and beneficial. This position may vary slightly between the snatch and clean because of the last two criteria, and it may vary again for the jerk—the jerk drive positioning will be discussed fully in the Jerk section of the book.

In theory, positioning the feet such that the legs are approximately vertical when the athlete is standing—feet directly under the hips—will allow maximal power production during the final stage of extension. This is simply because the force against the platform is being directed straight down, and therefore straight back up through the athlete, rather than some of the extension power being lost due to being at an angle from the desired direction of force. The more hip-dominant an athlete's pulling style is, the less this matters. Similarly, the small difference this makes can be easily eclipsed by limitations imposed by an uncomfortable position for a given athlete. Additionally, the more vertical the legs are during the pull of the snatch and clean, and the drive of the jerk, the higher the bar will be elevated at the point of complete knee and hip extension simply by virtue of the athlete's standing height. Again, while these are valuable, they are not so critical that non-traditional pulling or driving positions should not be considered if they better accommodate a given lifter's individual anatomical structure.

The feet will be turned out to whatever degree is comfortable for the athlete, within reason—generally approximately 10-20 degrees from center. Angles beyond about 20 degrees fall outside the range of advantageous alignment for maximal drive against the platform and will make the maintenance of balance more difficult because of an excessive shortening of the lifter's base. A foot angle too close to straight forward prevents proper thigh angles in the starting position and during the pulls. Research has shown a 2.5-5kg reduction in the snatch and clean with the feet straight forward in the pull (Glyadkovsky & Rodionov 1971/1992).

From this starting point, the athlete can adjust to accommodate for his or her unique anthropometry and how it dictates the starting position of the snatch and clean. Shorter-legged athletes may need to make no adjustments at all; longer-legged athletes may need to widen the stance and/or turn out the feet slightly more to bring the hips in closer to the bar—however, this positioning shift of the hips and trunk can also be made to a large extent simply by flaring the knees to the sides without affecting the placement of the feet. Modifications to foot placement should only be made to improve performance, not to circumvent correctible problems such as immobility.

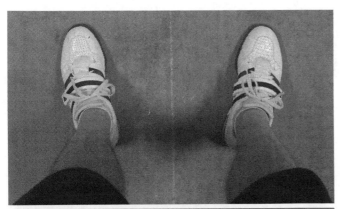

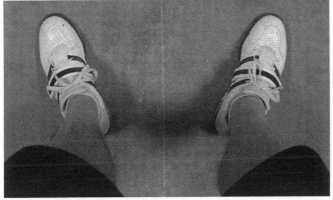

FIGURE 8.1 Typically the feet should be turned out between 10-20 degrees relative to the centerline in the pulling position. Each end of the range is pictured here.

Foot Transition

Because the pulling and receiving stances are distinct positions, it should be obvious at this point that the feet must transition from one to the other during the snatch and clean. There is a broad range of foot transition styles among even the elite weightlifters of the world—none is inarguably correct. How exactly a lifter transitions the feet should be determined based on what produces the best results for that particular lifter, and this will depend on a number of factors related to lift performance. Determination will require some time, experience and experimentation. Again, however, athletes should learn with conventional technique and only diverge when and if necessary.

There are two primary purposes for lifting the feet off the ground during the snatch or clean: repositioning them from the pulling position to the receiving position, and removing force against the ground to allow the athlete to move down under the bar faster. It is possible to keep the feet in contact

with the ground and remove any significant pressure, but zero contact guarantees zero pressure and consequently maximal downward speed. Even if a lifter uses identical stances for pulling and receiving, this lift of the feet will still be beneficial for this reason.

An additional reason for lifting the feet is that in the event of a lifter's balance shifting forward or backward inadvertently during the lift, the feet are able to move along with the rest of the body and bar and can be placed directly under the center of mass to improve the probability of the lifter being able to establish balance in the receiving position and succeed with the lift. If the lifter's balance moves forward or backward and the feet remain planted in the starting point on the floor, the lifter's base will no longer be directly under his or her center of mass upon receiving the lift, making the recovery anything from more difficult to impossible.

Greater elevation of the feet and the attendant increase in time during which the athlete is moving downward without being connected to the floor can mean more possibility of instability upon receiving the bar, both due to potential misplacement of the feet, and greater, more abrupt downward force of the bar onto the body upon reconnecting. However, the latter is also related to bar drop during the turnover, and is not necessarily a problem.

Jumping

Confusion with transitioning of the feet and jumping is common. It needs to be understood clearly that picking up the feet and jumping are two distinct and very different actions. Jumping is the action of elevating the entire body to a higher position by pushing off against the ground—*everything* moves up off the ground. Picking up the feet is actually the exact opposite action—it will cause the body to *fall down* toward the ground under the force of gravity. (Stand tall and pick up your feet and see what happens if you're confused about this.) No matter how aggressively or high an athlete lifts the feet like this, his or her body will absolutely not move up even the slightest amount. In other words, even dramatic elevation of the feet during the transition from the pulling to receiving position in a snatch or clean is not itself an indication that the lifter is jumping.

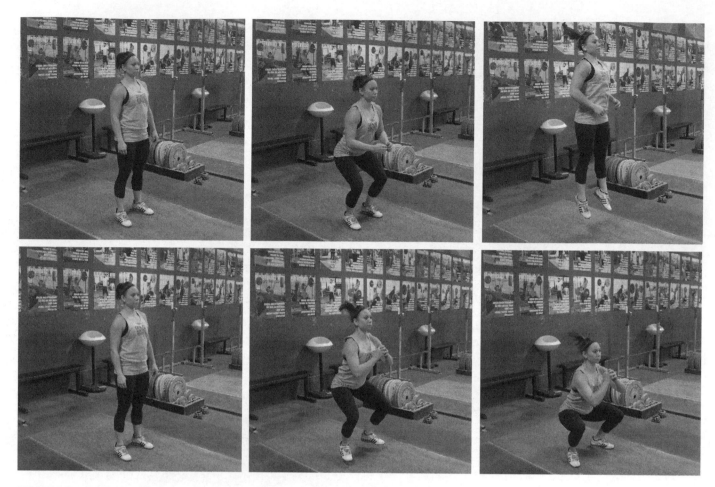

FIGURE 8.2 Jumping (top) is the action of elevating the entire body to a higher position through the action of pushing off against the ground. Lifting the feet (bottom), however, causes the athlete to drop.

Foot Transition Drill

With the foot positions established, the athlete can proceed to drilling the transition between them. The importance of footwork to the success of the lifts cannot be overstated, and a solid foundation built at this stage will encourage the speed, accuracy and consistency necessary for excellent technique.

Starting in the pulling position, the athlete will establish the proper balance over the front edge of the heel. From a position standing tall on the balls of the feet, the athlete will lift and transition the feet into the receiving position without further elevating the body as a whole, landing flat-footed in a quar-

ter-squat depth. This transition must be aggressive and the reconnection of the feet with the platform should produce an audible clap because of the viciousness of the movement and the foot hitting the floor flat—if a significant sound is absent, the athlete is likely landing on the balls of the feet and rolling down to flat feet.

Once the athlete is comfortable with this initial transition drill, the depth of the squat should be increased as gradually as necessary until it reaches full depth. Note that even when transitioning into a full squat in this drill, the athlete's feet will reconnect with

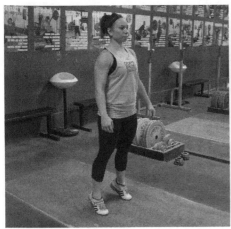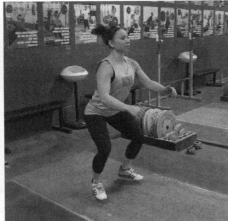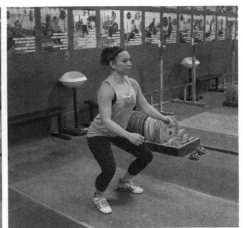

FIGURE 8.3 Foot transition drill into quarter squat

the floor before reaching full depth—this is proper, but the athlete needs to continue fluidly into the bottom of the squat without hesitation.

The deeper the athlete moves into the squat in this drill, the more important it will become to elevate the feet by lifting the knees—essentially performing a squatting motion by lifting the knees and feet. This focus on the knees will help prevent kicking the feet backward rather than lifting them straight up, which will be a serious technical problem later.

On every repetition of the drill the athlete performs, the squat stance should be corrected if needed. The more time the athlete spends in the correct positions, and sees the correct positions, the more quickly he or she will develop consistency.

3 Progression Summary

Foot Transition

Start with the feet approximately under the hips and turned out comfortably

Weight slightly more on the heels than the balls of the feet

Rise to the balls of the feet and then quickly lift and move the feet to the squat position, landing flat-footed.

Initially land in quarter-squat depth

On each subsequent transition, land in a deeper squat until finally transitioning into a full squat as quickly as possible.

The Hook Grip

The hook grip is a pronated (palms facing the lifter) grip in which the thumb is trapped between the bar and usually the first and second fingers, depending on hand size. For the pull of both the snatch and the clean, this method of gripping is an eventual necessity to maintain control of the barbell during the violent explosion of the second pull.

It's important to understand that the thumb is itself wrapped around the bar inside the fingers and not simply pinned parallel to the bar. With the thumb wrapped over the fingers as it would be in a conventional overhand grip, it will typically reach only the index finger and have a weak purchase on it due to being only partially flexed. By wrapping the thumb around the bar directly, we create a powerful hook on the bar, which can then be reinforced by

the grip of both the index and middle fingers. This allows the thumb to reach around the bar enough to significantly contribute to grip integrity without limiting the ability of the fingers to wrap around the bar adequately to grip it as well. Additionally, the fingers grasp the thumb ("hooking" onto it), creating a strong ridge to improve their purchase.

This also creates a system of balanced hooks on the bar. In a standard overhand grip, the bar is supported by the fingers, which all open in the same direction, creating a tendency for the bar to roll back-

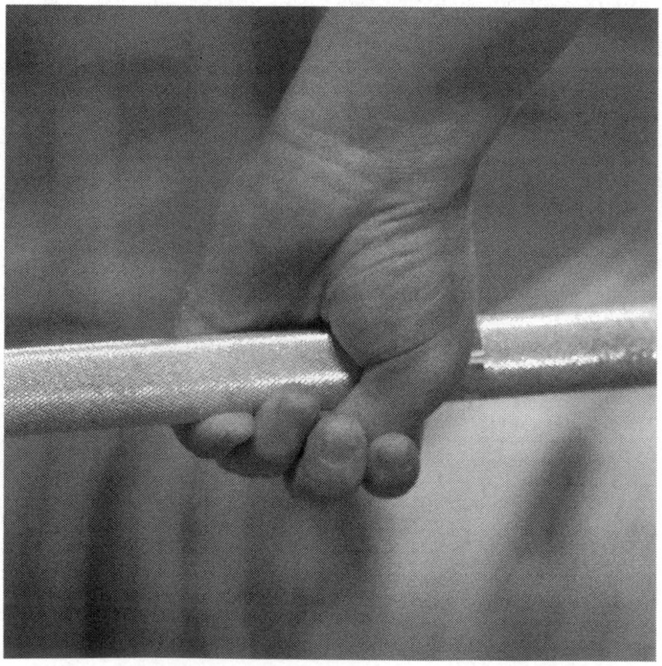

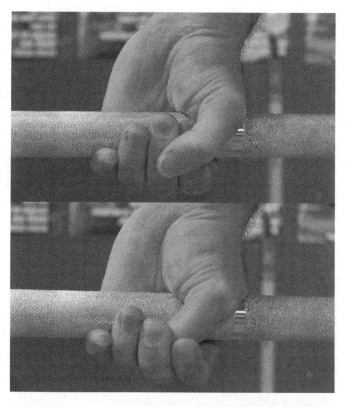

FIGURE 9.2 With the hook grip, the thumb is able to wrap farther around the bar than in a regular overhand grip, while the fingers are still able to wrap considerably, allowing more overall contribution to grip security. Additionally, the fingers hook onto the thumb, which acts as a ridge for greater purchase of the fingers.

FIGURE 9.1 The hook grip is a pronated grip in which the thumb is trapped between the bar and fingers.

Greg Everett

ward out of the hand. The mixed grip—one pronated and one supinated hand—is commonly employed in the deadlift by powerlifters because the backward rolling tendency on the pronated side is countered by a forward rolling tendency on the supinated side, thereby stabilizing the bar.

The hook grip creates a similar system of countering this tendency of the bar to roll while allowing the necessary movement and position of the hands and arms during the snatch and clean that a mixed grip precludes. The bar will try to roll out of the thumb in one direction, and out of the fingers in the opposite, eliminating to a great degree the spinning element of grip loss.

Finally, because of the increased security created by the hook grip for the reasons described above, the athlete can rely on lower levels of grip tension during a lift. This reduction in finger and wrist flexor tension allows a reduction in elbow tension during the pulling phases of the snatch and clean that improves the transmission of leg and hip power to the bar and the speed and fluidity of the transition between the second and third pulls. In short, the hook grip optimizes the anatomy of the hands for this application.

The more relaxed the athlete can keep the hands during a lift, the more relaxed the arms will remain, and the better the transmission of force from the legs to the bar will be. However, the hands can only relax so much before the grip begins slipping with the violence of the body's extension. Depending on grip strength and hand size and shape, athletes will be able to maintain different levels of gripping effort, but all should make it a goal to grip only as tightly as necessary.

In the snatch, because the wide hand placement of the lift results in the angle of the hand attachment to the bar being such that the origins of the two shortest fingers are the farthest from the bar, the third and fourth fingers will typically have little purchase for everyone but those possessed of fairly large hands. This being the case, the integrity of the grip of the first and second fingers in combination with the thumb is critical.

In order to ensure this integrity, the athlete needs to use the fingers to actively pull the thumb around the bar rather than simply pressing it against the bar. This hook of the thumb around the bar with the fingers hooking onto the thumb is what provides the primary grip power. However, the third and fourth fingers are still important contributors, and their slipping can initiate a complete grip failure, or at least enough of a psychological hit to prevent the necessary commitment to the rest of the lift.

The wrist can be flexed somewhat so that the back of the hand is in approximately straight alignment with the forearm, which will relieve the thumb of some pressure and shift it more into the fingers. For most lifters, this will increase the comfort and security of the grip both by reducing the discomfort of the thumb and by allowing the shorter fingers to wrap farther around the bar. However, this is a minimal degree of wrist flexion—it is certainly not

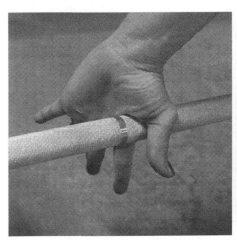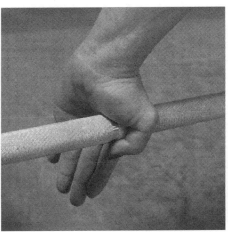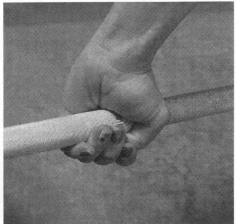

FIGURE 9.3 Setting the hook grip: Press the webbing of the hand between the thumb and index finger against the bar; wrap the thumb around the bar as far a possible; grab the thumb with the index and middle fingers; use these first two fingers to pull the thumb farther around the bar; grip the bar with the remaining fingers.

significant. Excessive wrist flexion in the pull will be similar in effect to partially flexed elbows; that is, it's a weak point in the system that can extend during the explosive final extension of the snatch or clean and create a loss of force transfer to the bar.

Typically the hook grip will be uncomfortable if not considerably painful initially. Consistent use will condition the offending structures appropriately over time and the grip will ultimately offer no trouble. It will, in fact, become more comfortable than a conventional overhand grip with experience. Covering the thumbs with flexible athletic tape can reduce the discomfort and, for some, improve the feeling of grip security by increasing friction. Lifters can submerge the hands in ice water for 5-10 minutes after training to help reduce pain and speed the adaptation.

If taping the thumb (or other fingers) across a joint, it's important to use elastic tape rather than conventional athletic tape. Non-elastic tape will limit the motion of the taped joint and create potential for sprains in the next joint up the chain. If elastic tape isn't available, non-elastic tape can be used if wrapped and/or cut in a manner that prevents it from covering the back of the joint.

New lifters should be taught and learn the hook grip early on so that they are familiar with it. However, it's recommended that they train without the hook grip for an initial period of time to help better develop grip strength (likewise, it's suggested they avoid using straps even for pulls and deadlifts during this early development period). There is no precise timing for beginning to use the hook grip—as weights increase and the lifter begins to feel less secure during the second pull of the snatch and clean, it can be introduced. Ideally, during this transition period, it's

reserved for only the heaviest sets of a given exercise.

In the long term, if grip is not a limiting factor for a given lifter, it can be used for all training sets of the snatch, clean and their variations. For lifters for whom grip strength is an issue, warm-up sets can be performed without the hook grip to encourage more grip strength development, and the hook grip employed only on heavier sets when it becomes necessary. In any case, the hook grip should be used with regularity once it's introduced to ensure the lifter is comfortable with it and setting it correctly, and that the hands adapt adequately.

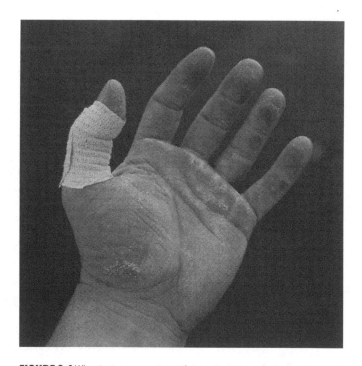

FIGURE 9.4 When taping across a joint, it's important to use elastic tape to prevent sprains of adjacent joints.

The Double Knee Bend

The double knee bend is a phenomenon that occurs at the initiation of the second pull of the snatch and clean. As the knees achieve partial extension as the bar reaches approximately the level of mid-thigh, the athlete initiates the final violent extension of the hips and knees. As this hip extension begins, the knees shift forward at this partially bent angle, bending more to a slight degree, and then finish their extension along with the hips. This is more a momentary cessation of knee extension as they shift forward than actual flexion of the knee—to what degree the knees actually bend again will vary among lifters and depends on the position the lifter is in when he or she initiates the final explosion effort, the relative strength of the legs and hips, and the leverage of

the lifter's build (i.e. shorter-legged, more leg-dominant lifters will typically demonstrate larger degrees of flexion upon entering the double knee bend and larger degrees of re-bending, as this will exploit their greater leg extension strength in the effort to elevate and accelerate the barbell). Ideally there is minimal flexion of the knees, which minimizes any reduction of bar speed during this transition phase—this is best achieved by initiating the second pull with the bar higher on the thigh and focusing on continuous aggressive leg drive.

This movement is the product of two elements: the bi-articular nature of the hamstrings and a need for the body to maintain balance. Because the hamstrings group crosses both the hip and knee joints,

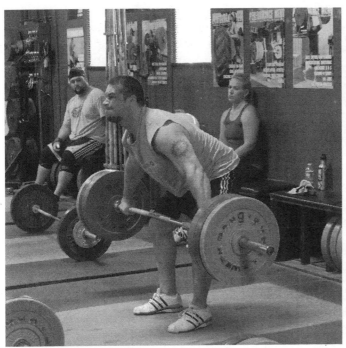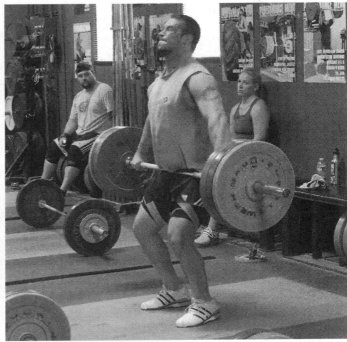

FIGURE 10.1 The double knee bend or transition is the temporary cessation of extension (and possibly very slight flexion) and shifting of the knees forward under the bar during the final extension of the snatch or clean.

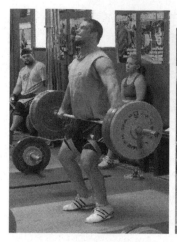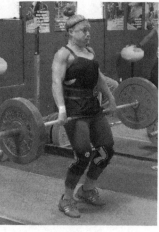

FIGURE 10.2 Final forward knee position of the double knee bend (Left: snatch; Right: clean). This position is commonly referred to as the Power Position.

the contraction of the hamstrings to help effect the aggressive extension of the hip also creates a pull to flex the knee; this prevents the knees from finishing their extension, maintaining the partially flexed angle they were in at the point the hip extension. As the trunk moves up and back as a result of hip extension, the hips and knees must move forward to maintain the balance of the bar-body system.

This forward shifting of the knees under the bar in a partially bent position is referred to as the *scoop* or *transition*. The maximal forward position of the knees occurs as the torso reaches approximately vertical, placing the athlete in a position in which the knees are forward of the bar and the hips under the shoulders. This position is often called the *power position*. As the trunk reaches approximately vertical, the athlete's continued effort to aggressively drive against the ground with the legs finalizes the knee extension along with the remaining hip extension.

This movement of the knees is unavoidable when executing the lifts with proper positioning and speed. It is a natural reaction to the body's action overall, just as plantar flexion of the ankle is a natural part of jumping—it is not an action the athlete has to intentionally perform.

Teaching the Double Knee Bend

Because the double knee bend is a natural and unavoidable action if position, balance and timing of the lift are correct, it does not require teaching. In fact, teaching the double knee bend—that is, teaching a lifter to intentionally shift the knees forward under the bar—invariably creates problems.

No lifter ever needs to even hear the term or know that the action is occurring to properly perform the snatch and clean. In fact, it's arguable that not knowing about it will improve lift performance as there will be no opportunity to attempt to perform it intentionally and alter what should be the natural mechanics of the movement. Multiple international elite lifters have stated, in fact, that they had never even heard of the concept before coming to the United States and hearing coaches discuss it—this alone should be adequate evidence that instruction is unnecessary.

Conscious attempts by an athlete to create the double knee bend nearly always result in an early scoop. This premature shifting of the knees under the bar is problematic for a number of reasons. At the most basic level, this movement will drive the bar forward through contact with the forward shifting thighs, often resulting in its swinging out away from the lifter. The movement will also shift the balance of the lifter's weight too far forward on the feet, and this weight shift is increased with a swinging bar. At the more complex level, this premature scoop pauses the knee extension before adequate extension has been achieved. This greater knee flexion angle means reduced tension on the hamstrings and a reduction of hip explosiveness in the final extension effort. Adequate hamstring tension upon entrance into the final explosion is imperative for maximal power production and the resulting speed on the bar. Finally, the shoulders moving behind the bar prematurely will cause the bar to drag on the thighs, reducing its speed directly and reducing the speed of the final hip and knee extension of the second pull.

In short, a genuine double knee bend is achieved only by allowing it to occur naturally through ensuring correct positioning and timing.

Demonstrating the Double Knee Bend

While teaching the double knee bend in the strictest sense isn't possible, because it can be a confusing concept for both athletes and coaches, it's helpful to have a way to demonstrate and observe the movement when appropriate—coaches should consider carefully whether or not the concept should be introduced to an athlete at all. Certainly this will be more appropriate for coaches than athletes.

A simple demonstration can be accomplished by performing a vertical jump from the optimal second pull position. With the feet in the pulling position, the athlete will bend the knees slightly and hinge at the hips, bringing the shins approximately vertical, the shoulders slightly in front of the knees, and the weight balanced over the front edge of the heel. From this position—without a countermovement and keeping the weight balanced where it starts—the athlete will simply jump as high as he or she can. While the complete extension of the hips is important, primary focus at this point should be on knee extension because it tends to be the neglected element in this case. If we focus excessively on hip extension, we nearly always see a failure to finish the drive with the legs, resulting in marginal vertical acceleration and an unproductive forward slide of the hips due to an absent base.

To anyone observing, such as a coach or other athletes, the knees should be the focus. It will be clear that as the athlete initiates the jump, the knees shift forward before extending—it's important that the athlete jumping not be given any instruction to shift the knees forward: only to jump straight up as aggressively as possible directly from the static starting position.

If this shifting of the knees is not evident, it can be made more visible by creating a reference line with a length of PVC. With the athlete in the starting position, the coach can hold a PVC bar vertically with the front edge in line with the front of the athlete's knee, standing as far behind it as possible to allow a clear view for the observers, who should be positioned directly to the athlete's side. When the athlete jumps, the knees will clearly travel in front of the bar. This natural, unintentional movement of the knees is exactly what occurs during the snatch or clean—with this demonstration, it should be evident that the motion does not need to be performed intentionally during the lifts.

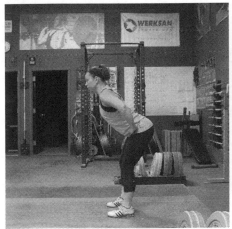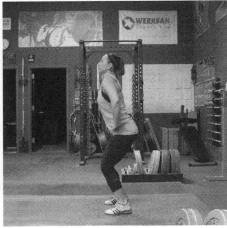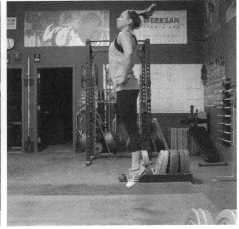

FIGURE 10.3 The natural forward movement of the knees that occurs in the snatch and clean pulls can be demonstrated by performing a standing vertical jump from a static start mimicking the beginning position of the second pull. With the effort to jump, the athlete's knees will naturally and unavoidably shift forward as the trunk moves vertically.

Starting Position Principles

The starting position of the snatch and clean is a topic that warrants independent discussion for a number of reasons, one of which is simply that it applies to both the snatch and clean. Additionally, the topic has generated a considerable degree of confusion within the broader strength and conditioning community (there is little disagreement, and of comparatively minor degree, within the weightlifting community). Because the criteria and the rationale for the proper starting position are the same for both the snatch and clean, they will be presented here as a universal element, and then details specific to each lift addressed in the respective sections of the book.

The primary requirement of the starting position is to create the optimal position, balance and positional relationship of the barbell and body throughout the first and second pulls of the lift. In other words, it must set the lifter up for the ideal mechanics later in the lift. The comfort of the position itself is irrelevant unless the discomfort is of such a degree that it in some way negatively affects the lift.

The second pull of the snatch and clean is the source of the most critical upward acceleration of the barbell—it is the heart of the lift, and the phase in which the barbell is imparted with enough upward momentum to allow the lifter time and space to relocate underneath it; its performance also dictates to a large extent the success of the third pull.

The optimal second pull position is defined by the ideal degree of knee and hip flexion and balance on the feet to generate maximal force against the ground and upward acceleration of the barbell in the correct path while also allowing the lifter to change directions and relocate under the bar as quickly and accurately as possible.

While our criteria will produce a very upright posture in the starting position, this does not mean forward inclination of the trunk is not important.

An angle on the torso is necessary to allow hip extension to contribute, along with knee extension, to the upward acceleration of the bar, as well as to help maintain the proper balance of the system's center of mass over the feet.

There are several reasons for beginning the lift with such an upright posture rather than one that places the hips higher and the shoulders farther forward of the bar. First, this more upright angle minimizes hip and lumbar torque and consequently fatigue of the spinal extensors during the first pull. Because the lower back is most easily fatigued relative to the other muscle groups involved in the lift, and these muscles must be able to maintain rigidity of the spine during the second pull in order to maximize the conversion of hip and knee extension power to acceleration of the barbell, more work by the lower back early in the lift will mean less rigidity and more of the hips' and legs' power being absorbed by the back's extension softening during the final extension of the hips.

Second, the reduced torque on the hips with a more upright back angle allows greater hip extension speed during the second pull because the lower degree of initial torque allows better acceleration and creates less fatigue.

Third, the shorter rotational distance during the second pull minimizes the demands on balance maintenance and allows the athlete to focus more on the power of execution rather than the balance of the system.

Fourth, such an upright posture encourages the bar to remain close to the body where it needs to be with less additional effort due to the angle of the arms being nearer to their natural loaded orientation.

Finally, athletes will generally feel more comfortable in a more upright position and consequently be better prepared psychologically for a successful lift.

This reason cannot be underestimated in terms of its contribution to lift success.

Understanding the Position

The starting position is dictated by two primary criteria. First, the barbell begins over approximately the balls of the foot. Second, the lifter assumes a posture that orients the arms approximately vertically when viewed from the lifter's side—that is, the shoulder joint is approximately directly above the barbell, placing the leading edge of the shoulders very slightly in front of it.

In addition to these criteria, the back must be fixed securely in a complete arch (i.e. the length of the spine from the sacrum to the base of the skull forms a single continuous arch), the head and eyes oriented forward with a focal point straight ahead or slightly above, the arms internally rotated (bony points of the elbows facing out to the sides) and extended passively, the shoulder blades approximately neutral in terms of protraction-retraction and depressed by the contraction of the lats being employed to help cre-

ate the arch of the back and maintain the barbell's proximity to the body, the knees over the bar and pushed outward inside the arms, and the feet turned out slightly with the weight balanced evenly across them. The height of the hips relative to the knees will range from slightly below to slightly above depending on the build of the athlete.

The starting position of the barbell over the balls of the foot creates space for the shins to incline forward adequately for the lifter to achieve the desired posture. Positioning the bar over the middle of the foot, as may make sense intuitively for the sake of establishing balance, prevents this necessary forward movement of the shin and forces the lifter to assume a position with the hips higher and shoulders farther forward. In some cases, lifters are built in a way that does allow the bar to be positioned slightly farther back than the balls of the foot without forcing the remaining criteria of the position to be violated, and without having problematic consequences in the first pull. In such cases, this bar position can be employed if the athlete finds it more effective. Generally, lifters with shorter legs will be able to start the bar slightly behind the balls of the foot, while lifters will longer legs will need to start the bar slightly in front.

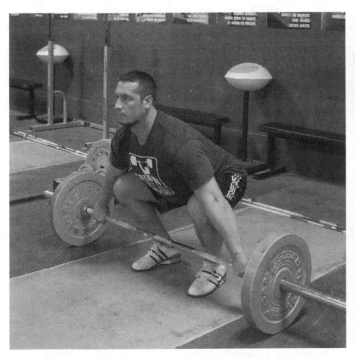 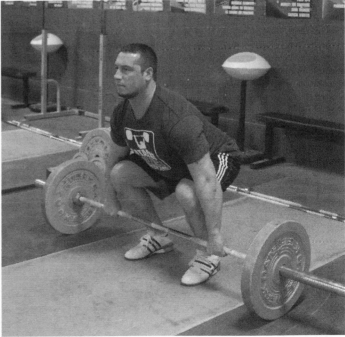

FIGURE 11.1 The snatch and clean starting positions adhere to the same criteria and vary only in the effects of the different grip widths on the bar.

Because the barbell begins over the balls of the foot, as a significantly heavy bar is separated from the platform, the lifter's weight will be farther forward over the foot than is ultimately desired. However, the shifting of the weight back to reposition the line of gravity at the proper location for the remainder of the pull is accomplished easily and quickly during the first pull.

The approximately vertical orientation of the arms ensures an upright posture in the starting position and creates a trunk angle that allows for an easier maintenance of the bar's proximity to the body during the pull. It's important to understand that this orientation is placing the shoulder joint, not the leading edge of the shoulder musculature, directly over the bar. How far forward of the bar the leading edge of the shoulder is in this position will depend on the shoulder mass of the athlete in question. If this criterion of the shoulder above the bar is misinterpreted to mean the front of the shoulder, the athlete's arms will be inclined backward rather than vertical.

The arch of the back is critical for maximizing the effectiveness of the pull. The failure to secure a solid back arch will result in the reduction of the force that is transferred to the bar from the extension of the knees and hips due to a portion of it being absorbed by unwanted softening of the back—up to a 15% reduction in force has been found to occur with a rounded back (Kanyevsky 1982/1992). The lifter is attempting to create a single, continuous arch along the entire length of the spine—from the base of the skull to the sacrum. While the cervical and lumbar sections of the spine are naturally arched in their neutral position, the thoracic spine is curved in the opposite direction. The goal is to flatten this curve to create the continuous arch. As a part of this, it's important the athlete maintains an upright head position. This does not mean extreme cervical spine hyperextension—it means that the head position contributes to the continuous back arch and allows the desired forward or slightly above forward focal point. Additionally, this upright head position has been demonstrated to improve the strength of the back muscles in holding this position by an average of 20kg relative to a more downward head orientation (Kanyevsky 1982/1992). The natural tendency for the body to assume this stronger position can be observed frequently with athletes struggling with

very difficult squatting or pulling efforts.

Aside from improving the strength of the back during the pull, an upright head position allows an optimal focal point during the lift straight forward or slightly above that point. A constant focal point throughout the duration of a lift maximizes a lifter's balance by providing a reference for orientation, but also minimizes the potential for distractions and can even help prevent the lifter from throwing the head backward excessively at the top of the extension of the snatch or clean.

Internal rotation of the arms—turning the bony points of the elbows out to the sides as much as mobility allows—is a critical position to establish in the starting position so that it can optimize the mechanics of the third pull by allowing the maintenance of the barbell's proximity to the body during the lifter's relocation under it. The extension of the elbows is also important primarily for a later portion of the lift—this ensures the elimination of any slack in this part of the system that can later be a source of power loss. However, this extension must be passive—that is, the elbows should not be actively extended, but should be extended due to the tension created by the pull between the shoulders and the barbell.

The position of the shoulder blades will largely be a consequence of actions that affect them rather than a direct intent to position them in a certain way. Due to the engagement of the lats in order to both keep the bar pushed back toward the body and reinforce the arch of the back, the shoulder blades will be depressed. Some lifters will find it effective to intentionally spread the shoulder blades—partial protraction—but in general, they should remain in an approximately neutral position with regard to protraction and retraction.

The knees should protrude over the bar to a degree consistent with the lifter's proportions. If this protrusion is extreme, it likely is an indication that the lifter's hips are too low and the shoulders are behind the bar. However, if the knees are not over the bar, it indicates that the shins are too near to vertical, preventing the lifter from achieving the proper posture and likely balancing the weight too far back over the feet. The knees also need to be flared out inside the arms, often to the point of light contact. Unlike in the squat, in which we want to maintain the knees' position over the corresponding foot, this flaring of the knees in the starting position will likely position them outside the feet.

This flaring of the knees is an important factor in the establishment of an upright pulling posture. The length of the upper leg will in part affect the angle of the back by dictating how far back the hips are positioned relative to the knees and bar. By flaring the knees to the sides, the length of the upper leg is in effect shortened, bringing the hips closer to the bar and allowing a more upright back angle.

The bar will not necessarily be in contact with the shins in the starting position, although contact is certainly acceptable. For many lifters, maintaining maximal proximity of the bar to the shins without allowing contact will produce better results by helping to avoid catching on the shins or the knee during the pull. In any case, the barbell scraping the shins during the first pull is an indication of a technical error—most commonly the shoulders being behind the bar rather than above it from the start of the lift, because the lifter is beginning to extend the hips prematurely or because the athlete is pushing the bar back toward the body too aggressively at that point of the lift (with the shoulders directly above the bar, maintaining the bar's proximity to the legs requires little effort—the effort will not need to be significant until the bar passes the knees).

The pulling stance has been discussed previously in detail—the feet will be approximately hip-width and the toes turned out to some reasonable degree. Again, the angle of the feet and the thighs will not necessarily align in the starting position like they will in the squat. Additionally, the lifter's weight should be balanced approximately evenly across the foot—it should not be on the heels. Attempting to balance toward the heels in the starting position creates a number of problems, including typically preventing the correct position and the resulting overcompensation as the lift begins, shifting the lifter's balance too far forward.

Finally, the height of the hips will vary among athletes in response to their builds. Their position will range from slightly below the knees to above the knees. The lift of the bar from the floor will be easier with the hips beginning above the knee because of the more advantageous joint angles (A hip position above the knees, along with the better leverage of shorter limbs, is responsible for the general ability

of shorter lifters to be capable of higher speeds in the first pull relative to their taller counterparts). If the athlete can achieve a hip position above the knee while meeting all other starting position criteria, this is preferable.

However, the ease of the lift from the floor is not the first priority; this ease will need to be sacrificed in some cases to achieve the desired position, as this will have a more positive effect on the lift overall. The greater mechanical difficulty created by a low hip position can also be mitigated with the use of a dynamic start (discussed later in this chapter).

Variation

Actual variation in the starting position for the snatch and clean—that is, divergence from the criteria presented here—will exist among athletes for reasons such as immobility and limitations from past injuries. These should be corrected to the greatest extent possible over time. Differences in the appearance of the starting position will also exist among athletes as a consequence of variation in stature and structure, which are not in need of correction (Figure 11.2). These differences include elements such as the angle of the back, the angle of the shins, the height of the hips, the degree to which the feet are turned out, the degree to which the knees are flared to the sides, the degree of back arch, the degree of internal rotation of the arms—in other words, any detail that is a product of the athlete's proportions or permanent anatomy (i.e. skeletal structure). It's important to be capable of distinguishing between these two types of variations in order to know if corrections will need to be made.

Entering the Starting Position

To some extent, how the athlete enters the correct starting position is inconsequential. If the starting position and lift that result from the entrance is consistently correct, that entrance can be left entirely to personal preference. Distinguishing between the starting position and the preparatory position is important here—the preparatory position (the position

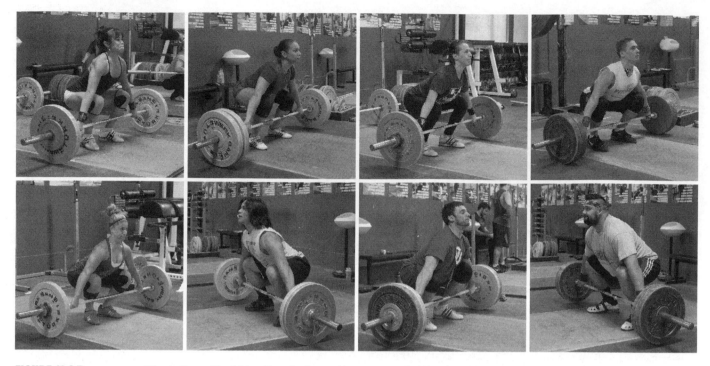

FIGURE 11.2 The appearance of the starting position (pictured here for the snatch) can vary considerably among athletes even when the same criteria for proper positioning are met due to differences in stature and structure. This includes elements such as the angle of the back, the angle of the shins, the height of the hips, the degree to which the feet are turned out and the degree to which the knees are flared to the sides—in other words, any detail that is a product of the athlete's proportions or permanent anatomy (i.e. skeletal structure). Additionally, mobility-related variations such as the degree of extension in any given region of the spine and the degree of internal rotation of the arms will be observable.

the athlete is in prior to assuming the starting position) is often confused for the starting position itself, particularly in cases of dynamic starts. As was established previously, the starting position is the position from which the lifter actually begins the lift; that is, it's the last position prior to the separation of the barbell from the platform.

With a static start, the athlete sets and holds the starting position for a moment before initiating the lift; in a dynamic start, the athlete moves in a number of possible ways into or often through and then back into the starting position, initiating the lift without ever holding the starting position.

Static Start

The static start should be taught to and employed by all beginning weightlifters. In the early stages of development, it's critical to establish technical consistency as well as kinesthetic awareness and familiarity with the positions involved in the lifts. The static

start aids in this by allowing a distinct position for the lifter to assume and practice, building a foundation that will support long term technical proficiency advances.

Employing a static start minimizes the number of variables in a given lift, improving consistency and reducing the number of details with which the lifter must be concerned during the lift. It also is helpful to the coach, who can, in real time, see the position clearly and provide corrections as necessary. With a dynamic start, problems with the starting position are more difficult to recognize for the coach because of the brevity of the position.

Additionally, the use of a dynamic start by beginners is unnecessary. The weights being lifted by beginners are limited by a lack of technical proficiency and often immobility. Consequently, there is no need to employ more complex strategies to make the separation of the bar from the floor and first pull easier. This will only become necessary—and not for all lifters—later in a lifter's career. Accordingly, lifters are encouraged to continue the use of a static start in the snatch and clean until a reasonable level of technical proficiency and consistency have been established.

Dynamic Start

A dynamic start will make the separation of the bar from the floor and the initial pull easier through the mechanism of either a stretch-shortening reflex or the generation of more muscular tension prior to separation. For lifters who quickly pump the hips down into position and immediately break the bar from the floor, there is usually sufficient speed to elicit a stretch-shortening reflex. For athletes who instead perform a movement such as sitting the hips down slowly and then lifting them back up into position to initiate the lift will be generating tension in the muscles prior to moving the bar so that more force will be developed by the time the lift begins. In either case, the separation of the bar will be made easier, incurring less fatigue, increasing the speed of the pull and generally increasing the lifter's confidence and consequently his or her commitment to the lift. Additionally, certain dynamic starts can make it easier improve the arch of the back in the pull. Experimentation by Glyadkovsky and Rodionov (1971/1992) showed that a dynamic start produced on average a 2.5 cm increase in snatch pull height relative to a static start.

For advanced lifters who are snatching and cleaning large percentages of their basic strength capacities, and in particular, those who are possessed of less advantageous proportions for this segment of the lift (i.e. longer-legged and/or taller), the dynamic start can essentially be a necessity for near-maximal and maximal lifts.

The type of dynamic start used will need to be determined by each athlete through experimentation. Lifters will tend to naturally gravitate toward the type of start most effective for them; if their selection appears to the coach to be problematic, he or she should intervene and help the athlete either modify it as necessary or select an entirely different style. For example, with a given style of dynamic start, an athlete may continually push the bar forward with his or her shins, creating imbalance as the bar breaks from the floor. This should be correctable with adjustments and practice; if it proves uncorrectable, a different style of start should be found.

The concern with the dynamic start, as discussed with regard to the static start, is the potential for inconsistency. Even athletes who have been employing dynamic starts for years are often in different positions at the moment the bar leaves the platform in each lift if they began employing such a start prior to establishing a solid enough foundation of technical proficiency. Athletes should be certain that introducing a dynamic start to their snatches and cleans (an athlete does not necessarily have to employ a dynamic start, or the same type of dynamic start, in both lifts) is appropriate for their level of development and needs.

Types of Dynamic Starts

Sit-Through In this start, the athlete will typically set the back arch with the hips in a high position, and then in one continuous motion, slowly lower the hips down past the starting position and into a deeper squat, often leaning the shoulders back behind the bar, and then bring the hips back up, separating the bar from the floor and beginning the lifts as the hips reach the starting position.

Hip Pump Typically with this start, the athlete will set the starting position momentarily, and then quickly lift the hips up and pump them back down into the starting position, breaking the bar from the floor with this downward pump. The lifter may perform a single pump or a series of pumps before lifting. The study by Glyadkovsky and Rodionov (1971/1992) found the "double pump" dynamic start (two consecutive hip pumps) to be the most effective; however, this style makes proper balance and position upon separation of the bar from the platform difficult.

Slow Descent Somewhat of a combination of the previous two, the lifter begins with the hips high, usually with the back already arched, and slowly lowers them into the starting position, generating tension throughout the legs and hips, and then breaking the bar as the hips reach the final starting position.

Low Sit The low sit can be considered a variation of the sit-through. Rather than starting in a high-hipped position and squatting through and then back up into the starting position, the lifter begins sitting in the low squat, and then creates tension and lifts the hips into position, breaking the bar from the floor as they reach the proper height.

The Rip This start is usually the sign of a very aggressive lifter. After sitting in a squatting preparatory position with the stance and grip set, the lifter will abruptly launch into the start of the lift, essentially yanking the bar off the floor (Bulgaria's Zlaten Vanev is probably the most recognizable user of this type of start). This start can make it a little more difficult to set a proper back arch, and also can create a problem with a reduction in bar speed after the initial acceleration.

Dive Start The dive start is a very rare style, mostly associated with David Rigert of Russia and Wes Barnett of the US. It's also more likely to be used in the clean than the snatch. In this start, the lifter begins in a fully standing position at the bar, and then simply reaches down, grabs the bar and immediately lifts. While this may make it easier for some athletes to set a better back arch, it's very difficult to ensure a secure grip and proper position and balance when separating the bar.

Preparatory Position

There are options for entry into both static and dynamic starts. Again, how the starting position is entered is less important than the position itself, unless the manner of entrance negatively influences the starting position and first pull, such as preventing the lifter from securing a proper back arch, creating an imbalance over the feet, or disrupting the proper

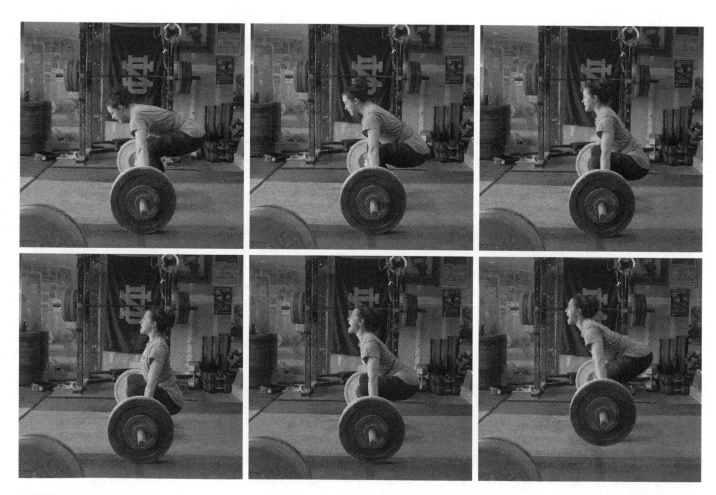

FIGURE 11.3 In a dynamic start, the athlete moves into or through and back into the starting position and initiates the lift without ever holding the starting position. Pictured here is the "sit-through" style dynamic start.

Greg Everett

speed, acceleration or timing of the pull.

Irrespective of each lifter's chosen entrance, consistency is imperative. The process should be ritualistic in many respects, both for the sake of encouraging the correct starting position and bolstering the athlete's confidence—the fewer variables in the system, the smaller the chance of mistakes, discomfort and doubt. In competition, in particular, the importance of this cannot be overstated.

There are two basic types of preparatory positions. In the first, the athlete stands with the feet in position and the grip set and leans forward over the bar. In the second, the athlete squats behind the bar with the feet and grip set. Which—or which variation of either—is used by each lifter is a matter of personal preference within the constraints of allowing a proper start.

When the lifter takes in the final pressurizing breath to stabilize the trunk will depend on the style of start. In all cases, this breath should be taken as near to the start of the lift as possible to avoid excessive durations of breath-holding, and should be taken in a position or at a stage in the movement that allows adequate expansion of the trunk for a full breath.

The more accurately this process is repeated for each lift, the greater control the athlete will have over the technical facets of the rest of the lift. Athletes should experiment and find the process that feels most comfortable and effective for them.

Introduction to the Snatch

The snatch is the first of the two lifts contested in weightlifting, in which the barbell is lifted from the floor to overhead in a single movement. With its unparalleled speed and extensive range of motion, it epitomizes mechanical power—the performance of maximal work in minimal time—as well as technical precision.

The fundamental pulling mechanics of the snatch apply to that of the clean, and learning the snatch is typically more difficult than learning the clean or jerk for new lifters. Additionally, the wide grip of the snatch improves the ease of learning the proper interaction of the barbell and body in the extension. For these reasons, teaching the snatch first is generally recommended—once a new lifter is reasonably comfortable with the snatch, the learning time for the clean and the jerk will be greatly reduced.

For the initial learning progression for the snatch, athletes can use a length of PVC pipe or wooden dowel as a substitute for a barbell. A 5-foot length of ¾" pipe or dowel will be of similar diameter to a bar, but will be light enough for any athlete to manage for large volumes of training drills, and for certain drills that will be difficult if not impossible for some athletes even with an empty 15 or 20kg barbell. The inexpensiveness of PVC also allows the teaching of many athletes simultaneously.

Even for strong athletes, some of the following drills will be impossible to perform correctly with a regulation barbell. A 5-10 kg technique barbell can be used with these athletes if one is available. Otherwise, PVC is the best starting point for these learning drills. Bear in mind that in the descriptions of these drills that follow, the "bar" refers to whichever implement is being used at that time by the athlete.

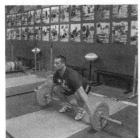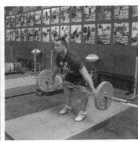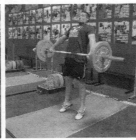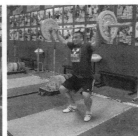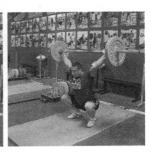

FIGURE 12.1 The snatch is the first of the two lifts contested in Olympic weightlifting in which the barbell is lifted from the floor to overhead in a single movement.

The Receiving Position

The overhead position in the snatch is critical for successful lifting, as it will be in the jerk. In preparation for receiving and supporting heavy loads, the athlete needs to establish a position with maximal structural integrity and develop consistency in achieving it.

Progression Overview

- Grip Placement
- Overhead Position
- Overhead Squat
- Pressing Snatch Balance
- Drop Snatch
- Heaving Snatch Balance
- Snatch Balance

This method will account for not only arm length and shoulder width, but also their relation to the proportions of the trunk and legs. The position of the bar relative to the hips is the priority—not how the grip width relates to the length of the arms or width of the shoulders directly. Other methods that rely on measurements of the upper body only—for example, the distance from elbow to elbow with the upper arms held horizontally to the lifter's sides—neglect the length of the torso and may place the bar too high or low relative to the hips.

This grip width will serve as a solid starting point from which small adjustments can be made later to accommodate each athlete's strengths, weaknesses, personal preference. Athletes with unusual propor-

Grip Placement

The wide hand placement for the snatch serves to reduce the distance the barbell must travel in its path from the platform to over the lifter's head. There are numerous ways to determine starting grip width for the snatch, ranging from simple to surprisingly complicated.

The ideal point of contact for the barbell with the body in the snatch is at the crease of the hips; consequently, the optimal grip width is that which places the bar in the crease of the hips in an extended body position. To quickly determine this hand placement, the athlete will stand upright and hold a bar with the hook grip at arms' length. From this position, the width of the hand position should be adjusted until the bar rests in the crease of the hips. The bar should contact the body just above the pubic bone to avoid painful collisions during the final extension.

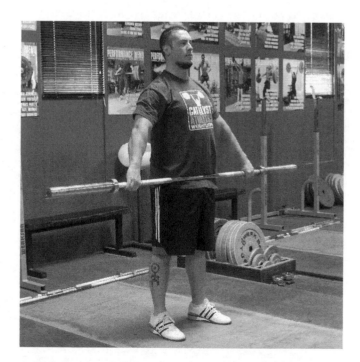

FIGURE 13.1 The placement of the bar in the crease of the hips. The bar should contact the body just above the pubic bone to avoid pain during the extension.

tions will find that this method can place them at a width far too wide or narrow. For example, athletes with unusually long legs and short torsos will find this method places their hands too wide because the bar has too little clearance overhead, the grip at that angle is insecure, the overhead position is painful for the hands and wrists, or the overhead position is simply too unstable due to the extreme angle of the arms.

Each end of the grip width spectrum is accompanied by its own benefits and drawbacks. Wider grips will reduce the distance the bar must travel, reduce the demands on shoulder mobility overhead, keep the center of mass somewhat lower when the bar is overhead and therefore improve stability slightly, and tend to increase the proximity of the bar and body and the speed during the third pull, but will make the starting position more difficult by reducing the knee and hip angles, generally place greater strain on the wrists and hands in the overhead position because of the extreme angle in which they're placed under the bar, make gripping the bar during the pull more difficult, reduce the structural integrity of the elbows and shoulders in the overhead position, and increase the likelihood of the lifter missing snatches behind.

Narrower grips will allow a stronger and more comfortable starting position and first pull, improve grip integrity and typically reduce wrist strain, and allow better structural integrity overhead, but will increase the time of the turnover and the distance the bar must travel, make the overhead position more demanding of mobility, increase the difficulty of maintaining the proximity of the bar to the body during the third pull, and can create problems in the second pull in terms of speed, balance and accuracy due to the bar contacting the body too low.

As the lifter progresses and his or her joints become better conditioned to the demands of training, variations in hand placement can be experimented with until a width that best suits each lifter is found. For example, if a lifter has great grip strength, the more difficult grip of a wider hand placement is not an issue, and this wider grip may improve the snatch with a quicker turnover and better point of bar contact with the body. On the other hand, a lifter with smaller hands whose grip integrity is consequently the weak point may not even have the choice to widen the grip.

Once a lifter has determined his or her ideal grip and has progressed to a barbell, it's important he or she note the hand placement relative to landmarks on the bar—either the breaks in the knurling or the insides of the sleeve flanges—in order to ensure consistent hand placement each time the bar is grasped. If the athlete and coach don't know where the grip is on each lift, the process of evaluating movement technique takes on an unnecessary element of speculation.

The Overhead Position

To quickly establish the correct overhead position, the athlete will hold the bar with a snatch-width hand placement with no hook grip on the bar and place it across the shoulders behind the neck as he or she would for a back squat. The shoulder blades should be squeezed together along their upper inside edges to create retraction and upward rotation. There should be no active elevation of the shoulder blades (shrugging), although there may be the appearance of shrugging in this position and a small degree of scapular elevation.

This bar placement should naturally cause the torso to lean forward very slightly and position the bar over the feet as it needs to be in order for the athlete to remain balanced with the addition of weight. From this position, the athlete will press the bar straight up with no change to the torso or shoulder blade positions. The bar should finish directly above the base of the neck.

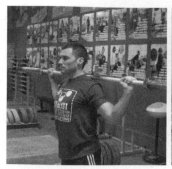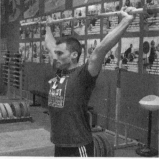

FIGURE 13.2 To find the correct overhead position easily, begin with the bar behind the neck and the upper inside edges of the shoulder blades squeezed together tightly. Press the bar straight up and maintain the same torso inclination and shoulder blade position.

The bony points of the elbows should be oriented approximately halfway between down and back (neutral internal-external rotation of the upper arm), the wrists and hands should be somewhat relaxed with the bar in the palm just behind the midline of the forearm, the grip no tighter than what is necessary to maintain control and position, and the arms oriented approximately vertically when viewed from the lifter's side.

The Overhead Structure

The overhead position is extremely active and a reduction in the effort to maintain it will result in sudden and unpredictable bar movement, which is magnified quickly with relatively minor movement of the lifter, often past the point of the lifter's ability to maintain control of the bar. Not only does this create the possibility for a failed lift, but for injury to the shoulders, elbows and wrists.

A solid overhead structure requires first a solid base, which must be established with the position of the shoulder blades. The shoulder is an extremely mobile joint by design, so the active creation of stability through proper positioning is necessary to establish a foundation capable of supporting the load overhead. This foundation is best achieved by forceful retraction and upward rotation of the scapulae—anchoring the arms securely to the body and preventing potentially injurious shifts in shoulder position. Essentially the athlete is securing the shoulder blades tightly to the ribcage for stability and orienting them

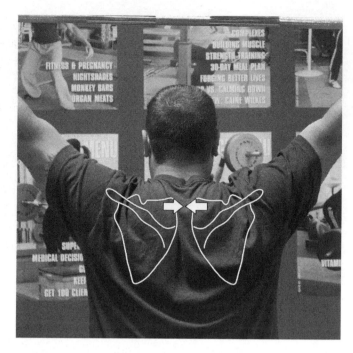

FIGURE 13.3 The ideal shoulder blade orientation for the overhead position is complete retraction with upward rotation. This can be achieved by squeezing the upper inside edges of the shoulder blades together.

in a way that allows the arms to achieve the necessary position to hold the bar. This action should not be confused with scapular elevation—upward shrugging of the shoulders—which will reduce stability.

In order to achieve this position of the scapulae and maintain the bar positioning over the feet, the head must be pushed forward through the arms and the torso inclined forward slightly. Attempts to maintain a completely vertical torso and head will prevent the scapulae from being able to reach proper retraction due to the demands of bar positioning over the feet and in the arms.

The arms will be oriented approximately vertically when viewed from the lifter's side, placing the bar over the top of the shoulder blades. Because the hands and bar are sitting behind the forearm slightly, the arms will be slightly in front of the vertical line passing through the barbell's center and the top of the shoulder blades or the base of the neck.

The arms in the overhead position are acting as static support columns. As such, their rigidity is imperative. A fully extended elbow in the correct orientation will create a remarkably solid structure able to withstand extremely great compressive forces. Attempting to support a similarly heavy load with even slightly flexed elbows will prove markedly more difficult and, with the exception of pre-approved anatomical issues preventing full elbow extension, any elbow flexion during the receipt and support of the snatch will prevent the lift from passing in competition, a rule that should be observed equally in training for the sake of maintaining consistent standards and accurate measurement of progress.

Some lifters will be fortunate enough to possess the particular anatomical structure to allow slight elbow hyperextension. This hyperextension allows a very secure overhead position because of the ability to rely on skeletal structure for much of the support. Without this, more muscular effort is required to maintain elbow extension.

In the overhead position, the bony points of the elbows should be directed approximately halfway between backward and down. In other words, this will be about the mid-point between full internal (elbow back) and external (elbow down) rotation of the upper arm. Some degree of variation is allowable here to account for individual anatomical peculiarities—the athlete should place the elbows in this initial neutral position and then adjust slightly into the position that feels most comfortable without a dramatic divergence.

This position will provide the greatest structural stability for two basic reasons. First, this elbow orientation encourages and allows correct positioning of the shoulder blades and opens the shoulder joint adequately to bring the arms overhead; second, if the elbows are oriented directly downward, the force of the weight must be resisted almost entirely by muscular strength—with the elbows turned back halfway, the elbows' articulation is no longer aligned with the downward force and the rigid structure of the skeleton can assist in supporting the load to a greater extent (this effect is not as dramatic for lifters whose elbows hyperextend, as this hyperextension will make it easier to keep the elbow extended in any orientation).

Elbow orientation can be manipulated during the recovery of a lift to save a barbell that has failed to come to rest precisely in the desired position. This manipulation will be minor and effect only minor change—it will not overcome the imbalance of a significantly misplaced barbell. This kind of repositioning will generally happen naturally during an effort to save a lift.

The grip on the bar will affect both the position of the hand and wrist in the overhead position, as well as the speed of the elbow lockout and degree of elbow extension at the end of the turnover. The hands overhead should be as relaxed as possible while maintaining control of the bar, cradling the bar rather than gripping it tightly, with the wrist allowed to extend back and the heel of the palm driven up aggressively. The bar should be in the palm, slightly behind the center of the forearm, with the fingers wrapped around it completely.

It's important to understand that the bar is in the palm, not farther up toward the joints of the fingers

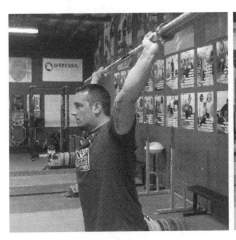

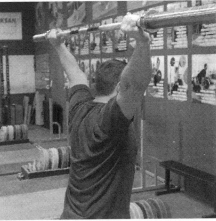

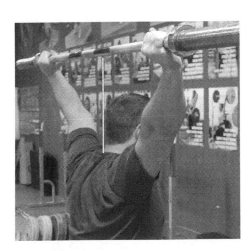

FIGURE 13.4 In the overhead position, the bony points of the elbows should be directed approximately halfway between down and back.

FIGURE 13.5 In the overhead position, the barbell should be over the base of the neck.

to the hand. Holding the bar this far back will place excessive strain on the wrists and limit how forcefully the elbow can be extended against the load, usually resulting in a soft and unstable overhead position.

The proper placement of the bar in the hand and the position of the hand and wrist results in a consistent slight tendency for the bar to move backward (or extend the wrist), making its stabilization simple; with the wrist and hand in a neutral position (hand in line with the forearm) and the barbell centered over the wrist, it becomes more difficult to stabilize the bar due to its tendency to shift both forward and backward equally—the attempt of lifters to maintain a neutral wrist overhead nearly always produces visible instability at the hands and wrists, which often travels dramatically into the overhead position as a whole. A neutral wrist position is also virtually impossible to maintain with significant weight.

An excessively tight grip overhead will prevent the bar from settling down into the hand as it should, with the hand and wrist somewhat relaxed and extended. Instead, the bar will be slightly more forward than can be supported well (the wrist closer to neutral), which places an additional burden on the

shoulders and elbows, and often is forward enough to shift the athlete's balance to a degree that disrupts the receipt and recovery of the snatch, or causes a failed lift. A single inch, as weights increase, is often more than enough to prevent success.

In addition to problems with positioning, a tight grip overhead will limit somewhat the degree of extension of the elbow and also the speed at which the lifter can achieve that extension when finalizing the turnover. Activation of the flexor muscles of the wrist and hand encourages activation of the flexor muscles of the elbow, which inhibits activation of the extensor muscles of the elbow. While a tight grip on the bar may improve pressing strength in slow, grinding movements like the bench press, this has essentially no relevance to the snatch turnover (or jerk lockout). This phenomenon is typically quite noticeable by an athlete if instructed to compare his or her overhead elbow extension with a tight grip versus a loose hand, and to compare the possible speed of elbow extension with a loose grip and tight grip using a simple movement like a snatch push press with an empty bar.

The issue of hand and wrist position and grip ten-

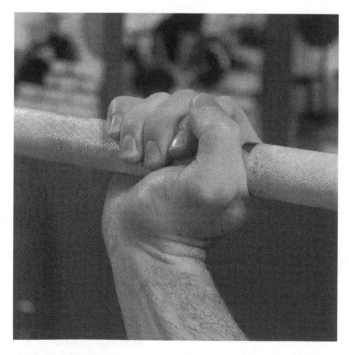

FIGURE 13.6 Correct snatch grip. The grip should be only as tight as needed to maintain control of the bar, and the hand acting as a cradle, with the bar in the palm slightly behind the midline of the forearm.

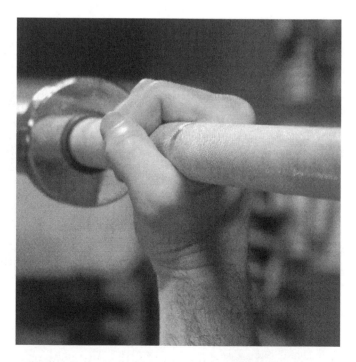

FIGURE 13.7 An excessively tight grip on the bar will prevent the proper hand and wrist position.

Greg Everett

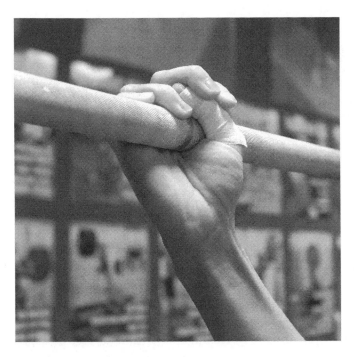

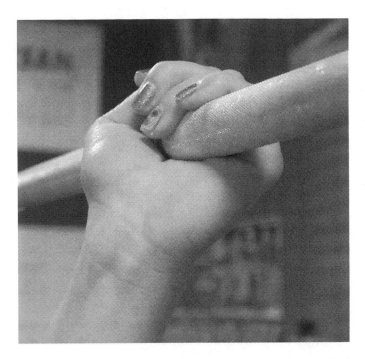

FIGURE 13.8 A neutral wrist position creates instability overhead because of the bar's equal tendency to move backward and forward, and places additional strain on the joints.

FIGURE 13.9 An example of a lifter who is capable of achieving the proper hand and wrist position overhead while maintaining the hook grip.

sion leads obviously to the question of whether or not a lifter should maintain the hook grip throughout the snatch and into the overhead position. The answer depends primarily on whether or not a given athlete is able to achieve the correct hand and wrist position, optimal grip tension and maximal elbow extension force and speed with the hook grip. If an athlete can, there is no reason to complicate the lift by forcing a release of the hook grip. This ability will be more common among female lifters, who tend to have more slender hands and better mobility, and who use barbells of a smaller diameter, and consequently are more likely to be capable of achieving the proper overhead position with the hook grip. Men, with typically thicker hands, less mobility and larger diameter barbells, are less likely to be capable of this. Generalities notwithstanding, the issue will need to be evaluated for each athlete individually.

The maintenance of the hook grip throughout the turnover of the snatch is ideal, in part because of its simplicity, but primarily because it makes it easier and more likely for the lifter to maintain a tight, uninterrupted connection to the barbell throughout the lift. However, these benefits do not outweigh the drawbacks of a problematic overhead position—it

does very little good to be capable of getting a bar overhead if it can't then be kept there. Learning to release the hook grip properly during the turnover of the snatch is an important skill to develop, and is recommended for all new athletes; it's very easy later on to keep the hook grip if it's determined to be acceptable, but learning to release it after having trained maintaining it for a significant period of time will prove very difficult. The mechanics of properly releasing the hook grip in the turnover will be described in detail in later chapters of the book.

For athletes who do choose to maintain the hook grip overhead, it's important to perform snatch assistance exercises accordingly, also using the hook grip with all snatch overhead work such as the overhead squat, snatch push press and snatch balance.

Horizontal & Vertical Action

The overhead position of the bar will often be thought of by newer lifters as the end of a rotation of the arms into place; that is, it appears in the snatch that the bar swings around the lifter and moves back into position at the end of this swinging motion.

In some cases, this actually does occur due to poor execution of the lift by inexperienced lifters. This concept can be further reinforced early on in lifters with poor flexibility as well, as they will naturally find themselves trying to "pull" the bar back into position against the resistance of tight joints.

The final phase of the third pull is actually a vertically oriented push up against the bar (this action pushes the lifter down under the bar more than it pushes the barbell up). Attempting to swing the bar back into place overhead will usually result in it continuing far past the correct position and being missed behind, or cause a compensatory dive forward of the chest and head, preventing the establishment of the proper structure needed to support the weight.

This being the case, it's important from the earliest stages of learning to encourage lifters to actively and aggressively push straight up against the bar in the overhead position and to make sure they conceptually associate the position with vertical action. This will also contribute to naturally better execution of the entire turnover phase of the lift by encouraging the lifter to minimize horizontal movement of the bar and body and focus on maintaining proximity of the bar to the body in order to feed into this proper overhead position.

The Overhead Squat

The overhead squat (Figure 13.10) is the position in which the lifter will receive the bar in the snatch. Until this position is both solid and consistent, the lifter will not be able to progress substantially with the lift. This is cause, during the earliest stages of an athlete's development, for a great deal of emphasis on establishing the mobility for and consistency in this position.

All of the position requirements described previously for the squat must be met in the overhead squat. Foot positioning should result in the thigh being approximately parallel with the foot when viewed from above and the knee approximately above the toes when viewed from the front of the foot. The hips should be pushed in over the heels as much as possible and the torso nearly vertical. Recall that the correct overhead position demands slight forward torso lean; violation of this will be impossible for the majority of athletes anyway due to its demands on mobility, but those who do possess this level of mobility need to ensure the proper inclination for ideal overhead structure.

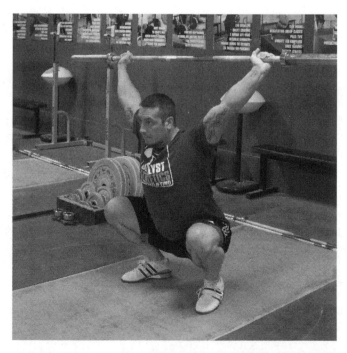

FIGURE 13.10 The overhead squat meets all the position criteria for the squat and the overhead position.

Greg Everett

It's rare for a new lifter to be capable immediately of a perfect overhead squat, although it's more common among female athletes due to their typically greater natural mobility. Mobility limitations should be immediately and actively addressed to ensure the athlete's progress is not delayed unnecessarily. Specific weightlifting mobility training is discussed in detail in its own section of the book.

The athlete's present mobility will determine the details of his or her lifting progression. The coach will need to adjust instruction accordingly. Typically the initial learning progressions can and should be attempted irrespective of mobility—the light or absent loading prevents any real injury risk, and attempting to achieve the various positions is itself excellent mobility training. The coach and athlete should remain vigilant, however, and avoid forcing any positions that may lead to injury in the extraordinarily immobile. In such cases, the power variations of the lifts may have to be used exclusively during the early stages of training.

Posture in the Overhead Squat & Snatch Recovery

There is a small range of possible arm and torso orientations during the overhead squat or recovery of the snatch that will allow control of the barbell to be maintained. The combined mass of the barbell and athlete must remain approximately centered over the foot in order for the system to remain balanced. Because any forward shift of body mass (within a reasonable limit) tends to be naturally accompanied by a countermovement, the body itself will generally remain balanced over the feet even through unintended postural changes. For example, if the torso leans forward, the hips will shift back, because people by nature prefer not to fall on their faces, and the body will react accordingly.

However, there is a limit to what compensation can account for. The farther forward the torso inclines, the greater the disruption of the structural integrity of the system due to the greater divergence from an essentially vertical stack of structural components between the barbell and the floor. In other words, the lifter's posture must remain as upright as possible throughout the movement to maximize strength and stability.

The hips will unavoidably move backward during the course of the recovery from the snatch, like they will during the overhead squat, reaching the farthest point back as the athlete's thighs reach horizontal. This backward movement needs to be minimized, just as it does during all squatting in weightlifting, to maintain an upright posture. As the hips move backward, the chest must lean forward in reaction to maintain balance; the farther back the hips move, the farther forward the chest leans. A small lean during

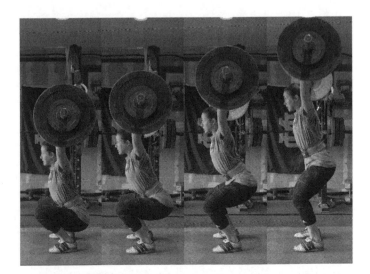

FIGURE 13.11 The bar and body system must remain balanced over the foot, and the posture kept as upright as possible, throughout the overhead squat or snatch recovery. The lifter can think of pushing up on the barbell and following it with his or her body.

the course of recovery is not a problem; an excessive forward lean due to uncontrolled squat or improper squat mechanics is a serious problem.

In the overhead squat or snatch recovery, maintaining this upright posture and bar position is often helped if the athlete focuses on leading with the bar during the recovery—that is, pushing up on the bar and following it with the body. If the bar is not the focus of attention, more often the lifter will lead with the hips in the squat recovery, shifting the trunk forward and diverging from the optimal overhead structure.

Pressing Snatch Balance

With the overhead squat positioning established, layers of complexity and speed can be introduced. The series of snatch balance exercises adds dynamic entry into the position with increasing complexity and speed in order to better prepare the athlete to receive the snatch successfully. In all of the following exercises, it's recommended that the athlete sit in the bottom position for three seconds before recovering to train stability and mobility. When used later as training exercises, this pause in the bottom can be removed and reintroduced to bolster receiving position strength, stability and confidence when athletes demonstrate the need.

The first exercise of the snatch balance series is the pressing snatch balance (Figure 13.12). This step serves simply to introduce the athlete to the basic

movement pattern, positioning and timing, and acts as well as an active stretching drill, which can be useful in later stages of training.

The lifter will begin with the feet in the receiving position and the bar racked across the back with a snatch-width grip in the same manner that was used to establish the overhead position earlier—that is, the shoulder blades should already be locked tightly into the correct position with the upper inside edges squeezed together—and the hands should be relaxed with the wrists allowed to settle back with the bar in

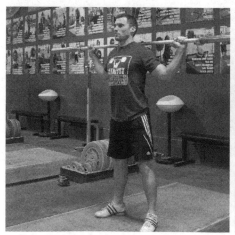
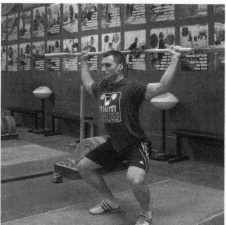
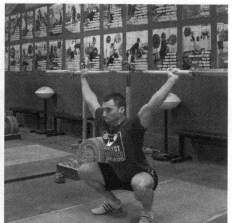

FIGURE 13.12 Pressing snatch balance

Greg Everett

the palm over the forearm. As discussed previously, the hook grip should only be used here if the athlete will be maintaining it in the snatch—new lifters for whom this is not yet determined should not use it at this stage. All the athlete needs to do now to achieve the correct overhead position is press the arms into the locked out position with the elbows properly oriented.

At a deliberate speed, the athlete will press him- or herself down under the bar without elevating it until reaching the bottom position of an overhead squat. The path of the bar is nearly non-existent—because it starts in the correct plane over the foot, and because the athlete is pressing him- or herself down without elevating the bar, it should travel only slightly downward, and in a straight vertical line when viewed from the lifter's side.

Once settled tightly into the bottom of the squat, the athlete will recover to the standing position while keeping the bar locked tightly overhead. Once standing again, the bar can be returned to the back for the next rep.

Drop Snatch

The drop snatch (Figure 13.13) introduces the elements of speed and the transition of the feet, and will become a valuable training exercise later for many lifters. The starting position will be identical to that of the pressing snatch balance with the exception of the feet, which will now be in the pulling position;

the bar is still racked on the back with a snatch-width grip and the shoulder blades already tightened into the correct position.

The name drop snatch is somewhat misleading—the athlete must actively push under the bar rather than simply dropping. After taking in a stabilizing breath, the athlete will settle with proper balance over the feet, then initiate the exercise by beginning to transition the feet from the pulling position to the receiving position. As the feet begin moving, the

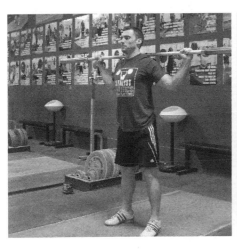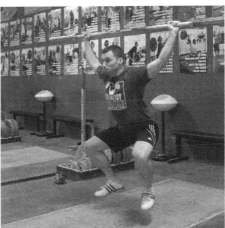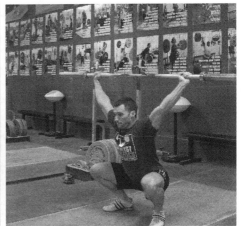

FIGURE 13.13 Drop snatch

athlete will aggressively punch under with the arms, driving him- or herself into a squat with the barbell locked out in the proper overhead position. The goal is to allow the bar to rise as little as possible, and instead to push the body underneath it. The feet must reconnect flat with the platform—the athlete should not land on the balls of the feet.

The athlete should attempt to achieve a locked-out overhead position at least slightly above the bottom of the squat and then continue to sit into the bottommost position in one continuous motion, stabilizing and holding this position for three seconds before standing again with the bar overhead.

The speed of the movement will be improved by the athlete attempting to achieve the overhead lock-out position at the same time the feet reconnect with the floor. This timing will be used in the snatch as well; beginning to focus on this early in the new lifter's training will improve results later.

Once settled tightly into the bottom of the squat, the athlete will recover to the standing position while keeping the bar locked tightly overhead. Once standing again, the bar can be returned to the back for the next rep.

Heaving Snatch Balance

The heaving snatch balance (Figure 13.14) is essentially an intermediate step between the drop snatch and the next exercise, the snatch balance. While it may not be strictly necessary in many cases when teaching new lifters, it will become a valuable training and remedial exercise later, making it useful to learn at this stage.

In this exercise, a dip and drive with the legs is

introduced to momentarily unload the bar and create an opportunity for the athlete to push down farther underneath it. This dip and drive is relatively small in magnitude—the goal is not to drive the bar up significantly, but to create a brief window of near-weightlessness.

Beginning with the bar on the back, the shoulder blades set in position and the feet in the receiving position, the athlete will bend at the knees smoothly, making sure the bar stays connected to the body and the trunk remains as upright as possible, then push against the ground with the legs to lift the bar very

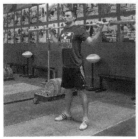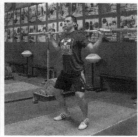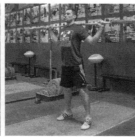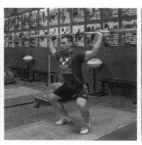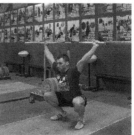

FIGURE 13.14 Heaving snatch balance

slightly. As the bar begins moving upward, the athlete will release the pressure against the floor with the legs and punch aggressively against the bar to move down into the bottom of an overhead squat as quickly as possible with as little elevation of the bar as possible.

The feet should remain flat on the floor throughout this movement. If the heels lift during the leg drive, that drive is too powerful. A relatively slow dip and drive will produce the best results, minimizing the upward movement of the bar and allowing the lifter to focus more on pushing down under the bar quickly and aggressively.

Once settled tightly into the bottom of the squat for three seconds, the athlete will recover to the standing position while keeping the bar locked tightly overhead. Once standing again, the bar can be returned to the back for the next rep.

Snatch Balance

The series is completed with the snatch balance (Figure 13.15), which combines elements of the preceding exercises. This will be the most commonly used snatch balance variation in training.

The athlete will start with the feet in the pulling position, dip at the knees while maintaining an upright trunk, push with the legs up against the bar just enough to unweight it momentarily, then lift and transition the feet to the receiving position, landing flat, while punching down under the bar into the overhead squat. Again, the athlete should lock the bar out into the overhead position at the same time the feet reconnect with the floor to ensure maximal speed and aggressiveness.

Like with all variations of the snatch balance, the

10 Progression Summary
Snatch Balance

Start with the feet in the pulling position and the bar behind the neck.

Hold the bar with a snatch grip and squeeze the upper inside edges of the shoulder blades together.

Pressurize and stabilize the trunk.

Bend at the knees smoothly and drive with the legs up against the bar enough to unweight it without elevating it significantly.

As the bar moves up, lift and transition your feet into the receiving position, landing flat.

As the feet move, punch against the bar to push yourself down into a squat, trying to lock the bar out overhead at the same time the feet reconnect with the floor.

Recover to the standing position with the bar locked tightly overhead.

goal is to elevate the bar as little as possible and move down under it as far and as quickly as possible, establishing security and balance in the receiving position immediately.

The snatch balance needs to be performed with maximal speed and aggression for success once heavier weights are introduced. As with all parts of the learning progression, establish position and proper movement first and foremost, and then increase the speed according to the athlete's present ability.

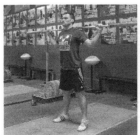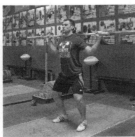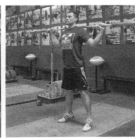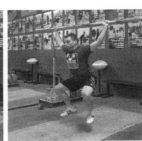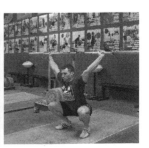

FIGURE 13.15 Snatch balance

Learning the Snatch

With the receiving position established, the athlete can learn the movement that will deliver the barbell there. This will be accomplished by breaking the whole movement into a series of brief sections to isolate elements of the lift. It's far easier and more productive to drill these elements individually than to simply attempt to teach the movement in its entirety—such drills allow the body to learn the constituent movements with less interference from the brain. The more the athlete can ingrain the positions and movements into the body without involving the conscious brain, the more quickly and easily the body will be capable of executing the entire movement accurately. These sections are eventually assembled to produce the entire movement, which will be performed remarkably well simply through the body's retention of the drills and positions with which it has been constructed.

Progression Overview

- Mid-Hang Position
- Mid-Hang Snatch Jump
- Mid-Hang Snatch Pull
- Tall Muscle Snatch
- Scarecrow Snatch
- Tall Snatch
- Mid-Hang Snatch

The Mid-Hang Position

The first step is establishing the mid-hang position (Figure 14.1), in which the bar is positioned at approximately the level of mid-thigh. This is the position from which the athlete will first learn to snatch

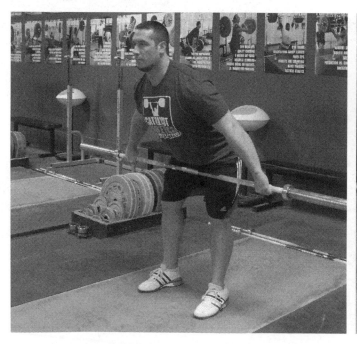
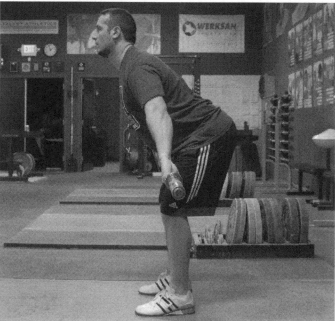

FIGURE 14.1 The mid-hang position is a critical position for the snatch and will be the initial starting position for the snatch in the first part of the progression.

Greg Everett

before learning the pull from the floor. The importance of the mid-hang position cannot be overstated—it is the position he or she will be in immediately prior to the initiation of the final explosion of the hips and knees. The precision and consistency of this position will have enormous influence on the successfulness of the lifter's snatches. Learning and ingraining it at the earliest stages of training will maximize the lifter's progress.

The mid-hang position begins familiarizing the athlete with the proper positioning and timing for the all-important second pull, and allows the double knee bend to occur naturally as it should with no specific instruction (other than perhaps the demonstration described in the Double Knee Bend section), creates the opportunity to learn the feeling of aggressive leg and hip extension to maximally accelerate and elevate the barbell, and builds confidence that adequate acceleration and elevation can be achieved from such a high position, laying the foundation for proper lift rhythm and timing from the floor.

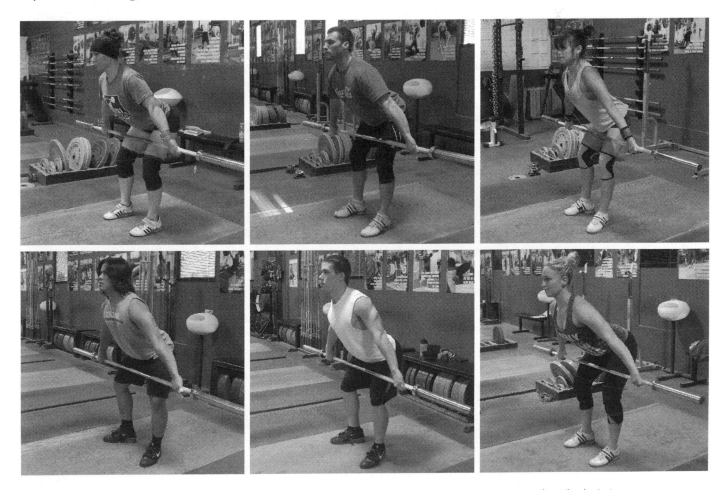

FIGURE 14.2 The mid-hang position will appear somewhat different among athletes based on their builds even when conforming to the outlined criteria.

With a snatch-width hand placement and the hook grip on the bar, the athlete will stand with the feet in the pulling position. The wrists should be neutral and the arms internally rotated to orient the bony points of the elbows out to the sides. This rotation of the arms does not involve any scapular protraction—the athlete's shoulders should not round forward. The shoulder blades should be held in a neutral position in terms of protraction-retraction and the rotation of the elbows achieved only with internal rotation of the arms.

The athlete will set a continuous arch in the back with the trunk pressurized and tight, hinge at the hips and bend the knees slightly, and, using the lats and shoulders to keep the bar in light contact with the legs, slide the bar down to the level of mid-thigh. The athlete should arrive in a position in which the shins are approximately vertical and the shoulders are slightly forward of both the bar and the knees.

The athlete's weight should be balanced over the front edge of the heel—slightly behind the middle of the foot—and the hamstrings, glutes and back under obvious tension. If the hamstrings and glutes are not tight, the knees are either too far forward or bent too much. The knees should be pushed out to the sides slightly rather than directed straight forward.

The arms should be passively extended—that is, the elbows remaining straight without being actively straightened. The shoulder blades will be depressed in this position by the contraction of the lats, which both aids in the extension of the upper back and the push of the bar back toward the body. The athlete's head should be up and the eyes focused on a point straight ahead or slightly higher.

The actual angle of the back and how far forward of the bar the shoulders are positioned will vary among athletes depending on their proportions. The key points are approximately vertical shins, slight knee bend, and the shoulders slightly ahead of the bar and knees.

Athletes will commonly want to move the bar farther down the thighs than they should, and over the course of a series of drills starting from the mid-hang position, the bar height will usually creep incrementally lower toward the knees. It's important in this early stage to establish and reinforce the correct position by preventing this divergence. The athlete will be able to achieve a far more explosive finish and

transition under the bar more quickly and accurately if he or she has the discipline (and the knowledge) to achieve this position in the snatch from the floor. Learning and practicing it at this point is far easier than attempting to correct problems related to this position later.

Mid-Hang Snatch Jump

The mid-hang snatch jump (Figure 14.3) provides an opportunity for the athlete to feel a violent, concerted explosion of the hips and knees from the proper position while controlling the bar's proximity to the body. The presence of this drill should not be misinterpreted to mean that the athlete should jump in the air when snatching, as has been discussed in previous chapters. Too often athletes fixate on either hip or knee extension and neglect the other; this drill helps establish the feeling of both contributing simultane-

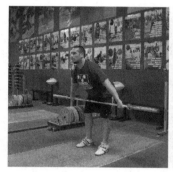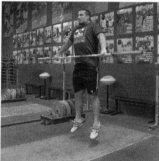

FIGURE 14.3 The mid-hang snatch jump is a simple drill to introduce the feeling of aggressive, vertically-oriented knee and hip extension.

12 Progression Summary
Mid-Hang Snatch Jump

Start in the mid-hang position with the weight properly balance over the front edge of the heel.

With no countermovement, jump vertically as high as possible.

Keep the bar in light contact with the body throughout the movement.

ously to the explosion effort, and also teaches the feeling of timing the explosion high on the legs. This movement will not look exactly like the finish of a snatch; the point is not to mimic the lift perfectly, but to create an extremely quick, sharp extension of the hips and knees together that imparts force to the bar in a vertical direction.

Starting in the mid-hang position, the athlete will simply jump vertically as high as possible while actively pushing the bar back with the lats and shoulders to maintain light contact with the body throughout the movement, preventing it from moving away from the body at any point. There should be no countermovement to begin the jump—it must be performed directly from the static mid-thigh position.

Prior to each jump, the athlete should be sure to have his or her weight balanced over the front edge of the heel, and to prevent a last-moment shift of balance to the balls of the feet before initiating the jump. It's equally important for the bar to start at the correct height on the thigh—this jumping motion must be extremely brief and violent like the second pull will be in the snatch.

Athletes will often perform what they believe the coach is looking for and attempt to execute a snatch pull rather than a vertical jump, which typically means excessive hip extension through the bar, soft knees, and a weak forward jump. It needs to be made clear that the intent at this time is literally a vertical jump—no need for interpretations—just an aggressive vertical drive against the floor with the bar kept against the body. The movement will be refined in the next drill and continue increasing in precision throughout the learning process.

the precision and speed of the transition and third pull. It can be difficult for athletes initially to feel the movement and perform it properly with the weightlessness of a PVC bar; if needed, an empty barbell can be used in this stage to provide some feedback, and the PVC returned to for the following drills.

Essentially, the athlete will perform the mid-hang snatch jump drill while keeping the balls of the feet connected to the floor at the top of the extension. The intent is still aggressive leg drive against the floor that continues into complete knee extension and the force of which naturally causes the athlete to rise onto the balls of the feet.

The hips should be slightly hyperextended at the peak of the pull, positioning the shoulders slightly behind the hips. The glutes must be activated to finalize the extension of the hips, or this hyperextension will naturally originate in the lower back rather than at the hip joint. The final extended position will have the lifter on the balls of the feet, the legs vertical when viewed from the side, and the shoulders slightly behind the hips.

The feet should remain in the same position on the floor from start to finish—if the athlete is sliding forward, he or she has the weight balanced too far forward over the feet during the pull and is ceasing to push against the floor with the legs prematurely; if the athlete is sliding backward, he or she has the weight balanced too far back over the feet—and is likely extending the hips and/or leaning back excessively at the top of the pull—and is also releasing the pressure against the ground prematurely by not continuing to push with the legs until the final extended position is achieved. Additionally, although the goal

Mid-Hang Snatch Pull

The mid-hang snatch pull (Figure 14.4) brings together the aggressive concerted hip and knee extension of the mid-hang snatch jump and the precision necessary to channel it into what will become the second pull of the snatch. The importance of learning and practicing this section correctly cannot be overstated. This movement—the second pull of the lift in isolation—is responsible for the most critical acceleration of the barbell, and will directly influence

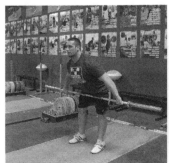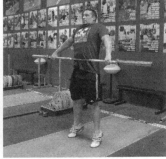

FIGURE 14.4 The mid-hang snatch pull refines the mid-hang snatch jump into a more precisely channeled extension of the body to accelerate and elevate the barbell;

is to mimic the leg drive of the vertical jump from the previous drill, the magnitude of the force needs to be controlled to prevent the athlete from actually leaving the floor. It's helpful for some athletes struggling with this to imagine the movement as stretching the body out.

During the extension, the bar should remain in immediate proximity to the thighs and then come into full contact at the hips. This proximity is created and maintained through the activation of the lats and shoulders, which push the bar back toward the body even when the shoulders are in front of the bar. Once in contact with the hips, the bar should remain in contact with the body for the remainder of the movement, never allowed to swing forward away from the body.

The arms should remain loose and passively extended during this extension—the elbows should remain straight not because the athlete is actively extending them, but because the athlete is *not* bending them. The distinction between these two actions is important—stiff elbows will both slow the transition between the second and third pull and force the bar to swing forward at the peak of the extension.

As the lifter reaches complete knee and hip extension, the shoulders should be shrugged up without being allowed to round forward. This shrugging motion plays a very simple role in the movement—it gives the bar somewhere to go other than forward away from the body. With the knee and hip extension, the athlete has given the bar upward momentum. That momentum will continue the bar's tendency to rise past the point of body extension. If the shoulders are not shrugged at this point, the bar will simply want to swing forward away from the body.

It should be understood at this point that the purpose is not to lift the bar with this shrugging motion directly; that is, the shrug is not part of the lifter's primary effort to upwardly accelerate and elevate the bar. It is a mistake to consider the shrug part of the primary lifting action, but an equally problematic mistake to attempt to prevent any shrugging motion in the lift or to eliminate it from this drill.

The shrug is primarily a part of the athlete's effort to move down under the bar following the upward extension—that is, the majority of the movement should be occurring during the third pull as the athlete's body is moving downward. However, the shrug

will span both the end of the second pull and beginning of the third pull—it is transitional and consequently needs to be present in the segments of the lift on either side of the peak of extension. The key is simply avoiding an effort to actively shrug the barbell up significantly as part of the effort to further elevate it and instead focus on knee and hip extension for the upward acceleration and elevation.

The mid-hang snatch pull can be performed as slowly as necessary initially for the athlete to master the motion. Again, the importance of correct positioning and movement here eclipses speed. Once the fundamental positioning and movement is established, speed can be increased as tolerated until the athlete is able to perform the movement at full speed.

Irrespective of the speed of any given rep at this stage, the athlete should not hold the extended position for any longer than is necessary to ensure it has been reached completely and properly. While it's important to ensure the athlete is learning to achieve this complete extension of the body, he or she also needs to avoid prolonging the extension or hesitating in the extended position during the snatch.

The final explosion at the top and the transition under the bar (the second and third pulls) should ul-

> **13** Progression Summary
> # Mid-Hang Snatch Pull
>
> Start in the mid-hang position with the bar hook-gripped at snatch-width.
>
> Push against the ground aggressively with the legs, using the lats and shoulders to keep the bar in immediate proximity to the thighs.
>
> Reach the final extended position with the legs vertical and the shoulders slightly behind the hips.
>
> Actively push the bar back into light contact with the hips.
>
> Shrug the shoulders up to allow the bar to continue traveling momentarily without swinging forward.
>
> Do not prolong this extended position.

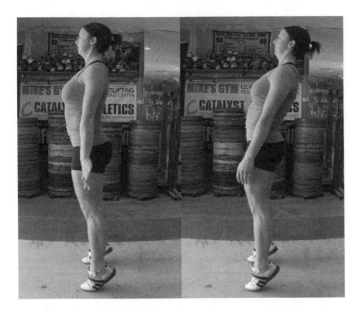

FIGURE 14.5 If lifter prolongs the extended position (left), the athlete's line of gravity will have to shift forward to match the center of pressure (the balls of the feet). If extension is not prolonged, i.e. is performed quickly (right), the athlete can maintain the line of gravity farther behind the center of pressure on the feet to achieve the desired position and balance.

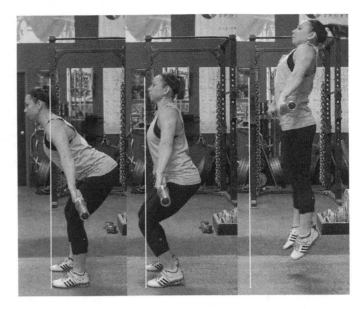

FIGURE 14.6 A mid-hang snatch jump that moves the lifter backward from the starting point is a simple demonstration of the ability to rise onto the balls of the feet without the center of mass and line of gravity shifting forward along with the center of pressure.

timately be considered a single fluid action without any hesitation. Time spent in the extended position after the peak of force application to the bar is merely time the bar has to lose its upward momentum and begin falling, reducing the already limited window the athlete has to relocate under the bar to receive it.

In addition to this, prolonging the extended position will force the lifter's line of gravity to shift forward from the desired position at the front edge of the heel to the balls of the feet to match the center of pressure. In other words, an extension with the proper timing can bring the athlete up onto the balls of the feet with the heels elevated (meaning the center of pressure is also on the balls of the feet) without the center of mass shifting forward—that is, the center of mass and line of gravity can be maintained in the same place while the center of pressure shifts forward. However, if the extension is prolonged, this cannot occur—in a static position, the line of gravity must pass through the center of pressure for the system to remain balanced (Figure 14.15).

It is often confusing to athletes, and even coaches, that the lifter can be on the balls of the feet with the heels elevated yet have the center of mass balanced farther back over the foot. The ability to do this can be easily illustrated by having the athlete perform the mid-hang snatch jump drill but land a few inches behind the starting point (Figure 14.6). This demonstrates the ability of an athlete to extend onto the balls of the foot with the line of gravity behind that point—so far back in this case that the lifter actually travels backward.

At this point, athletes should be expected to naturally extend the ankles as part of the effort to drive aggressively and completely against the ground through the finish of the pull. This drive should be the focus of instruction and practice and ankle extension not discussed directly unless it becomes clear that an athlete is either intentionally extending the ankles or preventing their extension.

Remedial Modification

If an athlete is struggling to correctly perform the vertical leg drive in this drill, a remedial modification can be used to help temporarily before returning to the standard exercise (Figure 14.7). Rather than beginning at the mid-hang position, the lifter will start in a dip position in which only the knees are bent, the

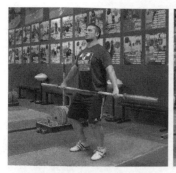
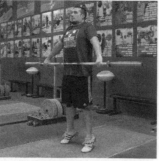

FIGURE 14.7 A remedial variation of the mid-hang snatch pull can be used for athletes struggling to properly perform the vertical leg drive component of the mid-hang snatch pull.

trunk vertical, and the bar in contact in the crease of the hips. From this position, the movement is greatly simplified and it will be easy for the athlete to focus on driving vertically against the ground with the legs. All other criteria for the lift remain the same, such as keeping the bar against the body and finishing with the shoulders slightly behind the hips with the balance still over the front edge of the heel.

Tall Muscle Snatch

The tall muscle snatch (Figure 14.8) introduces the isolated movement of the upper body during the third pull. At this point, the progression has diverged from strict reality by bending the arms to elevate the bar without any downward movement of the athlete.

In an actual snatch, the arms actively bend only to pull the lifter underneath the bar, and consequently, there should be no active elbow flexion without concurrent downward travel of the lifter's body to at least some degree. However, the mechanics of the upper body in the third pull are critical for successful lifting, and therefore isolated introduction and practice is warranted at this stage.

The athlete will begin in the tall position—standing straight up with the bar hanging at arms' length, the weight balanced over the front edge of the heel, and the arms internally rotated to orient the points of the elbows out to the sides. With no movement of the lower body, the athlete will lift the elbows as high as possible, moving them out to the sides and squeezing the shoulder blades back together to keep the bar in immediate proximity to the body. A shrug up of the shoulders will naturally accompany this movement of the arms; maximal elbow height will not be possible without it.

As the elbows reach their maximum height, which will vary somewhat depending on the athlete's build and present mobility, the lifter will turn the arms over to bring the bar overhead, still maintaining proximity of the bar to the body by squeezing the shoulder blades and elbows back as the arms flip over, and punch the bar up into the correct overhead position. During this turnover, the elbows should never drop from their elevated position.

As the hands turn over—that is, move from over to under the bar, the hand and wrist should be relaxed into the proper overhead position with the

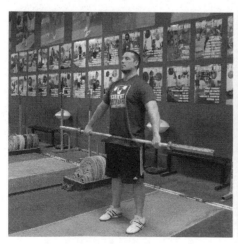
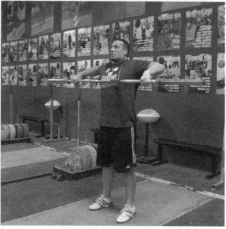
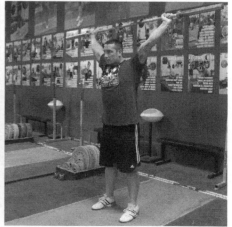

FIGURE 14.8 The tall muscle snatch introduces the upper body mechanics of the third pull.

Greg Everett

wrist and hand settled back and the bar in the palm just slightly behind the midline of the forearm. This is the point at which the lifter will need to release the hook grip. This release must be timed carefully to occur in the brief window as the hand is turning over during which there is neither pressure on the grip from pulling the bar maximally or from pushing up against it; in other words, it needs to occur in the quick transition from pulling to pushing. If the hook is released too early, the lifter has to relax the grip and will lose the necessary tight connection to the bar; if the hook is released too late, the bar will already be pushing down into the hand overhead and prevent the necessary movement of the thumb.

This turnover should be finalized with an aggressive and vertical punch up against the bar in the overhead position. It's critical athletes understand this point and perform it properly. The turnover is not simply the action of swinging the bar around the head and back into its final position—it is an active pull of the elbows up and out, then a rotation of the arms to bring the bar overhead, and then an aggressive, vertical push up against the bar exactly like what was performed in the snatch balance, but over

a much shorter distance.

The importance of internally rotating the arms to orient the elbows outward from the start of the lift should become apparent in this exercise. This orientation is what allow the elbows to travel up and to the sides as the athlete pulls with the arms to move down, which allows the bar to remain close to the body as it travels up. During the snatch, this upward and outward pull of the elbows is imperative to maintaining proximity of the barbell and body to maximize mechanics, speed and accuracy. If the arms are allowed to hang in their neutral position, the elbows will naturally remain close to the lifter's sides and move backward, causing the bar to move forward away from the body and limiting the ability to actively pull the body down.

The initial action of pulling the elbows up and out is a critical element of the snatch—this is the movement that truly accelerates the lifter down under the bar following the second pull. The turnover of the bar itself is just a follow through and requires existing momentum and correct positioning to occur. Think of shoulder external rotation exercises and the loading possible with them—this external rotation is not a strong or powerful movement. Without the action of the elbows being pulled up and out aggressively first to bring the bar and body into the ideal position with adequate momemtum, that turnover will be impossible.

This drill should be initially performed slowly to allow the athlete to ensure maximal elbow height and bar proximity prior to the turnover. Once the movement is sound at low speeds, it can be executed quickly, at all times emphasizing proximity, elbow height, and an aggressive, vertical punch up against the bar overhead.

Scarecrow Snatch

The scarecrow snatch (Figure 14.9) drill is an abbreviated variation of the tall snatch exercise in which the bar begins in a higher position to focus on the most important principle of this section—learning the action of pulling under the bar with the proper upper body mechanics—before adding another layer of complexity.

The athlete will begin the exercise with the feet in the pulling position and standing tall with the arms in the scarecrow position—the elbows maximally elevated and out to the sides with the bar in light contact with or immediate proximity to the body. This is the same upper body position the athlete reached immediately prior to the turnover in the tall muscle snatch. It's important that the athlete focus on elbow height rather than bar height—if bar height is the focus, athletes will often drop and pull the elbows backward to elevate the bar farther.

Commonly the tall snatch, of which the scarecrow snatch is a variation, is started with the lifter on the balls of the feet. While this may be the ideal way to perform this exercise for a lifter with established lift technique, in this learning progression, a flat-footed start is employed for two basic reasons: primarily, it removes the balance component and an additional element of complexity and allows the athlete to focus on the most important components of the drill. Secondarily, it forces the lifter to lift the feet somewhat more, emphasizing this motion. In short, the flat-footed start removes only a minor element, and its benefits outweigh its drawbacks in this application.

From this starting position, with no upward movement from the lower body, the athlete will turn the bar over as aggressively as possible just as he or she did in the tall muscle snatch while lifting the feet and placing them flat into the receiving position, attempting to lock the bar in the overhead position at the same time the feet reconnect with the floor. The

movement of the arms is identical to that practiced in the tall muscle snatch.

The goal is maximal downward movement of the lifter and minimal upward movement of the bar, just as in the snatch balance exercises. To achieve this, the timing of the foot movement is critical—the feet need to lift from the floor at the same time the arms begin turning the bar over, or the lifter will be lifting the bar rather than pulling down under it. Often it's easier to achieve this timing by actually attempting to lift the feet first. In any case, the bar will (especially when using a PVC pipe or dowel) move up somewhat even when the exercise is performed correctly.

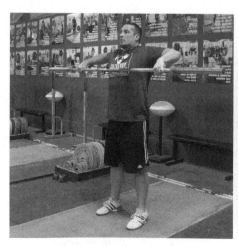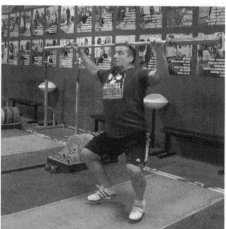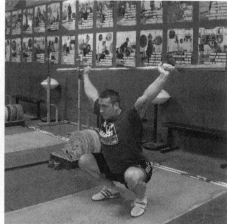

FIGURE 14.9 The scarecrow snatch introduces the athlete to the third pull in an abbreviated fashion to reinforce the proper upper body position and mechanics.

Greg Everett

The movement of the feet is identical to that practiced in the drop snatch and snatch balance. While the athlete should avoid excessive elevation of the feet, the feet do need to be lifted completely off the floor and moved aggressively into the receiving position, reconnected flat with the floor. This will result in a sharp clap. This noise is an indication of three important elements: the feet being removed entirely from the floor, aggressive movement, and a flat-footed reconnection. If noise is absent in this drill, it indicates that the lifter is failing to correctly perform one or more of these elements.

Once the athlete reaches the bottom of the receiving position, he or she will recover to a standing position with the bar still locked securely overhead. Again, it's recommended that athletes hold this bottom position for three seconds at this stage.

This drill can be performed initially into a partial squat depth like a power snatch. Once comfortable, it should be performed into a full squat; however, even in this case, the bar should still be fixed in the overhead position as quickly as possible. This should occur before the athlete reaches the bottom of the squat, but there should be no hesitation—the athlete will turn the bar over and sit into a full squat in one continuous motion.

A common mistake when performing this drill with a full squat is allowing the speed of the turnover to slow. The lifter will often not complete the turnover and fix the bar in the overhead position until reaching the bottom of the squat. The turnover needs to be as quick as possible irrespective of the ultimate depth of the receiving position—in short, the bar should be secured in the overhead position at the same time and height in both the power and squat receiving position variations of this drill. Again, attempting to make the lockout of the overhead position coincide with the reconnection of the feet to the floor will help maintain the proper speed and aggression.

Tall Snatch

The tall snatch (Figure 14.10) is identical to the scarecrow snatch but begins with the bar at arms' length rather than in the scarecrow position. Like the muscle snatch, the tall snatch will have application later as a training exercise to help improve the athlete's third pull speed and accuracy, although it will remain primarily a technique drill with relatively little utility for strength development.

The athlete will begin the exercise with the feet in the pulling position and standing tall with the bar hanging at arms' length and in light contact with the body. From this starting position, with no upward movement from the lower body, the athlete will pull the elbows up as high as possible and turn the bar over aggressively while lifting the feet and placing them flat into the receiving position, attempting to lock the bar in the overhead position at the same time the feet reconnect with the floor. The movement is identical to that practiced in the scarecrow

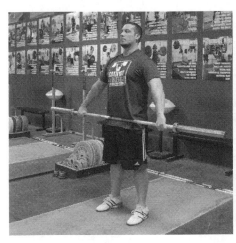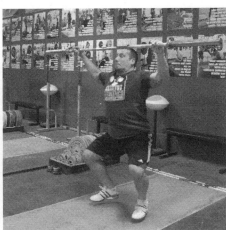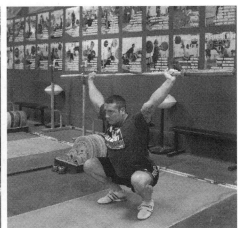

FIGURE 14.10 The tall snatch is the third pull of the snatch in isolation, teaching the athlete the mechanics, precision and aggression needed in the movement.

snatch with the exception of the arms in the starting position.

Because this drill begins prior to the elbows' elevation, athletes will have a tendency to stiffen the elbows and swing the bar away from the body. The elbows must be turned out completely in the starting position, the arms relaxed as much as possible, and focus directed on pulling the elbows up as high as possible before the arms are turned over, maintaining the proximity of the bar to the body throughout the movement.

Just as in the scarecrow snatch, the intent is to minimize the elevation of the bar and maximize the movement of the athlete down under it. Of course, with a PVC or empty barbell, it will be impossible to prevent any upward movement of the bar, and some upward movement will have to occur for the athlete to get under the bar (even in a snatch, the pull against the bar to move down under it will produce some elevation of the bar). However, the focus needs to remain on the aggressive pull down of the body.

Initially, the tall snatch can be received in a quarter squat depth if needed, and then in a full squat depth. In all cases, the goal again is to lock out the overhead position at the same time the feet reconnect flat with the floor to encourage speed.

Once the athlete reaches the bottom of the receiving position, he or she will recover to a standing position with the bar still locked securely overhead. Again, it's recommended that athletes hold this bottom position for three seconds at this stage.

Mid-Hang Snatch

The final step of the snatch progression from the hang assembles all the previous drills into a snatch from mid-thigh, or a mid-hang snatch (Figure 14.11). This is the first snatch the athlete will perform, and with the previous drills learned, it will very likely be done well with little or no additional instruction. The mid-thigh position is important here—athletes will tend to creep the bar lower and lower down the thigh with successive reps and sets to reach a more comfortable starting position. It's important to prevent this and reinforce the higher starting position.

Once setting the mid-hang position as described previously and holding it for a couple seconds to ensure proper position and balance, the athlete will initiate the lift by pushing against the floor with the legs, then snap the hips open to achieve the final ex-

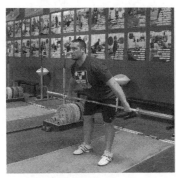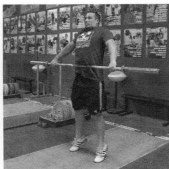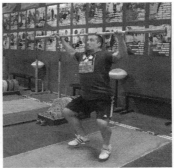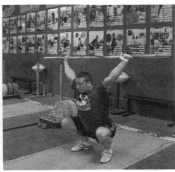

FIGURE 14.11 The mid-hang snatch is the first snatch variation the lifter will learn, focusing on the core of the movement without the complications of the first pull.

tended position we have described above: the legs approximately vertical, the shoulders slightly behind the hips, the arms long and loose, the bar in contact with the body at the hips, and the heels naturally lifted off the floor with the effort to drive aggressively with the legs. Throughout this extension, the athlete needs to be actively maintaining the bar's proximity to the body with the lats and shoulders, and then ensuring full contact as it reaches the hips. Note that full contact with the hips does not mean significant pressure against the body—it simply means that the bar and body are completely touching.

Once the athlete completes this upward extension, he or she will lift the feet to move them into the receiving position while aggressively pulling the elbows as high as possible and out to the sides to accelerate him- or herself down, turning the arms over and attempting to lock out the bar in the proper overhead position at the same time the feet reconnect flat with the floor. An adequately aggressive third pull will mean the bar is secured in the overhead position before the athlete reaches the bottom of the squat—regardless of the height the bar is fixed overhead, the athlete should continue sitting into the bottom position fluidly and without hesitation.

This entire movement should be considered a single, continuous action; that is, there should be no pausing or hesitation in the final extension position prior to the athlete pulling under the bar. At the same time, however, the athlete must reach complete extension before moving down.

The mid-hang snatch can be performed initially as a power snatch, with the receipt of the bar at quarter squat depth. This can be helpful for the athlete's confidence, reducing the number of elements in the ath-

lete's mind, and encouraging a faster third pull. Once the athlete is comfortable with the mid-hang power snatch, he or she should progress to a full squat, but without any reduction in speed of the third pull. In other words, the bar should be fixed in the overhead position at the same time and same height in both the power and squat variations of the exercise.

If the athlete has been performing these drills with PVC or a dowel, some practice with the barbell should be undertaken before moving to the next stage of learning the pull from the floor. In order to snatch from the floor, the athlete will need to be capable of handling at least a light technique barbell loaded with light technique plates—usually a minimum of about 15kg.

This practice can be comprised of overhead squats, snatch balances and mid-hang snatches to progressively move the lifter into snatching the barbell and build confidence with the new weight. Once the athlete is comfortable with the mid-hang snatch with an empty barbell, or at least a light technique barbell, he or she can move to the pull from the floor.

Missing Snatches Safely

Before progressing to snatching with considerable weight, it's important to familiarize the athlete with strategies for escaping immanent doom. Bailing out of a failed snatch isn't complicated, but it does require commitment and a strategy that has become second nature before its employment is needed—under a heavy bar that's threatening to split the athlete in half or injure a shoulder, elbow or wrist is neither a good time nor place to consider exit strategies.

There are two directions to dump the bar with a failed snatch: forward or backward. The most important point to understand about missing snatches is that the location and present direction of travel of the bar determines the dumping location, not the lifter's preference. The athlete is simply guiding the bar and body safely away from each other; heavy weights with momentum in such positions cannot be controlled more than this. Inexperienced athletes will often, for example, try to drop bars forward when they and the bar are falling backward, which can bring the bar down right onto their shins.

It's also important to maintain clear lifting areas of adequate size. Bumper plates, change plates, other bars, squat racks, the raised edge of a platform and the like can all be objects onto which a bar may

fall and off of which it may subsequently bounce unexpectedly, setting up some potentially ugly collisions. Platforms should always be cleared of unused weights prior to lifts, and all athletes should be taught from day one to be aware of their surroundings when lifting and when around lifting.

Lifters can practice missing snatches with a lightly loaded bar from full and partial overhead squat positions to get comfortable with the movements.

Missing Forward

Dumping a bar forward is the easiest direction because it will require the least movement of the lifter, flexibility is not an issue, and the bar will be in the lifter's field of vision. Typically this happens invol-

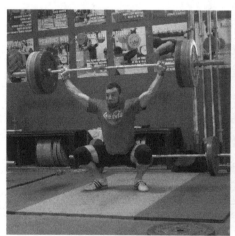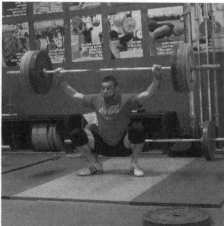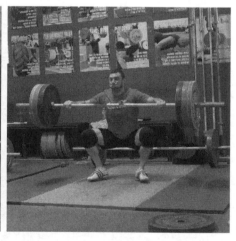

FIGURE 14.12 To miss a snatch in front, guide the bar forward away from the body and jump the body back away from the bar.

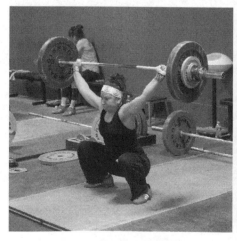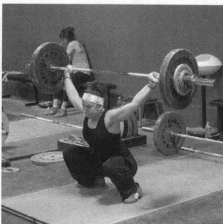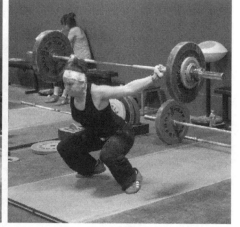

FIGURE 14.13 To miss a snatch behind, guide the bar back as far away from the body as possible and jump the body forward out of the way.

Greg Everett

untarily when a lifter leaves the bar out front during the pull or fails to turn it over aggressively enough—it will simply come to rest overhead in front of the lifter's base and promptly fall right back to the floor.

More of a concern are the instances in which the bar lands correctly in the slot directly overhead, but for one reason or another, one or both of the lifter's arms fail to lock and the bar begins descending. In these cases, the lifter must actively push the bar forward, keeping the arms as long as possible, and jump backward (Note that this is assuming the bar is directly overhead or slightly forward. If when an elbow or the elbows break the bar begins to favor the back, that's the direction in which it must be dumped.). Attempting to jump the feet backward and guiding the bar forward is important to avoid having the bar fall onto the knees or thighs.

Missing Backward

Three things are critical when dumping a bar behind: keeping the arms as long as possible, loosening the grip on the bar, and jumping forward out of the way. Extending the arms or keeping them extended will maximize the radius of the falling bar's arc, creating more safe space for the lifter. However, not all athletes will have the shoulder mobility to maintain their grip on the bar throughout said arc—it's therefore important that they open their grip on the bar as it travels down, ideally letting it go at the farthest possible point behind them. At the same time, the lifter must jump forward as far as possible to prevent the bar from dropping onto his or her back.

The Power Snatch

The power snatch is simply a snatch in which the athlete receives the bar in a relatively high position rather that sitting into a full squat. Most commonly, the requirement is that the lifter remain higher than a parallel squat (above a horizontal thigh position, or even more simply to observe, the crease of the hips above the top of the knee). Some coaches will accept lifts stopped at parallel rather than above, and others require a knee angle no smaller than 90 degrees.

Coaches and athletes should choose the definition that best suits their present training needs and goals, and that may vary somewhat even within a single training cycle.

A frequent point of confusion that arises with new lifters is that in order to qualify as a power snatch, the lifter must stop before reaching the depth threshold. That is, even if a lifter fixes the snatch overhead well above a parallel squat, but then continues to sit into a full squat, the lift is a snatch, not a power snatch. The lifter must receive the bar and stop the downward movement before reaching the depth threshold for the lift to qualify as power. This requires an immediate and forceful resistance of the legs upon receipt of the bar.

Generally speaking, the power snatch should be no different from the snatch with regard to the movement with the obvious exception of the ultimate squat depth. In other words, the two are really just a single lift with different depths.

This means that ideally the power snatch is performed with the same receiving position of the feet as the snatch—the squat position. If the athlete is unable to either elevate the bar adequately or arrest the downward movement soon enough, the failed power snatch attempt becomes a successful snatch attempt. Often athletes are taught the power snatch with an extremely wide receiving stance, or are allowed or encouraged to use it when it occurs naturally. The primary advantage of this wide stance is that it's easier to support the receiving position because there is less knee flexion at any given depth. If the exclusive goal for the power snatch is to get as much weight overhead at a power receiving height, this makes sense.

However, for the weightlifter, the power snatch must serve purposes beyond itself. That is, it's a tool to develop certain elements of the snatch, not an end itself. These elements include things like extension speed, turnover speed and aggression.

There are two potential problems with an extremely wide receiving stance in the power snatch. The first is simply that it makes consistency in the receiving position of the snatch more difficult by reducing the volume of practice in the normal snatch receiving position, and creates a competing motor pattern. This is a concern largely exclusive to novice lifters not yet technically proficient; more advanced lifters will be less susceptible to negative influences in snatch technique.

The second issue with a wider receiving position is the inability of the athlete to continue sitting into a full depth squat if adequate height hasn't been achieved, as he or she would be when using the same receiving position. This creates a few potential problems. For example, being forced into an unexpected depth with an excessively wide stance can expose the hips and knees in particular to injury.

Additionally, one of the benefits of the power snatch or power clean is the training of the ability to absorb force and brake with the legs rapidly. This contributes to the lifter's ability to receive and recover from snatches and cleans more successfully, and even to the elasticity and ultimate power of the dip and drive of the jerk. Using the same receiving position for power snatches and power cleans as for their squat counterparts means more reliance on the muscles to brake rather than resistance in the hip joint, and a greater transfer of that ability to the snatch, clean and jerk because of the similarity of positions.

As was discussed early in the book, a power lift occurs when the weight on the bar allows it with a maximal attempt at upward acceleration. The lighter the weight is, the more it will be accelerated during the second pull and the higher it will travel under the resulting momentum. As the athlete executes the third pull and continues pulling on the bar with the arms, the athlete will begin descending while the bar continues to rise. The degree to which each object descends or rises depends on their masses relative to each other, assuming constant effort by the athlete. The lighter the barbell relative to the athlete, the higher it will rise and the less the athlete will descend with a given magnitude of force application. If the bar is light enough, the athlete will be able to elevate it high enough to receive the lift with the thighs above horizontal, thus performing a power snatch. Otherwise, the movements of the snatch and power snatch are identical.

Benefits & Uses

The power snatch is used by weightlifters for a number of different reasons. One is as a substitute for the snatch on lighter training days—this allows the athlete to continue performing essentially the same snatch motion with less taxing loads (even at maximal effort), but still with a demand for speed and precision. Another use is as a tool for improving certain aspects of an athlete's snatch performance—the power snatch forces an extremely violent second pull, abrupt transition at the top, and a vicious turnover of the bar, all because of the need to elevate the bar higher and secure it overhead in less time and space. The power snatch can also be used as an early variation of the snatch for new lifters who are not yet mobile enough to snatch with a full squat, or as an abbreviated movement in the learning progression to reduce the number of elements for the athlete to consider.

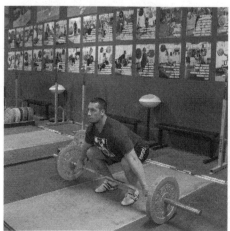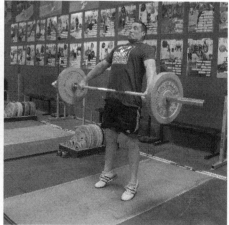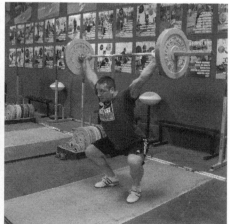

FIGURE 14.14 The power snatch is identical to the snatch with the exception of a shallow receiving depth.

Greg Everett

The Split Snatch

The split snatch was the dominant lift style prior to the modern squat style. As the lifting technique and equipment (shoes) evolved through the efforts of athletes to continually lift heavier weights, the squat became the dominant style and the split faded into obsolescence within competitive weightlifting, with the exception of some master lifters.

While the great splitters of the era were capable of receiving depths comparable in some cases to a squat, the dramatic displacement of the feet still requires more time and space, which as a consequence requires more elevation of the bar, ultimately limiting the weights that can be lifted in the split style.

While not ideal for lifters at the highest levels of competition, the split snatch certainly has utility in some situations. The most obvious is as a snatch style for masters lifters or others who are, due to extreme immobility or injury-related mobility limitations, unable to squat. The split will typically allow these lifters to achieve somewhat greater depth than they would be capable of with a power snatch, and specifically reduces the demand on shoulder and thoracic spine mobility. The split snatch allows the athlete to keep the torso vertical, and even behind vertical in some cases, to accommodate extreme upper body immobility. All of this being said, switching to the split snatch is not a substitute for addressing correctible mobility limitations—it should be a last resort.

Another use of the split snatch for the typical competitive weightlifter is as a drill to train the split footwork and position for the jerk. While this may seem like an oddly indirect approach, it makes sense for some lifters to address multiple goals without overloading the training program. If a lifter would normally be power snatching in the program, using a split snatch (with a receiving depth and stance comparable to the lifter's jerk split position) is a way to train essentially the same thing the power snatch is likely being used for (assuming it's not being used for footwork) while also giving the athlete an opportunity to work on split jerk footwork.

The technique of the split snatch differs from the squat snatch only in the movement of the feet during the third pull. In a full split snatch as performed by the top lifters of the split era, the lead knee will be fully closed or close to it and the hips nearly as low as they would be in a squat. This is a different position than the split used for the jerk; it requires that the front foot not be as far forward and demands a great deal of mobility in the hips. For athletes of the present era who employ the split in order to snatch, the absence of such mobility is likely the reason for splitting, so the split position used will likely be higher and more similar to the jerk.

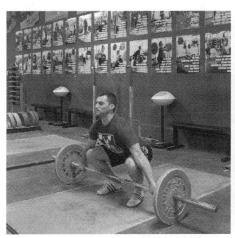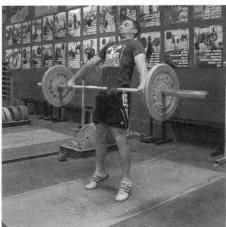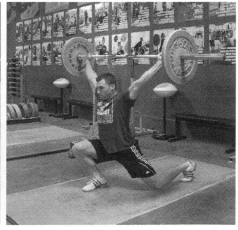

FIGURE 14.15 The technique of the split snatch differs from the squat snatch only in the movement of the feet during the third pull.

Pulling from the Floor

At this point, the athlete is able to perform a snatch and power snatch from the mid-hang position with at least an empty barbell. To complete the snatch progression, the pull from the floor must be introduced. The addition of the first pull often proves surprisingly difficult for many athletes and may temporarily disrupt their technique; however, with a smart progression and proper attention to the principles, this section of the movement can be learned quickly and correctly. As was discussed in the previous section, it's important for the athlete to be comfortable snatching from mid-thigh the minimum weight that will have to be used from the floor before beginning this stage.

The following progression will teach the lifter the correct positions throughout the pull that are critical for successful lifting, as well as introduce valuable training exercises that can be implemented in the program later.

Progression Overview

- Starting Position
- Snatch Segment Deadlift
- Halting Snatch Deadlift
- Segment Snatch + Snatch
- Snatch

Starting Position

Our first step in teaching the pull from the floor is of course the starting position (Figure 15.1). Universal details of the position have been covered in a previous chapter, and additional details specific to the snatch will be discussed in the following section. At this stage, instruction for the athlete should be kept as simple and concise as possible while still ensuring correct execution.

Mobility will be a limiting factor for many athletes at this point and a considerable number of them will be unable to achieve the correct position initially. In this early stage it's more important to work on learning the basic position with regard to knee and hip angles, bar position and balance over the feet than to have a perfectly arched back, which may be physically impossible for some adult lifters at this point. However, correcting any mobility limitations for such athletes needs to be made the first priority, as this is a

---

18 Progression Summary
Snatch Starting Position

Place the barbell over approximately the balls of the foot.

Turn the feet out slightly and balance the weight evenly across them.

Hold the bar with the hook grip at snatch-width.

Assume an upright posture that orients the arms approximately vertically when viewed from the side.

Pressurize the trunk and fix the back securely in a continuous arch.

Keep the head up with a focal point straight ahead or slightly above.

Push the knees outward inside the arms and over the bar.

Internally rotate the arms and keep them passively extended.

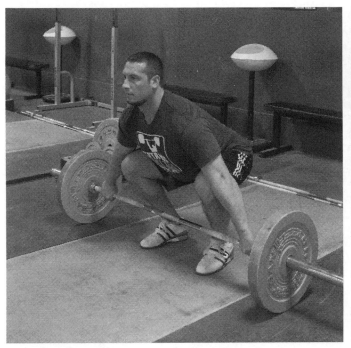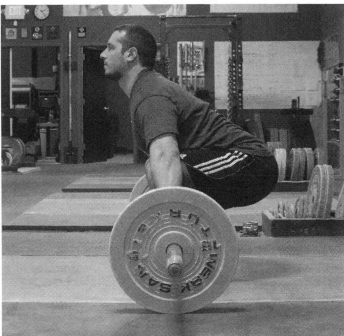

FIGURE 15.1 The starting position for the snatch

major limiter of performance and cause of increased injury potential.

For this stage of learning, the barbell should be loaded lightly—the weight should be the same or very similar to what the athlete was capable of easily snatching from mid-thigh, as these drills will ultimately progress again into snatching. A technique barbell and/or technique plates can be used if needed.

With the bar loaded on the platform, the lifter will place the feet in the pulling position with the balls of the feet under the bar. Holding the bar with a hook grip and the hand width determined previously, the athlete will arch the back tightly and bring the hips down to assume a posture that places the hips anywhere from slightly below to above the knees and orients the arms approximately vertically when viewed from the side. The arms should be extended passively with the tension created by the athlete lifting the chest, and internally rotated to orient the bony points of the elbows out to the sides. The knees should be pushed out to the sides to help improve the arch of the back and allow a more upright posture—they can be out as far as being in light contact with the arms. The knees should be over the bar somewhat and the shins either in light contact with or very close to the

bar. The athlete's head should be upright and the eyes focused straight head or slightly above.

Snatch Segment Deadlift

The first step in the progression is the snatch segment deadlift (Figure 15.2). This exercise is a way to both teach and reinforce the proper positions at different critical points in the pull. The segmented movement allows athletes to better feel and correct posture and balance during the lift.

After setting and holding the starting position momentarily, the lifter will begin the deadlift by pushing with the legs against the floor, separating the bar smoothly without jerking or yanking. This should be a deliberate, controlled movement, and the lifter should maintain the same approximate back angle from the starting position. Once the bar reaches a height of 1 inch off the floor, the lifter will pause and hold for 3 seconds. This position should be nearly identical to the starting position but with the weight over the foot shifted backward very slightly from the even balance in the starting position. The bar can be

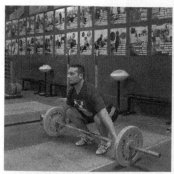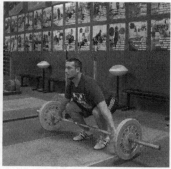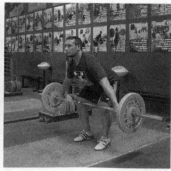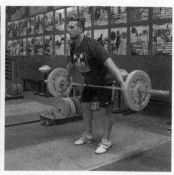

FIGURE 15.2 The snatch segment deadlift teaches and reinforces the most critical positions in the pull from the floor.

in very light contact with the shins, but should not be pushed back into them forcefully.

This 1-inch height is much lower and is reached much sooner than athletes typically expect—they will commonly not pause until the bar is several inches up. The simplest way to instruct proper timing of this first pause position is to have the lifter stop as soon as they feel the bar separate from the floor.

After holding this position for 3 seconds, the lifter will resume standing by again pushing with the legs, still with a controlled, deliberate speed, until the bar reaches the level of the knees and pause again with the bar in light contact with the kneecaps. During this movement, the lifter should continue shifting the center of balance back until it reaches the front edge of the heel where it should stay for the remainder of the lift. The lifter will then pause again with the bar in light contact with the kneecaps for 3 seconds.

At this second pause position, the shoulders should be very slightly farther forward than they were in the starting position—that is, very slightly forward of the bar. However, this is minor and the back angle should have changed only slightly from the first position. Any dramatic change in the back angle or with the shoulders' position in front of the bar at this point indicates that the athlete is elevating the hips too much relative to the shoulders and bar. Likewise, it's important the athlete not move the shoulders behind the bar.

After holding this position at the knees for 3 seconds, the lifter will proceed to the final position at mid-thigh by again pushing with the legs against the floor at a controlled speed and using the lats and

shoulders to keep the bar in immediate proximity to the thigh. This final movement should bring the lifter into the same mid-hang position he or she has already practiced, with the bar in light contact with the mid-thigh, the shins approximately vertical, the knees pushed out to the sides slightly (less than in the starting position), the back still arched completely, the shoulders in front of the bar and the knees, the weight balanced over the front edge of the heel, and the head and eyes directed forward.

Overall there will be a slight change in the back

---

19 Progression Summary

Snatch Segment Deadlift

Set the starting position tightly and hold momentarily.

Push with the legs to separate the bar from the floor 1 inch and pause for 3 seconds.

Push with the legs and shift the weight back to the front edge of the heel to bring the bar to the kneecap, maintaining a similar back angle, and hold for 3 seconds.

Push with the legs to move into the mid-hang position and hold for 3 seconds, maintaining balance over the front edge of the heel.

Return the bar to the floor at a controlled speed, trying to move through the same correct positions on the way down.

Greg Everett

angle and the position of the shoulders between the starting position and mid-hang position, but again, it will be relatively minor—no more than is necessary to achieve the correct mid-hang position for a given athlete.

Frequently athletes will shift their weight too far back toward the heels, particularly at the knee position. The full foot should remain in contact with the floor throughout the movement—if the athlete's toes are lifting from the floor, the balance is too far back. This kind of excessive backward balance will typically cause subsequent excessive forward rocking in the snatch.

After holding the mid-hang position for 3 seconds, the athlete will return the bar to the floor at a controlled speed, attempting to reverse the movement accurately to pass through the same correct positions on the way down. The starting position should be reset with the bar resting completely on the floor before subsequent reps.

Sets of 3 reps will allow practice without excessive fatigue of the back from holding the pause positions. Once this exercise can be performed with the athlete consistently reaching the correct positions immediately at each point—that is, the lifter does not have to make adjustments at each pause to find the correct position—he or she can proceed to the next step.

Halting Snatch Deadlift

When the segment deadlift can be performed correctly, the athlete will progress to the halting snatch deadlift (Figure 15.3), which simply removes the first two pause positions so the lifter is pausing only at mid-thigh. Although the first two pauses have been removed, the athlete should still be passing through the positions with the same postures and balance over the feet practiced in the segment deadlift.

This exercise should also be performed at a controlled, deliberate speed like the segment deadlift.

Rushing the lift not only makes it less likely that the athlete will achieve the correct positions and balance, but reduces the effectiveness of even correct positions. This is an exercise intended to train and reinforce positional awareness and stability, not speed.

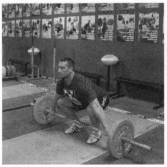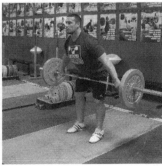

FIGURE 15.3 The halting snatch deadlift teaches the lifter how to properly move the bar from the floor to mid-thigh, where the second pull will begin.

Segment Snatch + Snatch

When the athlete is capable of consistently performing the halting snatch deadlift correctly, the first pull, in terms of position and balance, has been learned. What remains is for the athlete to learn to transition from the first pull into the second pull seamlessly and confidently—in other words, to combine the halting snatch deadlift and mid-hang snatch into a single, continuous lift.

In order to make this transition easier and less intimidating, the athlete will use a complex that allows the lifter in the first rep to perform two movements he or she is already comfortable with: the halting snatch deadlift and the mid-hang snatch, and then follow it immediately with a snatch (Figure 15.4). This helps improve confidence and reduce unwanted thinking, as well as continuing to reinforce the proper positions and timing.

Each set will consist of 2 reps: 1 segment snatch and 1 snatch. For the first rep, the athlete will perform a halting snatch deadlift at a controlled speed, hold the mid-hang position for 3 seconds, and then perform a mid-hang snatch directly from that pause position (no countermovement to begin). After returning the bar to the floor, the lifter will perform a snatch with no pause on the way up. However, at this stage, the lift from the floor to mid-thigh should remain at a deliberate speed to ensure proper positioning, balance, and timing of the final explosion. The

Set the starting position tightly and hold momentarily.

Perform a halting snatch deadlift to the mid-hang position and hold for 3 seconds.

Directly from this pause position, perform a mid-hang snatch.

Return the bar from the floor and reset the starting position.

Perform a snatch with no pause, but keep the lift from the floor to mid-thigh slow to ensure correct positions, balance and timing.

lifter can control this speed easily by keeping the pull from the floor to mid-thigh timed to a count of 3.

As the lift improves and the lifter's confidence increases, this first pull speed can be increased slightly, although it should still remain relatively slow. The speed of the first pull will be increased later as the lifter becomes more technically proficient and loading increases. Once the snatches in the second rep of this complex are consistent, it's time for the final step of the process: the snatch.

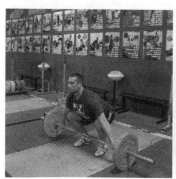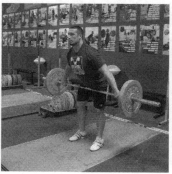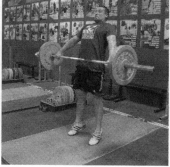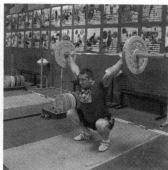

FIGURE 15.4 The segment snatch + snatch complex progresses the athlete to the first snatch from the floor while continuing to reinforce the critical mid-hang position.

Snatch

At this point, the athlete is capable of performing the classic snatch (Figure 15.5). Practice should consist of sets of 2-5 repetitions with weights that allow correct and safe execution. In the early stages of development, large volumes of very lightweight practice is appropriate and most effective; partial lifts and assistance exercises will be used to develop strength for the snatch. For practice of the snatch as part of the earliest training program, weights should be approximately 40-50% of bodyweight, or what the athlete and coach feel could be lifted without trouble for 5-6 repetitions (Medvedyev 1986/1995). Of course, lighter weights should be used if needed and the initial practice stage extended as much as needed for each athlete prior to beginning a more structured training program. This process is discussed in detail in the Program Design & Training section of the book.

If the athlete is having difficulty in particular aspects of the snatch, he or she should practice the exercise or exercises from the progression process that best address the position or segment of the movement in question for remediation in addition to the snatch. Always keep in mind that the quality of repetitions is of greater priority than the quantity.

22 Progression Summary
Snatch

Set the starting position tightly and hold momentarily.

Initiate the lift by pushing with the legs against the floor.

Shift the weight back to the front edge of the heel by the time the bar reaches knee height.

Continue pushing with the legs until reaching the mid-hang position, maintaining the balance over the front edge of the heel.

Execute the final upward explosion by pushing with the legs against the ground and extending the hips aggressively, actively maintaining the proximity of the bar to the body.

As you reach the final extended position with the legs vertical, bar against the hips, and shoulders slightly behind the hips, lift the feet and pull the elbows high and out.

Keep the bar as close to the body as possible, turn the arms over and bring the bar into the overhead position, locking it out at the same time the feet land flat on the floor in the receiving position.

Continue sitting into the bottom of the squat fluidly with the bar secured tightly overhead.

Recover to a standing position by pushing straight up against the bar and following it with your body.

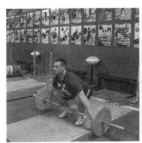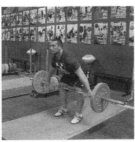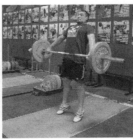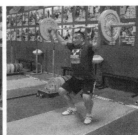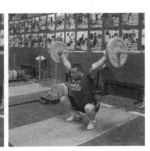

FIGURE 15.5 The snatch from the floor finalizes the snatch progression.

Understanding the Snatch

This chapter expands on the information presented in somewhat simplified fashion during the snatch learning progression. For athletes at this point who are not yet comfortable with their technical performance of the snatch, it's advised to skip this section and focus on practicing the lift and its basic variations (e.g. hang and power) along with basic assistance exercises such as squats and pulls until a reasonable level of consistency is developed.

Prior to this point, additional information is more likely to be overwhelming and confusing than helpful. From a coaching perspective, it's generally ideal to present as little conceptual information to the athlete as possible and focus on the practical aspects of execution primarily until athletes are more advanced and beginning to experiment with more idiosyncratic technical modifications to best suit their individual peculiarities.

The Starting Position

The importance of the starting position is often underestimated and the resulting lack of attention it receives leads to unnecessary difficulty with technical proficiency. As was discussed previously, the hierarchy of technical aspects will remain sound guiding principles throughout both the learning process and the athlete's training career. At the top of this hierarchy—or possibly more appropriately viewed as the base—is position. It is impossible to generate a correct movement from an incorrect position, and neglect of this principle is responsible for a great deal of frustration and wasted training time and energy.

Distilled to its essence, the primary purpose of the starting position is to allow the proper execution of the lift as a whole. This means that, while it may

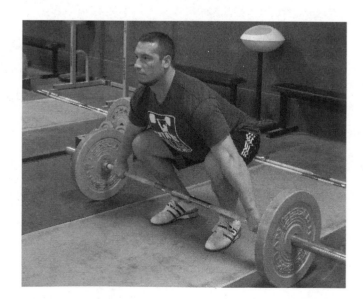

FIGURE 16.1 The proper starting position for the snatch allows optimal execution of the lift.

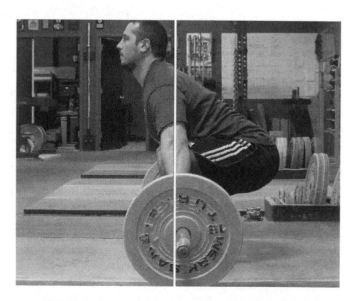

FIGURE 16.2 The arms should be approximately vertical, placing the front of the shoulders slightly forward of the bar, with the bar over the balls of the feet and the hips from slightly below to slightly above the knees. This position will change slightly to accommodate each lifter's proportions and relative strengths and weaknesses.

Greg Everett

seem counterintuitive, the position does not necessarily make the initial separation of the bar from the floor or the first pull optimal in the way it would be expected to if the first pull were the entirety of the lift. In other words, compromises of various natures and degrees, depending on the lifter, may need to be made in order to optimize the entire lift. For example, the initial separation of the barbell from the floor may be easier with a larger knee angle in the starting position, but such an angle will require a compensatory shift in the athlete's posture that disrupts the optimal mechanics later in the lift and reduces the effectiveness of the lift to a greater extent than the deviation from this easier starting position does. In other words, the compromise may make a particular segment of the lift less than optimal in isolation, but creates a net benefit when the lift is considered as a whole, which it must be.

Much of the individual variation in the starting position will consist of the adjustments necessary to accommodate problematic characteristics of the proportions or the relative strengths and weaknesses of a given lifter to create the position that optimizes the movement for that specific individual. However, such variation will rarely be dramatic.

In slower movements such as the deadlift, athletes can typically compensate to a fairly large degree for a poor starting position through continual adjustments in reaction to sensory feedback during the lift. However, if we consider the ability to make such adjustments in terms of the time available, the degree to which such adjustment is possible is dramatically reduced in lifts as fast as the snatch, clean or jerk. The execution time of a snatch is a fraction of that of a deadlift even with a far greater amplitude; it's clear the opportunity for correction during the lift itself is extremely limited, and arguably impossible to any significant degree. This being the case, it's imperative that consistency of a proper starting position be a priority for all lifters.

Universal Elements

There are a few elements of the starting position that can be considered universally accepted irrespective of contention regarding other points of technique: feet turned out moderately, the back arched com-pletely, the barbell over the foot, the arms extended, and the arms internally rotated. Recommendations vary somewhat for other elements, although typically, at least among experienced weightlifting coaches and weightlifters, to a negligible degree.

The feet will be placed in the pulling position, discussed in detail in the Foot Positions chapter. In short, the heels should be approximately hip-width (creating vertical orientation of the legs in a standing position) and turned out approximately 10-20 degrees relative to straight forward (Figure 16.3). This position creates the optimal mechanics for the acceleration and elevation of the barbell, but does not take into account the anatomical peculiarities of individual lifters that may affect the final optimized position.

The width of the stance determines multiple facets of the pull. The closer the legs are to a vertical orientation at the top of the pull, the larger percentage of the force against the platform generated by the lifter is directed into the vertical movement of the barbell rather than being displaced horizontally. A stance wider than this (or narrower, although this is very uncommon) results in a portion of the generated force to be dissipated horizontally, reducing the force available to accelerate and elevate the bar. Additionally, vertical leg orientation allows the greatest possible height of the athlete in the extended position, and consequently the greatest possible height of the barbell by virtue of its connection to the shoulders.

Of course many other factors contribute to the acceleration and elevation of the barbell, and divergence from this ideal stance may maximize factors that improve the lift to a greater extent than a change in the stance detracts from it. Similarly, changes may be necessary to accommodate certain issues related to anatomy and proportions that make this ideal stance impossible to achieve in the starting position, or in some way create problems of a magnitude that exceeds the benefit of the ideal stance. A simple example of this is a widening of the stance by a superheavyweight lifter to accommodate the need for more space between the thighs for the upper body; this may reduce the ultimate height the bar achieves directly through the extension of the body, but a narrower stance may force a serious divergence from the optimal starting position that limits the lift to an even greater degree.

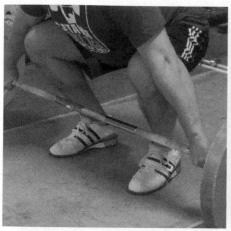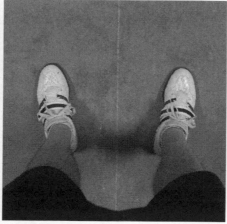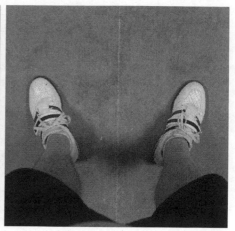

FIGURE 16.3 The basic starting position will place the heels directly under the hips to orient the legs vertically when extended, and rotate the feet outward between approximately 10-20 degrees from center.

The rotation of the feet out from the centerline helps the athlete move the thighs into a position that allows the desired posture—by allowing the necessary mobility in the hips and a shortening of the fore-aft distance between the barbell and hips—in the start and first pull without creating problematic torque or tension in the legs. Angles greater than approximately 20 degrees create problems as well. Primarily, there is too significant a reduction in the depth of the lifter's base—the distance between the front and back edges of the feet—which reduces the lifter's ability to establish and maintain balance. Additionally, excessive outward rotation can disrupt the mechanics of the knees and hips to the point of limiting strength during the pull.

Typically athletes will, without interference, turn their feet out naturally to a degree that suits them well. Unless a given athlete's chosen foot placement exceeds the range of acceptable angles, there is no reason to modify it unless it is later discovered to be negatively affecting another element of the lift.

Initially effort should be made to use the ideal starting position described and gain experience with the lifts from this position before experimenting with significant variations. Without this initial period of consistency, it will be impossible to legitimately evaluate the stance and make informed decisions regarding alteration. There will be more than enough inconsistency in technique further along in the movement to create frustration—the more variables

can be reduced, the more easily and quickly effective technique changes can be made. In the early stages of a lifter's development, mobility limitations may force divergence from the optimal position in terms of both the width of the stance and the degree of foot rotation. As mobility is actively improved, the pulling position should be incrementally moved back toward the ideal. In the long term, the foot position should be whatever proves with experience to be most effective for each athlete when considering the lift as a whole.

Barbell Placement & Leg Position

The bar should begin approximately over the balls of the feet. This is an approximation of the metatarsophalangeal joints (the joints of the toes to the foot), the five of which will angle back slightly, and the outer of which may be behind that of the first toe due to the outward rotation of the feet. Using the balls of the feet as the landmark will place the bar over the collection of them on average with most focus near the first and second toes as it should be. Generally speaking, lifters with relatively long legs and short torsos may need to start the bar slightly farther forward, while lifters with relatively short legs and long torsos may need (or prefer) to start the bar slightly farther back. Lifters should begin with the bar over the balls of the feet and adjust as needed to accom-

Greg Everett

modate their proportions to create the ideal overall starting position in consideration of all criteria.

Because during the pull the bar will be intentionally moved farther back over the foot in order to bring the lifter-barbell system's center of mass into the desired balance over the base, the obvious question is why the bar is started farther forward over the foot. The rationale is simple: In order to create the relatively upright posture in the desired starting position, the shins must be inclined forward to a degree that prevents the bar from being positioned closer to the middle of the foot. However, as mentioned above, lifters with more dolichomorphic proportions may be capable of starting the bar farther back due to the more upright shin angle that naturally accompanies their proportions.

Over the balls of the feet is approximately as far forward as the barbell can begin while still allowing the athlete to maintain and readjust balance over the base during the initial pull from the floor. Note that this is true only for significant weights—the lighter a weight relative to the lifter, the less its beginning position matters because the less of an influence it has on the system's balance due to being a smaller fraction of its total mass. Lifters who have the good fortune of proportions that accommodate an optimal starting position while allowing the bar to begin closer to mid-foot can position the bar accordingly.

The lifter's weight should be balanced approximately evenly across the length of the foot; some lifters may have slightly more weight on the balls of the foot than the heel when in the optimal starting position. Attempts to shift the balance toward the heels will force improper positioning, moving the

lifter behind instead of above the bar, and should be avoided. The shifting of the balance toward its ultimate point will occur early in the pull from the floor.

The bar may or may not be in contact with the shins in the starting position. If it is not, it should remain in close proximity. If it is in contact, care must be taken to ensure that this contact is not a result of the shoulders being too far behind the bar. Some lifters have an uncanny ability to trace the legs with the bar without ever allowing it to drag against them; most lifters will find it easier and more effective to begin with the bar as close to the shins as possible without touching.

The knees should be flared out to the sides to further open the hips and shorten the fore-aft distance between the hips and bar, which allows a more upright posture without affecting the shoulder or barbell position (Figure 16.4). The knees can be pushed out as far as the boundaries of the arms allow, with even light contact between the thighs and arms. However, the knees should not be out so far that the arms are forced to bend to accommodate the thighs. This will, for most lifters, move the knees outside the feet to some degree; unlike with the squat, this is not a concern for the pull from the floor.

The knees will be over the bar to an extent commensurate to the athlete's proportions, like the knees move forward over the toes in the bottom position of a squat. A common error for new lifters is the attempt to keep the knees behind the bar with a shin angle close to vertical, ostensibly to ensure a clear path for the bar. This notion neglects, however, the fact that the shins and knees will naturally move back out of the way as the legs are extended during the

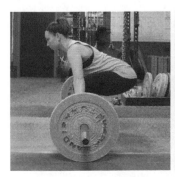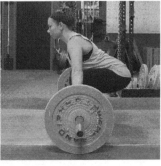

FIGURE 16.4 The knees should be pushed out to the sides (right) inside the arms to open the hips and allow a more upright posture than with the knees forward (left).

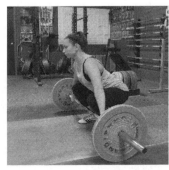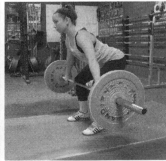

FIGURE 16.5 The knees should be over the bar in the starting position. The shins and knees will move out of the way of the bar as the legs are extended in the first pull.

first pull. Additionally, the outward flaring of the knees reduces the extent to which the knees would otherwise protrude over the bar in the starting position, and consequently, the extent to which they need to move out of the way of the bar as it rises.

Back Arch

The back should be set in complete extension—effectively a single continuous arch from the lumbar to cervical spine. The natural lordotic curve of the lumbar spine should be exaggerated slightly and the kyphotic curve of the thoracic spine flattened as much as possible. The latter is often limited in new lifters with the prevalence of thoracic immobility and stiffness, while the former is often prevented by limited hip mobility. Both need to be addressed and correct-

ed as soon as possible in a new lifter's development, as the ability to establish a proper back arch is one of the most important fundamental elements in successful lifting. (Figure 16.6)

This arch of the entire back creates the most rigid lever arm possible to transmit the force generated by the legs and hips to the barbell. Such an arch shortens the length of the back slightly, reducing the length of the lever arm the musculature must support and move, and creates the best possible position for the spinal extensor muscles to act on the spine—reduced extension increases their mechanical disadvantage. As was mentioned in the Starting Position chapter, rounding of the back can reduce the force to the bar by as much as 15%. In addition, the slight hyperextension acts as a buffer against inadvertent lumbar flexion, which is the position that creates the greatest risk for injury for the lower back.

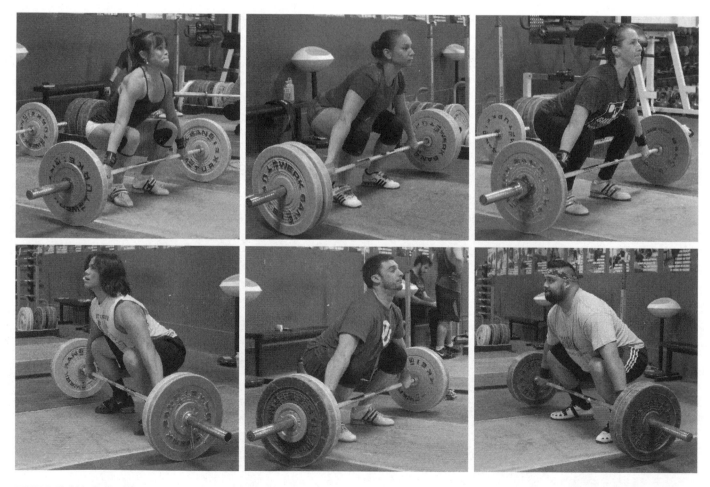

FIGURE 16.6 Ideally lifters have the mobility and strength to establish a single continuous arch along the length of the back, but there will be variations in the degree of extension, particularly in the thoracic region, due to mobility restrictions.

Greg Everett

The proper back arch should be reinforced, and maximal rigidity of the trunk ensured, with pressurization and aggressive circumferential muscular tension as described in the Breathing & Trunk Rigidity chapter. It will generally be easier to take this breath before entering the final starting position, in which the abdomen will usually be compressed to some degree. This is another advantage of a dynamic start—such starts usually naturally create opportunities to take in an unrestricted breath.

The shoulder blades should remain in an approximately neutral position fore and aft, although for some lifters, the shoulder blades will protract to some degree unavoidably in order to allow the lifter to reach the bar in the starting position. The lats should be engaged naturally with the effort to extend the upper back, which will create depression of the shoulder blades. This activation of the lats will also keep the bar in close proximity to the body during the pull when the shoulders are in front of it rather than allowing it to swing away.

Arm Orientation

The arms should be oriented approximately vertically when viewed from the athlete's side. This will place the leading aspect of the shoulders slightly forward of the bar because of the shape and mass of the shoulders themselves. The precise location of the shoulder joint relative to the bar can be adjusted within a small range to best suit each lifter's proportions, but in no case should be significantly forward of the bar, and never behind it.

The arms should be internally rotated maximally (the bony points of the elbows turned out to the sides). This rotation of the arms should not affect the position of the shoulders; many athletes will roll the shoulders forward and protract the shoulder blades when internally rotating the arms. This may be a result of immobility or simply inadequate control of the movement without practice. Mobility limitations should be addressed and corrected immediately, and the action of internal rotation can be practiced in isolation by standing with the arm out to the side at an approximately 45 degree angle and turning the palm to face as far backward as possible without allowing the position of the shoulder to change (Figue 16.7).

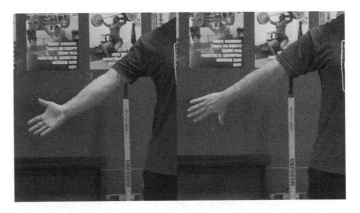

FIGURE 16.7 If athletes struggle to internally rotate the arms without moving the shoulders, they can practice the internal rotation in isolation by standing with the arm out to the side at an approximately 45 degree angle and turning the palm to face as far backward as possible without allowing the position of the shoulder to change. Left: externally rotated; Right: internally rotated.

The importance of this orientation of the elbows cannot be overstated. Most athletes will find it awkward and avoid committing fully to the position, while others may not initially have the specific strength to maintain the position during heavy pulling movements. The internal rotation of the arms will primarily allow the lifter to properly execute the third pull with maximal bar and body proximity.

Head Position

The lifter's head should be upright and the eyes focused approximately straight forward or slightly higher. Because of the great range of motion and diversity in positions throughout the lift, the ideal direction of vision is one that can be consistent from start to finish. Shifting the focus of the eyes during such a rapid and violent movement is disruptive at best. The focal point should be fairly distant to minimize any movement relative to the lifter. Beginning the lift with the eyes focused on the floor encourages unwanted forward shifting of the lifter's balance and excessive tipping of the shoulders forward because of the body's tendency to follow the eyes.

Concerns occasionally arise regarding extension of the cervical spine in the starting position. Because of the upright posture in the start, and the flattening of the thoracic spine, an upright head position should not hyperextend the cervical spine to a significant degree, and accordingly, no concern is necessary. Additionally, cervical extension has been shown to strengthen overall spinal extension force considerably; however, excessive hyperextension should be avoided in order to prevent any undue strain.

The First Pull

The first pull brings the barbell from the floor to the point at which the final explosion of the hips and knees begins—approximately the level of mid-thigh. The purpose of this initial movement is primarily positioning and secondarily acceleration—that is, the priority is bringing the bar and lifter into the most advantageous position from which to perform the second pull, the source of the majority of the power delivered to the barbell (at least in lifts heavier than 70-75% of maximum—the acceleration in the first pull is typically greater than in the second pull with lighter loads (Zehkov 1976/1992) due to the reduced effect of the smaller joint angles in the first pull).

While seemingly a relatively simple movement, the first pull commonly presents many problems for even experienced lifters because of the interaction of the knees with the bar and the shifting of balance and posture that must occur. Establishing the optimal starting position for a lifter and developing consistency with it will contribute significantly to the success of the first pull, but the motion of the pull itself must also be learned and practiced.

The framework of the first pull can be considered as moving the lifter from a position at the floor with the shoulders above the bar and the weight somewhat in front of the center of the base to a position with the shoulders over the bar and the bar-body system balanced properly over the base. The essential motion will remain the same among lifters, while the observable movement will vary in appearance based on the lifter's proportions, relative strengths and minor stylistic peculiarities.

The gross movement of the first pull is knee extension—pushing against the platform with the legs, or as it is often helpful for athletes to think of it, pushing the floor away. That is, there should be no net hip extension during the movement. The angle of the back relative to the floor should not increase until the second pull is initiated. While there will be a slight shift of the trunk (leaning farther over the bar) to a degree that will vary among lifters, it should remain at approximately the same angle until the second pull is initiated and the hips begin to extend.

Combined System Balance

In the starting position, the lifter and barbell are two separate objects whose masses are each supported individually by the floor. At the moment of bar separation from the platform, the lifter and barbell become a single system that must remain balanced over a single base—the lifter's feet. Because in the starting position the lifter is balanced over the whole foot and the bar is over the balls of the feet, at the moment of separation, the lifter-barbell system will be balanced over the forefoot to a degree commensurate to the portions of the total mass the barbell and lifter each

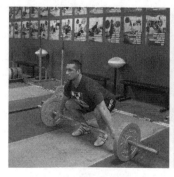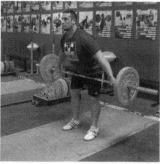

FIGURE 16.8 The first pull of the snatch brings the barbell from the floor to the point at which the final explosion begins, approximately mid-thigh.

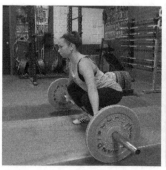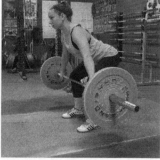

FIGURE 16.9 Because it starts over the balls of the feet and must move farther back over the feet to establish balance of the combined bar-body mass, the bar will move back toward the body as it leaves the floor.

Greg Everett

represent. That is, the heavier the barbell relative to the lifter, the closer the balance point will be to the location of the bar over the foot as the two join into a single mass over a single base.

Because we want to balance the system slightly behind mid-foot during the pull, the system needs to be rebalanced during the initial movement of the bar from the floor. This is accomplished primarily through moving the barbell back toward the lifter as it leaves the platform and the shins move out of the way with the extension of the knees. Depending on the lifter's proportions, the starting position, and to some degree, the weight on the bar, the lifter's center of mass will shift back slightly as well. However, this is not a dramatic movement and should not be exaggerated, as it will shift the balance too far toward the heels.

This need to rebalance the system over the feet is what prevents the possibility of a perfectly vertical bar path—the initial movement of the first pull to lift and shift the bar back toward the lifter creates a slight backward angle on the path of the barbell. If the barbell moves directly vertically, the balance of the bar-lifter system will be too far forward over the feet, and the forward pull of this imbalance will increase the higher the barbell travels. In short, the lifter must rebalance the system as quickly as possible to establish and maintain control of the lift. The proper balance over the feet should be established before the bar reaches the height of the knee.

If the weight is forward during the first pull, it will be exaggerated as the athlete extends and the combined center of mass is elevated. At best this will result in the athlete being forced to jump forward to receive the bar—a precarious feat and one that places unnecessary strain on the joints—and at worst will result in the lift being missed entirely. Such forward imbalance will typically disrupt the second pull, limiting the speed and height of the bar, and the timing and speed of the third pull.

Separation of the Barbell

The separation of the barbell from the floor should be relatively smooth—that is, it should not be jerked abruptly from its static position on the floor. This kind of separation creates two potential problems:

first, it significantly increases the likelihood of an unwanted shift in balance or position; second, if the initial speed off the floor reaches a certain threshold, the lifter will have to actually slow the bar down somewhat to maintain tension against it and continue applying force effectively. The heavier the weight, the more the first issue is a concern, but the less the second issue is probable or possible because the lifter will simply be unable to achieve that level of speed.

This should not be misinterpreted to mean that the separation of the bar should be slow, but simply that there needs to be continuous tension and force application without the allowance of slack, and inadvertent shifts in balance and position need to be avoided.

As with nearly everything in weightlifting, there are exceptions to this general rule—some world class lifters are able to consistently execute successful lifts with a vicious yank of the bar from the floor. However, like most things, experimentation with this approach to the start should be reserved for after a solid base of technical proficiency has already been established and significant training experience accumulated.

Barbell Proximity

As the lifter pushes with the legs against the floor to continue lifting the bar toward the knees, the barbell should remain as close to the lifter's legs as possible without dragging. If the shoulders are directly above or slightly forward of the bar while the bar is in light contact with the shins, any friction will be negligible unless the lifter is aggressively pushing the bar against the shins; however, contact will be problematic when the bar reaches the protrusion of the knee, which will be an obstacle for the bar to catch on. If the athlete is wearing knee sleeves, the bar will hook the bottom edge. In either case, this interruption may be significant enough to reduce bar speed and possibly cause unwanted position shifts. This being the case, ideally the bar remains as close to the shins and knees as possible without actually contacting them.

Continuing to flare the knees outward until the bar passes them will allow the maintenance of the desired posture and ease the navigation of the bar past the knees by keeping the knees back out of the way in a manner that doesn't force the shoulders down and forward. After the bar passes the knees, the active effort to flare the knees can cease, and the legs will naturally move as needed into the most advantageous position for the second pull.

Once past the knees, immediate proximity of the bar to the thighs should be maintained, ideally without contact; again, however, very light contact is preferable to any considerable distance between the bar and body. The engagement of the lats that was begun in the starting position will become most important in this stage, as the shoulders will be moving forward of the bar, requiring the lifter to actively push the weight back toward the body to prevent it from swinging forward naturally from the shoulders in a pendular action. Again, this action of the lats to push the bar toward the body is to maintain immediate proximity, not to create contact with the thighs that would cause the bar to drag up the body.

It needs to be understood that the action of pushing the bar back toward the body does not involve significant backward movement. The intent is to maintain the proximity of the bar and the body during the adjustment of the combined barbell-lifter balance after the barbell separates from the floor, and as the shoulders move in front of the bar. If the lifter does not actively push the bar back toward the body as the shoulders move forward, it will naturally swing forward away from the lifter with the shoulders. In other words, the action is really to maintain the barbell's course rather than to actually alter it.

If the lifter pushes the barbell too far back toward the hips while the shoulders are still in front of the bar, it will shift the combined weight too far back over the feet and cause either an excessive backward jump, unwanted backward movement of the feet, or an incomplete extension in compensation. Additionally, the bar will contact the hips prematurely and gather excessive forward momentum as it's pushed forward by the extending hips.

The goal is to bring the hips and barbell together in a balanced position over the feet as the trunk is reaching an approximately vertical orientation during the scoop of the second pull. In other words, the barbell and the body come together over the base rather than one being brought to the other exclusively.

Back Angle & Rigidity

As the bar rises and moves back, the lifter's trunk will shift slightly to bring the shoulders slightly forward of the bar. How much of a shift occurs will vary depending on factors such as the posture of the starting position, the lifter's proportions, the relative strength of the legs and hips, and how well controlled the movement is.

If a lifter uses a starting position with the shoulders forward of the bar rather than directly above, there should be no changing of the back angle in the first pull, as the ultimate position of the shoulders has already been established. If a lifter begins with the shoulders directly above the bar, there will be a slight shifting of the back angle as the bar moves back and the shoulders move forward, but in all cases, this should be tightly controlled and consistent to establish the optimal position. The stronger the lifter's legs are relative to the hips, and the shorter the legs are relative to the trunk, the more upright the lifter will tend to remain in the first pull, potentially maintaining the same shoulder position and posture throughout the movement. In contrast, lifters with longer legs relative to their trunks, and with weaker legs relative to hips, will tend to shift farther over the bar. (Figure 16.10)

This latter type of athlete is susceptible to excessive tipping over the bar. Technique instruction and practice will need to be geared toward preventing this, and a focus on leg and postural strength to sup-

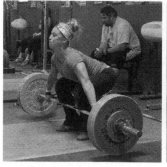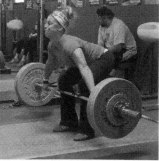

FIGURE 16.10 The back angle will change slightly in the first pull, bringing the shoulders slightly forward of the bar. The closer the shoulders begin in the starting position to this ultimate location, the less this shift will occur.

Greg Everett

port the proper positions made a priority.

Rushing the pull from the floor will typically result in the hips leading the shoulders and the lifter tipping excessively over the bar. Tension and postural control in the starting position and first pull are critical for all athletes to prevent this.

Some lifters have been very successful—to world championship levels—with a first pull that actually swings the bar slightly forward around the knees during the first pull in order to maintain a very upright posture. For a lifter with extremely strong legs, this style can be effective if done well, although ideally the shoulders remain directly above the bar rather than ever moving behind it prior to the second pull. Like with any technical idiosyncrasies, lifters should diverge from more conventional technique only after establishing technical proficiency and demonstrating a need to do so.

The spine will be responsible for transmitting the force of the legs and hips to the bar through the arms. Accordingly, its rigidity during the pull is critical, as any movement will divert force from the bar. While the acceleration during the first pull is not as rapid as in the second pull, the moment on the hips and spine will be at its greatest, so the arch established in the starting position will need to be actively and forcefully maintained to ensure the back is properly arched and rigid to resist the violent force of the subsequent second pull.

Arm Activity

The arms during the first pull serve as connections from the trunk to the barbell, and as such should remain passively extended in order for force to be transmitted as completely as possible through the body. This passive extension of the elbows can be viewed as simply allowing the weight of the bar to stretch the arms long. In other words, the arms remain straight not because they are being actively straightened, but because they are not being actively bent. Intentionally locking the elbows will encourage forward swinging of the bar during the second pull and interrupt the transition between the second and third pulls when the arms must immediately engage powerfully to pull the athlete under the bar.

While the arms remain extended and relaxed, they are by no means inactive, although their activity is indirect. The arms will remain internally rotated maximally to orient the bony points of the elbows to the sides and continue pushing the bar, through the action of the lats and shoulders, toward the body to whatever degree is necessary to maintain immediate proximity to the legs as the leg and shoulder positions change through the lift.

Speed

The position of the athlete in the first pull is one of great mechanical disadvantage—the knees and hips flexed as much as they'll be in the pull, creating the weakest leverage for the muscles responsible for extending the joints—preventing this segment of the lift from ever reaching the same speed as the second pull. The speed developed by a given lifter in the first pull, relative to the first pull of other lifters as well as to the same lifter's second pull, will vary considerably. Most of this variation is the product of the mechanics of each athlete due to their proportions and the angles created at the knee and hip joints. Generally speaking, the smaller the joint angle in the starting position and first pull, the slower the pull will be due to the poorer leverage of the muscles extending the joints. This translates in a practical sense to lifters with relatively short legs typically being capable of generating higher speeds in the first pull, all other elements being equal, in the same way that lifters with such proportions tend to demonstrate greater squat strength and speed due to the leverage advantage.

However, other factors such as the type of start employed (i.e. static or dynamic and type of dynamic), the exact starting position, and the lifter's intent to move the bar at a particular speed or at a particular level of effort will also determine the ultimate speed of the first pull at any given weight.

The first pull can remain relatively slow (compared to the second pull) without detriment to the lift. However, aside from beginning lifters still establishing technical proficiency or light warm-up weights, the first pull should not be slowed intentionally—the closer the barbell's movement is to none at all, the more force must be applied to create a given magnitude of acceleration and speed. However, as bar speed increases, the ability for the athlete to apply force decreases because the generation of force requires time—more speed means less time to generate force. In other words, if the weight is light enough, a maximal effort first pull will produce a speed at the beginning of the second pull that actually limits the athlete's ability to apply maximal force. Additionally, excessive speed in the first pull dramatically decreases the likelihood of the athlete establishing the proper position from which to initiate the second pull.

Essentially the goal is to find the ideal balance between optimal positioning, overall bar speed and the ability to maximally accelerate the bar in the second pull. That is, to move the barbell through the first pull as fast as possible without interfering with proper positioning or disrupting the acceleration and maximal bar speed of the second pull.

Conveniently, with heavy weights, excessive speed in the first pull is essentially impossible because of the natural limitations of the mechanics. Controlling the speed of the first pull is really only an issue for beginning lifters and warm-up lifts. The beginning lifter is limited by technique and consequently even his or her heaviest lifts are not heavy in terms of actual strength capacity, meaning the weights can be accelerated past a speed that allows proper positioning. This is the rationale for encouraging a relatively deliberate first pull speed for new lifters. The speed of the first pull should be gradually increased after the early learning stages once the athlete's technique is well established.

As weights begin approaching the lifter's strength capacity, the speed of the first pull will be naturally limited by the combination of the disadvantaged mechanics of the movement and heavy loading; that is, even maximal or near-maximal efforts to accelerate the bar in the first pull will result in relatively low bar speeds, eliminating the need to actively limit the speed of the first pull.

The acceleration of the bar during the first pull should never drop below zero—that is, the speed of the bar should always be increasing (early in the pull) or remaining static (later in the pull). This is a function of proper timing and positioning, as well as the constant effort to keep the bar moving. In a practical sense, this can be accomplished with a continued drive of the legs through the floor, avoiding any reduction in this effort prior to the second pull.

The Second Pull

The second pull is the final, vicious explosion of the hips and knees beginning at approximately the level of mid-thigh. This segment of the lift is the source of the highest power during the pull—as much as 150-250% of the power in the first pull (Zhekov 1976/1992). While the second pull is the final and most significant source of barbell acceleration and elevation, it should be continuous with the pull under the bar. That is, the final acceleration of the bar is as much about allowing the athlete to pull under it than it is about elevating the bar; elevation of the bar itself is meaningless without the lifter's transition underneath it. This should not be misinterpreted to mean that elevation of the barbell is unimportant—the higher the bar is elevated, the more time and space the lifter has to reposition him- or herself underneath it. The barbell's speed actually peaks approximately halfway through the second pull, not at its completion (Zhekov 1976/1992); accordingly, the final segment of the second pull must be already seamlessly feeding into the third pull. The more abrupt the final explosion in the second pull, the more easily the athlete will be able to lift and relocate the feet in the third pull—this is more related to the leg drive against the platform than the hip extension. The athlete needs to "punch" the legs through the floor with the same explosiveness with which the hips are extended to produce the optimal effect.

The athlete should consider the final explosion upward as the first stage of a single fluid movement

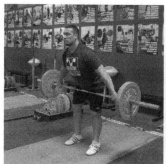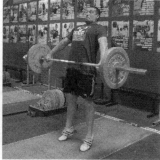

FIGURE 16.11 The second pull is the final, vicious explosion of the hips and knees at the top of the lift and begins at approximately the level of mid-thigh.

Greg Everett

also involving the pull under the bar; in other words, the second and third pulls should be considered a single continuous action rather than two distinct stages in practice. The two are separated only for the sake of instruction and analysis.

While the second pull is dramatically faster than the first, the transition between the two pulls should be seamless. Many novice lifters will mistakenly slow, pause or even reverse the bar's movement briefly as the bar reaches the thighs. Any cessation or reversal of the bar's upward movement—termed *hitching*—during the pull is in the most practical sense wholly counterproductive, and in competition is illegal. The speed of the bar will unavoidably slow during the double knee bend, but if performed properly, this reduction of speed will not be dramatic or problematic, or even observable in real time. Slowing the bar before the final acceleration is analogous to slowing a car from 60 mph to 40 mph so you can accelerate to 80 mph.

While it's not possible in the strictest sense to delineate the precise moment at which the first pull ends and the second pull begins, we will define it in a practical manner as the moment the lifter intentionally initiates the final upward explosive extension of the body. In practice, this may occur for some lifters in certain lifts as soon as the bar has passed the knees; ideally, however, it is delayed until the bar is nearing approximately mid-thigh.

Posture

In any case, the posture at the beginning of the second pull should resemble the mid-hang position discussed in detail throughout the book—the hips and knees are back with the shins approximately vertical, the shoulders are in front of the bar, the bar is in immediate proximity to the thighs, the back is forcefully and completely arched, the arms are passively extended and internally rotated, the head and eyes are directed forward, and the weight is balanced approximately over the front edge of the heel.

The patient maintenance of this posture to approximately mid-thigh is critical for maximal explosiveness, timing and balance. By waiting until the bar is at approximately the level of mid-thigh with the shoulders over it and the knees back properly before

initiating the final violent hip and knee extension of the second pull, the athlete ensures greater hamstring tension, better balance, and an uninterrupted bar path, all of which will maximize the explosiveness of the final pull. This timing is usually difficult for lifters, who will often feel they are waiting far too long to initiate the explosion. However, with practice and discipline, and specific strength work to reinforce the necessary posture as needed, the correct timing can be learned and perfected. This being said, the precise timing of the second pull will still vary among lifters; the coach simply needs to ensure that such variation is the product of the body's natural tendency to calibrate movement to maximize effectiveness based on its present state and abilities, and not a technical failure or a significant correctable weakness preventing the athlete from maintaining the ideal position.

Double Knee Bend

As the lifter initiates the second pull, the knees will begin shifting forward under the bar with the natural action of the double knee bend discussed previously in its own chapter. With proper timing and position, the double knee bend will be subtle and extremely quick. If the knees are shifting forward relatively slowly or with a dramatic degree of flexion, it's likely the lifter is initiating the second pull prematurely rather than waiting to hit the optimal position. It will be common for athletes—particularly those with legs stronger than their hips and with relatively short legs—to begin shifting the knees forward and raising the shoulders as soon as the bar passes the knees, as this transfers more of the role of elevation and acceleration of the barbell to the stronger legs.

Bar-Body Contact

Throughout the second pull, the bar should remain in immediate proximity to the thighs. This requires the lifter actively push the bar back toward the body while the shoulders remain in front of it, as well as properly time the movement and adjust the backward push of the bar to avoid dragging it on the thighs as they move forward during the double knee bend. While light contact of the bar with the thighs is preferable to significant distance between the two, dragging will both slow the bar and push it out of position.

The bar should come into full contact with the body at the crease of the hips at approximately the time the trunk reaches a vertical orientation and the knees reach their farthest forward position in the double knee bend (Figure 16.12). This position will be the farthest point back in the barbell's path, which should be approximately over the middle of the foot. If the barbell contacts the body significantly earlier, it will gain excessive horizontal force as it's driven forward by the thighs and hips. Additionally, this will typically indicate that the lifter has pushed the barbell back too far relative to the feet, which disrupts the system's balance and the mechanics of the final extension.

Maintaining immediate proximity of the bar and body prior to the bar's contact with the hips will help prevent excessive horizontal force being imparted to the bar as the hips extend violently. Considerable distance between the bar and hips prior to their contact will result in a collision with greater horizontal reactive forces, even if the extension of the hips is performed properly, while proximity will mitigate the horizontal forces of contact. A simple analogy

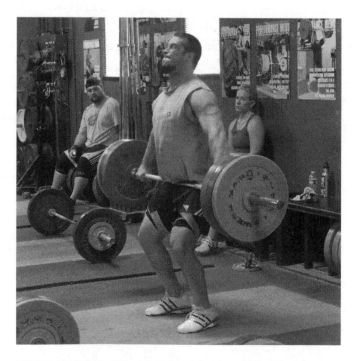

FIGURE 16.12 Ideally, the barbell achieves full contact with the body at the crease of the hips as the trunk reaches an approximately vertical orientation.

to illustrate this point is two cars facing each other: if the cars begin with their bumpers touching, even with maximal attempts to accelerate, little will occur; if the cars are backed up to create distance between them and then accelerated toward each other, the reactive forces of the resulting collision will cause each to bounce away from each other. In the same way, the bar will bounce away from the lifter's hips to a greater extent as the distance between them prior to their contact increases.

However, even if the athlete mistakenly allows the bar to move too far from the hips, or the hips are hyperextended excessively, and it is consequently bumped forward, the athlete should be actively resisting any forward movement of the bar with the same lat and shoulder tension used to maintain the bar's proximity to the body throughout the pull.

Additionally, the correct motion of the third pull will prevent the bar from moving away from the body. The same internal rotation of the arms that was set in the starting position must be maintained throughout the second pull to ensure the correct bar path during the third pull. If the elbows are not correctly oriented going into the third pull, it's unlikely the athlete will be able to make the necessary adjustment in time.

If the barbell does not contact the body at all, it is a clear indication of an error in the lift, such as a failure to extend the hips adequately, a significant forward imbalance, an attempt to pull the bar up with the arms, a failure to actively keep the bar close to the body after it has passed the knees, or, most likely, a combination of these.

This is the point of the snatch at which the width of the grip and the lifter's proportions will significantly influence the movement. Ideally the bar comes into contact with the body directly in the crease of the hips, as was described earlier in the book. This will allow the optimal movement of the knees, hips and barbell and the lifter as a whole without disruption.

If the bar connects with the upper thighs rather than the hips, it is more likely to drag against the thighs and be pushed forward somewhat as the knees move forward in the double knee bend, which will reduce the bar speed and prevent the correct motion and balance of the final extension. To some degree, the problem can be avoided, or at least mitigated, by properly timing the initiation of the second pull to

Greg Everett

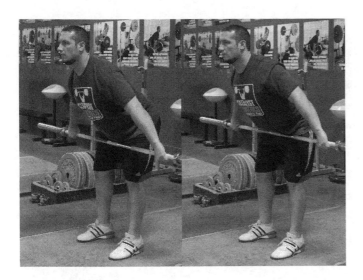

FIGURE 16.13 Lifters with long arms and short trunks, or unavoidably narrow snatch grips, can achieve a higher point of bar contact by partially shrugging the shoulders back and up during the second pull, reducing the need for arm bending.

occur with the bar higher on the thigh.

However, lifters with long arms and short torsos—or those who for whatever reason are forced to use a narrower than ideal grip—may fall outside the range of being able to avoid the problem through timing alone. The lifter can achieve a higher contact point for the bar on the body through partial retraction and elevation of the shoulder blades early in the second pull. This backward and upward shrugging action will improve the interaction of the bar with the body without requiring a bend of the arms; such a position can be maintained against the forces of the explosion more easily than a bend in the arms, resulting in less force reduction due to movement in the chain. (Figure 16.13)

Arm Activity

The arms during the second pull function as connections between the body and the bar to transmit leg and hip power. Accordingly, any extension of the arms from a partially flexed position during the explosion absorbs a portion of that force and reduces what actually reaches the barbell. Complete extension of the arms is the only way to avoid any loss of this force, and consequently such extension throughout the second pull should be the goal.

Again, this extension should be passive, with the arms remaining as relaxed as possible. If the elbows are actively extended, and the arms consequently stiff, the athlete will encounter problems when finalizing the extension. Once the bar has been accelerated upward by the extension of the legs and hips, it possesses momentum has to continue travelling somewhere. Stiff arms will delay the transition into the pull under the bar because of the additional time required to begin bending the arms (this itself is a problem because of the need for immediate transition from elevating the bar to pulling the body under it); if the arms are not bending and the bar still has upward momentum, the only option is for the bar to swing forward away from the body. For this reason, passive elbow extension is critical.

Unfortunately, neither the lifter nor the system itself is perfect, and a small degree of elbow flexion during the second pull is common (Figure 16.14). There are two basic potential causes for this. First is that such a movement is a natural way for the body to avoid early contact of the bar with the thighs; the longer the lifter's arms, shorter the lifter's trunk, and narrower the lifter's grip, the more pronounced this bending of the arms will naturally be. Lifter's with ideal proportions will likely never bend the arms unless in response to another technical error.

The second possible cause is that the body is naturally trying to preserve the barbell's speed during the movement of the knees forward under the bar, which unavoidably results in a reduction of bar speed; this bending of the arms (up to approximately 10 degrees) may cause a loss of acceleration in the final explosion, but will maintain a higher speed of the movement as a whole (Zhekov 1976/1992). To be considered acceptable, any such bending of the arms must be natural rather than intentional, and not accompanied by any other technical errors to which the bending may be a reaction.

Contributions of Legs & Hips

The second pull should be a concerted extension of the hips and knees, or described in a more practical way, an effort to push against the ground with the legs while opening the hips. Generally, based on relative strengths and proportions, athletes will be some-

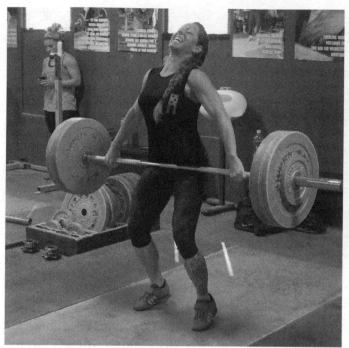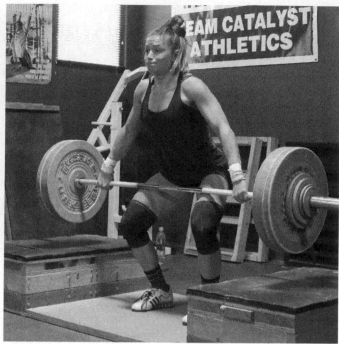

FIGURE 16.14 A small degree of elbow flexion during the second pull is acceptable if all other technical points are correct and it occurs naturally.

what more hip or knee dominant in this motion, sometimes to a degree detrimental to the lift. That is, athletes with powerful hips will tend to focus on hip extension, while athletes with stronger legs will tend to focus on pushing against the ground.

An excessive reliance on leg extension will typically result in forward imbalance, reduced bar speed, and a delayed transition under the bar. An excessive reliance on hip extension will typically result in limited bar height and forward barbell movement.

Each athletes needs to learn to coordinate knee and hip extension optimally to maximize potential barbell acceleration and elevation. This means exploiting natural strengths, mitigating the negative effects of natural weaknesses and avoiding limitations created by excessive disparity. In cases of severe disparity, specific strength work to improve the weaker of the two motions will be necessary.

While not a perfectly accurate description of the mechanics in question, in practical terms hip extension can be considered to be the primary source of speed and leg extension the primary source of elevation in the second pull. Accordingly, the optimal lift must rely on the coordinated summation of the two.

The forceful drive against the ground with the legs not only contributes acceleration and elevation

to the bar directly, but, as importantly, creates the solid foundation for the explosion of the hips. Without active extension of the knees during the extension of the hips, the force generated by the hips that is imparted to the bar will be reduced through absorption by knee flexion, and will be directed partly forward rather than completely vertically. This can be thought of as similar to jumping off of a hard, solid surface compared to jumping off of a soft, compliant surface; the former will result in maximal force being used to elevate the jumping body, whereas in the latter case, some of the generated force will be lost as the surface sinks in response to the downward force. Legs actively driving against the floor will create that solid surface, while inactive legs will absorb force like a soft surface.

Note that extension of the knees during this leg drive against the floor does not mean that the knees are extended into a locked position; "complete" leg extension in the context of the snatch (and clean) pull means the maximal degree of extension that is proper for the movement. In a well-executed lift, the knees will not reach absolute maximal extension (which for most athletes will actually be some degree of hyperextension).

Similarly, emphasizing the importance of active

and aggressive leg drive against the ground does not imply any particular timing at the top of the lift; this action must be as violent and abrupt as the explosion of the hips to prevent unwanted prolonging of the extended position. The athlete must attempt to explode the hips and knees together to achieve maximal bar speed and elevation, and then transition fluidly without hesitation into the pull under the bar.

This active leg drive also ensures that pressure is maintained between the feet and platform throughout the extension of the body. This pressure anchors the lifter in place and prevents undesired shifts of the feet and body, usually forward, but also potentially a backward sweep of the feet, that can occur as a result of powerful hip extension. For this reason, it's important this pressure be maintained until the lifter has actively begun pulling under the bar. Said another way, the leg drive must continue throughout the completion of hip extension.

The more vicious and abrupt—while remaining complete—this final burst of leg extension is, the better will be the lifter's ability to lift and relocate the feet into the receiving position. An inability to properly move the feet and plant them flat again on the platform is often related to a failure to achieve an adequately explosive drive of the legs in the final extension.

Elevation & Jumping

The purpose of the second pull is to vertically accelerate and elevate the barbell, not for the sake of elevation itself, but expressly to allow the lifter to successfully relocate under the bar. The elevation of the barbell and elevation of the body are distinct pursuits; the bar must be elevated as much as possible *relative to the body*, not the platform. That is, how high above the platform the bar is lifted is incidental; the only criterion for height is that it must be adequate for the lifter in question to move under it into the receiving position, which is dependent not just on the lifter's total height, but proportions, mobility, timing, speed, precision and overall technical proficiency.

Any elevation of the body as a whole beyond a position of maximal hip, knee and ankle extension with the feet in contact with the platform does not increase the net elevation of the bar—it is additional distance the athlete must travel back down to get under the bar. Put simply, the athlete must not jump off the platform; separation of the feet from the platform should only occur during the third pull as the lifter is traveling down and repositioning the feet into the receiving position.

This should not be misinterpreted as an implication that the term *jump* is universally inappropriate for weightlifting instruction, or that the motion of the body in the second pull is not similar in many respects to a vertical jump. The second pull does, in fact, share many similarities to the action of a vertical jump (and the term can be very useful in many cases of instruction and remediation), but there are three primary and very simple reasons the second pull does not actually produce a jump (that is, an elevation of the body's center of mass above its location in a standing position).

First, and most obviously, the athlete is attached to a heavy weight—this of course limits how much any amount of driving against the ground will elevate the athlete. Even the most powerful lifters in the world cannot meaningfully elevate the barbell-body complex with any significant weight on the bar. Second, the ultimate orientation of the body's extension is slightly backward rather than completely vertically. Third, and most importantly, once the athlete has accelerated the barbell maximally through the extension of the body (the motion of which in isolation would cause him or her to jump off the ground), he or she is immediately and aggressively pulling the body down to move under the bar. That is, at the moment in a vertical jump in which the athlete's feet would separate from the floor to allow the center of mass to move upward, the athlete is using the inertia of the barbell as an anchor to arrest and reverse any continued upward motion of the body.

The elevation of the feet specifically is not necessarily tied to the elevation of the body as a whole, as was discussed in the Foot Positions & Transition chapter of the book, and will be further discussed in the following section regarding the third pull.

Final Extension Position

At the finish of the second pull, the athlete should not be extended perfectly vertically. If a lifter standing vertically with a barbell at arms' length is viewed from profile, it can be seen that the bar is not directly above the center of the base—it must rest against the hips or thighs, which places it in front of the middle of the foot. Such a position will create a forward imbalance of the bar-body system due to the barbell's necessary location over the front of the foot; the forward imbalance will be proportional to the portion of the system's total mass the barbell represents. That is, the heavier the barbell is relative to the lifter, the more the lifter's body will need to be oriented in a way that both brings the bar farther toward the middle of the foot and places more of the body's mass behind it (Figure 16.15).

If the second pull is performed properly, the lifter will finish in a position in which the legs are oriented approximately vertically and the hips are hyperextended to some degree, bringing the shoulders behind the hips and maintaining the balance of the system over the front edge of the heel, even with the heels elevated off the platform (Figure 16.17). This position will both ensure maximal hip extension power and balance over the feet.

It's important to distinguish between vertically- and horizontally-oriented hip extension. Vertically-oriented hip extension will ensure that the force imparted to the bar is overwhelmingly vertical rather than reduced with a competing horizontal force, which will also misdirect the barbell.

If a standing lifter is viewed from the side, an imaginary vertical line can be drawn through the ankle, hip and shoulder. This line represents a convenient boundary for the hips during the pull—the hips should move forward into this line and then up along it as the second pull is performed. If the hips cross through the line, they will impart excessive horizontal force on the bar (Figure 16.17). Note this refers to the area of the hip joint, not the front of the body.

Primarily this is an issue of adequate contribution from the legs in the second pull rather than allowing the hips to dominate the movement. If the leg drive against the floor is inadequate or is ceased prematurely, the hips will likely be pushed forward of the vertical plane in which the legs should finish, pushing the bar away, reducing the vertical force and speed, and shifting the lifter's balance too far forward.

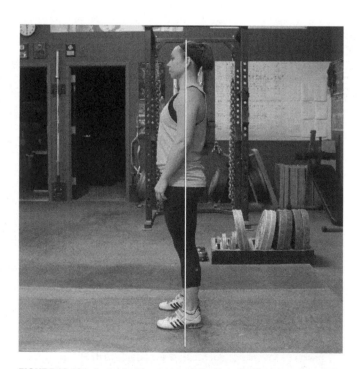

FIGURE 16.15 A barbell hanging at arms' length in a vertical standing position will be near the front of the foot. The greater the portion of the barbell-lifter system the barbell represents (i.e., the heavier the weight), the more the lifter will have to lean back (with the trunk or body as whole) in order to maintain the system's balance over the base. This is what prevents a perfectly vertical extension in the pull from being possible.

FIGURE 16.16 In the finish of the second pull, the hips should not cross through the vertical plane in which they would be with the athlete standing—a vertical line that passes approximately through the lifter's ankle, hip and shoulder. During the second pull, the hips should move forward into this plane and then up along it. Allowing the hips to cross through this plane will impart excessive horizontal force on the barbell.

Greg Everett

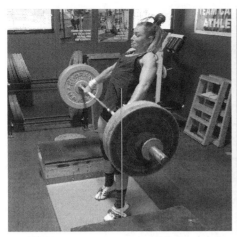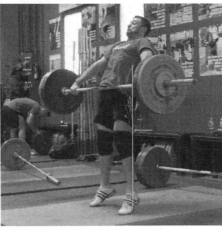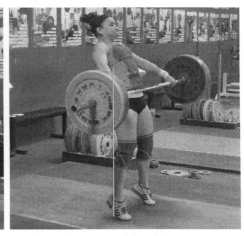

FIGURE 16.17 Vertically-oriented hip extension, the result of continue leg extension during hip extension and preventing the hips from driving forward through the bar excessively, will ensure the force imparted to the bar is overwhelmingly vertical.

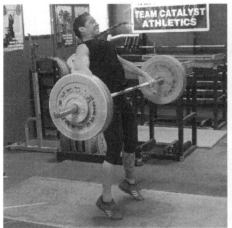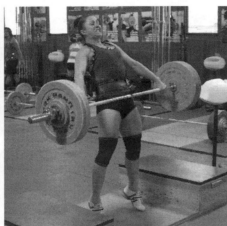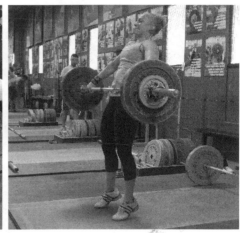

FIGURE 16.18 The precise position will vary somewhat among lifters with regard to the degree of hip and ankle extension, but the basic position should be the same: the legs oriented approximately vertically and the hips hyperextended to bring the shoulders behind the hips while maintaining balance over the feet.

Over-Extending

This desired hyperextension of the hips can be considered a backward-leaning of the body as whole, despite the legs being vertical, in the sense that the center of mass is shifted backward relative to a vertically standing position. It's important the lifter achieve the degree of hyperextension that maximizes the speed and force of the second pull and creates the optimal balance of the system.

Extending beyond this point creates two basic problems: first, the system's weight is shifted too far back over the base, directing the mass backward to some extent as well as upward; and second, excessive extension of the hips can delay the transition into the third pull, missing the window of maximal upward barbell momentum and reducing the time the lifter has to relocate under the bar. This does not mean that lifters can't be successful with sometimes extreme hip extension, but caution should be exercised to ensure this is actually benefitting the lift and not limiting it.

Because a lifter cannot actually see his or her own final extended position, this cannot be used directly as a reference except in video review. What can be evaluated by any lifter is the pressure across the foot, the approximate degree of hip extension, the speed of the transition between second and third pull, and the relative difficulty and successfulness of the lift. Additionally, the lifter will be capable of feeling where the pressure on the foot is during the earlier part of the pull, and whether or not he or she receives the bar in the same place versus jumping forward or backward during the lift; these things will provide the feedback regarding balance and indirectly, the degree of backward leaning or hip extension (Technical errors in foot movement can complicate this evaluation somewhat; that will be addressed in the third pull section.).

As the weight of the barbell increases relative to the lifter's body, how far back the body must be during the pull and in the extended position will increase to keep the combined center of mass, which is increasingly located nearer the bar, over approximately the middle of the foot or slightly farther back. This will only be true to a point, however; eventually the barbell will be essentially directly in the line of gravity once it's heavy enough, and will not ever continue farther behind this point, or the entire system would be imbalanced backward.

Jumping Backward

It is possible for a lifter to shift the system's balance too far back over the foot during the pull. This can happen through a number of different scenarios. For example, the lifter who mistakenly shifts the weight too far over the heel during the first pull will then increase this backward imbalance as he or she extends and moves more of the body's mass behind the bar; if the lifter is balanced in the first pull, an excessively extended finish position in the second pull can shift the balance backward excessively. In any case, the entire bar-body system will be directed backward rather than directly vertically over the feet, causing the lifter to jump backward during the third pull.

A backward jump in the snatch is not necessarily problematic, and in fact, some of the world's most accomplished weightlifters have used such a balance and backward jump in their snatches and cleans. Lifters for whom this backward movement is optimal will discover it naturally—there is no need to teach it explicitly. However, new lifters should work to main-

tain their original base—that is, keep the feet in the same area in which they begin—until such a habit naturally begins to develop in a way that demonstrates its effectiveness.

If this style does in fact allow an athlete to perform better, it should be allowed; however, vigilance should be continued to prevent it from becoming excessive and passing the threshold of productivity. There will be a point after which any further backward shifting of balance over the feet or increase in extension or backward leaning at the top of the pull will fail to improve the lifter's performance. Usually this is due to the body, or at least the feet, moving farther backward than the bar does, making it impossible to secure the bar overhead (the same basic effect of the bar moving forward away from the lifter). Such a backward imbalance can be considered excessive if the distance of the resulting backward jump is greater than can be reasonably compensated for by the slight backward trajectory of the bar and the power of the athlete's third pull. A general idea would be a maximum of approximately 3-4 inches of backward foot movement.

As will be discussed with regard to the third pull, backward movement during the lift may actually be the result of an error in foot placement, rather than direction of the entire system's center of mass slightly backward. It will be important to distinguish between the two so errors can be corrected before they become habit.

Jumping Forward

While a moderate backward jump, if all else is correct, can be acceptable and effective, a forward jump is invariably indicative of an error in the lift. There are a multitude of possible causes for this that can be found in the first, second or third pulls. In the second pull specifically, it will typically be the result of inadequate hip extension that fails to balance the system at the top of the pull, excessive horizontally-oriented hip extension that moves the bar forward from its ideal upward trajectory, or inadequate leg drive against the floor in the presence of adequate hip extension. Possible causes and corrections are discussed in detail in the Error Corrections section of the book.

Grip Security

The security of the grip on the bar during the second pull in particular is critical for successful lifting. The wide grip of the snatch directly increases the amount of force the hands must resist. With the arms hanging vertically, the weight of the bar and the forces created during the pull are shared by each hand as 50% of the weight or force. As the arms move away from vertical (with a widening grip) and the effect of vector forces become involved, the amount of force increases with the same weight on the barbell, and the force increases further beyond the actual weight of the bar with the effort to accelerate it. With a full snatch-width grip, the force each hand needs to resist at the peak of acceleration can increase to as much as 150% of that in a vertical arm orientation (Zhekov 1976/1992).

Add to this unfortunate fact of physics the problem of the hands' reduced connection to the bar because of the angle—that is, the third and fourth fingers for most lifters will have much less purchase on the bar relative to the clean grip—and the security of the grip is being tested to an extreme degree.

Because the body will respond to grip weakness or insecurity naturally by reducing the speed of the barbell to reduce the forces the grip must resist, grip weakness can significantly limit a lifter's performance in the snatch. This is one of the reasons many lifters are capable of snatching significantly more weight with straps than they are without—the dramatically increased grip security removes the body's self-limiting response to grip insecurity.

For this reason, developing and maintaining excellent grip strength is critical for all new lifters, and the use of straps for snatching in training must be judicious.

Ankle Extension

In the final extended position of the second pull, the lifter's ankles will be extended to some degree, lifting the heels and bringing the lifter onto the balls of the feet. Two points are critical to understand with regard to ankle extension in the pull. First, the lifter's line of gravity should remain in the same position throughout the pull (approximately running through the front edge of the heel when the lifter is flat-footed) despite the center of pressure shifting forward to the balls of the foot; this concept was discussed earlier in the Learning the Snatch chapter with regard to the mid-hang snatch pull drill. Second, this ankle extension should not be performed intentionally as an isolated action.

There are a few of considerations with regard to the extension of the ankles (plantar flexion) during the second pull of the snatch or clean. The structure of the ankle is one that is able to produce great magnitudes of force due to the class-two lever created with the insertion of the calf muscles behind the ankle joint. That is, the force lever arm—from the fulcrum of the balls of the foot—to the point of force application—the insertion of the calf muscles—is longer than the resistance lever arm from the fulcrum to the point of loading—the attachment of the body and barbell at the ankle joint.

This unusual mechanical advantage allows heavy loads to be lifted through ankle extension; however, it simultaneously results in less potential speed. In any case of mechanical advantage, the end of the force lever arm must travel farther than the end of the resistance lever arm; that is, the calf muscles must contract a great deal to produce relatively little motion, and consequently that motion will naturally be slower relative to another joint in which the mechanics are opposite (i.e. a shorter contraction produces a longer movement). In short, plantar flexion is not a significant contributor to the speed of the barbell directly.

However, this does not mean that plantar flexion does not play an important role in the pull of the snatch (or clean). Ankle extension is naturally coupled with an aggressive drive of the legs against the ground. A simple way to illustrate this idea is to instruct an athlete to perform a standing vertical jump without extending his or her ankles—the resulting jump will not only be remarkably awkward, but its height not even measurable on the same scale as a natural vertical jump effort. This is why, in the pull of the snatch, plantar flexion is expected—not because the athlete is intentionally extending the ankles directly to contribute speed or elevation to the bar, but because the athlete is driving aggressively against the ground with the legs until reaching full extension, and plantar flexion is a natural part of this action; attempting to prevent it will reduce the power of the leg extension.

The actual degree of plantar flexion will vary among lifters, depending largely on their relative reliance on hip and leg extension: a lifter who is more hip-dominant will typically demonstrate less ankle extension that a lifter who is more leg-dominant. However, this can be altered somewhat by the lifter's timing of the transition into the third pull or inadequate power in the legs at certain weights.

As has been discussed previously, there are individual variations in lift technique among lifters for numerous reasons from anatomical to pedagogical, and such variations are not necessarily incorrect or problematic. These are idiosyncrasies that should be allowed to develop after the stage of basic technical proficiency attainment; in the early stages of learning, significant plantar flexion in the second pull of the snatch should be expected in all lifters.

An absence of plantar flexion is often an indication that a lifter is failing to drive aggressively enough or is ceasing that leg drive prematurely. Similarly, it will occur with maximal snatch attempts in which the lifter may simply not have the strength and power capacity to produce adequate leg drive.

Ankle extension should generally occur late in the second pull. Ideally, the lifter remains flat-footed through the double knee bend, and the ankles extend with the final explosive drive through the floor with the legs. However, some lifters will naturally lift the heels to a small degree earlier (during the double knee bend) without negatively affecting the lift—this is acceptable if proper balance and timing is maintained in the lift. For such lifters, attempting to force flat feet longer through the pull will typically have more of a negative than positive effect.

The Shrug & Third Pull Continuity

Again, because it warrants repetition, the second pull should be considered continuous with the third pull. There should be no hesitation or delay between the completion of the final explosion of the hips and knees and the violent pull of the athlete under the bar. Time spent in the extended position of the second pull only reduces the time available for the lift-er to relocate under the bar; it does not contribute any further speed, which peaks approximately halfway through the final upward explosion, when the trunk is approximately 10-15 degrees short of vertical (Zhekov 1976/1992). Continuing to pull upward on the bar in the fully extended position will achieve more barbell elevation (such as in a snatch high-pull), but such elevation will be occurring with rapidly diminishing bar speed, reducing and eventually eliminating the very small window of opportunity the lifter has to move under the barbell.

As was discussed in the context of the snatch learning progression, the acceleration and elevation of the bar is achieved overwhelmingly through the violent and concerted extension of the knees and hips, and the follow-through of ankle extension (incidentally, the extension of these three joints is the basis for the term *triple extension*, often used to describe the correct final position of the second pull).

The upward shrug of the shoulders is not a direct contributor to this acceleration and elevation of the bar. It occurs considerably later than the point of maximal bar speed in the second pull and consequently can't contribute meaningfully to bar speed, but more importantly, the shrug is largely a transitional movement, and while started in the second pull, should be completed during the third pull. It is in practical terms part of the arms' movement to pull the lifter under the bar, which begins in the last moment of the second pull. In other words, if the shrug is completed while the athlete is in a fully extended position at the top of the second pull, the transition under the bar is too late.

In the final upwardly extended position of the second pull, the lifter should be on the balls of the feet with the heels elevated, the legs straight and approximately vertical, the hips hyperextended to bring the shoulders behind the hips, and the shoulders partially shrugged up and arms beginning to bend as they pull against the bar. This initiation of the arms' pull against the bar (which naturally includes the shrugging motion) will ensure continuity with the third pull, help avoid any delay in the transition and excessive reduction of bar speed, and prevent unwanted shifts in balance or foot position during the third pull by maintaining pressure of the lifter's feet against the floor.

The Third Pull

The third pull is the athlete's relocation under the barbell after having accelerated and elevated it with the extension of the body in the first and second pulls—the movement from the fully extended position into the receiving position (overhead squat). Many athletes and coaches misunderstand this final part of the snatch or clean as *dropping* under or *catching* the bar. The third pull must be just as active and vicious as the second, and passivity or a lack of connection to the bar will prevent success as weights increase—as the term suggests, this segment of the lift is an aggressive *pull* under the barbell.

In order to execute lifts with maximal loading—in which, as weights increase, the maximum possible upward speed and elevation decrease—the lifter must increase the speed of his or her descent under the bar beyond what will occur naturally by falling strictly under the influence of gravity.

The third pull can be considered a series of three phases, defined by the basic motions occurring in each: the initial pull down against the barbell, the turnover of the arms from above to below the bar, and the push up against the bar by the arms.

Momentum & Acceleration

The violent explosion of the hips and knees in the second pull has maximally accelerated the barbell up-

ward. In addition to the elevation it has gained simply by virtue of being attached to the arms as the body extended upward, at this point the bar possesses momentum from the force applied to it and will continue its upward movement temporarily even with the removal of all external force application. The distance and time the bar will continue traveling upward under this momentum decreases as the weight of the barbell increases because maximal force application will have accelerated the bar less. This being true, the heavier the barbell, the sooner its upward travel will be arrested and reversed by the force of gravity, and the more critical the active, aggressive third pull becomes.

After finalizing the extension of the hips and knees in the second pull, the lifter will immediately retract the hips and bend the knees to begin a squatting movement. However well-timed and quick this may be, this movement alone will not reposition the lifter under the bar. Unless the feet are attached to the ground, the lifter cannot pull his or her body down significantly faster than the speed of gravity by simply flexing the knees and hips (the lifter will get some downward acceleration beyond the pull of gravity through this action because of the inertia of the legs, but it will be minimal and the effort will elevate the feet as it lowers the rest of the body).

Because objects fall under the force of gravity at the same rate irrespective of their masses (assuming no interference of friction), it should be clear that the athlete cannot simply drop after the second pull and expect to arrive underneath the barbell—at the

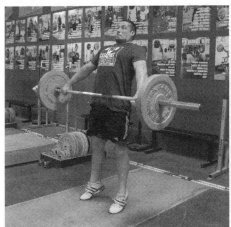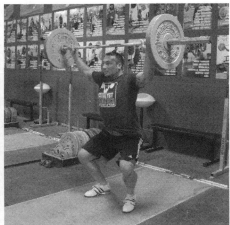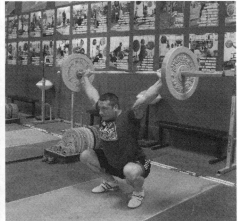

FIGURE 16.19 The third pull brings the lifter from the fully extended position into the receiving position under the barbell.

peak of the second pull, the barbell is near the level of the abdomen and must finish at arms' length overhead, meaning the athlete's body must travel a great distance relative to the barbell. Even in consideration of the momentary continued upward travel of the bar under its own momentum and the small degree of downward acceleration possible from flexing the hips and knees in the squatting motion, it's impossible to rely entirely on gravity to accomplish this repositioning underneath the bar.

Barbell Inertia as Anchor

During the first and second pulls, the inertia of the earth itself is used as the anchor against which the athlete applies force with the lower body to move the barbell. After upward acceleration of the bar has occurred, the barbell's inertia in its elevated position becomes the new anchor against which the athlete must apply force. This is accomplished by removing the pressure of the feet against the platform—they do not necessarily need to lose contact, but the force against the ground must be less than the force being applied to the bar. The closer the force against the ground is to zero, the less resistance to the downward movement of the lifter there will be, and the faster the pull under the bar can be.

In other words, there is no real difference in the force application to the bar during the three pulls—the real difference is that in the first and second pulls, the lifter is using the ground as the anchor for force application, and in the third pull, the lifter is using the barbell as the anchor for force application. Additionally, the lower body is responsible for the force generation in the first and second pulls, while the upper body is responsible for the force generation in the third pull.

The Arms & Barbell Elevation

The commonly expressed notion that the barbell is not lifted by the pulling of the arms is not entirely accurate. Insisting arm bend doesn't contribute to the elevation of the barbell is more of a coaching cue than a statement of fact—it's intended to discourage rowing the barbell up with the arms as a substitute

for hip and knee extension.

While the net effect of the continued effort to pull the barbell with arm flexion following the completion of knee and hip extension is the movement of the athlete under the bar, the bar is in fact further elevated simultaneously to a degree consistent with its relative mass and upward momentum. The heavier the barbell is relative to the athlete, and the greater its relative inertia, the farther the athlete will move down relative to the barbell as a result of any given magnitude of pulling force against it.

Assuming the force applied by the athlete during the entire lift remains constant among attempts (maximal in this case), the height at which the barbell is received will be determined by the relative masses of the athlete and the barbell. The heavier the barbell, the less it will be accelerated in the first and second pull, the lower its upward speed, the less it will be elevated by that upward momentum, and the sooner it will change directions and begin falling. This is the first element determining the relative magnitudes of the barbell and lifter movements.

With a maximal effort in the third pull—that is, the athlete pulling with the arms against the barbell to move down—how far the lifter travels down and how far the barbell continues traveling upward as a result of this force will depend on the relative masses of the bar and body. A heavier barbell will result in less upward travel of the barbell, more downward travel of the athlete, and a lower receiving position; a lighter barbell will result in more upward travel of the barbell, less downward travel of the athlete, and a higher receiving position. In other words, if the efforts of the lifter remain constant and maximal, it is the relative masses of the barbell and lifter that dictate the height at which the bar is fixed overhead. This can only be altered through the manipulation of force application or timing at some point during the lift.

Pulling Down

The first of the three phases of the third pull is the change of direction and downward acceleration of the body. This reversal of direction by the athlete must be as vicious as the explosion of the second pull in order to capitalize on the barbell's temporary upward inertia. The motion is the result of the lifter's active pull against the bar with the arms in the absence of resistance against the ground from the legs. This motion is a pull of the elbows up and out to the sides (the latter will happen naturally if the arms are internally rotated as they should be during this pulling motion). The points of the elbows must remain oriented to the sides as much as possible prior to and during this motion to ensure the proper mechanics, as learned and practiced with drills like the tall muscle snatch and tall snatch.

This pull of the elbows up and out will naturally be accompanied by a shrugging motion, both of which began in the last moment of the second pull. The shrug of the shoulders does not need to be performed directly as its own motion, and doing so will only slow the movement. Pulling the elbows up and out as high as possible will naturally result in the elevation of the shoulders—attempting such a motion without a shrug is an awkward action that must be done intentionally. However, the shoulder blades should be intentionally retracted.

The need for this initial pull of the elbows up and out to be aggressive and complete should be underscored. The turnover of the arms—external rotation—is not a strong movement. The strongest athletes can move very little weight in this motion. The key to executing this portion of the pull under is generating momentum during the initial pull down with the arms—that is, for the athlete to accelerate the body downward as much as possible. If this movement is fast and the body and bar are moving past each other with adequate momentum and proximity to each other, the turnover can occur quickly and smoothly. Without that speed and proximity, the athlete will be attempting to externally rotate the arms against a great deal of force, and will be unsuccessful.

This orientation of the arms and elbows is critical for maintaining the proximity of the barbell to the body while simultaneously accelerating the lifter down. Proximity can be maintained by pulling the elbows back instead of up and out (which is common in both the snatch and clean), but this prevents the maximal downward acceleration of the lifter by transforming the third pull into what is in essence single continuous external rotation of the arms—the weakest way to achieve the movement.

Clarification is necessary regarding this upward movement of the elbows, as it is frequently misinterpreted, misrepresented and misunderstood. First, the direction up is relative to the lifter's trunk, not an imaginary vertical line. In other words, the reference is the current angle of the trunk—up means moving toward the shoulders and head. If the trunk is angled backward as it will be in the finish of the second pull and during the initial phase of the third pull, the elbows will be moving back to a proportional degree relative to a vertical plane.

Further, the movement is not perfectly upward—there is a slight backward inclination as the shoulder blades are shrugged up and back to aid in the effort to maintain the barbell's proximity to the body during the third pull. The important point is that the elbows must first move primarily up toward the head and shoulders, and ideally reach approximately the level of the shoulders, before the arms are turned over. In a snatch, this will be a very brief movement, but that action will have a dramatic influence on the subsequent movement of the barbell and body.

The extent to which the elbows can be elevated directly toward the shoulders will be governed by the lifter's shoulder mobility—the less mobile the lifter's shoulders in internal rotation, the more the elbows will be forced to move backward during an effort to lift them upward while maintaining the bar's proximity to the body. In no case will the forearms be parallel with the trunk, as this would require that the shoulders be protracted significantly to bring the shoulders directly above the bar (Figure 16.20).

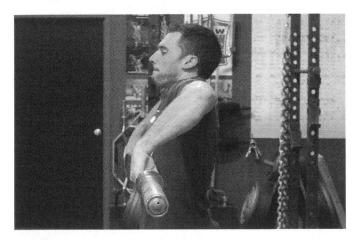

FIGURE 16.20 Even with ideal shoulder mobility and arm movement in the third pull, the forearms will not be parallel with the trunk, as this would require that the shoulders protract significantly and the lifter's trunk be inclined over the bar.

Additionally, the elbows will not reach the maximum height possible within the limits of mobility and structure for that athlete. This maximum height will be used during certain related learning, remedial and training exercises, such as high-pulls, but because of the requirements of timing, it will not be achieved during the snatch itself and other exercises with similar timing requirements and limitations, such as the tall snatch. However, the maximum height possible during the lift in question is the goal, and even more important is the intent to aggressively elevate them accordingly, as this again is the basis of the lifter's combined downward acceleration and maintenance of bar-body proximity.

The action of the pull under will also include retraction of the shoulder blades in the finalization of the upward pull of the elbows and the transition into the turnover phase.

Repositioning of the Feet

The repositioning of the feet, as discussed in the Foot Positions & Transition chapter of the book, serves two primary purposes: to move the feet into a stance better suited for the squat, as this is for most lifters different from their pulling stances, and the elimination of any resistance against the ground that could reduce the lifter's downward acceleration under the barbell.

As was mentioned previously, in order to pull under the bar, the feet do not actually have to lose contact with the platform—the pressure on them simply needs to be reduced dramatically, and ideally removed completely during the initial pull down. The only way to ensure zero pressure is to establish zero contact; consequently, the way to maximize potential downward speed is to lift the feet completely from the platform.

Elevation of the feet has additional benefits. If the lifter's balance is not maintained perfectly during the pull and the system's center of mass is traveling forward or backward as a result, the elevation of the feet will allow the lifter's base to move along with the rest of the system and be re-established in a position that can support the new location of the center of mass. If the feet remain planted on the floor, any movement of the center of mass forward or backward will result in the system not being supported directly by the base.

Further, more elevation of the feet will allow the lifter to plant the feet flat on the platform as desired more easily. Naturally the toes will be below the heels during the initiation of the third pull due to the extension of the ankles in the second pull. In order for the feet to reconnect flat with the floor, this needs to be adjusted. If the feet as a whole are inadequately elevated, the balls of the feet will reconnect with the floor before the athlete has the opportunity to reposition them properly. Even if the feet happen to land in the correct position relative to the body, this is not the ideal way to reconnect with the floor, but it is also likely that in such an event, the feet will actually be too far back relative to the system rather than directly underneath it as they need to be.

Finally, an aggressive reconnection of the feet with the platform helps the muscles of the lower body prepare to productively absorb the impending downward force.

Elevation of the feet is not without its potential drawbacks, however. Most notably, excessive elevation can create the potential for the bar-lifter system to "fall" in a way that creates a crashing effect, which then makes stabilizing the barbell overhead more difficult. However, this is related more to the interaction of the lifter and the barbell during the turnover and the timing of the reconnection of the feet; it is not a necessary a product of foot elevation.

Many world-class lifters are successful with everything from no elevation of the feet, to dramatic elevation; which best suits a given lifter will depend on a number of factors. New lifters are encouraged to learn and practice elevation of the feet during the third pull until it can be determined reliably that a different method is more effective for them.

The timing of the separation of the feet from the floor will have numerous effects on the lift from the barbell's ultimate elevation to the balance in the pull to the final placement of the feet in the receiving position. Ideally the feet are lifted a split second after the lifter begins pulling under the bar. This ensures maximal pressure against the ground during the final explosion and the accompanying bar elevation and balance of the system. At the earliest, the feet should be lifted at the moment the final explosion of the second pull is completed—that is, at the moment the greatest point of hip, knee and ankle extension is reached. Separation prior to this will result in a reduction of barbell acceleration and elevation, a reduced window for the successful execution of the third pull, unwanted shifts in the balance of the system, and improper positioning of the feet relative to the bar-body center of mass.

It's important during the third pull to elevate the feet by performing a squatting motion rather than isolated knee flexion, which will be more natural for most athletes. That is, the lifter needs to intentionally flex the hip and lift the knees in order to simultaneously elevate the feet and move the body downward. This motion will help maintain the position of the feet relative to the rest of the body, as well as help orient the soles of the feet parallel to the floor to allow a flat reconnection. If the knees are not actively lifted, the feet will likely be elevated primarily through knee flexion, which will bring the feet backward as well as up as the lower leg rotates around the knee, and will naturally angle the soles of the feet even more relative to the floor, rather than bring them into a horizontal orientation.

The feet should be reconnected flat on the floor with aggression, which will produce an audible stomping noise. This noise should not be a goal in and of itself, but can be used as a diagnostic to evaluate the execution of the movement. If a sharp clap is absent, it indicates either a lack of aggression, inadequate elevation, or a reconnection of the balls of the foot before the heel rather than the whole sole of the foot together.

The issue of jumping versus elevating the feet is discussed in detail in the Foot Positions & Transitions chapter of the book. In short, elevation of the feet during downward movement of the body as occurs in the third pull does not constitute jumping and should not be misinterpreted as such.

The Turnover

The second phase of the third pull is the turnover of the arms, bringing them from above the bar to below it. This is the actual external rotation of the arms at the shoulders that follows the initial upward and outward pull of the elbows to accelerate the lifter down and create the momentum and proximity necessary for a successful turnover.

The turnover needs to accomplish three basic tasks: bringing the bar and body into their final relative fore-aft positions, bringing the lifter and bar to the relative heights necessary for the athlete to fix the bar in the overhead position, and maintaining the tightest proximity possible of the bar and body.

As the elbows reach their maximal height during the first phase of the third pull, the athlete will turn the arms over, retracting the shoulder blades and bringing the elbows back slightly in the process to maintain the minimal possible distance between the bar and body. The elbows should remain at approximately the same height relative to the shoulders during the turnover, which will require the athlete continue to actively pull the elbows up relative to the shoulders throughout the turnover rather than allowing them to drop as they will naturally be inclined to (Figure 16.21).

The speed and success of the turnover will be dependent on three primary factors: the proximity of the bar to the body, the existing downward momentum of the body and upward momentum of the barbell, and the aggression of the lifter.

The lifter's aggression during the movement

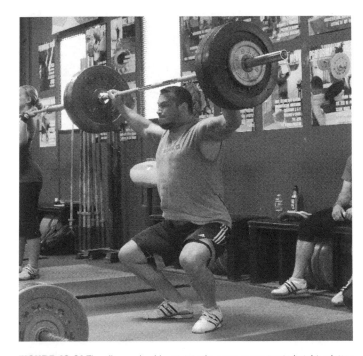

FIGURE 16.21 The elbows should maintain the same approximate height relative to the shoulders (approximately shoulder height) throughout the turnover rather than being allowed to drop from their highest position.

should, of course, be maximal in order to preserve as much of the existing speed of the barbell and body through this relatively weak phase of the lift. This will allow the lifter to complete the movement as quickly as possible, which means more time and space in which to establish an effective receiving position under the bar and prepare to absorb its downward force.

The closer the barbell is to the body, the better the mechanics will be due to reduced lever arm length, and the less resistance the upper body will encounter in the necessary motion of the arms and shoulders. This proximity will also help maintain the balance of the system over the base by concentrating the combined mass it rather than allowing it to spread and potentially shift balance.

The existing downward speed of the lifter and upward speed of the barbell will allow this relatively weak motion to occur with two massive objects it otherwise would not be capable of influencing to any meaningful extent.

The bar will reach its maximal height and begin its downward travel during this phase of the third pull. Without adequate upward momentum of the bar and downward momentum of the lifter, the lifter will be incapable of completing the turnover in time to establish a position under the bar from which to push up against it. The faster the turnover can be completed, the sooner the lifter can establish this position and begin resisting the bar's downward force, and the more easily stability and security can be established.

Along with speed, accuracy is necessary for a successful turnover. This involves the precision of the barbell's location horizontally relative to the lifter's body—that is, movement of the bar behind the lifter's head and over the lifter's base, which of course involves also the movement of the body relative to the barbell—and the vertical location of the body relative to the bar—that is, the body must remain connected to the bar so that at the point of achieving the correct overhead position, the barbell does not drop down onto the lifter, but is secured tightly and absorbed by the lifter's squatting legs.

The latter is an issue primarily of maintaining the grip on the bar long enough through the turnover; a premature loosening of the grip coupled with an indiscriminate drop down into a deep squat creates the opportunity for the barbell crashing. The depth of the squat should be governed by the height of the bar exclusively. In other words, the lifter must pull under the bar, not simply squat down as deep as possible irrespective of the height of the bar. Maintaining this relationship with the bar will ensure a solid receipt at any height and weight.

Push Up

The final phase of the third pull, following the initial pull down and the turnover, is a push up against the bar. This is a critical movement, as it is what truly secures the bar in the overhead position and establishes the controllable vertical orientation of force; without it, the bar may arrive in or near the final position, but will not remain there except with a perfect combination of relatively light weights and luck.

The distance of this pushing motion will be very short; in most cases, it will not be observably distinct from the rest of the third pull in real time. The key is its vertical orientation and aggressiveness—punching straight up against the bar to finalize the lifter's movement into the necessary squat depth and resist the downward momentum the barbell has gained during the final moments of the turnover phase.

The lifter should attempt to complete the turnover of the bar and be pushing straight up against it at the same time the feet reconnect flat with the platform. In reality, the feet will nearly always reconnect with the platform prior to the completion of the turnover, but the attempt to time the two actions together will encourage greater speed and aggression. The turnover of a well-performed lift viewed in real time will appear to finish at the same time the feet reconnect; this is a more important criterion than the actual timing that can be observed in slow-motion analysis of the lift. To the observer, the sound of the feet meeting the platform again should coincide with the lifter's punch up against the bar overhead.

The reconnection of the feet with the floor means that the athlete's push up against the bar is both driving him or her down into a deeper squat, but also beginning to slow the barbell's descent. The resistance applied in this squat position must balance the need to support and stabilize the bar while simultaneously allowing enough downward movement of the athlete to achieve a complete lockout position overhead. In other words, the athlete needs to fluidly and immediately sit into a squat of the depth necessary to achieve the locked out overhead position, but with enough control and resistance to arrest the downward movement and prevent the barbell from crashing down. This will require a smoothly increasing degree of tension in the legs as the athlete reaches the bottom of the squat.

As the arms transition from pulling to pushing, the hands are flipped over into their final position with the wrist extended and the hands relaxed enough to allow a quick and complete extension of the elbows while tight enough to maintain control of the bar. This motion must occur after the pulling motion against the bar is complete—if the grip is relaxed to flip the hand over too early, the athlete will lose the necessarily tight connection to the bar in the turnover and typically the bar will end up too far forward overhead.

Many athletes, particularly males, will not be able to turn the hand over and achieve a stable hand and wrist position while maintaining the hook grip. With the exception of individuals who have adequate mobility and slender enough fingers (female lifters most commonly meet these criteria, the effects of which are then magnified by the smaller barbell diameter), the hook grip will limit the mobility of the hand and wrist.

Those with adequate mobility can maintain the hook grip as long as the speed of the turnover of the hand is the same and final hand and wrist position are correct, solid and comfortable. If maintaining the hook grip appears to be the correct choice for a given lifter, but some discomfort is present in the overhead position, it may simply require some time for the hands and wrists to become conditioned. The hook grip should be used in all snatch-related overhead work (such as overhead squats and snatch push presses) to ensure this conditioning occurs.

The release of the hook grip is more of a passive movement than an intentional action—that is, the hook grip is not released because the athlete is pulling it out through significant movement of the hand, but because the athlete is not attempting to maintain it while simultaneously flipping the hand and wrist over. If the hook grip is not held tightly, this turnover of the hand and wrist should allow the

thumb to slide out from under the fingers. As part of this turnover, the athlete should think of driving the heel of the palm straight up—because the bar will be slightly behind the heel of the palm, this action will encourage the wrist to turn over and the bar to settle into the hand properly, as well as feed into the action of punching up against the bar to secure it overhead.

Bar Path & Proximity

The backward lean of the torso achieved at the end of the second pull will be continued in the initial phase of the third pull to allow the athlete to complete the pull under the bar with minimal disruption to its desired path. This layback should be as minimal as possible in order to keep the combined center of mass concentrated over the base to reduce extraneous movement and limit the potential for imbalance, as well as ensure optimal mechanics. As the athlete pulls under, the torso will begin coming forward again so that as the trunk and head pass the bar, the torso can continue into its final position in the squat, which will be one of slight forward inclination as learned in the context of the overhead position.

The athlete will be attempting to maintain as direct of a bar path as possible. It will never be perfectly straight due simply to the mechanics of the body, but the closer it is within the constraints of those mechanics, the more effective the movement. The bar will travel slightly forward during the third pull and then back into its final position overhead. The layback initiated in the second pull and continued in the third pull will open a clear path for the bar (and balance the combined center of mass), while the efforts of the third pull will guide it, and the body, to their final positions relative to each other. This path is impossible with a vertical torso, as can be easily demonstrated with a muscle snatch viewed from the side (Figure 16.22)—the bar must travel forward around the chest and then back into position overhead. The athlete leans back away from the bar to counterbalance it during this movement rather than allowing the bar to drift forward.

Occasionally athletes will intentionally flex the wrists during the snatch and clean in the mistaken belief (or according to the request of a coach) that it's a necessary action to keep the bar close to the

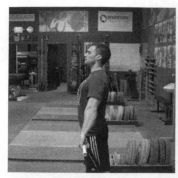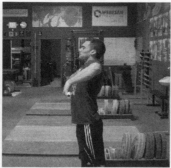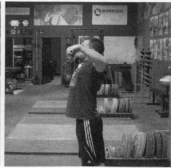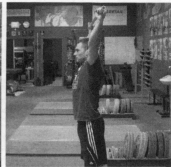

FIGURE 16.22 If the lifter's trunk is vertical, the barbell must travel forward to move around it into the overhead position, shifting the combined barbell-body center of mass too far forward when significant weights are being lifted. The backward lean of the trunk established in the finish of the second pull will continue during the initial downward movement of the lifter in the third pull, clearing a more direct path for the barbell and helping to maintain a balanced combined center of mass.

body. It should be understood that wrist flexion will occur naturally during the third pull of both lifts due to the activation of arm flexor groups, and that the wrists should be allowed to remain neutral during the first and second pulls (or very slightly flexed as described in the Hook Grip chapter). This wrist flexion is unnecessary to maintain barbell proximity, and is similar in effect to premature elbow flexion in that it creates a component in the chain that can be re-extended by the power of the knee and hip extension, reducing the transfer of power to the bar. The proximity of the barbell to the body should be maintained through the action of the arms and shoulders, and begin with the correct movement of the barbell and body leading into the third pull.

Receiving the Bar

At the point at which the lifter has finished turning the bar over and is pushing vertically against it, the lifter will be in some degree of squat with the body and bar positioned in accordance to the description provided previously with regard to the overhead squat. Movement of the bar and lifter must now be arrested and the system stabilized in a balanced position over the feet. Just as with each prior segment of the lift, successful receipt of the bar must be active and aggressive.

Failure to actively secure the correct overhead position immediately and aggressively will cause the bar to drop in front or behind the lifter, or possibly the collapse of the support structure, resulting at best in

illegal elbow flexion. At this point, the lifter should be focused on confining all movement to the vertical plane. That is, the lifter should be actively punching up vertically against the bar while sitting in vertically to the bottom of the squat. This vertical alignment is what allows stability. Significant horizontal movement of the barbell or body at this point will usually be impossible to control. This vertical alignment is possible only with the delivery of the barbell to the correct position overhead, the correct position of the body in relation to the bar, the proper placement of the feet on the platform, and the correctly timed and positioned movement of the athlete down into the squat during the third pull. None of these things can be manipulated to any considerable degree by this point in the lift.

The air pressure being used to stabilize the torso should be maintained. Release of the breath at this point will reduce structural integrity and potentially result in either a missed lift or injury. This is the point of the lift at which the torso will be managing the greatest compressive forces, and consequently the added rigidity from pressurization is critical to prevent unwanted flexion of the spine or other shifting in positioning.

The depth of the squat at the moment of receipt will never be absolute bottom in even the deepest receiving position, although extremely proficient snatchers will manage to come remarkably close. This distance above absolute bottom, however minimal, allows the athlete to absorb the downward force of the bar with the legs and make microadjustments to establish stability. The heavier the barbell, the clos-

Greg Everett

er to the bottom of the squat the third pull will be completed; lighter snatches will be received at higher levels commensurate with the weights and the greater maximal height the barbell is able to reach. As was discussed above, lifters must always stay tightly connected to the bar and move under it accurately, meeting it at the height to which it has been elevated, rather than dropping indiscriminately into the bottom of the squat.

While the athlete will obviously need to apply effort during the bar's receipt to begin resisting its downward force, it's important that he or she not attempt to lock up the legs abruptly as one would when arresting a power snatch. The athlete should allow the bar to push him or her down into the bottom of the squat and finalize the tightness of this receiving position there. Attempts to lock up too much too soon will limit the ability to stabilize the bar and result in a more jarring receipt, which itself can decrease stability and is certainly harder on the body in any case.

While in the clean, it's critical for the athlete to utilize the bounce effect to recover from the squat with weights that may be very near a maximal front squat effort, the priority in the snatch is stability and security of the bar. Premature recovery attempts with an unstable overhead position will most often simply magnify such instability and push the bar farther to whatever direction it's shifting; for example, an attempt to rush a recovery with a bar that is slightly forward will typically push it even farther forward to the point at which it can't be supported.

It should be obvious that the more precise the lift, the more accurately placed the barbell and body will be and the less effort will be necessary to establish stability and security (and the greater the chance of the lift being successful). That said, perfection is rare, and some degree of effort, however minimal, will usually be required to stabilize the bar. It's critical this stabilization take place before the athlete attempts to recover from the squat. Often athletes will rush the recovery and lose a lift that should have otherwise presented no problem. Exceptions are cases in which movement of the feet is necessary, which will be facilitated by at least partial recovery from the squat. Of course, in the event the bar is obviously

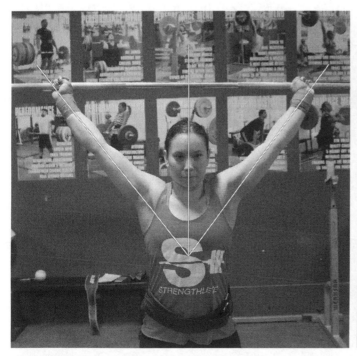 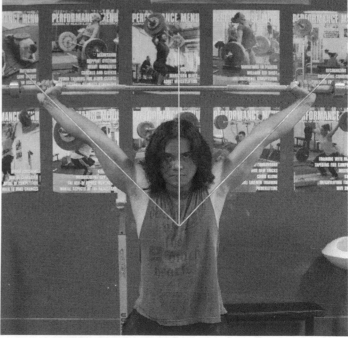

FIGURE 16.23 Any increase in the angle of the arms relative to vertical creates vector forces that increase the load each arm must support. With vertical arms, each would support a force equal to 50% of the weight on the barbell; the farther from vertical, the greater the force (as a percentage of the weight on the barbell) each arm has to support. One lifter pictured has an arm angle of 75 degrees; at this angle, each arm must support a force equal to 63% of the weight of the barbell. The other lifter has an arm angle of 90 degrees; at this angle, each arm must support a force equal to 71% of the weight of the barbell.

stable upon receipt, the athlete can and should recover immediately.

The width of the lifter's grip will affect this segment of the lift to some degree. The wider the grip, the lower the combined center of mass will be, and consequently, the easier it will be to stabilize the balance of the system over the base. However, wider grips also reduce the structural integrity of the overhead position and make misses behind more likely, as well as typically being harder on the wrists and elbows. With the arms vertical, each supports 50% of the total weight on the barbell; as the width of the grip increases, the actual downward force each arm must resist increases beyond 50% of the total weight due to the introduction of vector forces (Figure 16.23).

As the vector forces increase with the increasing internal angle between the arms, the structural integrity also decreases due to the positions of the shoulders and elbows, magnifying the effect. The internal angle of the arms will vary among lifters with their different grip widths. For example, if the internal angle of a lifter's arms is 75 degrees, each arm will be resisting a force equal to 63% of the weight on the barbell—in practical terms, this means that if the barbell weighs 100kg, each arm is supporting a 63kg force rather than 50kg. A 90-degree internal angle of the arms will mean that each arm is supporting a force equal to 71% of the weight on the barbell. ("Vector Forces," 2011) These factors need to be balanced to create the optimal circumstances for each lifter, with additional consideration of all the effects of grip width on previous phases of the lift.

Recovery

Once the bar is secured and stabilized overhead, the athlete will recover from the squat to a standing position, keeping the bar secured overhead. As mentioned previously, there may be times in which movement of the feet is necessary to achieve balance. This stepping, however minimal, is more easily accomplished the closer to standing the athlete is. Duck-walking under a heavy unbalanced snatch offers great potential for knee injury and should be discouraged outside of the most clinch competition situations.

Occasionally the athlete will feel the bar moving out of position forward or backward and will be able to begin standing and re-establish the base under the shifted center of mass to regain control. This typically looks like one or more short, quick steps as the athlete is standing from the squat, although at times dramatic steps may be taken. This is an acceptable practice within reason, but athletes should never be allowed to chase poorly executed lifts at the risk of injury. Instead, they need to improve their technique and consistency to avoid placing themselves in such situations.

Commonly such imbalance is unnecessary and simply the result of the athlete rushing the recovery or recovering with improper mechanics at the expense of stability. A simple diagnostic and often effective correction of this habit is to force the athlete to stay at the bottom of the squat for 3 seconds before recovering on every snatch. It will quickly become clear whether the source of the imbalance is the manner of recovery itself or an error earlier in the lift.

The lifter should lead the recovery with the bar rather than with the body. That is, instead of simply standing from the squat, it will be more effective to actively push up against the bar and follow it with the body. Too often simply standing from a squat will result in the athlete's hips rising too quickly relative to the shoulders and bar, tipping the trunk forward and undermining the integrity of the structure supporting the weight. By consciously and actively leading with the bar, athletes are more apt to stand with the necessary upright posture and maintain the proper supporting structure.

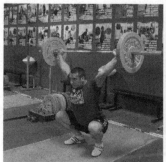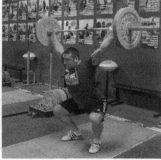

FIGURE 16.24 The recovery from the snatch must be as active and aggressive as the rest of the lift to ensure continued security of the barbell overhead.

Additionally, this will help ensure that the shoulders and arms remain fixed tightly throughout the recovery. Actively maintaining the overhead position is critical during this recovery period, as the movement of standing introduces new destabilizing forces that need to be continuously resisted to prevent their shifting of the barbell's position.

Once the athlete has returned to a standing position, the bar should be held overhead for a moment before it's dropped to the platform. Dropping the bar immediately upon standing—or as some athletes do, prior to even reaching a fully standing position—often masks imbalances and prevents the recognition and correction of the causative faults. Holding the bar overhead momentarily will not only ensure its stability, but will improve the athlete's strength in this position and help condition the joints. An exception to this practice is periods of time when an athlete is experiencing wrist, elbow or shoulder injuries, pain or similar problems that would be aggravated by holding the bar overhead for an extended period of time.

Athletes intending to compete will need to be prepared to hold the bar overhead until receiving the down signal from the officials, which occasionally can be a significant wait. A lift is not complete until the lifter is standing fully with the feet in line parallel with the barbell and stability is obvious. Following this rule in training is the best way to ensure preparedness for competition physically, and to avoid embarrassing failures to secure a successful lift judgment due to premature dropping of the bar.

The Barbell's Path

As has been alluded to in previous sections, the path of the barbell during the snatch is not a straight vertical line, but describes a slight *S* shape (when viewed from the lifter's profile). This minimally curved path is not a goal itself, but is the result of optimal pulling mechanics due to the body's interaction with the barbell and the maintenance of balance over the base. It would be convenient to be able to lift a barbell in a perfectly vertical line, but this is not how the body functions mechanically; additionally, a straight vertical line would not allow the bar-body unit to remain correctly balanced over its base with the necessary movements of the body during the course of the lift and the end point of the barbell.

The term *S-pull* has recently become unfashionable because of its association (fairly or not) with more pronounced bar path curvature. In truth, the ideal bar path does not describe a perfect *S* shape, but the point is that it conveniently describes in a basic sense the horizontal deviation pattern of the bar path. The term itself is immaterial; however, the understanding that the bar path is neither perfectly vertical nor straight is important, as attempts to achieve either will compromise optimal lifting mechanics and balance.

The newly increased accessibility to software that allows easy bar path tracing on video has led to a commensurate increase of its use and arguably to over-analysis with insufficient understanding. Viewing bar paths and using them effectively as diagnostic tools is impossible if the viewer is unaware of what should be expected.

Two points regarding bar path are important to keep in mind. First, the exact path will vary among lifters based on the minutiae of their technical styles, body types, anatomical peculiarities, and relative strengths and weaknesses. Second, the degree of horizontal deviation will decrease as the weight of the barbell increases relative to the bodyweight of the lifter.

All technically proficient lifters will have bar paths that share certain universal characteristics. On average, the bar will move backward between its starting point on the floor and approximately the height of the hips, forward between the hips and near its ultimate height, and then backward again into its final position overhead, finishing slightly behind its starting point (in cases of lifters who jump backward, significantly behind). Exactly how the bar achieves this movement will vary somewhat among lifters, particularly in its initial movement from the floor, but generally all proficient snatching will fit into this basic description.

As the weight of the barbell increases relative to the lifter's bodyweight, it will comprise a greater portion of the combined barbell-body mass. In consequence, the barbell will need to remain closer to the center of the base in order for the combined center of mass to remain balanced. Additionally, the lifter's body will naturally move around the barbell more in reaction to the same efforts during the lift because of the greater inertia of the bar relative to the lifter. This results in the curvature of the bar naturally being reduced somewhat as the barbell weight increases, even with the lifter performing the same actions.

In all cases, the goal is to lift the bar in a way that allows optimal mechanics for accelerating the barbell upward, maintaining balance of the system over the base, and optimal mechanics for moving the body under the bar. In short, the intent is to minimize horizontal deviation of both the barbell and the body without compromising the ability to lift with maximal effectiveness.

Viewing the diagram of the bar path during the snatch (Figure 16.25), we can associate points of the curve to moments of the lift. The beginning of the path represents the center of the barbell's diameter in its starting position approximately over the balls

of the athlete's feet. As the bar is separated from the floor and the athlete begins extending the legs, the bar moves back farther over the feet, bringing the athlete into better balance over the base while maintaining the desired posture for the remainder of the pull. The bar reaches its farthest point back during the upward pull at approximately the height of the hips when the bar and body meet.

Once the athlete has extended the body completely, the bar moves slightly farther forward in reaction to the body extending backward, the need for the bar and body to pass each other, and the horizontal force, however minimal, of the contact of the barbell and hips. The bar reaches its maximal height near the finalization of the turnover. As the bar is received, the athlete completes the squat under and extension of the arms under the bar and settles into the bottom position, the bar continuing to move back slightly into the correct overhead position and approximately

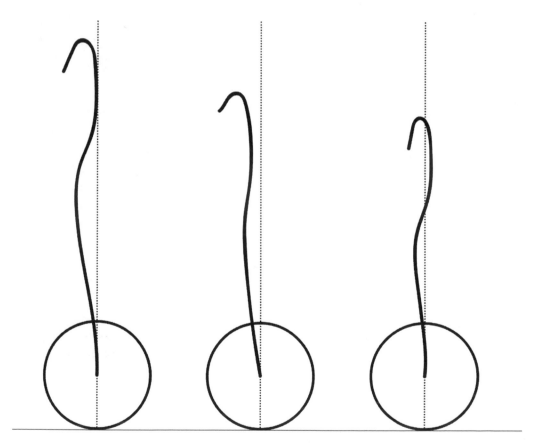

FIGURE 16.25 Pictured are the bar paths of successful snatches by three different technically proficient world-class lifters from three different weight classes. What should be immediately obvious is that, while they differ very slightly, they all conform to the same basic shape. (Lifters facing to the right side of the page.)

Greg Everett

over the middle of the foot.

How far the bar drops from its maximal height into its lowest point in the receiving position is some indication of how efficient a lifter is. That is, less bar drop indicates that the lifter has been able to move under the bar with minimal elevation. However, this alone is really only a reflection of the lifter's ability to quickly move under the bar; it provides no information on whether or not the lifter was maximally accelerating and elevating the bar within the limits of his or her physical capacity. If we view a maximal snatch attempt and see minimal bar drop, it demonstrates the lifter has been successful in moving under the bar well; but it may be that the lifter is forced to do so because he or she is unable to elevate the bar any farther at this weight, and a greater ability to elevate the barbell will translate into heavier snatches with the same capability of moving under the bar.

The bottom line is that bar path analysis must be undertaken with the consideration of other data. In isolation, it provides an incomplete picture and can be misleading.

Bar Drop

Bar drop is the distance the barbell travels downward from its maximal height in the pull to its lowest position when received overhead in the snatch, seen in Figure 16.25 as the section of the bar path that moves down from the highest point. Minimal bar drop is commonly used as a marker of efficiency in a lift—that is, the lifter was able to relocate under the bar with only as much elevation as absolutely necessary. While this is true in the strictest sense, it's important to understand this concept more completely to avoid potential mistakes that can arise from using efficiency as a goal itself.

Bar drop distance should progressively decrease from lighter weights to heavier weights. The degree of this change will vary among lifters, and may be small for some, but the pattern will remain generally reliable. Minimal bar drop with maximal weights is the result of a lifter's ability to move under a bar that cannot be elevated considerably due to its weight; it should never be the result of a lifter artificially limiting barbell elevation with lighter weights in an effort to minimize bar drop for some sense of efficiency. In other words, with maximal lifts, minimal bar drop indicates a lifter is capable of moving under the bar even with extremely limited time and space, an absolutely necessary skill for heavy lifts; with lighter lifts, minimal bar drop more likely indicates the lifter has reduced the effort to accelerate and elevate the barbell to artificially produce the minimal bar drop of heavier lifts. This reduces the development of the critical ability to accelerate and elevate the bar, which can have a negative impact on the athlete's lifts. If an athlete is in need of developing a stronger, faster third pull with minimal bar drop for heavier weights, exercises to train this specifically can be used without forcing a reduction in second pull effort in the snatch itself (e.g. tall snatch, high-hang snatch or high block snatch).

Introduction to the Clean

The clean & jerk is a two-part lift, contested after the snatch in competition. The bar is lifted first from the floor to the shoulders with the clean and then driven from the shoulders to overhead with the jerk. Because of this segmentation into shorter distances of travel for the bar and body, and the stronger positions of the body, lifters are able to handle significantly greater loads in the clean and jerk than in the snatch.

For most athletes, the clean is more easily learned than the snatch, particularly when already familiar with the snatch, but it is not without its own technical subtleties. The clean is also generally less demanding of mobility than the snatch, and consequently more quickly accessible to more athletes.

The clean learning progression should be performed with an empty barbell or a light technique barbell if necessary. PVC pipe or dowel will be problematic due to the impossibility for most athletes to establish a clean rack position with a virtually weightless implement. However, if a lightweight technique barbell is needed and not available, it will be preferable to use PVC or dowel initially to familiarize the athlete with the drills before moving to a barbell.

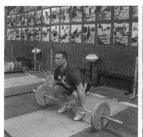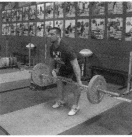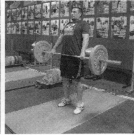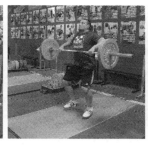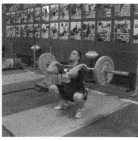

FIGURE 17.1 The clean is the first phase of the clean & jerk, in which the barbell is lifted from the floor to the shoulders.

The Receiving Position

The receiving position for the clean will determine to a great extent the successfulness of the lift. Failure to establish and maintain the necessary posture and security of the barbell on the shoulders will prevent a successful clean even with weights a lifter may be capable of pulling to the shoulders relatively easily. Just as in the snatch, the goal is to create a position that provides maximal structural integrity in both the initial receipt and recovery.

Progression Overview

· Grip Placement
· Rack Position
· Front Squat

Grip Placement

There is considerable variation among lifters in terms of grip width for the clean to account for disparities in proportions, mobility and anatomical peculiarities. The higher on the thigh toward the hip that the bar comes into contact with the body, the better, just as in the snatch the ideal point of contact is the crease of the hip rather than the thighs. However, the narrower grip of the clean will necessarily cause the bar to hang lower than in the snatch; the goal is to mitigate the drawbacks of this lower bar position while ensuring a strong receiving position and sound turnover.

The basic starting point for hand placement is approximately half a fist-width to a fist-width outside the shoulders. With this hand placement, and the bar held up against the shoulders, the forearms should be approximately vertical when viewed from the front of the lifter. In any case, the hands should not contact the shoulders at all.

For most athletes, this grip width will allow a strong rack position and also a reasonable point of contact on the thighs, while also allowing a strong grip on the bar during the pull. Additionally, this same grip will be a good starting point for the jerk, although that of course can be adjusted later as needed.

The wider the grip, the higher the bar will contact the body, which will improve the mechanics and

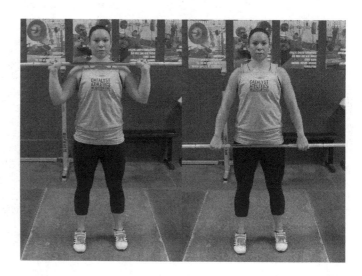

FIGURE 18.1 The grip width should be half a fist-width outside the shoulders or slightly more, allowing a secure rack position and creating a contact point for the bar on the upper thighs.

---

23 Progression Summary
Clean Grip

Hold the bar half a fist-width to a fist-width outside the shoulders more with the hook grip.

Adjust from this starting point to accommodate unusual proportions as needed.

timing of the extension and to some degree the pull under the bar. It can also improve the speed and ease of the turnover. However, it will also make the rack position more difficult and less stable (sometimes impossible for certain lifters due to their builds and mobility limitations), and will make gripping the bar somewhat more difficult. The wider the grip, the lower the hips and shoulders will be in the starting position as well, making the first pull somewhat more difficult.

A narrower grip will typically allow a stronger and more comfortable rack position, reduce the difficulty of gripping the bar during the pull, and keep the hips and shoulders higher in the starting position, making the pull from the floor somewhat easier. However, it will cause the bar to contact lower on the thighs, which can increase the difficulty of a proper and explosive second pull and change of direction into the third pull, and make it somewhat more likely that the lifter will swing the bar away during the lift.

Ultimately, grip width will need to be experimented with by each athlete to find the position that best suits his or her individual proportions, strengths and weaknesses.

As in the snatch, the hook grip is used during the first and second pulls of the clean. Unlike in the snatch, the thumb is invariably released as the barbell reaches its destination on the shoulders. Although some athletes will have the particular anthropometrics in addition to the mobility needed to rack a barbell on the shoulders with a hook grip, it is neither necessary nor helpful as it may be in the snatch for some athletes. The release of the grip will be discussed further in later sections.

The Clean Rack Position

The clean rack position secures the bar on the lifter's trunk and allows for the proper posture in the receiving position. It can be a difficult position for some athletes due to the demands on mobility and may take time to develop fully.

The most important point to understand with regard to the rack position is that the barbell is supported directly by the lifter's trunk, not by the arms. While the hands and arms contribute ultimately to

the security of the bar's position, they are not directly responsible for supporting the weight.

For an initial introduction to this idea of direct support of the bar by the trunk and to establish the proper shoulder position, the lifter will bring the bar to the shoulders, push the shoulders forward (protract the scapulae) as much as possible while keeping the upper back extended to be as flat as possible, and elevate the shoulders slightly (Figure 18.2). The bar should rest in the channel created between the throat and the highest point of the shoulders. Once this position is established, the lifter should be able to let go of the bar and reach the arms straight forward without the bar moving.

It's important to distinguish between scapular protraction and thoracic spine flexion—they are neither the same thing nor necessarily coupled. However, for many athletes the attempt to push the shoulders forward in order to create the shelf for the bar will result in simultaneous rounding of the upper back. If this becomes apparent for a particular athlete, the movement of the scapulae without spinal flexion can be practiced in isolation as needed before returning to the barbell by having the athlete stand with

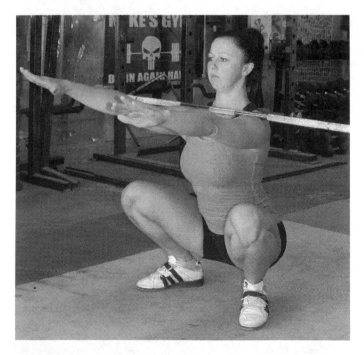

FIGURE 18.2 This position can help the athlete find the proper shoulder position and barbell placement, and understand that the bar is supported directly by the trunk rather than the arms.

the upper back flat against a wall or lying flat on the back and reaching the shoulders forward. The ability to protract the shoulder blades while maintaining a strong, extended thoracic spine is critical for successful cleans.

Once the athlete is able to secure the bar with the shoulders only, we can progress to establishing the actual rack position. Holding the bar in the clean width grip, the athlete will bring it to the shoulders, pushing the shoulders forward and slightly up and securing the bar in the channel between the throat and the peak of the shoulders. Keeping the bar in place, the lifter will elevate the elbows as much as possible while maintaining as close to a full grip on the bar as possible, although not gripping the bar tightly.

Some lifters will not possess the mobility or have the proportions to be capable of maintaining a full grip on the bar when racked properly. These athletes will need to open the hands and allow whatever length of the hand necessary to move off the bar, resulting in a position in which potentially only the last joints of the fingers are under the bar. In extreme cases, a lifter may be able to keep only two or three fingers under the bar.

A full grip in the rack position is ideal for two primary reasons. First, maintaining a full grip during the third pull keeps the lifter and bar connected tightly throughout the movement, improving the accuracy and fluidity of the turnover. This means a more precise meeting of the bar and body when receiving the

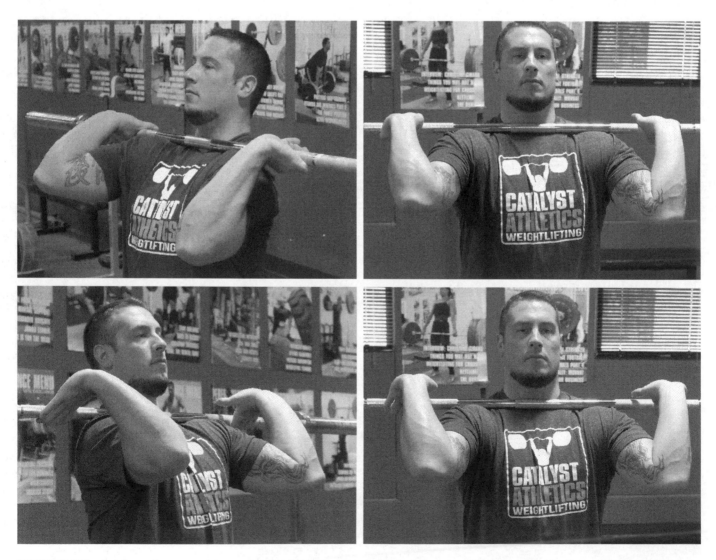

FIGURE 18.3 The ideal clean rack position maintains a relatively full but loose grip on the bar (top). However, some athletes will be forced to use an open grip with only the fingers under the bar (bottom).

Greg Everett

clean, improving the lifter's ability to establish stability and recover immediately and aggressively.

Second, maintaining a full grip in the rack position will assist in the strong extension of the upper back in the front squat. With the grip set on the bar, the angle between the upper arm and upper back is essentially fixed; the effort to elevate the elbows in the rack position then will force the upper back to extend. With an open grip, the elbows can be elevated through shoulder flexion with no effect on the thoracic spine position.

A full grip, however, does not mean a tight grip. If the lifter's grip remains too tight on the bar during the end of the turnover, it can slow the movement of the elbows up into their final position, and even prevent their complete movement into that position. Releasing the hook grip and maintaining the proper grip on the bar during the turnover will be discussed later.

A full grip is not advisable if it prevents the necessary protraction and elevation of the shoulders and adequate elevation of the elbows to create a secure rack position. In other words, a full grip should only be employed if it improves the rack position, not if it disrupts it.

If an open grip is used, the athlete should still attempt to keep as much of the hands or fingers under the bar as allowed by his or her proportions and mobility.

In addition to contributing to creating the channel in which the bar rests between the peak of the shoulders and throat, the slight elevation of the shoulders will do two important things. First, it will keep the bar from actually resting on the collarbones. Light contact is not necessarily problematic, but such a position means that in a less than perfect clean turnover, there will be at least some direct impact of the bar against the collarbones. This can be painful, and over time will likely develop nearly permanent bruising above the bone and scar tissue build-up under the skin, making the collarbones in effect higher profile and even more apt to be hit by the bar, further exacerbating the problem. Second, this elevation of the shoulders helps prevent the carotid arteries from being occluded—enough pressure on these arteries for only a couple seconds can cause unconsciousness.

The elbows should be elevated as much as possible in the rack position. This will reinforce the position, increase the security of the bar on the shoulders, and help keep the elbows away from the knees in the bottom of the squat. While the shoulder position is primarily responsible for securing the bar, the elevation of the elbows is an important contributor. With an open grip, the elevation of the elbows becomes even more important.

The placement of the barbell must be as far back as possible—it should be in light contact with the throat (Figure 18.4). In addition to this being the most secure position, it will reduce the distance between the load and the spine and consequently the length of the moment arm, minimizing the torque on the back and hips and allowing the athlete to maintain the upright posture more easily. If there is uncomfortable pressure against the throat, the athlete can reduce it by flattening the curve of the cervical spine slightly, which will bring the throat back slightly.

Some athletes will find it literally impossible to achieve a proper clean rack position initially. This can be due to a number of factors, such as large disparities in upper and lower arm lengths, excessive upper arm mass, and immobility. These athletes will need to immediately and aggressively address any limiting factors that can be improved. In the meantime, and for issues like proportions that can't be improved, the

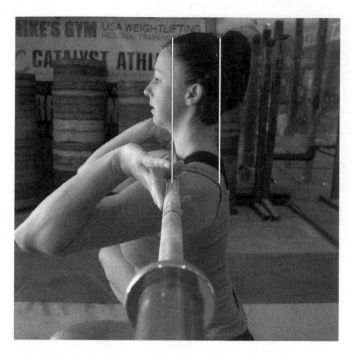

FIGURE 18.4 The farther back the barbell is placed toward the throat, the shorter the distance between the load and the spine, and the more easily the lifter will be able to maintain the upright posture in the squat.

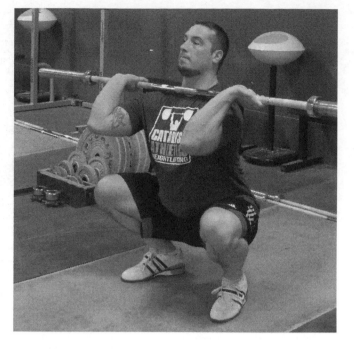

FIGURE 18.5 The front squat meets all the position criteria for the squat and the clean rack position.

athlete should experiment with different grip widths to find the hand position that allows the most secure rack possible. Typically this means a wider grip, but occasionally a narrower grip will work as well.

The Front Squat

The front squat is the position in which the lifter will receive the bar in the clean. Just as with the overhead squat for the snatch, the athlete's progress in the clean will be limited according to his or her level of proficiency in the front squat. This is a foundational position and movement that must be emphasized with new lifters.

All of the position requirements described previously for the squat must be met in the front squat. Foot positioning should result in the thigh being approximately parallel with the foot when viewed from above and the knee approximately above the toes when viewed from the front of the foot. The hips should be pushed in over the heels as much as possible and the torso nearly vertical. The bar will rest securely in the clean rack position.

Although it's more common for a new lifter to be capable of a better front squat position than overhead squat position initially, many athletes will not be capable of a proper, full-depth front squat immediately. Mobility limitations should be immediately and actively addressed to ensure the athlete's progress is not delayed unnecessarily. Specific weightlifting mobility training is discussed in detail in its own section of the book.

If the lifter is incapable of sitting into a full-depth front squat with proper positioning of the back in particular, the early lifting progression will need to be modified by the coach to account for this. Like with the snatch, the learning progressions can still be performed with full squats because of the inconsequential loading as long as there is no pain associated with the squat, but the early stages of loaded training may need to be restricted to power cleans until the front squat position can be improved enough to be safe.

Posture in the Front Squat & Clean Recovery

While the rack position is critical for securing the bar, the posture of the front squat is the foundation for that position. Without the proper upright posture in the squat, the rack position cannot be established.

As was discussed in the Squat chapter and with regard to the receiving position of the snatch, the movement of the squat should minimize horizontal movement of the hips and as a consequence, maintain a relatively constant angle of the trunk that never deviates considerably from its upright posture. This requires the simultaneous flexion and extension of the knees and hips, rather than one leading the other.

The farther backward the hips travel, the farther forward the lifter must lean the trunk.

The importance of maintaining an upright trunk will become extremely clear to the athlete who fails to adhere to this positioning and quickly finds the back rounding forward, the weight of the barbell driving the arms down, and with heavy enough loads, the bar dropping to the floor. A constant effort to maintain proper back extension and an upright trunk must be made throughout the movement.

The recovery out of the bottom of the front squat is aided greatly by the effort to drive the elbows and shoulders up. Leading with the elbows and shoulders in the front squat or clean recovery has a similar effect as leading with the bar in the overhead squat or snatch—it reinforces the extension of the upper back and the upright posture, reducing the tendency of most lifters to allow the hips to rise faster than the shoulders and tip forward.

The transition out of the bottom of the clean must be vicious in order to capitalize on the effects of the bounce described in the Squat chapter and minimize fatigue of the legs to ensure greater available power for the subsequent jerk. This aggressive transition and rapid recovery should nearly always be practiced with front squats in training. At times during the learning process and later training, a pause at the bottom of the front squat can serve a specific training purpose, but the rapid transition and recovery should be the default.

Learning the Clean

After having established the receiving position, the movement of the clean can be learned in the same manner as the snatch. The lifter will learn and practice a series of drills that teach and reinforce the elements of the clean to eventually produce a technically sound lift. These drills follow the same fundamental pattern as the snatch progression.

If the athlete has already learned the snatch, typically the time needed to learn the clean is reduced because of the similarities. However, coaches and athletes should be cautious of rushing or abbreviating the process, as the clean is in its own ways technically nuanced and deserves attention equal to the snatch. What will seem initially to save time can result in more total time spent on instruction as the athlete progresses and technique flaws become more evident and their influence on lift success increases. It's more effective to teach technique in a rational order that addresses the details as they arise than to attempt to later correct technique faults that have already become habit.

Because of the overlap of many of the details with the snatch, some information has been left out of the clean progression to avoid redundancy. Familiarity with the snatch progression is important for ensuring the effectiveness of the clean progression.

Progression Overview

- Mid-Hang Position
- Mid-Hang Clean Jump
- Mid-Hang Clean Pull
- Rack Delivery
- Tall Muscle Clean
- Scarecrow Clean
- Tall Clean
- Mid-Hang Clean

The Mid-Hang Position

The mid-hang position of the clean (Figure 19.1), like for the snatch, positions the barbell at mid-thigh. The criteria used to position the athlete is also the same: the shins are vertical, the bar in light contact with the thigh, the shoulders slightly in front of the bar and the knees, the back arched completely, the head and eyes forward, the elbows turned out to the sides and passively extended, and the weight balanced over the front edge of the heel.

Although these criteria are identical for the snatch, the narrower grip in the clean will result in a somewhat different body position—the lifter's trunk will be more upright and the angle at the hip larger.

---

26 Progression Summary
Clean Mid-Hang Position

The feet are in the pulling position with the weight balanced over the front edge of the heel.

The shins are approximately vertical.

The knees are bent slightly, and the back is set tightly in complete extension with the trunk pressurized.

The shoulders are slightly in front of the bar and knees.

The bar is held in light contact at the mid-thigh.

The arms are long and loose with the elbows turned to point to the sides.

The head and eyes are directed forward.

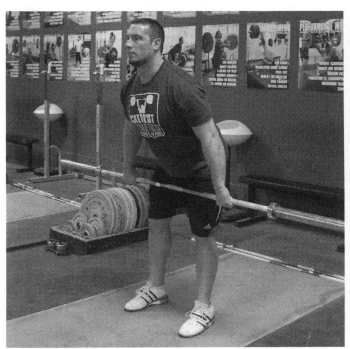

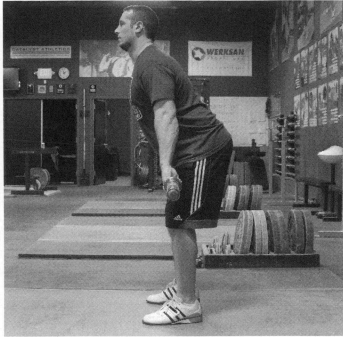

FIGURE 19.1 The mid-hang position is a critical position for the clean and will be the initial starting position for the clean in the first part of the progression.

Because of this, athletes will be even more likely in the clean to move the bar closer to the knees during the following drills from mid-hang because of what they perceive as being too little distance and time to accelerate and elevate the bar. However, just like in the snatch, this mid-thigh position needs to be reinforced in these early stages of training.

Mid-Hang Clean Jump

The mid-hang clean jump (Figure 19.2) is again a drill for the athlete to feel aggressive, concerted leg and hip extension to accelerate and elevate the barbell. The narrower grip in the clean and the consequently lower contact point on the thighs rather than in the crease of the hip will create a significant difference in feel and for most athletes make completing the hip extension somewhat more difficult. Becoming comfortable with this drill will improve the lifter's consistency with the movement.

After setting and holding the mid-hang position and ensuring the proper balance over the front edge of the heel, the lifter will jump vertically as high as

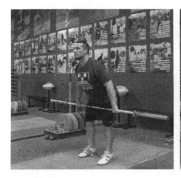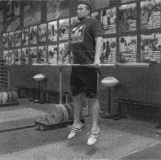

FIGURE 19.2 The mid-hang clean jump is a simple drill to introduce the feeling of aggressive, vertically-oriented knee and hip extension.

27 Progression Summary
Mid-Hang Clean Jump

Start in the mid-hang position with the weight properly balance over the front edge of the heel.

With no countermovement, jump vertically as high as possible.

Keep the bar in light contact with the body throughout the movement.

possible while actively keeping the bar in light contact with the body. Again, it's important this jump begin from a static mid-hang position without any countermovement. The athlete should be landing in the same position in which he or she started—movement forward or backward indicates improper balance or incomplete leg drive.

Mid-Hang Clean Pull

The mid-hang clean pull (Figure 19.3) brings together the aggressive hip and knee extension of the mid-hang clean jump and the precision necessary to produce what will become the second pull of the clean, the final upward explosion. The importance of learning and practicing this section correctly cannot be overstated.

After setting and holding the mid-hang position and ensuring proper balance, the athlete will essentially perform the mid-hang clean jump while keeping the balls of the feet connected to the floor. This will require extending less forcefully, but the goal is still a quick and powerful movement. As the athlete reaches extension, he or she will shrug the shoulders up to give a path for the bar to continue moving without swinging forward and to help keep his or her feet on the floor.

At the top of the pull, the hips should be slightly hyperextended to bring the shoulders slightly behind the hips rather than directly above. The glutes must be activated to finalize the extension of the hips, or this hyperextension will naturally originate in the lower back rather than at the hip joint. The final extended position will have the lifter on the balls of the feet, the legs vertical when viewed from the side, and the shoulders slightly behind the hips.

The feet should remain planted in the same position on the floor; if the athlete is sliding backward, he or she has the weight balanced too far back over the feet—and is likely extending the hips and/or leaning back excessively at the top of the pull—and is also releasing the pressure against the ground prematurely by not continuing to push with the legs until the final extended position is achieved.

During the pull, the bar should remain as close to the thighs as possible and then contact the upper thigh as the trunk reaches a vertical orientation. This proximity is created and maintained through the activation of the lats and shoulders, which push the bar back toward the body even when the shoulders are in front of the bar. Once in contact with the upper thighs, the bar should remain in light contact with the body for the remainder of the movement, never allowed to swing away from the body.

Because the narrower grip places the barbell against the upper thighs instead of in the crease of

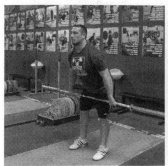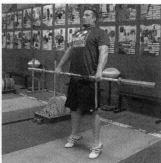

FIGURE 19.3 The mid-hang clean pull refines the mid-hang clean jump into a more precisely channeled extension of the body to accelerate and elevate the barbell; it is the second pull performed in isolation.

28 Progression Summary
Mid-Hang Clean Pull

Start in the mid-hang position with the bar hook-gripped at clean-width.

Push against the ground aggressively with the legs, using the lats and shoulders to keep the bar in immediate proximity to the thighs.

Reach the final extended position with the legs vertical and the shoulders slightly behind the hips.

Actively push the bar back into light contact with the hips.

Shrug the shoulders up to allow the bar to continue traveling momentarily without swinging forward.

Do not prolong this extended position.

the hips as it was in the snatch, it's important the lifter not drag the bar up the thighs or bring the shoulders behind the bar prematurely, as this will cause the bar to be pushed forward by the thighs as the knees shift forward in the double knee bend. This is one of the primary reasons that the timing of the second pull is so critical in the clean and why the mid-thigh position is a useful starting position for early clean instruction.

The arms should remain loose and passively extended during the pull. Again, this means that the arms are straight because they are being allowed to hang, not because the athlete is actively extending the elbows. Stiff arms will increase the likelihood of the bar swinging forward in the lift and typically slow the transition into the third pull.

As the lifter reaches the completely extended position, the shoulders should be shrugged up to keep the bar moving up and against the body rather than swinging forward under its momentum. Again, this shrugging motion is not a direct part of the effort to accelerate and elevate the bar in the clean, but part of the transition into the third pull, and in this drill, a way to maintain the bar's proximity to the body.

If needed, the mid-hang clean pull can initially be performed slowly to ensure the lifter is balanced and extending properly. The positions, movement and balance are more important than the speed, although the athlete should progress to full speed in the drill before moving to the next step.

Rack Delivery

The purpose of the rack delivery drill (Figure 19.4) is to teach and practice the proper and accurate turnover of the barbell into the rack position on the shoulders. The precision of this movement in the clean is imperative—a smooth and accurate delivery of the bar to the shoulders will often be the deciding factor in the success of heavy cleans by allowing the lifter to meet the bar and establish stability more effectively. Such an extreme abbreviation of the movement may seem excessive initially, but the importance of this segment of the clean is frequently underestimated.

The key point in this drill, as in the clean turnover, is that the athlete must actively bring the bar to the shoulders (and the shoulders to the bar), not simply accelerate the bar upward and drop down underneath it indiscriminately. This involves an acute awareness of bar and body positions and consistent movement regardless of the weight on the bar. The athlete needs to bring the elbows around as quickly as possible and correctly time the relaxing of the grip to allow the barbell to arrive in the proper position without crashing down onto the trunk. In order to learn, this segment of the clean is isolated and practiced without any distractions before integrating it into the whole movement.

The athlete will begin standing tall and holding the barbell with the hook grip in the clean hand placement established earlier, and the elbows lifted as high as possible and directed to the sides. In this position, depending on arm segment length and mobility, the barbell will be resting around the lower chest. There will be a tendency to bring the bar higher by dropping the elbows back and raising the hands—this should be avoided by focusing exclusively on elbow elevation rather than bar elevation. The goal is to elevate the elbows to approximately shoulder height or above if possible. This is an awkward position and may be difficult for some athletes with the weight of a barbell. These athletes should use a lighter technique barbell for this drill.

From this scarecrow position, maintaining the bar's proximity to the body, the athlete will pull the elbows up and back, squeezing the shoulder blades together, to bring the bar to the shoulders, then spin the elbows around the bar, pushing the shoulders forward and slightly up to establish the rack position as the bar meets the shoulders.

The grip on the bar should be maintained as long as possible to ensure a tight connection throughout the turnover and a smooth delivery to the shoulders without any crashing. The release of the hook grip and the transition to an open grip if necessary should occur only when the elbows lifting into the final rack position forces the transition—in no case should the grip be released before the elbows move around in front of the bar and are beginning to move up.

The most important point to understand here is that the barbell is the axis around which the elbows pivot primarily (Figure 19.5); that is, the barbell is near the shoulders and moving continually nearer in what is as close to a fixed position as possible,

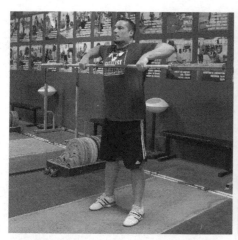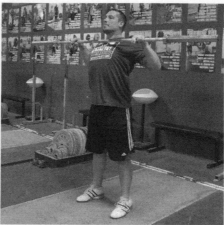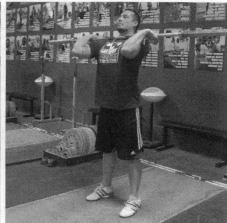

FIGURE 19.4 The rack delivery drill teaches the smooth and precise delivery of the bar into the rack position.

and the arms move around it, rather than the arms remaining essentially fixed and the barbell pivoting around the elbows' position (with a loaded barbell, this motion will require the spinning of the barbell's shaft while the plates remain close to motionless in terms of rotation).

The constant proximity of the bar to the body is absolutely critical for a smooth delivery—distance will mean a collision of the bar against the body, which will with heavier loads cause unwanted rounding of the upper back and forward leaning of the trunk. Actively bringing the bar back toward the throat and maintaining the grip on the bar as long as possible will contribute to this.

The goal for this drill should be to feel and see a

29 Progression Summary

Rack Delivery

Begin standing tall with the elbows in the scarecrow position—elevated as much as possible, above the bar, and pulled out to the sides.

Pull the bar up and back toward the throat and spin the elbows around the bar quickly.

Push the shoulders forward and slightly up to establish the clean rack position as the elbows move up into position, bringing the bar smoothly into position.

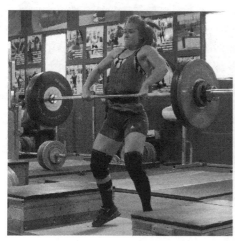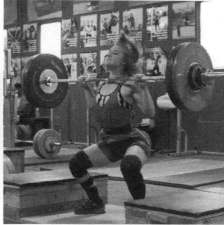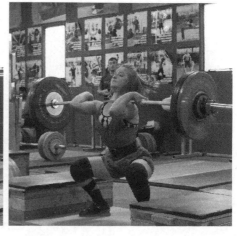

FIGURE 19.5 In a properly executed clean turnover, the elbows primarily pivot around the barbell in a position increasingly nearer the shoulders. This is the opposite of what occurs in a curl, in which the barbell pivots exclusively around the elbows.

Greg Everett

fluid movement with no crashing or bouncing of the bar on the shoulders, and its delivery directly into the channel created between the peaks of the shoulders and the throat, rather than the bar initially contacting farther forward on the shoulders and then being pushed backward.

With a light enough bar, this movement can be performed slowly initially to lay the movement pattern, and the speed increased gradually until the elbows are whipping into place as quickly as possible without the bar shifting and crashing onto the shoulders.

Tall Muscle Clean

The tall muscle clean (Figure 19.6) is essentially the same as its snatch counterpart—the isolated upper body movement of the third pull. As was discussed with regard to the tall snatch, the tall muscle clean is not exactly a segment of the clean, as this motion in a clean would be accompanied by downward movement of the athlete under the bar rather than exclusive elevation of the bar. However, it is an accurate representation of the upper body mechanics used in the relocation of the lifter into the receiving position.

The athlete will begin in the tall position—standing straight up with the bar hanging at arms' length, the weight balanced over the front edge of the heel, and the arms internally rotated to orient the points of the elbows out to the sides. With no movement of the lower body, the athlete will lift the elbows as

high as possible, moving them out to the sides and keeping the bar in immediate proximity to the body. A shrug of the shoulders will naturally accompany this movement of the arms; maximal elbow height will not be possible without it.

Once the elbows have reached the maximal height possible for the athlete based on build and mobility, he or she will turn the bar over and bring it smoothly into the rack position in the same manner practiced in the Rack Delivery drill previously. The entire movement should be a single, fluid motion with no hesitation between the initial upward pull of the elbows and the turnover.

The importance of the pull of the elbows up and out before the turnover deserves to be underscored

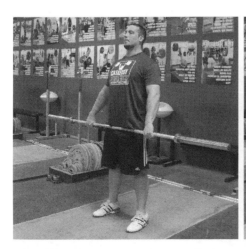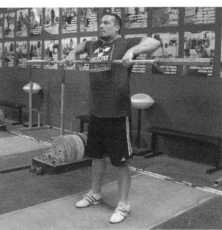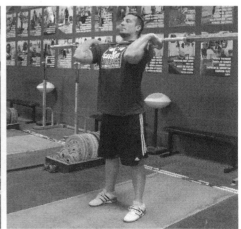

FIGURE 19.6 The tall muscle clean introduces the complete upper body movement of the third pull.

again as it was for the snatch. This movement maximizes the lifter's downward acceleration in the third pull, and is responsible for bringing the barbell to the shoulders so that the arms can be spun around it and into the rack position. Without this initial pull, the turnover is reliant on a weaker movement that reduces precision and increases the likelihood of the bar crashing onto the lifter.

As in the snatch, the internal rotation of the arms is necessary to orient the elbows to the sides and maintain the proximity of the bar to the body during the third pull. If the elbows are not turned out, they will naturally move back and the athlete will be unable to perform the turnover properly.

Again, this movement can be performed slowly initially to ensure correct movement of the bar and elbows and a smooth connection of the bar with the shoulders before increasing to full speed.

Tall Clean

The tall clean (Figure 19.7) is identical to the scarecrow clean but begins with the bar at arms' length rather than in the scarecrow position. Like the tall muscle clean, the tall clean will have application later as a training exercise to help improve the athlete's third pull speed and accuracy, although it will remain primarily a technique drill with relatively little utility for strength development.

The athlete will begin the exercise with the feet

31 Progression Summary
Tall Clean

Begin standing tall with a clean-width grip on the bar, and the bar hanging at arms' length in light contact with the body.

Simultaneously lift and move the feet into the receiving position and pull the elbows up and out, then turn the bar over into the clean rack position to move down into a squat.

Secure the bar in the rack position at the same time the feet reconnect flat with the floor.

Recover to standing by leading with the head, shoulders and elbows.

in the pulling position and standing tall with the bar hanging at arms' length and in light contact with the body. From this starting position, with no upward movement from the lower body, the athlete will pull the elbows up as high as possible and turn the bar over aggressively while lifting the feet and placing them flat into the receiving position, attempting to secure the bar smoothly in the clean rack position at the same time the feet reconnect with the floor.

Because this drill begins prior to the elbows' elevation, athletes will have a tendency to stiffen the elbows and swing the bar away from the body. The elbows must be turned out completely in the starting

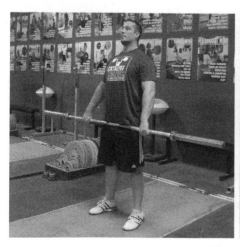
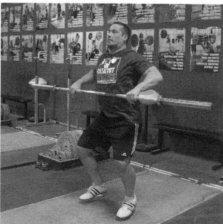
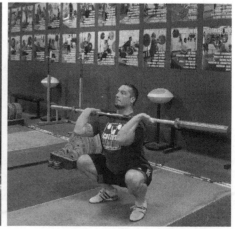

FIGURE 19.7 The tall clean is the third pull of the clean in isolation, teaching the athlete the mechanics, precision and aggression needed in the movement.

position, the arms relaxed as much as possible, and focus directed on pulling the elbows up as high as possible before the arms are turned over, maintaining the proximity of the bar to the body throughout the movement.

Just as in the tall snatch, we want to minimize the elevation of the bar and maximize the movement of the athlete down under it. Of course, with an empty barbell, it will be impossible to prevent any upward movement of the bar, and some upward movement will have to occur for the athlete to get under the bar (even in a clean, the pull against the bar to move down under it will produce some elevation of the bar). However, the focus needs to remain on the aggressive pull down of the body.

Initially, the tall clean can be received in a quarter squat depth if needed, and then into a full squat depth. In all cases, the athlete is again attempting to fix the bar in the rack position at the same time the feet reconnect flat with the floor to encourage speed. In practical terms, this means that the bar should be racked on the shoulders at approximately the same height whether the lifter is receiving in a partial or full squat.

The lifter should rebound immediately from the bottom of the squat and recover as quickly as possible to a standing position, leading with the head, shoulders and elbows to ensure proper posture and maximal security of the bar in the rack position.

Mid-Hang Clean

The final step of the clean progression from the hang assembles all the previous drills into a clean from mid-thigh, or a mid-hang clean (Figure 19.9). This is the first clean the athlete will perform, and with the previous drills learned, it will very likely be done well with little or no additional instruction. The mid-thigh position is important here—athletes will tend to creep the bar lower and lower down the thigh with successive reps and sets to reach a more comfortable starting position. This is even more common in the clean than in the snatch, as the narrower grip means even less bend at the hips and knees with the bar at mid thigh. It's important to monitor the lifter and reinforce the mid-thigh starting position.

Once setting the mid-hang position as described previously and holding it for a couple seconds to ensure proper position and balance, the athlete will initiate the lift by pushing against the floor with the legs, then snap the hips open to achieve the final extended position we have described above: the legs approximately vertical, the shoulders slightly behind the hips, the arms long and loose, the bar in contact with the body at the upper thighs, and the heels naturally lifted off the floor with the effort to drive aggressively with the legs. Throughout this extension, the athlete needs to be actively maintaining the bar's proximity

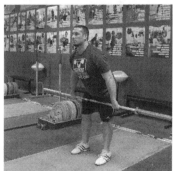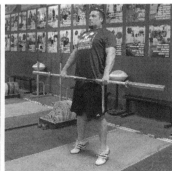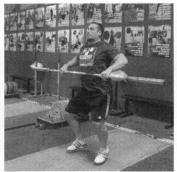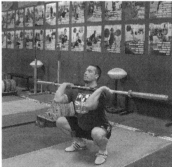

FIGURE 19.8 The mid-hang clean is the first clean variation the lifter will learn, focusing on the core of the movement without the complications of the first pull.

to the body with the lats and shoulders, and then ensuring full contact as it reaches the upper thighs.

Once the athlete completes this upward extension, he or she will lift the feet to move them into the receiving position while aggressively pulling the elbows as high as possible and out to the sides to accelerate him- or herself down, turning the arms over and attempting to secure the bar smoothly in the rack position at the same time the feet reconnect flat with the floor. An adequately aggressive third pull will mean the bar is secured on the shoulders before the athlete reaches the bottom of the squat—regardless of the height the bar is fixed in the rack position, the athlete should continue sitting into the bottom position fluidly and without hesitation.

This entire movement should be considered a single, continuous action; that is, there should be no

32 Progression Summary

Mid-Hang Clean

Begin in the mid-hang position with a clean-width grip.

Initiate the movement by pushing with the legs against the floor.

Maintain the bar's proximity to the body with the lats and shoulders.

Snap the hips open and continue to drive with the legs to achieve complete extension with the legs vertical, shoulders slightly behind the hips and bar against the upper thighs, naturally moving up onto the balls of the feet.

Lift the feet and pull the elbows as high as possible and to the sides to move down, maintaining the bar's proximity to the body.

Turn the bar over and bring it smoothly into the clean rack position at the same time the feet reconnect flat with the floor.

Rebound immediately from the bottom of the squat and recover to a standing position by leading with the head, shoulders and elbows.

pausing or hesitation in the final extension position prior to the athlete pulling under the bar. At the same time, however, the athlete must reach complete extension before moving down.

Because the narrower grip of the clean results in a lower contact point with the body, lifters are more likely to push the bar away with the thighs in the clean than in the snatch. Again, it's important to maintain the proper mid-hang starting position and to actively maintain the bar's proximity to the body throughout the extension and pull under the bar.

The mid-hang clean can be performed initially as a power clean, with the receipt of the bar at quarter squat depth. This can be helpful for the athlete's confidence, reducing the number of elements the athlete is thinking of, and encouraging a faster third pull. Once the athlete is comfortable with the mid-hang power clean, he or she should progress to a full squat, but without any reduction in speed of the third pull. In other words, the bar should be fixed in the rack position at the same time and height in both the power and squat variations of the exercise.

Once the athlete is comfortable with the mid-hang clean with an empty barbell, or at least a light technique barbell, he or she can move to the pull from the floor.

Missing Cleans Safely

As with the snatch, there will be occasions when a clean is not completed successfully for any number of reasons and the athlete must safely discard the barbell. Unlike in the snatch, however, there is only one desirable option for missing a clean—dumping the bar forward.

With a lightly loaded bar, the lifter can practice this procedure as he or she did for the snatch. From the bottom of the squat, the athlete will need to be the most aggressive in his or her exit. Pushing the bar forward, the athlete will attempt to jump the feet and hips back out of the way as far as possible. In the bottom of a clean, it's unlikely the lifter will be able to move the feet, or at least do so quickly enough. More likely, the bar will be falling too quickly and suddenly, with too much weight on the feet for them to be moved. Instead, the lifter will need to rely on

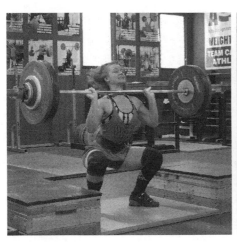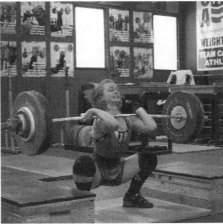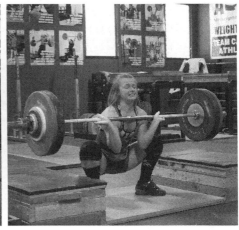

FIGURE 19.9 A missed clean or front squat is ideally dropped forward while the leans forward to guide the bar away from the legs and moves the elbows away from the knees to avoid collision.

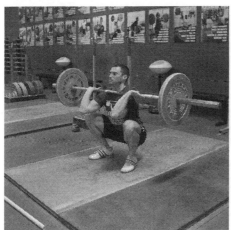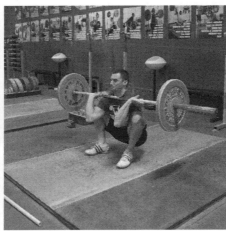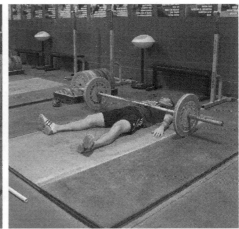

FIGURE 19.10 In rare cases, the athlete is falling backward in a clean and cannot drop the bar in front. In these cases, it is best to lie flat and keep the elbows away from the floor to prevent wrist injury.

leaning forward and guiding the bar forward away from the legs.

When pushing the bar away, the athlete should bring the elbows in toward the midline to prevent their colliding with the thighs as they drop—this collision can easily injure the wrists. (Depending on the position of the arms in the rack position and the position of the legs in the squat for, the elbows may need to be directed outward instead to avoid the knees.)

Occasionally a clean will be received with the athlete's balance too far backward on the feet. Ideally, the athlete will respond immediately and dump the bar forward while jumping back. If the athlete fails to react quickly enough or the weight is too far back

to allow it, however, he or she will fall backward. In this case, the best course of action is to lie flat—the height of the bumpers will keep the bar safely off the throat and most likely over the face. The lifter should not attempt to hold up the bar—if the weight of the bar comes down in the hands with the elbows in contact with the platform, serious wrist, hand and arm injury is likely. It's best to try to maintain the rack position to keep the elbows away from the floor, or if the bar is released, to get the hands away from the bar as quickly as possible. Incidentally, this is why it's recommended to never use straps for the clean, as they tie the lifter too much to the bar and make the potential for injury during a backward miss too great.

The Power Clean

The power clean, like the power snatch, is simply a clean in which the athlete receives the bar in a relatively high position rather that sitting into a full squat. Most commonly, the requirement is that the lifter remain higher than a parallel squat (above a horizontal thigh position, or even more simply to observe, the crease of the hips above the top of the knee). Some coaches will accept lifts stopped at parallel rather than above, and others require a knee angle no smaller than 90 degrees. Coaches and athletes should choose the definition that best suits their present training needs and goals, and that may vary somewhat even within a single training cycle. Again, the lifter must stop before reaching the depth threshold. That is, even if a lifter racks the bar well above a parallel squat, but then continues to sit into a full squat, the lift is a clean, not a power clean.

The motion of the power clean should be the same as for the clean with the exception of the receiving depth. The same problems with an excessively wide receiving stance for the power snatch apply to the power clean, and to a greater extent because of the significantly heavier loading possible in the power clean.

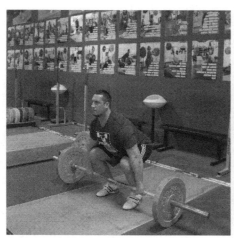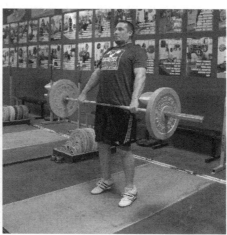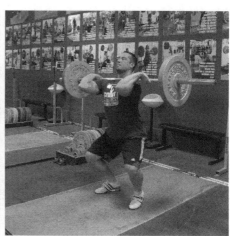

FIGURE 19.11 The power clean is identical to the clean with the exception of a shallow receiving depth.

Benefits & Uses

The power clean has uses similar to the power snatch, such as a way to train the clean with reduced loading, and to train the speed and aggression of both the second and third pulls. Additionally, the power clean is useful to train athletes to meet the bar more accurately in the turnover rather than allowing it to crash down onto the shoulders, and to more quickly establish tightness to resist the downward force of the bar.

The Split Clean

The split clean, like the snatch, pre-dates the squat clean. It has the same limitations described with respect to the split snatch, as well as the same benefits. Again, it offers an option for masters and other lifters possessed of inadequate mobility or working around limitations of injuries, and can be used to train split jerk footwork in some cases when it proves an efficient use of limited time or work capacity. Like the split snatch, the technique for the split clean does not vary from the squat clean with the exception of the foot movement in the third pull.

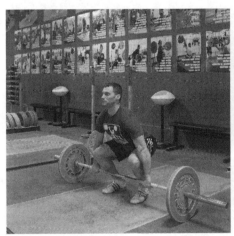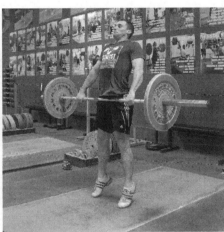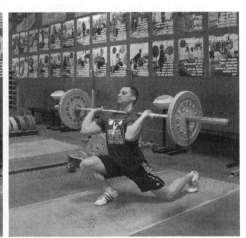

FIGURE 19.12 The technique of the split clean differs from the squat clean only in the movement of the feet during the third pull.

Pulling from the Floor

At this point, the athlete is able to perform a clean and power clean from the mid-hang position with at least an empty barbell. To complete the clean progression, the pull from the floor needs to be introduced. The addition of the first pull often proves surprisingly difficult for many athletes and may temporarily disrupt their technique; however, with a smart progression and proper attention to the principles, this section of the movement can be learned quickly and correctly.

The following progression will teach the lifter the correct positions throughout the pull that are critical for successful lifting, as well as introduce valuable training exercises that can be implemented in the program later.

Progression Overview

- Starting Position
- Clean Segment Deadlift
- Halting Clean Deadlift
- Segment Clean + Clean
- Clean

Starting Position

The first step in teaching the pull from the floor is the starting position (Figure 20.1). Universal details of the position have been covered in a previous section, and additional details specific to the clean will be discussed in the following section. At this stage, instruction for the athlete should be kept as simple and concise as possible while still ensuring correct execution.

Mobility will be a limiting factor for many adult athletes at this point, although generally to a lesser degree than in the snatch. In this early stage it's more important to work on learning the basic position with regard to knee and hip angles, bar position and balance over the feet than to have a perfectly arched back, which may be physically impossible for some lifters at this point. However, correcting any mobility limitations for such athletes needs to be made a priority.

For this stage of learning, the barbell should be loaded lightly—the weight should be the same or very similar to what the athlete was capable of easily cleaning from mid-thigh, as these drills will ultimate-

---

33 Progression Summary
Clean Starting Position

Place the barbell over approximately the balls of the foot.

Turn the feet out slightly and balance the weight evenly across them.

Hold the bar with the hook grip at clean-width.

Assume an upright posture that orients the arms approximately vertically when viewed from the side.

Pressurize the trunk and fix the back securely in a continuous arch.

Keep the head up with a focal point straight ahead or slightly above.

Push the knees outward inside the arms and over the bar.

Internally rotate the arms and keep them passively extended.

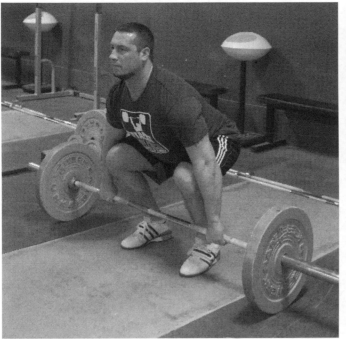
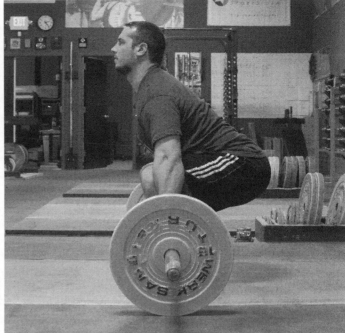

FIGURE 20.1 The starting position for the clean

ly progress again into cleaning. A technique barbell and/or technique plates can be used if needed.

With the bar loaded on the platform, the lifter will place the feet in the pulling position with the balls of the feet under the bar. Holding the bar with a hook grip and the hand width determined previously, the athlete will arch the back tightly and bring the hips down to assume a posture that places the hips slightly above the knees and orients the arms approximately vertically when viewed from the side. The arms should be extended passively with the tension created by the athlete lifting the chest, and internally rotated to orient the bony points of the elbows out to the sides. The knees should be pushed out inside the arms to help improve the arch of the back and allow a more upright posture, although this flaring of the knees will be limited relative to the snatch due to the narrower grip. The knees should be over the bar somewhat and the shins either in light contact with or very close to the bar. The athlete's head should be upright and the eyes focused straight ahead or slightly above.

Essentially the only difference in the clean starting position relative to the snatch starting position is that the lifter's hips and shoulders be will slightly higher due to the narrower grip that will place the shoulders farther above the bar. Whereas in the snatch, some lifters' hips may be level with or even slightly below the knees, nearly all lifters' hips will be above the knees in the clean starting position.

Clean Segment Deadlift

The first step in the progression is the clean segment deadlift (Figure 20.2). This exercise is a way to both teach and reinforce the proper positions at different critical points in the pull. The segmented movement allows athletes to better feel and correct posture and balance over the foot during the lift.

After setting and holding the starting position momentarily, the lifter will begin the deadlift by pushing with the legs against the floor, separating the bar smoothly without jerking or yanking. This should be a deliberate, controlled movement, and the lifter should maintain the same approximate back angle from the starting position. Once the bar reaches a height of 1 inch off the floor, the lifter will pause and hold for 3 seconds. This position should be nearly identical to the starting position but with the weight over the foot shifted backward very slightly from the even balance in the starting position. The bar can be in very light contact with the shins, but should not be pushed back into them forcefully.

This 1-inch height is much lower and is reached much sooner than athletes typically expect—they will commonly not pause until the bar is several inches up. The simplest way to instruct proper timing of this first pause position is to have lifters stop as soon as they feel the bar separate from the floor.

After holding this position for 3 seconds, the lifter will resume standing by again pushing with the legs, still with a controlled, deliberate speed, until the bar reaches the level of the knees. During this movement, the lifter should continue shifting the center of balance back until it reaches the front edge of the heel where it should remain for the rest of the lift. The lifter will then pause again with the bar in light contact with the kneecaps for 3 seconds.

At this second pause position, the shoulders should be very slightly farther forward than they were in the starting position—that is, very slightly forward of the bar. However, this is minor and the back angle should have changed only slightly from the first position. Any dramatic change in the back angle or with the shoulders' position relative to the bar at this point indicates that the athlete is elevating the hips too much relative to the shoulders and bar.

After holding this position at the knees for 3 seconds, the lifter will proceed to the final position at mid-thigh by again pushing with the legs against the floor at a controlled speed and using the lats and shoulders to keep the bar in immediate proximity

34 Progression Summary
Clean Segment Deadlift

Set the starting position tightly and hold momentarily.

Push with the legs to separate the bar from the floor 1 inch and pause for 3 seconds.

Push with the legs and shift the weight back to the front edge of the heel to bring the bar to the kneecap, maintaining a similar back angle, and hold for 3 seconds.

Push with the legs to move into the mid-hang position and hold for 3 seconds, maintaining balance over the front edge of the heel.

Return the bar to the floor at a controlled speed, trying to move through the same correct positions on the way down.

to the thigh. This final movement should bring the lifter into the same mid-hang position he or she has already practiced, with the bar in light contact with the mid-thigh, the shins approximately vertical, the knees pushed out to the sides slightly (less than in the starting position), the back still arched completely, the shoulders in front of the bar and the knees, the weight balanced over the front edge of the heel, and the head and eyes directed forward.

Overall there will be a slight change in the back angle and the position of the shoulders between the starting position and mid-hang position, but again, it

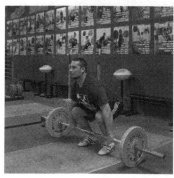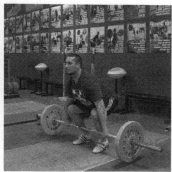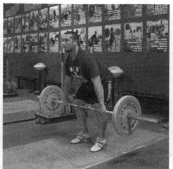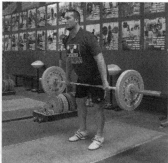

FIGURE 20.2 The segment clean deadlift teaches and reinforces the most critical positions in the pull from the floor.

will be relatively minor—no more than is necessary to achieve the correct mid-hang position for a given athlete.

Frequently athletes will shift their weight too far back toward the heels, particularly at the knee position. The full foot should remain in contact with the floor throughout the movement—if the athlete's toes are lifting from the floor, the balance is too far back. This kind of excessive backward balance will typically cause subsequent excessive forward rocking in the clean.

After holding the mid-hang position for 3 seconds, the athlete will return the bar to the floor at a controlled speed, attempting to reverse the movement accurately to pass through the same correct positions on the way down. The starting position should be completely reset with the bar resting completely on the floor before subsequent reps.

Sets of 3 reps will allow practice without excessive fatigue of the back from holding the pause positions. Once this exercise can be performed with the athlete consistently reaching the correct positions immediately at each point—that is, the lifter does not have to make adjustments at each pause to find the correct position—he or she can proceed to the next step.

Halting Clean Deadlift

When the segment deadlift can be performed correctly, the athlete will progress to the halting clean deadlift (Figure 20.3), which simply removes the first two pause positions so the lifter is pausing only at

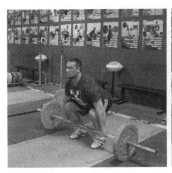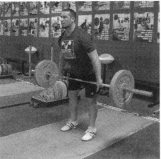

FIGURE 20.3 The halting clean deadlift teaches the lifter how to properly move the bar from the floor to mid-thigh, where the second pull will begin.

mid-thigh. Although the first two pauses have been removed, the athlete should still be passing through the positions with the same postures and balance over the feet practiced in the segment deadlift.

This exercise should also be performed at a controlled, deliberate speed like the segment deadlift. Rushing the lift not only makes it less likely that the athlete will achieve the correct positions and balance, but reduces the effectiveness of even correct positions. This is an exercise intended to train and reinforce positional awareness and stability, not speed.

Segment Clean + Clean

When the athlete is capable of consistently performing the halting clean deadlift correctly, the first pull, in terms of position and balance, has been learned. What remains is for the athlete to learn to transition from the first pull into the second pull seamlessly and confidently—in other words, to combine the halting clean deadlift and mid-hang clean into a single, continuous lift.

In order to make this transition easier and less intimidating, the athlete will use a complex that allows the lifter in the first rep to perform two movements he or she is already comfortable with—the halting clean deadlift and the mid-hang clean—and then follow it immediately with a clean (Figure 20.4). This

helps improve confidence and reduce unwanted thinking, and continues to reinforce the proper positions and timing.

Each set will consist of 2 reps: 1 segment clean and 1 clean. For the first rep, the athlete will perform a halting clean deadlift at a controlled speed, hold the mid-hang position for 3 seconds, and then perform a mid-hang clean directly from that pause position (no countermovement to begin). After returning the bar to the floor, the lifter will perform a clean with no pause on the way up. However, at this stage, the lift from the floor to mid-thigh should remain at a deliberate speed to ensure proper positioning, balance, and timing of the final explosion. The lifter can control this speed easily by keeping the pull from the floor to mid-thigh timed to a count of 3.

As the lift improves and the lifter's confidence increases, this first pull speed can be increased slightly, although it should still remain relatively slow. The speed of the first pull will be increased later as the lifter becomes more technically proficient and loading increases. Once the cleans in the second rep of this complex are consistent, it's time for the final step of the process: the clean.

> **36** Progression Summary
> ## Segment Clean + Clean
>
> Set the starting position tightly and hold momentarily.
>
> Perform a halting clean deadlift to the mid-hang position and hold for 3 seconds.
>
> Directly from this pause position, perform a mid-hang clean.
>
> Return the bar from the floor and reset the starting position.
>
> Perform a clean with no pause, but keep the lift from the floor to mid-thigh slow to ensure correct positions, balance and timing.

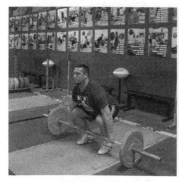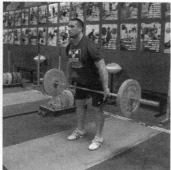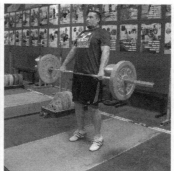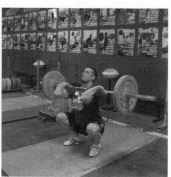

FIGURE 20.4 The segment clean + clean complex progresses the athlete to the first clean from the floor while continuing to reinforce the critical mid-hang position.

Greg Everett

Clean

At this point, the athlete is capable of performing the classic clean (Figure 20.5). Practice should consist of sets of 2-5 repetitions at the most with weights that allow correct and safe execution. In the early stages of development, large volumes of very lightweight practice is appropriate and most effective; partial lifts and assistance exercises will be used to develop strength for the clean. For practice of the clean as part of the earliest training program, weights should be approximately 50-60% of bodyweight, or what the athlete and coach feel could be lifted without trouble for 5-6 repetitions (Medvedyev 1986/1995). Of course, lighter weights should be used if needed and the initial practice stage extended as much as needed for each athlete prior to beginning a more structured training program. This process is discussed in detail in the Program Design & Training section of the book.

If the athlete is having difficulty in particular aspects of the clean, he or she should practice the exercise or exercises from the progression process that best address the position or segment of the movement in question for remediation in addition to the clean. Always keep in mind that the quality of repetitions is of greater priority than the quantity.

37 Progression Summary

Clean

Set the starting position tightly and hold momentarily.

Initiate the lift by pushing with the legs against the floor.

Shift the weight back to the front edge of the heel by the time the bar reaches knee height.

Continue pushing with the legs until reaching the mid-hang position, maintaining the balance over the front edge of the heel.

Execute the final upward explosion by pushing with the legs against the ground and extending the hips aggressively, actively maintaining the proximity of the bar to the body.

When complete extension is reached with the legs vertical, bar against the upper thigh, and shoulders slightly behind the hips, lift the feet and pull the elbows high and out.

Keep the bar as close to the body as possible, turn the arms over and secure the bar in the rack position at the same time the feet land flat on the floor in the receiving position.

Continue sitting into the squat fluidly and rebound immediately from the bottom.

Recover to a standing position by leading with the head, shoulders and elbows to maintain bar security and upright posture.

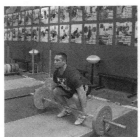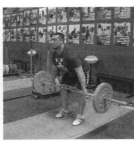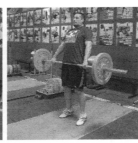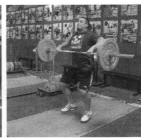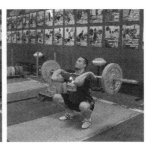

FIGURE 20.5 The clean from the floor finalizes the clean progression.

Understanding the Clean

This chapter expands on the information presented in somewhat simplified fashion during the clean learning progression. For athletes at this point who are not yet comfortable with their technical performance of the clean, it's advised to skip this section and focus on practicing the lift and its basic variations (e.g. hang and power) along with basic assistance exercises such as squats and pulls until a reasonable level of consistency is developed. Prior to this point, additional information is more likely to be overwhelming and confusing than helpful. From a coaching perspective, it's generally ideal to present as little conceptual information to the athlete as possible and focus on the practical aspects of execution primarily until athletes are more advanced and beginning to experiment with more idiosyncratic technical modifications to best suit their individual peculiarities.

Much of the information regarding the technical details of the clean is identical to that of the snatch, and in such cases it has been omitted or greatly abbreviated to avoid redundancy. Reading the Understanding the Snatch chapter will be necessary for a complete understanding of the material, as its presentation here will be minimal.

The Starting Position

The starting position for the clean is in its essence identical to that of the snatch—both adhere to the same principles discussed in the Starting Position and Understanding the Snatch chapters. The only differences are the width of the grip and the consequent changes in the heights of the hips and shoulders, angle of the trunk relative to the floor, and degree to which the knees can be pushed out to the sides. Some athletes may also prefer a slightly different pulling stance than they use in the snatch, although dramatic differences are unusual. The basic principles guiding positioning do not change.

Barbell Placement & Leg Position

Because the narrower grip will position the shoulders slightly higher above the bar, the shins will be slightly more upright relative to the snatch starting position, creating more space for the barbell. Consequently, a given lifter may be able to start the barbell slightly farther back over the foot in the clean than in the snatch. Generally speaking, this should make the first pull simpler by reducing the extent to which the barbell needs to move back horizontally to establish balance of the combined center of mass over the base. The lifter must choose the starting position that produces the best result.

Similarly, the knees will not protrude forward over the bar as much as they do in the snatch starting position, although they will still be over the bar to some degree.

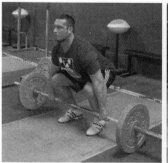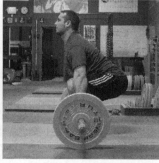

FIGURE 21.1 The starting position of the clean differs from the snatch only in the changes resulting from the narrower grip: the height of the hips and shoulders, angle of the trunk relative to the floor, and degree to which the knees can be pushed out to the sides. The basic principles guiding positioning do not change.

Because the narrower grip on the bar creates less space between the arms, the lifter will not be able to push the knees out to the sides to the same degree as in the snatch starting position. Conveniently, the higher position of the hips and shoulders in the clean will achieve the same basic purpose of moving the knees out in the snatch. The knees should, however, still be pushed out to the degree allowed by the position of the arms.

The First Pull

As we've established previously, the first pull brings the barbell from its starting position on the floor to the point at which the second pull is initiated, approximately the level of mid-thigh. This barbell position in the clean will involve larger joint angles than in the snatch, and as a consequence, lifters will often be more likely to initiate the second pull early. However, it's arguably even more important in the clean to achieve the proper timing, as the barbell's path will be disrupted to an even greater degree by the thighs moving forward due to the narrower grip.

The first pull of the clean does not differ in any significant way from that of the snatch; the movements share the same purposes, goals and methods. The separation of the bar from the floor should be controlled enough to ensure the preservation of proper balance and posture, and to avoid excessive initial acceleration that results in any subsequent slowing of the bar, all without unnecessarily limiting bar speed.

The initial movement needs to re-establish balance over the feet approximately over the front edge of the heel as the barbell and body become a single combined system with the bar's separation from the floor, while maintaining the optimal posture. As in the snatch, this will mean a slight forward inclination of the trunk from its original angle as the shoulders move from directly above the bar to slightly in front of it, while the bar moves back slightly farther over the foot.

The tendency for the lifter to tip forward over the bar excessively will typically be greater in the clean due simply to the greater loads being lifted, despite the somewhat improved mechanics due to the larger joint angles. This needs to be monitored and avoided through both technical work and development of appropriate postural strength.

Following this repositioning, the angle of the trunk and balance over the foot should remain approximately the same until the bar reaches mid-thigh and the second pull is initiated.

The Second Pull

The second pull begins with the initiation of the final hip and knee explosion effort. Just as in the snatch, this is the source of the highest power in the upward pull of the bar, and the motion of the hips and legs are identical in essence. However, the final movement is briefer than in the snatch, at least in terms of angular joint motion, because the same barbell position (mid-thigh) will occur with larger joint angles

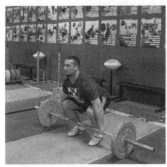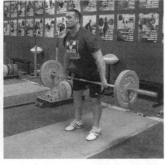

FIGURE 21.2 The first pull brings the barbell from its starting position on the floor to the point at which the second pull is initiated, approximately the level of mid-thigh.

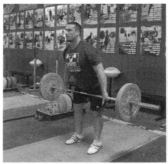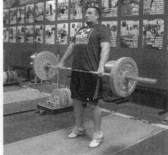

FIGURE 21.3 The second pull is the final, vicious explosion of the hips and knees at the top of the lift and begins at approximately the level of mid-thigh.

due to the narrower grip.

This segment of the clean differs from its snatch counterpart in two consequential ways. First, the narrower grip results in the bar contacting the body on the thighs rather than in the crease of the hips as it is in the snatch. Second, the distance the bar must travel to its final position on the body, and the distance the body must travel to its final position under the bar, are dramatically shorter.

Timing & Barbell Contact

Because the point of contact of the bar is the upper thigh, the forward knee movement in the double knee bend will have potentially more of a direct effect on the path and velocity of the barbell. Contact with the thighs too early in the second pull will reduce the upward speed of the bar, add horizontal momentum to it, and disrupt the motion of the legs and hips to some degree. Just as in the snatch, the goal is to avoid contact between the barbell and body until the trunk is approximately vertical. In this position, the barbell will be high enough on the thighs to avoid being pushed forward significantly and will be properly positioned relative to the feet. This is accomplished through correct posture leading into the second pull, proper timing of the initiation of the second pull, and vigilant maintenance of immediate proximity of the bar to the body without contact through the efforts of the lats and shoulders.

Narrower grips and longer arms relative to the trunk will exacerbate this natural difficulty. Widening the grip is typically the simplest method to improve this segment of the lift and should be attempted unless impossible due to limitations relating to the starting position or rack position. Additionally or alternatively, the method discussed with regard to the snatch of shrugging the shoulders up and back slightly during the second pull to bring the bar higher on the thighs can be employed.

Arm Activity

As was described with regard to the snatch, lifters will commonly bend the arms slightly during the second pull as an unconscious attempt to preserve the exist-

ing speed of the bar during the double knee bend, when bar speed will naturally decrease somewhat.

Arm bend in the second pull of the clean is more prevalent and pronounced than in the snatch, however, due to the additional problem of the lower barbell contact point on the thighs relative to the snatch. Bending the arms during the second pull brings the bar higher toward the hip and into a more advantageous position in terms of its interaction with the body during the final extension.

However, this bending of the arms may also be in reaction to a premature initiation of the second pull, which causes the knees and thighs to move forward excessively and with the bar too low. It's important the coach distinguish between these causes.

Like in the snatch, the more hip-dominant a given athlete's pulling style, the less of a potentially negative effect such arm bending will have on the lift. It will also create somewhat less of a problem due simply to the reduced distance the bar and lifter must travel relative to each other, which creates a larger margin for error.

As in the snatch, the athlete can achieve similar elevation of the bar's contact point toward the hips by shrugging the shoulders slightly back and up during the explosion phase (Figure 21.4). This motion can move the bar significantly enough to reduce the tendency and need for bent arms to improve interaction

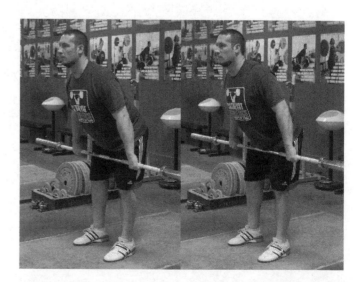

FIGURE 21.4 Lifters with long arms and short trunks, or unavoidably narrow clean grips, can achieve a higher point of bar contact by partially shrugging the shoulders back and up during the second pull, reducing the need for arm bending.

Greg Everett

of the barbell and thighs during the second pull.

As in the snatch, such bending of the arms during the second pull is acceptable if it's determined it is not in response to a correctible technical error (such as a premature initiation of the second pull), the extent is minimal (up to approximately 10 degrees of elbow flexion), and it's occurring naturally rather than as an intentional action by the lifter.

Reduced Travel

In the snatch, the barbell and body have to each cover a great distance to move from their respective starting positions to ending positions. In the clean, while the distances are not insignificant, they are approximately half those of the snatch. This fact is the primary source of athletes' ability to lift more weight in the clean than in the snatch, and also reduces the demand on both the elevation of the barbell and the downward acceleration of the lifter.

What this means in practical terms is that there is a significantly larger margin for error in the clean, and technical errors will affect the outcome of the lift to a smaller degree. For example, the extension of the knees and hips in the second pull of the clean typically will not need to be as complete as in the snatch to achieve a successful lift. This doesn't mean that a more complete extension may not be more effective, but simply that the athlete can get away with less in many cases. Many lifters do in fact display less knee and hip extension in the clean than in the snatch.

A related effect of these shorter distances is a somewhat reduced demand for barbell speed in the final explosion. A reduction in bar speed will already unavoidably occur in the clean due to the heavier weights being lifted relative to the snatch, so in large part, this is naturally balanced. However, in the same way lifters may still be successful with somewhat less extension in the clean than in the snatch, they may also be capable of succeeding with somewhat less acceleration in the second pull by making up for it with a more aggressive third pull.

As in the snatch, the final upward explosive effort in the second pull must be continuous with the third pull, and its purpose is largely to feed into the downward acceleration under the bar. The bar will reach its maximum upward speed before the final ex-

tension of the body; the intent of the final degrees of hip and knee extension as a consequence must be to squeeze out additional barbell elevation while preserving as much speed as possible, and creating maximal upward barbell inertia against which the lifter can pull down.

Ankle Extension

Extension of the ankles (plantar flexion) should be allowed to occur naturally as a part of the vicious drive against the platform with the legs, just as it is in the snatch. However, a given lifter will typically exhibit a smaller degree of ankle extension in the clean than in the snatch. This is the product of the heavier weights of the clean limiting the possible upward acceleration somewhat, and the slightly reduced degree of upward extension commonly seen in the clean.

The Third Pull

The third pull of the clean is the point at which the lift diverges considerably from the movement of the snatch. In principle, however, it remains identical: It is the lifter's relocation under the barbell after having accelerated and elevated it with the extension of the body in the first and second pulls—the movement from the fully extended position into the receiving position (front squat). Just as in the snatch, this movement is as active and aggressive as the rest of the lift—it is not simply dropping or falling under the bar.

The third pull of the clean can be considered as two basic phases: the initial pull down of the body, and the turnover of the arms into the rack position.

Pulling Down

The initial effort to pull under the bar is executed in the same manner as in the snatch—the athlete pulls aggressively with the arms, directing the elbows up and to the sides in order to ensure the barbell and body remain as close to each other as possible. It is this vicious pull with the arms against the bar in the

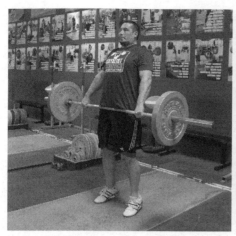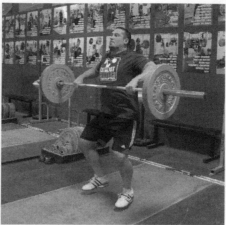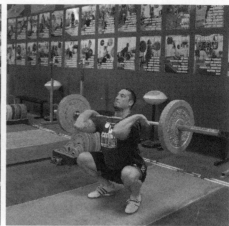

FIGURE 21.5 The third pull brings the lifter from the fully extended position into the receiving position under the barbell.

absence of pressure against the platform that changes the athlete's direction and accelerates him or her down under the bar. This immediate and aggressive acceleration is what allows the turnover of the arms to be completed successfully as soon as possible—the turnover itself is not a particularly strong movement and generally cannot be relied upon to directly move the athlete and barbell to any significant degree, nor can it happen properly without the pivot point (the barbell) being close to the shoulders.

Note that some lifters can successfully move under a clean with an immediate backward pull of the elbows rather than a pull of them up and out as described—this is possible because of the very short distance the lifter and bar must travel relative to each other and the greater ease of generating downward momentum with the initial change of direction at the top of the pull. However, such a motion is very likely to create subsequent problems such as crashing of the barbell into the rack position.

The elbows will not reach their maximal possible elevation in this orientation—that is, they will begin moving backward and down before they reach the level at which the athlete placed them during the initial learning progression. Generally they will rise only to approximately chest level (although there are a number of lifters who are able to elevate the elbows remarkably high). At this point, the barbell will have enough upward momentum, the athlete will have enough downward momentum, and the athlete and barbell will be enough within the range of rela-

tive positions that the turnover of the elbows can begin. The athlete will need to aggressively retract the shoulder blades and pull the elbows back to initiate their path around the bar to ensure the bar and athlete remain in close proximity. This can be thought of as pulling the bar back into the shoulders rather than simply pulling the body down. This will also ensure the maintenance of the correct upright squat posture and prevent the lifter from reaching with the chest to the bar.

In the clean, the bar and lifter have to travel fairly short distances in the third pull relative to the snatch—from about the waist to the shoulders compared to the waist to overhead. Additionally, the narrower hand placement on the bar places the arms in a stronger pulling position, allows a more secure grip around the bar, and means that each hand only has to resist about 50% or slightly more of the total force generated because of the more vertical orientation of the arms. These factors combined result in a greater ability of the athlete to move under significantly heavier weights with less bar speed relative to the snatch.

The Turnover

The path of the elbows during the turnover is critical for the success of the clean attempt. The barbell is the pivot point for the arms as they move into the rack position, and violation of this will shift either the bar or the athlete from their respective desired paths and slow the movement. If the elbows, instead of traveling up and to the sides, travel back prematurely, it's likely the athlete will fail to accelerate downward adequately due to the misdirection of the force of the arm flexion.

In addition, the elbows traveling back before the barbell and athlete have achieved their appropriate relative levels makes more likely the elbows becoming the point around which the arms pivot instead of the bar in its correct proximity to the shoulders. This results in excessive distance between the barbell and the athlete from a combination of the bar swinging away from the body and the athlete being pushed back away from the barbell.

Further, unless the bar is pulled up and back into the shoulders, the pivot point is in the wrong position, and the chances of the barbell crashing onto the lifter's shoulders increase. This correct positioning of the bar is achieved, again, by the effort to elevate the elbows as high and to the sides as possible during the first phase of the third pull, and then the active retraction of the shoulder blades and pull back of the elbows to initiate their spin around the bar.

The elbows must whip around the barbell to enter their orientation for the rack position as quickly as possible. The aggressiveness of this turnover is what ensures that the elbows are high enough and the shoulders protracted and elevated to create a solid rack in time for the delivery of the bar. An incomplete turnover of the elbows presents a number of potential problems. First, and most obviously, is the reduction of the shoulders' ability to support the bar. This will result in the load being placed in the arms, which will not be able to support heavy weights. If the bar is delivered too far forward on the shoulders due to the low position of the elbows, the upper back of the athlete will likely round forward under the weight, causing at best an unnecessarily difficult recovery and at worst a failed lift due to an inability to rise from the squat or the loss of the barbell. If the shoulders are creating a sufficiently secure rack for the bar, but the elbows are low, it's possible they will collide with the thighs as the athlete hits the bottom of the squat, producing anything from minor pain to serious wrist injury.

The lifter must attempt to finish the turnover and secure the bar in the final rack position as quickly as possible—that is, to meet the bar with the shoulders and bring the elbows up into their final position in as high of a squat as possible. The sooner the rack position is established, the more secure it will be when the lifter hits the bottom of the squat and must resist the abrupt downward force that will try to pull the chest and bar down.

The feet will begin their transition from the pulling to receiving position as the third pull is initiated. Depending on the lifter's individual style, they may reconnect very quickly—before the elbows move around the bar—or may be lifted higher and not reconnect until the elbows are nearly around the bar and in the rack position. In any case, however, just

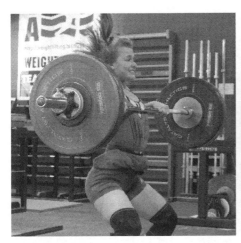 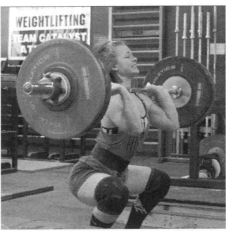 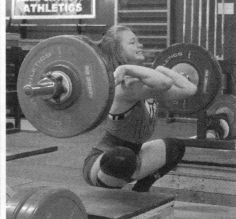

FIGURE 21.6 An effective turnover is accomplished when the barbell is in close proximity to the shoulders and acts as the pivot point around which the elbows rotate, rather than the barbell pivoting around the elbows. This can only occur if the first phase of the third pull is performed correctly.

as in the snatch, the attempt to finish the turnover of the bar at the same time the feet reconnect with the platform will help improve the speed of the third pull. Even with the quickest foot transition, in real time, it should appear to observers that the turnover is completed at the same time the feet are heard hitting the platform.

Grip

As was discussed with regard to the clean receiving position, ideally the lifter can maintain a full grip around the bar throughout the turnover and into the rack position—this will allow the most accurate turnover possible, and the smoothest connection of the bar and body in the receiving position, and typically the strongest upper back extension in the front squat. However, even if a full grip on the bar is maintained, the hook grip should be released, and will need to be released in nearly all cases.

Obviously during the first phase of the third pull—the aggressive pull against the bar with the arms—a tight grip on the bar is critical. During the turnover of the elbows around the bar, the grip on the bar is important for maintaining the lifter's connection to the bar to ensure optimal positioning and timing. Premature release of the grip will result in the bar and lifter drifting away from each other and the consequent crashing of the barbell onto the lifter's shoulders, typically in a position farther forward than is ideal.

The grip should be intentionally maintained tightly on the bar until the elbows have come around the bar and are beginning to move up into the rack position. At this point, the bar will be in contact with the shoulders, or at least in very close proximity, and releasing the grip will not have any significant effect on its movement or final position. The hook grip can be slid out and the grip relaxed as the elbows move up into position. This relaxation of the grip and the effort to lift the elbows into place will naturally cause the hands to open to the necessary degree for each lifter—that is, lifters who must rack the bar with open hands and only the fingers under the bar will naturally achieve this position by simply loosening the grip and driving the elbows up into place, while those who can maintain a full grip will find that

their thumbs will slide out of the hook grip but their hands remain around the bar appropriately with the same effort.

It's important the lifter not attempt to maintain a fuller grip on the bar than he or she is capable of in terms of mobility and proportions, as this will slow the movement of the elbows and limit their ultimate position. Similarly, even those able to maintain a full grip on the bar should not grip it excessively tightly, as the same result is likely to occur. In both cases, the lifter will end up with a rack position that is not as solid and secure as it needs to be.

Meeting the Bar

Pulling under a clean, while a vicious, aggressive action, also requires precision. It's important the athlete not simply attempt to pull down indiscriminately. Rather, he or she needs to pull him- or herself down accurately into a position to meet the barbell. The maintenance of the grip on the bar long enough through the third pull and the attempt to bring the barbell back to the shoulders and the shoulders up into the barbell will help ensure a tight and smooth connection rather than a crash of the bar onto the athlete.

This kind of precision also requires confidence, which requires experience. A lifter not confident in his or her technical ability will typically respond by pulling excessively deep into the squat, not believing the bar will be elevated adequately, and consequently causing the bar to crash down into the rack.

Receiving the Bar

The completion of the third pull will place the lifter in a front squat of a depth dependent on how high the barbell was elevated in the second pull and how quickly the athlete relocated him- or herself under the bar. With all cleans, the athlete should make an effort to rack the bar as quickly as possible. The sooner the bar is secured on the shoulders, the more time is available to tighten up the position and prepare for the force at the bottom of the squat. This means a greater eccentric segment, more potential for the stretch-shortening reflex element of the bounce, more stability, and a far greater chance of successful recovery from the bottom.

The placement of the feet in the correct receiving position as previously established will play a large role in the success of the clean. Misplaced feet can considerably reduce the squatting power of the athlete and place joints at undue risk of injury. Positioning of the feet in the correct fore-aft location to support the mass of the athlete and barbell is key, although the potential for this type of misplacement is significantly less than in the snatch due to the generally smaller relative foot movement and elevation during the transition between the second and third pulls. However, it's quite possible for the athlete to place the feet too far forward, or more likely too far backward, and create an immediate imbalance upon the receipt of the bar due to the center of mass not being directly over the base. As in the snatch, the feet should reconnect flat with the platform, not on the balls of the feet first. Attempting to lift the knees rather than the feet while pulling under will often help ensure this flat reconnection, as well as proper placement.

One of the most critical elements of receiving a clean successfully is the stability of the trunk. Even with the smoothest delivery of the barbell to the shoulders, the athlete will need to arrest the downward force of the barbell and change its direction abruptly as the body hits the bottommost position of the squat and the weight on the barbell tries to continue moving downward. The position of the bar on the shoulders creates a considerable lever arm on the spine with even the most upright torso, and the force of the barbell will encourage the upper back to round forward, increasing the length of the lever on the back and hips and pulling the athlete forward. This structural collapse can very quickly exceed the athlete's ability to compensate and result in a dropped barbell or a failed recovery.

The first key to preventing this collapse of the trunk is a correct pull and receiving position—that is, the more in balance the bar-lifter system, the closer the bar remains to the body during the lift, the more accurately it's placed on the shoulders and the more upright the posture in the receiving position, the less disruptive force the athlete will need to contend with in order to recover successfully and the more balanced the system will remain over the base in the re-

ceiving position.

The next is pressurization and aggressive muscular stabilization of the trunk—this is an absolute necessity irrespective of the technical accuracy of the lift. This pressurization needs of course to take place prior to the initiation of the lift. If anything, the athlete will involuntarily release a small amount of air during the second pull; there will be no chance to take in air during the lift itself.

Finally, a focus on maintaining the extension of the spine, especially in the thoracic region, is an important contributor to a successful receipt of the clean. Much like the pressurization of the trunk, this is largely a product of the starting position and first pull of the lift. Because the third pull is so rapid, it's unlikely the athlete will be able to achieve adequate spinal extension to receive the clean if that extension doesn't already exist to a large extent—in other words, it's more an issue of maintaining back extension during the lift than creating it in specific preparation for the receipt of the barbell. However, during the turnover, the effort to arch the upper back should be made as part of the effort to lift the chest and push the shoulders up to meet the bar.

The elbows at this point will already be elevated to support the rack position—they must be actively and aggressively lifted, and the shoulders actively elevated, to maintain a solid, secure rack position that will successfully resist the downward force of the bar without shifting as the athlete hits the bottom of the squat.

Although we want the athlete to catch the bounce out of the bottom of the squat to facilitate recovery, this does not mean the athlete can relax or allow the bar to continue its downward path uncontrolled. The athlete, once the bar is racked on the shoulders, must actively resist the downward force of the bar to establish control. With heavy cleans, no amount of resistance to the bar's downward force will be capable of actually stopping it above the bottom of the squat (there have been a few elite lifters who defy this rule, but they are anomalies), and a considerable degree of downward speed will be unavoidable. This being the case, the lifter can resist this downward force in an effort to stabilize and control the weight without concern for sacrificing the opportunity for the bounce out of the bottom.

Recovery

The recovery of the clean is in essence no different than that of the front squat. Where it diverges is the entry into the bottom position—a much shorter, but generally quicker, eccentric phase, and a potentially quicker transition from a greater bounce effect if the positioning is sound due to the barbell's downward speed. The receipt and recovery of the clean is extremely violent with heavy weights, and athletes need to be prepared in terms of strength, mobility, posture, timing and aggression.

All of the criteria discussed in regard to the front squat apply. The athlete's weight should be balanced over the feet approximately over the front edge of the heel (the weight may shift farther forward over the feet in the absolute bottom of the squat but should shift back quickly as the athlete recovers); the trunk must be kept as upright as possible with the spine held in complete extension with specific effort made to flatten the thoracic spine in particular; the bar must be racked securely with the shoulders protracted and slightly elevated and the elbows driven up actively; and the trunk must remain pressurized with air and stabilized through aggressive circumferential muscular action.

Actively driving the elbows up, particularly when reaching the bottom of the squat and during the recovery will encourage a quicker recovery and the maintenance of proper posture. In addition, immediately forcing the elbows up will discourage premature elevation of the hips by placing the elbows and consequently shoulders in a leading position. This movement must be aggressive and through practice should become a reflex associated with hitting the bottom of the squat. Always coupled with this lifting of the elbows should be the active elevation of the shoulders to maintain the security of the barbell and further encourage the proper upright posture. This shoulder elevation in the rack position will also help prevent pressure on the carotid arteries that can cause dizziness or lightheadedness.

The lifter should attempt to accelerate upward throughout the recovery effort. This will ensure momentum from the bounce is taken advantage of fully and will minimize slowing during the mechanically difficult mid-point of the squat, maximizing the chances of a successful recovery. Any reduction in speed will dramatically increase the difficulty of the recovery effort—this can mean a failed clean, or a failed jerk because of the excess of work in the clean recovery.

As was discussed with regard to the front squat, there may be times when air must be released during the recovery of the clean to avoid dizziness or possible unconsciousness. Again, this release should be limited to only the absolute minimum volume necessary. Forcing the release to be audible is typically a reliable way to ensure it's not excessive, as this requires the outflow to be restricted to some degree. Some lifters may find they feel stronger and faster making a habit of releasing air in this manner during all clean recoveries, in which case, this may be allowed to become a habit.

Occasionally a failure of timing or positioning will prevent the athlete from recovering immediately as intended. This of course should be avoided as much as possible, but its occurrence should not be necessarily accepted as failure before attempts at recovering are made. For athletes with comparatively weak legs, recovery without the advantage of the bounce may prove impossible, but it can still be attempted, and for those with stronger legs, it may pose little trouble at all.

Some degree of the bounce effect can be harnessed in this situation, although to a limited extent relative to what can be achieved with a proper clean. From the bottom position, the athlete can initiate a series of progressively larger bounces by performing quick activation of the quads and glutes, building on

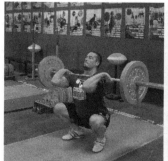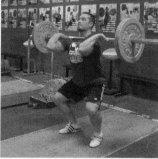

FIGURE 21.7 The recovery of the clean must be aggressive in order to maintain posture, catch the bounce out of the bottom, and drive through the sticking point of the squat.

Greg Everett

the momentum from each previous bounce with the following one. Once the athlete has generated adequate momentum and height with these bounces, he or she can attempt to initiate a full recovery, which may or may not be successful. Again, this recovery method is a last-ditch option and should be avoided by correct performance of the clean.

The Barbell's Path

As was discussed with regard to the snatch, the path of the barbell in the clean naturally and necessarily diverges from a perfectly vertical path as a result of optimal body positioning to impart force on the barbell and the need to maintain balance of the barbell-lifter system over the base. The path of the bar in the clean is in its essence the same as in the snatch, although, as a result of the different grip width and receiving position on the body, the curve is shorter, generally slightly flatter, and the distance between its maximal height and final position in the bottom of the squat is often considerably longer.

The start of the curve again represents the center of the barbell's diameter in the starting position of the lift, with the bar over the balls of the athlete's feet. As the lifter initiates the first pull, the bar shifts farther back over the feet and reaches its farthest backward point in the pull at approximately mid- to upper-thigh level (the practical equivalent to the hip position in the snatch). As the lifter finalizes the second pull, the bar is driven forward slightly, and continues in the slight forward deviation during the pull under as bar and body must pass by each other. The barbell reaches its maximal height as the lifter is squatting under it. Shortly thereafter, the lifter is bringing the elbows into place and the bar settling onto the shoulders as the squat under is completed and the bottom of the squat reached.

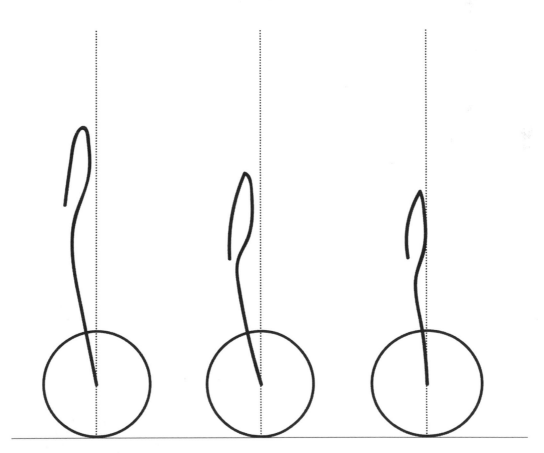

FIGURE 21.8 Pictured are the bar paths of successful cleans by three different technically proficient world-class lifters from three different weight classes. What should be immediately obvious is that, while they differ very slightly, they all conform to the same basic shape.

Again, just as with the snatch, the goal is not intentionally creating a curved bar path; the lifter is concerned only with ensuring balance of the system over the base of support and optimal postures for each phase of the lift while attempting to maintain maximal proximity of the barbell and body. That is, the lifter is attempting to minimize the curvature of the bar path without compromising balance and proper positioning.

As is the case with the snatch, the heavier the barbell is relative to the lifter, the flatter the curve of the bar path will be because the lifter's body will naturally move around the barbell more than the barbell moves around the lifter's body as a result of their respective inertia and the percentage of the total system mass they each represent.

Figure 21.8 shows three examples of slightly different bar paths from three successful cleans by three different elite weightlifters. While they differ somewhat, the basic shape is the same, and will remain essentially the same among any proficient lifters. Bar paths will deviate from this type of trajectory with less technically proficient athletes, or during poor lift execution.

Introduction to the Jerk

The jerk is the second and final phase of the clean & jerk in which the barbell is lifted from the shoulders to overhead. Although appearing with a cursory look to be entirely different from the more obviously similar snatch and clean, the jerk is in essence identical to these two lifts with regard to the actions performed by the lifter and the interaction between the lifter and barbell.

The athlete initially creates force against the platform with the lower body to accelerate and elevate the barbell, and then pushes him- or herself down underneath the barbell to fix the weight in the receiving position overhead. Conceptually this means that there is much in common among the three lifts, although in practical terms the jerk will require learning a collection of specific positions and movements. However, the learning progression for the jerk is the same in principle.

An empty barbell or light technique barbell should be used for the following drills. A PVC pipe or dowel will not allow the lifter to establish the proper jerk rack position.

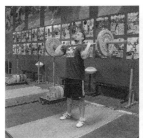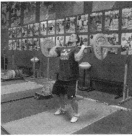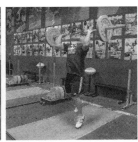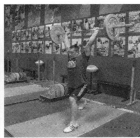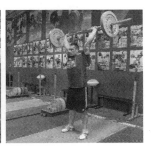

FIGURE 22.1 The jerk is the second phase of the clean & jerk, in which the barbell is lifted from the shoulders to overhead.

The Receiving Position

Just as in the snatch and clean, the first step in learning the jerk is to establish the proper receiving position to allow the lifter to receive and support maximal loads safely and effectively.

There are three styles of the jerk that rely on different receiving positions: the power jerk (or push jerk), squat jerk and split jerk. The split jerk is by far the most common competitive jerk style, and will be the end of the jerk learning progression. However, the power jerk will also be learned as a part of that progression. The squat jerk will be discussed in more detail in the following section of the book.

Power Jerk The power jerk is named such because the receiving position is identical to those of the power snatch and power clean—feet in the squat stance and thighs above horizontal. (The name *push jerk* is often used synonymously for power jerk; the two can be distinguished by defining a push jerk as a power jerk in which the feet remain connected to the platform rather than being lifted and replaced.)

While the power jerk is a fairly common training exercise, it's a comparatively rare competitive jerk style because of its great demand on bar elevation. Additionally, there exists little margin for error in bar position—the bar must be driven quite precisely into position overhead in order for the athlete to maintain its stability.

Squat Jerk The squat jerk is identical in foot position to the power jerk, but as the name implies, the ultimate receiving position is a squat. This clearly requires less elevation of the bar than the power jerk, but also introduces a few unique elements of difficulty. Mobility is an immediate limiting factor for most athletes—a relatively narrow-grip overhead squat is out of reach for lifters outside of the most mobile end of the spectrum. Additionally, there exists the need for precision in bar placement seen in the power jerk—little can be done to stabilize a bar that is even slightly out of position. Finally, consider the difficulty of recovering from the bottom of a

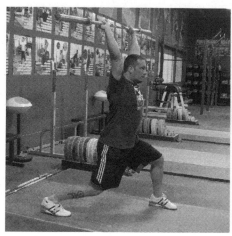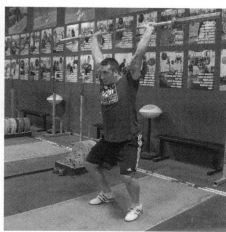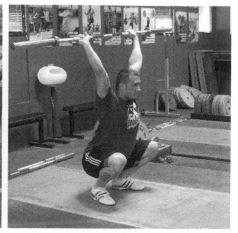

FIGURE 23.1 There are three jerk styles: split jerk, power (or push) jerk and squat jerk. The split jerk is the most commonly used by competitive weightlifters.

Greg Everett

close-grip overhead squat, often from a dead stop, particularly immediately following the effort to clean the weight. It is an extremely rare individual who possesses the mobility, precision and leg strength to make this jerk style successful.

This said, there will likely be an increase in the frequency of squat jerking in coming years, particularly among the smaller weight classes, as coaches and lifters find that jerk weights cannot keep pace with increases in the clean, and find ways to better train lifters from the start of their careers to receive and recover from squat jerks more effectively. This will allow larger weights to be jerked without having to be elevated farther, much like the squat style in the snatch and clean allowed greater weights than the split, not by increasing the ability to elevate the bar, but by moving the body lower under it. However, the likelihood of the squat jerk taking over as the dominant competitive style is still small.

Split Jerk The split jerk is the most common style used by competitive weightlifters for very simple reasons—it allows relatively great receiving depth while keeping recovery from such depths relatively easy, accommodates much greater imprecision in the overhead position of the bar than the power or squat jerk, and provides greater stability in all directions than the power or squat jerk.

The split stance, at its most extreme in the jerk, allows about the same hip depth as a parallel squat. Such a position is extremely difficult in a power jerk simply because the knee joint is at its weakest position in terms of leverage, and this depth is the point at which the hips must be farthest back, meaning there is significant forward inclination of the torso and consequently huge demand on shoulder and upper back mobility. Additionally, an athlete can recover if necessary from such a split depth by wedging up under the bar through alternating between very small movements inward by each foot rather than being forced to simply drive straight up in a single effort. It's rare that such depth is actually achieved, but the position will allow it.

The split also offers great stability in all directions by expanding the lifter's base. The width of the feet is at least that of the squat, and the length is extensive. Such a broad base, particularly in the fore-aft direction, not only improves the immediate stability

of the system, but allows for much more corrective adjustment to stabilize the bar overhead. That is, unlike with a power or squat jerk in which bar position overhead must be remarkably precise, the split allows the athlete to quickly and relatively easily shift forward and backward, and even to either side, in order to better position the support structure under the weight.

Over time, each lifter will find the jerk style that will allow the greatest weights to be lifted and spend the bulk of his or her effort developing technical proficiency and strength in that style. However, all lifters would be well served to become at least moderately competent in all three styles; each will have value as training exercises, and experience with them will allow proper evaluation of their viability as the lifter's chosen jerk style. New lifters are encouraged to learn, practice and train the split jerk until good reason is found to adopt another style.

Progression Overview

- Grip Placement
- Overhead Position
- Split Position
- Jump to Split

Grip Placement

Just as with the snatch and clean, there are a range of possible grip widths for the jerk, each end with its own benefits and drawbacks. Wider grips will reduce the distance the bar must be elevated and the depth the lifter must move under it, as well as lower the center of mass of the bar-lifter system, but will also produce more disadvantaged pressing mechanics for the arms and shoulders past a certain point, reduce the structural integrity of the overhead position somewhat, place greater strain on the wrists and elbows, increase the amount of the load each arm must bear due to increasing vector forces, and typically create more difficulty establishing a secure rack position on the shoulders.

A narrower grip will typically allow a more comfortable and secure rack position, optimize the pressing mechanics for the lifter's drive under the bar, minimize vector forces to limit how much of the load each arm is supporting, and maximize the structural integrity of the overhead position. It will, however, require more elevation of the barbell and greater depth in the receiving position, and raise the center of mass of the bar-lifter system.

Another consideration with regard to grip width in the jerk is its effect on the elastic whip of the barbell during the dip and drive. A narrower grip maintains a narrower area of support for the barbell, which allows greater deformation and rebound, potentially improving the speed and elevation of the bar. If held tightly, a wider grip expands this area of support and

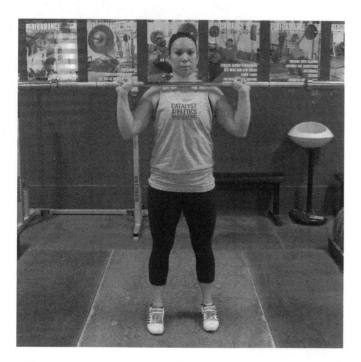

FIGURE 23.2 The grip width should initially be the same as used for the clean—half a fist-width outside the shoulders or slightly more, allowing a secure rack position.

reduces the whip of the barbell; in cases of very wide grips, it's important the lifter maintain relative looseness in the arms during the dip and drive to allow the bar to whip freely. With a narrow hand placement, a tight grip and tight arms will have negligible effects on the bar's reaction to the dip and drive.

At this stage, athletes can simply use their clean hand placement for the jerk—about half a fist-width to a fist-width outside the shoulders. After becoming more experienced with the movement, they can experiment with different hand widths to find what best suits their particular strengths and weaknesses.

Overhead Position

The overhead position for the jerk is identical to that of the snatch with the exception of the narrower grip. Accordingly, the athlete can use the same method to initially establish the proper position.

The athlete will take a jerk-width hand placement with no hook grip on the bar and place it across the shoulders behind the neck as he or she would for a back squat. The shoulder blades should be squeezed together along their upper inside edges to create retraction and upward rotation. There should be no active elevation of the shoulder blades (shrugging), although there may be the appearance of shrugging in

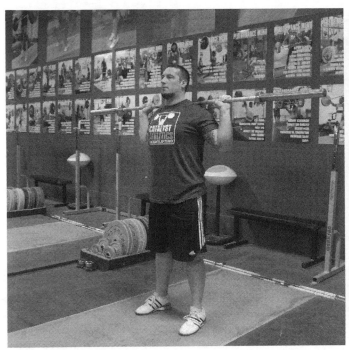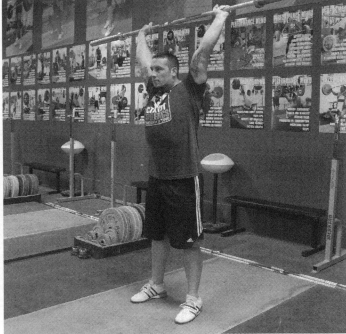

FIGURE 23.3 To find the correct overhead position easily, begin with the bar behind the neck and the upper inside edges of the shoulder blades squeezed together tightly. Press the bar straight up and maintain the same torso inclination and shoulder blade position.

this position and a small degree of scapular elevation.

This bar placement should naturally cause the torso to lean forward very slightly and position the bar over the feet as it needs to be in order for the athlete to remain balanced with the addition of weight. From this position, the athlete will press the bar straight up with no change to the torso or shoulder blade positions. The bar should finish directly above the base of the neck.

Relative to the snatch overhead position, the arms will be slightly more externally rotated in the jerk overhead position. That is, the bony points of the elbows will be oriented closer to pointing straight out away from the lifter, but not entirely. A proper degree of arm rotation for the jerk overhead position is generally more natural for athletes than it is in the snatch. The wrists and hands should be somewhat relaxed with the bar in the palm just behind the midline of the forearm, the grip no tighter than what is necessary to maintain control and position.

The details of the overhead structure are the same as in the snatch, and are left out here to avoid redundancy. The snatch overhead position can be reviewed in the Learning the Snatch chapter if these details are required.

Split Position

In teaching the athlete the receiving position for the split jerk, the first step is determining which leg the athlete will lead with. There are a number of ways to do this, and most are unnecessary and overly complex. Nearly invariably athletes will know intuitively which leg they'll feel more comfortable with in front before ever having performed a split jerk. If an athlete does not, he or she can simply stand in a basic split position with each foot forward and it should be immediately obvious which is more comfortable.

If this is not the case with a certain athlete, the coach can simply instruct him or her to perform walking lunges and provide no further detail. Athletes will naturally step out with the preferred forward leg to start the exercise. Following this, it's always wise to have the athlete stand in a split with each leg forward to compare the two; if he or she is an exception to this rule, it should be immediately obvious.

Once the lead leg is selected, the athlete will step into a shallow lunge position from which we can adjust to achieve the proper split position.

The width of the feet should be approximate-

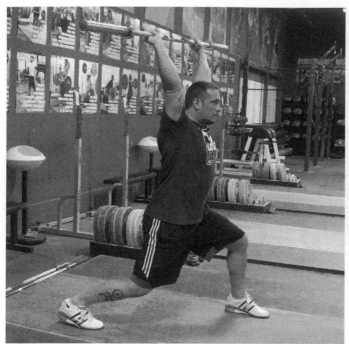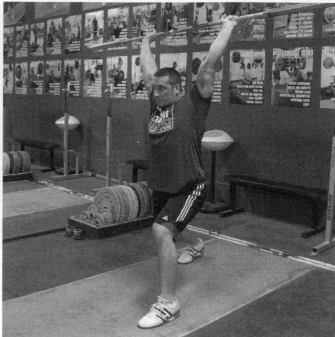

FIGURE 23.4 The split position for the jerk

ly the same as it is in the athlete's squat stance or even slightly wider in some cases. Lateral stability in the split is critical with the very high center of mass of the jerk and the consequently greater potential for instability.

The athlete's lead foot will be flat on the floor with the weight balanced across it with a slight preference for the heel, and the foot either straight forward or the toe turned in very slightly. The heel of the back foot will be elevated and the pressure on the balls of the foot; the heel should not be elevated dramatically and the weight shifted onto the toes.

The toes of the rear foot will be turned in somewhat in order to keep the foot in line with the lower leg as it would be if standing or squatting (Figure 23.5). Because the leg will be oriented at an angle away from the body, if the foot is straight forward, the ankle will not be aligned with the force traveling down that leg. Such misalignment limits structural integrity and opens the ankle for rolling out under the loading of the jerk.

The length and depth of the split should be ad-

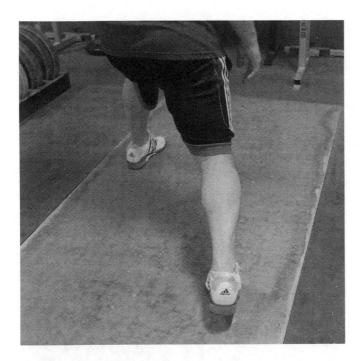

FIGURE 23.5 The rear foot should be turned in to remain in line with the leg to maintain the structural integrity of the ankle.

justed until the shin of the lead leg is approximately vertical (the knee above or slightly behind the ankle) with the front thigh at an approximately 20-40-degree angle relative to the floor. The back knee must remain unlocked—primarily this helps relieve tension on the hip flexors of the rear leg to help avoid lumbar hyperextension, and also allows the maintenance of balance under the bar in the split at any depth. Allowing the back knee to bend along with the front when driving under the weight will ensure the athlete moves straight down and remains in a supporting position under the bar. If the back knee locks while the athlete is bending the front knee to settle in under the bar, he or she will be pushed forward, which will push the bar forward as well, beyond a position that can be supported in most cases. This bend in the back knee does not need to be significant, but needs to be established in every jerk to allow better position under the bar as needed.

This split depth can be considered a default position for jerking and should be adjusted according to the demands of increasing weight. The depth of the hips in the split during an actual lift will be determined by how high the lifter is able to elevate the bar and consequently how far underneath it he or she

must push him- or herself in order to receive it with fully extended arms. While athletes will obviously be able to get away with much shallower and shorter splits with light weights, this can lead to trouble getting into an adequately long and deep split later with maximal jerk attempts. Because of this, it's suggested that even with light weights, the athlete split to approximately the same length, even if the depth is somewhat shallower.

The torso should be essentially vertical, although inclined forward very slightly as required by the correct overhead positioning. Once the barbell is added to the system, the correct position will place the hips directly underneath it. The spine should remain in neutral curvature with the trunk pressurized and tight. If the lower back is hyperextended with the trunk vertical, either the back knee is not flexed enough, the athlete's hip flexors need to be stretched, the abs are not tight enough, or a combination of the previous.

The lifter's weight should be balanced approximately equally between the two feet. Note that with the weight centered over the base, there will be slightly greater pressure on the lead foot than the back because of its greater proximity to the center of mass. However, this is generally not a significant enough difference to be noticeable by the athlete, and consequently the goal should be to feel approximately equal weight on each foot.

Jump to Split

Once the athlete has become familiar with the correct split position, we will perform the jump to split exercise without a barbell. This is a very simple way to practice the transition of the feet into the split position allowing focus on speed, precision, posture and balance without any concern for a barbell overhead.

The lifter will start standing tall with the feet in the pulling position used for the snatch and clean—the heels under the hips to orient the legs approximately vertically. With a shallow bend of the knees and then a slight jump straight up, the lifter will quickly reposition the feet in the split position.

The goal is to move the feet as quickly and accurately into the split position as possible and land immediately with the proper balance and upright posture. That is, eventually, no adjustments should need to be made to the lifter's position following the feet reconnecting with the floor.

Commonly athletes will leap forward into the split position, diving the chest forward and placing far too much weight on the lead leg. It's important that athletes attempt to maintain the same upright trunk they begin with and move only the feet.

In a proficient split jerk, the rear foot should connect with the platform just slightly before the lead foot. This will create a base against which the athlete will push as he or she completes the drive under the barbell, allowing the hips to move in under the bar as necessary. This will happen naturally if the athlete is balanced during the dip and drive of the jerk, and if the hips are moved in under the jerk properly.

Additionally, the front foot should be lifted somewhat more than the rear foot—the rear foot should remain close to the floor as it moves back into position, while the front foot must be lifted and stomped flat against the floor, producing the same sharp clap heard in the reposition of the feet for the snatch and clean. If the lead foot is elevated inadequately, the downward drive under the bar will cause it to recon-

nect with the platform prematurely, resulting in too short of a foot placement to achieve the necessary split depth or establish balance, and a failure to lock out the bar overhead. While elevation beyond what is necessary is preferable to insufficient elevation, considerable excess is also undesirable.

If an athlete tries to dive the chest forward through the arms, usually as a result of thinking of the slight forward torso lean of the overhead position, this will tend to cause the rear foot to lift excessively and reach too far back—often so far back that it actually pulls the hips back with it, preventing the lead foot from moving far enough forward, causing the lead foot to reconnect with the platform before the rear foot, and the lifter to be too far behind the bar to support it.

For this reason, the athlete will need to focus on maintaining his or her balance far enough back over the feet in the start, keeping the back foot as close to the floor as possible during its movement backward, and pushing the hips forward into position. The lead foot will need to be elevated higher than the rear foot in order to allow the athlete to drive under the barbell deeply enough.

The athlete should hold the split position for 3

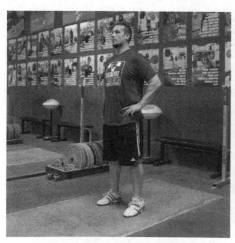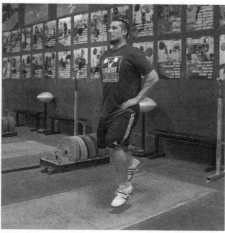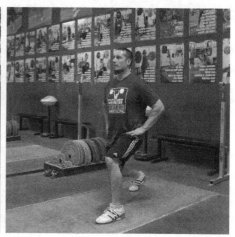

FIGURE 23.6 The jump to split allows the lifter to practice the quick and precise transition of the feet into the split receiving position while maintaining proper balance and posture following an upward drive of the legs.

Greg Everett

seconds before recovering to a standing position. If the initial position is not correct, the lifter should adjust until it is and hold that position. The more time spent in the correct position, the sooner the lifter will learn it. Repeatedly jumping into an incorrect split position will simply reinforce that incorrect position.

To recover from the split, the athlete will first step back about a third of the split distance with the front foot, and then bring the back foot up to meet it, being careful to maintain the upright trunk position and balance. This sequence should be the default for all jerks.

The jerk is the lift that will result in the greatest amount of weight in the highest position—this means the highest center of mass and the most opportunity for instability. By moving only part of the distance with each step and maintaining the same approximate location of the bar—essentially "wedging" up under it—the athlete minimizes movement of the bar overhead and limits the potential for instability. A complete forward or backward step pushes the bar a considerable distance forward or backward and generates momentum that will be very difficult to control. This recovery sequence should be employed in every exercise or drill the athlete performs involving the split position.

Stepping back with the front foot first is more stable than the reverse simply because the rear leg will be stiffer and less prone to collapsing unexpectedly than the front. By stepping the rear foot forward instead, the entire weight of the system is supported by a knee likely bent significantly, meaning it's in a position in which forward shifting is very likely, creating horizontal movement of the barbell and body that may not be recoverable.

---

41 Progression Summary

Jump to Split

Stand tall with the feet under the hips.

Bend slightly at the knees only and drive up in a slight jump.

Keeping your trunk upright, move quickly into the split position to land with equal balance between the feet.

Adjust the position and balance if needed and hold for 3 seconds.

Step a third of the split length back with the front foot, then bring the back foot up to meet it.

Learning the Jerk

Just as with the snatch and clean, the receiving position has been established first, and the athlete is now prepared to learn the technique of the jerk itself. As was the case with learning the clean, an empty barbell or light technique bar should be used for the following learning progressions.

Progression Overview

- Rack Position
- Stance & Dip
- Press
- Push Press
- Tall Power Jerk
- Power Jerk
- Split Jerk Behind the Neck
- Jerk Balance
- Split Jerk

Jerk Rack Position

The first step in the jerk progression is establishing a rack position specific to the jerk. This rack position will be used for all jerk-related exercises, both during the learning progression and in subsequent training, such as the press and push press.

As for the clean, the first priority of the jerk rack position is to connect the barbell directly to the trunk—that is, to support it on the shoulders completely rather than in the arms. This ties the bar to the legs and ensures maximal force transfer from the legs into the bar during the upward drive.

However, where the rack differs from the clean is in the position of the hands and arms, which need to be in the most advantageous position for the active

push of the body under the barbell without sacrificing the security of the bar on the shoulders during the preceding dip and drive. This position will allow optimal power in the push under the bar as well as encourage the proper bar path.

Questions occasionally arise regarding the use of the jerk rack position for the press, as it is often not clear why the bar must be connected the same way to the body, and because such a position places the bar slightly farther back in the hand than some lifters have been taught is ideal for pressing (in particular bench pressing). While it may be arguable that a bar placement closer to the heel of the palm is ideal for pressing in terms of the actual movement itself, there are two basic reasons this is not used. First, the athlete needs to be able to support the weight prior to

42 Progression Summary

Jerk Rack Position

Hold the bar in a jerk-width grip.

Extend the upper back.

Push the shoulders forward as much as possible and up slightly.

Place the bar in the channel between the throat and the highest point of the shoulders.

Keep as full of a grip around the bar as possible without squeezing tightly.

Bring the elbows down until slightly in front of the bar and spread them to the sides without changing the shoulder or bar positions.

and following the press—it's difficult to support this much weight in the arms alone. A rack on the shoulders creates a base from which to press. (It should be noted that typically during multiple-rep pressing sets, the rack position is not reset, and reps after the first completed as "touch and go".). Second, and far more important, the press in this particular context is nothing more than part of a teaching progression and an assistance exercise for the jerk. This being the case, the positions and movements must reflect those of the jerk for greatest utility; however, all athletes should aim to sink the palm as deeply as possible under the bar without sacrificing its placement on the shoulders.

The shoulders need to be elevated slightly and protracted to create a channel in which the bar can rest securely between the highest point of the shoulders and the throat just like in the clean rack position. Again, the slight elevation of the shoulders is important not just for the security of the bar, but also to keep pressure off of the carotid arteries and collarbones. The upper back also needs to be extended maximally.

The grip should be as full as possible—that is, the bar as close to being in the palms as it can be without the shoulders being moved from the proper position. However, no matter how full the grip is around the bar, it should be relatively loose—a tight grip can move the bar prematurely from the secure position on the shoulders, and it will also slow and possibly limit the extension of the elbows.

The elbows should be lowered and spread to the

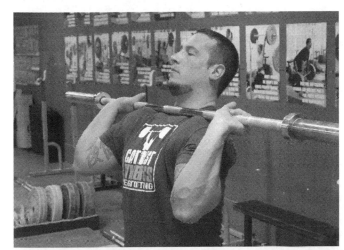
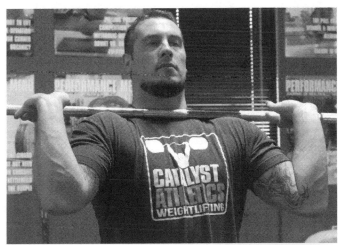
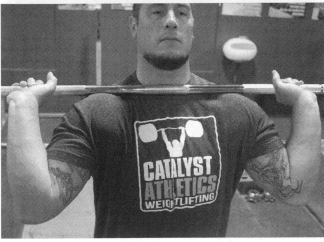
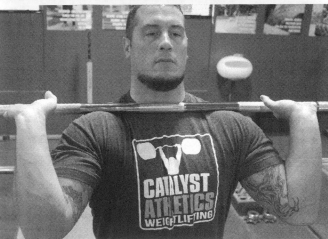

FIGURE 24.1 The jerk rack position, like the clean rack position, connects the bar directly to the trunk, but also prepares for the push under the bar by keeping the hands deeper under the bar and the elbows down and out.

FIGURE 24.2 Athletes with certain proportions or limited mobility may need to use an open grip with the bar on the fingers instead of a full grip, and may need to lift the elbows higher. Different grip widths should be experimented with to bring the athlete to the rack position closest to ideal allowed by the existing limitations.

sides. The lower the elbows are without being directly under the bar (they should always remain at least slightly in front of the bar), the better the mechanics will be for pushing under the bar after its upward drive with the legs. Spreading the elbows to the sides will also help with the pressing mechanics, as well as allow the lifter to better pressurize the trunk with air and create a strong position from which to drive the bar up. The lats should be spread to the sides to support the arms and shoulders in their proper positions.

The actual arm and hand positions achievable will vary with each athlete's individual anatomy and mobility. Again, the priority is the security of the bar on the shoulders—the athlete needs to achieve the best hand and arm positions possible at any given stage without sacrificing the proper shoulder position and placement of the bar.

Athletes unable to achieve the desired position should first experiment with different grip widths. Generally, wider grips will accommodate unusual proportions and limited mobility best. Occasionally, however, a narrower grip will be better. Athletes will have to experiment with the range of grip widths to find what works best, and this will change over time with improving mobility. The shifting of the grip between the clean and the jerk will be discussed in the Clean & Jerk chapter.

If a reasonable change in grip width still fails to allow a proper position of the bar, shoulders and arms, the athlete will need to open the grip somewhat and move the bar from the palms to the fingers. Likely an elevation of the elbows will need to accompany this, but not necessarily.

Stance & Dip

Just as in the snatch and clean, there will be two foot positions for the jerk—the drive position and the receiving position, which will depend on the jerk style, as discussed in the previous chapter.

The basic starting point for the drive position is essentially the same as the pulling position for the snatch and clean: the feet slightly wider than hip width and turned out about 10-20 degrees. Again like the pulling position for the snatch and clean, athletes will need to experiment to find the drive position

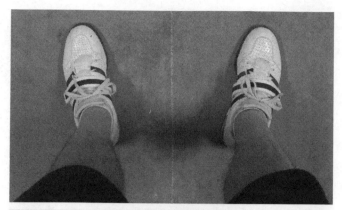

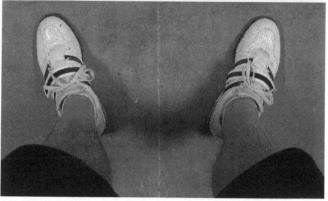

FIGURE 24.3 The feet in the jerk drive stance should typically be between 10-20 degrees from the centerline.

that feels most comfortable and allows them to be most effective in the jerk.

Theoretically, the stance that aligns the legs vertically will allow for the greatest barbell elevation in the drive both because it creates the greatest height for the body when extended upward and because the force of the legs is oriented directly down and back up rather than being dispersed through any angle of the legs.

However, numerous other factors contribute to the effectiveness of the drive of the jerk, some of which have a significantly greater effect than the previous. Accordingly, athletes must find the stance that allows the best possible dip and drive for their particular builds, strengths and weaknesses.

It's fairly unusual, although certainly not unheard of, for an athlete to prefer a significantly narrower foot placement, but slightly wider stances are common. These wider stances are typically similar to the athlete's squat width—the feet are simply left unadjusted following the recovery from the clean. This generally reduces the disadvantages of longer legs somewhat and may also reduce knee discomfort during the dip.

Dip Position

Initially, the athlete will be practicing a basic dip position to learn the fundamentals primarily with regard to position and posture, and secondarily to depth. These things may change for some lifters over time as experience and experimentation guide modifications to best suit each lifter.

The most important element of the jerk dip for the athlete to understand is that it involves the knees only. Most athletes are accustomed to hinging at the hips, and this is a natural movement when also bending the knees to drive against the ground (such as in a jump). While this may remain a relatively uncomfortable movement indefinitely, and feel weaker than a dip in which the hips are pushed back, the key is that the knees-only dip will keep the lifter positioned and move the bar properly—the lifter's comfort is essentially irrelevant, but it will improve over time with practice. This feeling of awkwardness can make learning the movement of the dip and drive very difficult for some new lifters—teaching and enforcing a proper dip position from the first day is the most effective way to avoid problems.

The athlete will hold an empty barbell in the jerk rack position and place the feet in the drive stance. When viewed from the side, a vertical line can be drawn through the front of the athlete's shoulder, hip and ankle. The knees should be straight but not locked in hyperextension. The weight should be primarily on the heel but with full contact of the foot on the floor—that is, the athlete's weight should never be so far back that the balls of the feet are not connected completely to the floor. The weight should be toward the heels, but the entire foot flat on the floor. The spine should be in its neutral position because of the essentially direct vertical loading, the thoracic spine extended, and the trunk pressurized with air and tightened circumferentially to create maximal rigidity.

To enter the dip position, the athlete will slowly bend at the knees only, making sure the knees travel in line with the feet as they would in a squat, which will mean moving outward to some degree, and maintaining constant tension in the quads. The barbell and hips should travel straight down through the vertical line described above, and the weight distribution remain unchanged across the feet. The starting point

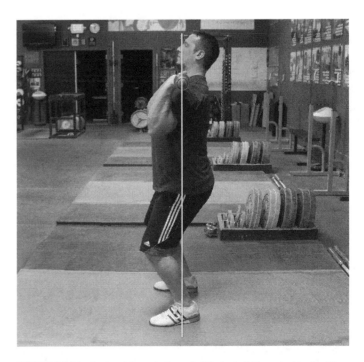

FIGURE 24.4 In the dip of the jerk, the end of the barbell, hip and ankle should remain within the same vertical line that passes through these points in the starting position. The starting point for dip depth is approximately 8-10% of the lifter's height.

---

43 Progression Summary

Jerk Dip

The feet are slightly wider than hip width and turned out 10-20 degrees, with the weight primarily on the heels but with full foot contact.

The knees are bent to lower the athlete 8-10% of his or her height.

The knees are pushed out to remain aligned with the feet.

The trunk is vertical with the barbell, hips and ankles remaining in the same vertical plane when viewed from the side.

---

for dip depth is approximately 8-10% of the lifter's height. Once the lifter has reached this depth, he or she should hold this bottom position for 3 seconds to ensure balance and proper posture—the weight still primarily on the heels with full foot contact and the trunk vertical.

Once the athlete has established his or her dip position, it can be drilled briefly before moving on. From standing, the athlete should slowly enter the position, hold it for further familiarization, and recover to standing at the same low speed. This deliberate speed will allow for the coach to observe and provide feedback for the lifter to adjust during the movement, as well as allow the lifter to actually feel the correct position. The quads and glutes should remain tight throughout the movement; in the standing position, the knees should not be locked.

Press

As in the snatch and clean learning progressions, the next step is to learn the upper body mechanics of the lifter's movement down under the bar following the drive. The lifter has learned the jerk rack position and overhead position, and now will learn how to properly move the bar between them, which will later translate into moving the body beneath the bar.

The primary element in this exercise is learning to move the bar past the face and into the overhead position in as direct a line as possible with the arms

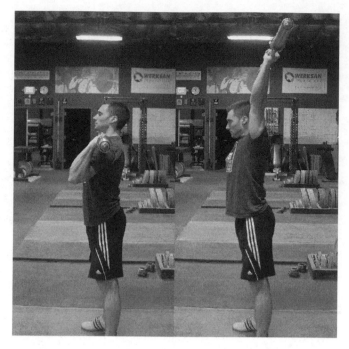

FIGURE 24.5 The barbell begins in front of the trunk and ends behind it, while the trunk begins behind the barbell and ends in front of it. This means that in the press and jerk, the bar and trunk must both move horizontally somewhat to remain in balance.

in the most mechanically advantageous position as possible. This requires some horizontal movement of the trunk, bar and head.

In the rack position, the barbell is in front of the trunk, while in the overhead position, it will be behind it. This means that during the press (and the push under the jerk) that the bar and trunk must switch places with slight horizontal movement (Figure 24.5). This will happen fairly naturally in the press as the

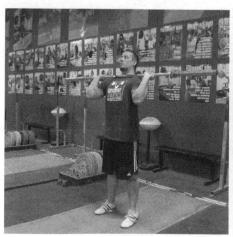
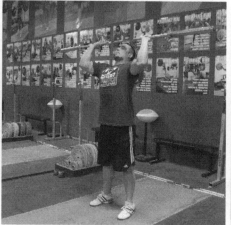
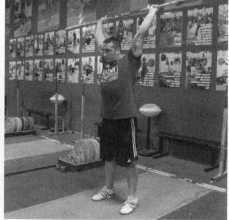

FIGURE 24.6 The press introduces the mechanics of the upper body for the drive under the barbell in the jerk.

Greg Everett

body adjusts to remain in balance in each position.

From the jerk rack position with a pressurized and tight trunk, the athlete will initiate the drive of the bar up by placing a very slight backward angle on it as it leaves the shoulders. This effort to press the bar through the face will ensure better positioning and prevent the common error of pushing the bar away from the body and leaning backward excessively, or of moving the bar out and around the head.

The athlete must press the bar in as direct a line as possible into its final position. In order to do this, the face must be pulled back out of the way. Generally, the athlete should pull the face back more than tilt the head back as the bar nears the chin. This repositioning of the face can be started while the bar is still racked on the shoulders to reduce the magnitude of the shift that will be necessary as the bar passes. This partial pull and tilt back of the face is naturally coupled with the lifted chest position that helps rack the bar correctly on the shoulders. The same focal point straight ahead should be easily maintained during this movement.

As the bar leaves the shoulders, the elbows should begin to be spread out to move under the bar rather than remaining in front of it. This helps with the proper bar path and improves the mechanics of the pressing motion. Again, spreading the lats in the rack position will help improve the position and the initial drive off the shoulders.

The torso may also need to lean back very slightly as the bar passes in front of the face, although usu-

ally such leaning of the torso is performed unnecessarily. Any layback should remain restricted to what is absolutely necessary. Excessive distance between the body and the bar simply increases the mechanical disadvantage of the pressing motion.

Once the bar has passed the head, the lifter will push his or her head forward again through the arms in order to achieve the proper overhead position, which will place the bar over the back of the neck. The lifter should hold the bar tightly in the correct overhead position, actively squeezing the shoulder blades together and the elbows in complete extension.

The grip should remain relatively loose—only as tight as necessary to maintain control of the bar and keep it positioned properly in the hand—just as with snatch overhead exercises. Again, while a tight grip may improve strength in slow lifts, it will limit elbow extension speed and the completion of full elbow extension in explosive movements like the jerk.

The press should be practiced until the bar path and elbow movement are smooth and consistent and the overhead position is correct and stable.

Push Press

The push press is an intermediate movement combining elements of the press and the jerk. As a lift itself, it's an excellent strength builder, allowing the athlete to press greater loads overhead by using the legs to assist the arms and shoulders, as well as training the position and timing of the dip and drive. As a progression toward the jerk, it introduces the athlete to the idea of initiating an upward drive of the bar with a dip and subsequent drive of the legs, as well as the timing of the transitioning between driving with the legs to pressing with the arms.

First and foremost, athletes need to understand that the leg drive is responsible for the majority of the barbell's elevation, just like in the jerk; the arms perform what is in effect a follow-through, using the existing momentum of the barbell to press it into the final overhead position. This should not be misunderstood to mean that the arms don't perform significant work, particularly in a heavy push press, but that complete and aggressive leg drive to accelerate and elevate the bar needs to be the focus of every push press rep.

The athlete will begin standing in the drive position with the bar secured in the jerk rack position and pressurize the trunk with air. This pressurization and rigidity of the trunk is critical for success—an unstable torso will succumb to the tendency for the spine to collapse forward, protracting the braking period at the bottom of the dip and reducing the elastic effects of the bar and muscles, reduce the transfer of leg drive into the bar, and typically shift the athlete's weight forward and misdirect the bar.

After filling the torso with air and tightening down the surrounding musculature circumferentially, the athlete should pause a second or two to ensure stabilization and balance has been established. Often a rush to commence the lift immediately after the breath or even as the breath is being finished will greatly reduce stability and typically pull the lifter's balance forward. This pause will allow the body to settle into this solid position, and as has been discussed previously, a correct movement is impossible from an incorrect position. At this point, the lifter should tighten the quads with the knees straight but unlocked to ensure a smooth initiation of the dip.

Once the lifter is stable, he or she will dip by bending at the knees only. The actual depth will vary among athletes depending on their particular strengths and proportions, but a starting point is 8-10% of their height—dip depth and speed will be discussed in detail in the following chapter.

For now, the speed of the dip must balance the need to generate a stretch-shortening cycle to increase the power of the subsequent concentric movement, the ability to transition powerfully, and the need to maintain a connection between the bar and the

45 Progression Summary

Push Press

Stand with the feet in the drive position, the bar secured in the jerk rack position, and the trunk pressurized and tight.

Keep the weight balanced primarily on the heels with full foot contact on the floor and the quads tight.

Dip smoothly at the knees to about 8-10% of height and drive back up immediately and aggressively.

As the legs finish extending, keep the knees straight and quickly push the bar up and back off the shoulders with the arms.

Move the head back out of the way of the bar and spread the elbows out and under the bar as it rises.

Bring the head back through the arms and secure the bar tightly in the correct overhead position.

shoulders. The initial acceleration into the dip must be controlled enough to prevent separation of the bar from the shoulders—too abrupt of an initiation of the dip, and the lifter will drop out from under the bar, and the bar will bounce or crash on the shoulders, disrupting the rhythm and the natural elasticity that plays an important role in the movement, and typically the balance and posture of the lifter.

The transition between dip and drive must be immediate and powerful, and the lifter's trunk remain

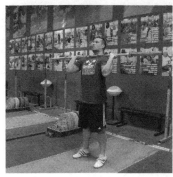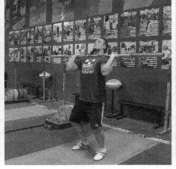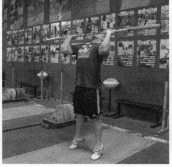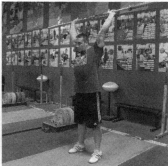

FIGURE 24.7 The push press introduces the dip and drive to accelerate and elevate the barbell.

rigid and vertical, without any forward shifting of balance over the feet. The tighter the lifter and more quickly the dip is stopped and reversed, the more powerful the subsequent drive can be.

The athlete will drive straight up with the legs, attempting to achieve maximal upward acceleration of the bar. As the legs near extension and the speed on the bar is maximal, the arms must be brought in to continue the bar's path upward. Timing this transition is key—pressing too early with the arms will prevent the full transfer of leg power to the bar, while waiting too long before initiating the press will mean loss of upward momentum from the powerful leg drive. Keeping the grip relatively loose during the dip and drive will help prevent premature engagement of the arms.

Athletes will naturally rise onto the balls of their feet at the end of the leg drive just as they do with the final extension of the snatch and clean. As with the snatch and clean, even with only the balls of the feet in contact with the platform, the center of mass must remain in its original position to prevent the balance of the system from shifting forward. Prolonged ankle extension will result in a forward weight shift. If a lifter remains flat-footed throughout a push press, it's a clear indicator of inadequate or incomplete leg drive.

Once the legs finish their extension, the quads should remain tight to keep the knees straight and provide a solid platform to support the press with the arms. Soft knees will limit the driving force transmitted to the bar, and any bending of the knees following the drive technically makes the movement a jerk rather than a push press.

As the bar leaves the shoulders, the lifter will perform the same movement practiced in the press—move the head back out of the way, push the bar at a slight backward angle, spread the elbows out and under the bar, bring the head back into position, and lock the shoulder blades and elbows forcefully in the proper overhead position. An active and aggressive overhead position should be practiced in every single rep to develop habits that will ensure proper structure and aggression in the jerk.

If an athlete is struggling with the timing of the push press, it can be split into two distinct movements by holding the bottom of the dip position for a moment before driving and pressing. Once the

transition between the leg drive and press has been learned, the lifter can return to performing the push press as a single continuous movement.

Tall Power Jerk

Now that the athlete has learned to accelerate the barbell upward with the legs and transition to pushing with the arms, the movement of driving the body down under the bar needs to be introduced. As in the snatch and clean progressions, an abbreviated movement will allow the athlete to feel this portion of the lift in relative isolation before integrating it with the entire lift.

Standing in the drive position with the bar in jerk rack position, the athlete will press the bar to the top of the forehead to set the starting position for the drill. In this position, the head should be pulled back out of the way of the bar as it would be during this segment of a jerk or push press, and the bar approximately above the shoulders with the elbows spread and nearly under the bar (Figure 24.8).

Once the athlete has set this starting position and

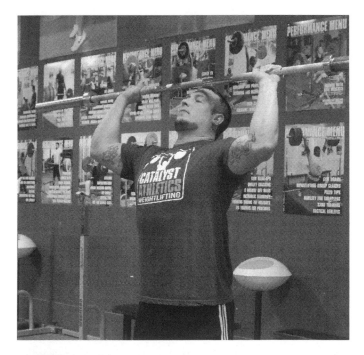

FIGURE 24.8 In the starting position for the tall power jerk, the head needs to be pulled back to allow the bar to be over the shoulders with the elbows nearly under the bar.

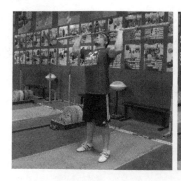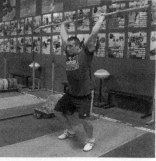

FIGURE 24.9 The tall power jerk is an abbreviated movement to introduce the feeling of driving aggressively under the bar into the receiving position.

pressurized and stabilized the trunk, he or she will lift and aggressively replace the feet flat in the power receiving position while punching down against the bar to fix it in the overhead position. Like in previous drills for the snatch, the goal is to attempt to lock the elbows into position at the same time the feet hit the platform.

In reality, the feet will reconnect prior to elbow lockout in the jerk, just as in the snatch, but also as in the snatch, extremely quick elbow extension is a critical component of a successful lift, and the attempt to achieve this timing will encourage greater speed. A sense of viciousness must be instilled in the athlete at the outset, whether working with little weight or maximal loads.

The athlete should hold the power receiving position for 3 seconds, aggressively locking the overhead position. A habit of forceful overhead lockout maintenance needs to be created from the outset.

Once the bar has been stabilized in the proper position, the lifter will recover to a standing position with the arms remaining extended actively—the lift does not end until the athlete is standing fully again and the bar is stabilized overhead. This is another habit that must be instilled early on. At this point, the bar may be lowered for a subsequent rep.

If an athlete is having trouble with the idea of pushing under the bar, this drill can be performed a slowly. Starting with the bar in the same half-press position, but with the feet already standing flat in the receiving stance, the lifter can slowly press him- or herself down into a quarter squat while locking out the elbows. The bar should remain at approximate-

ly the same height. Once the athlete is comfortable with this simplified movement, he or she can return to the original drill.

Power Jerk

Whereas the snatch and clean involve first an upward acceleration of the barbell with the lower body followed by pull of the body under the bar with the arms, the jerk begins with an upward acceleration of the bar with the lower body followed by a push of the body under the bar with the arms; the principle is the same—elevating and accelerating the bar as much as possible with the lower body before rapidly and actively relocating the body into a lower position in which to receive the weight with the arms.

The power jerk is used by some weightlifters in competition, although its use is less common than the split jerk because of its relative fore and aft instability and the limitations on possible depth. In order to be a successful power jerker, a lifter must be able to produce a very consistently precise dip, drive and bar path and be able to elevate the load relatively high.

Outside of a competitive jerking style, the power jerk is an important drill in the jerk learning progression, and will be a valuable training exercise later. The press has introduced the athlete to the motion of the upper body, the push press has taught the athlete the dip and drive of the legs and the transition between leg and arm drive, and the tall power jerk introduced the relocation of the body under the bar. The power jerk now assembles all of these elements into a complete jerk, but without overcomplicating it with the split receiving position.

The lifter will begin standing with the feet in the drive position and the bar in the jerk rack position, taking in a deep pressurizing breath and tightening the trunk musculature circumferentially to create maximal rigidity. Following this pressurization, the lifter should finalize the balance over the feet—most of the weight over the heels but with full foot contact on the floor.

Often athletes will maintain the initial standing position with a passive lockout of the knees in the same way they naturally stand. This means there is little tension in the quads, and if the dip is initiated from this passive knee lockout, there will be slack in the system and consequently a brief moment during which the athlete is essentially free-falling; this abrupt drop creates separation between the bar and body and disrupts the ideal eccentric loading of the legs to create the optimal elastic qualities of the dip and drive movement. To prevent this, the athlete should begin all jerks with the knees straight but unlocked and tension already generated in the quads. This will

prevent any slack and ensure a smooth acceleration into the dip.

Keeping the trunk tight and the knees moving in line with the feet, the lifter will dip at a speed that allows constant connection with the bar and a strong bottom position with no unwanted shifting of balance or posture. At the bottom of the dip, the tendency for most lifters will be to allow the balance to shift forward. The rack position needs to remain static with the bar secure and unmoving—the lifter will need to actively maintain the proper shoulder position by predicting and resisting the downward force of the bar, which will reach maximum and well beyond the weight of the bar at the bottom of the dip. Any dropping of the shoulders will result in a reduction of the possible elastic energy and the transfer of force into the bar, as well as typically shift the bar out of position forward.

Often a shifting rack position is the result of the athlete beginning to engage the arms for the pressing motion prematurely, producing a tightening of the grip and dropping of the elbows. This disrupts the balance and transfer of power to the bar, and can remove the support of the bar enough to cause it to visibly slide down the lifter's shoulders somewhat.

The arms and shoulders must remain in the same position throughout the dip and drive to ensure the bar's security on the shoulders. Again, this can best be encouraged by keeping the grip relatively relaxed during the dip and drive.

After braking as quickly as possible at the bottom of the dip, the lifter will immediately drive straight up as aggressively as possible with the legs, maintaining the same balance over the foot. The path of the bar during the dip and drive should describe a straight vertical line or even move very slightly back-

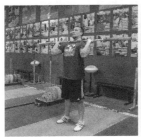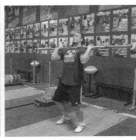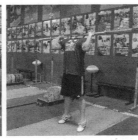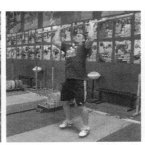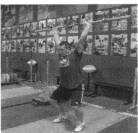

FIGURE 24.10 The power jerk introduces the lifter to the complete jerk motion with reduced complexity by avoiding the dramatic foot movement into the split receiving position.

ward in the drive—any deviation forward indicates a problem.

Most commonly the lifter's weight will shift forward because the chest drops to engage the hips more, or because the lifter has failed to maintain an adequately rigid trunk or secure rack position. Any imbalance in the dip or drive will redirect the bar out of its very limited allowable path.

While in the starting position and during the dip, the athlete will be able to feel more pressure on the heels than the balls of the feet, the center of pressure will naturally shift toward the balls of the feet during the drive, increasingly so as it progresses. However, just as in the snatch and clean pull, this change in the center of pressure over the foot is the result of the natural plantar flexion of the ankle that accompanies aggressive leg extension against the floor, and does not indicate a forward shifting of the center of mass. In other words, despite the pressure moving from the heel toward the balls of the feet during the drive, the combined barbell-lifter center of mass should remain balanced over the same point throughout the lift.

It's important when setting the starting position that the athlete not shift back excessively onto the heels as well. Such excessive balance on the heels will usually result in a compensatory rock forward as the lift is initiated, shifting the balance even farther forward. Again, maintaining contact of the full foot on the floor is important to avoid this.

At the top of the drive, the athlete should intentionally create a final, maximal effort against the bar much like would occur in the final pull of the snatch or clean, using this final explosion as the initiation of the arms' push against the bar and the transition of the feet into the receiving position.

As the bar separates from the shoulders at the top of the drive, the lifter will quickly pull his or her head back out of the way to allow the bar an uninterrupted line of travel past the face, after which it will be brought back into its final overhead position and locked forcefully. At the same time, the feet will need to be transitioned to the receiving position as quickly and powerfully as possible, and planted flat directly under the bar. An audible clap as the feet reconnect with the platform indicates a proper flat connection and adequate speed and aggression; it should not be the product of excessive elevation of the feet during

47 Progression Summary

Power Jerk

Begin with the feet in the drive position and the bar secured in the jerk rack position.

Pressurize and stabilize the trunk, settle the balance over the heels with full foot contact with the floor, and keep the knees straight but unlocked.

Dip at the knees only while maintaining connection with the bar, brake quickly, and drive straight up aggressively.

As the legs near complete extension, push against the bar with the arms to begin moving it into the overhead position, moving the head back out of the way.

As the arms push against the bar, lift and move the feet to plant them flat in the power jerk receiving position.

Lock the bar forcefully in the overhead position at a quarter squat depth at the same time the feet reconnect with the platform.

Hold the receiving position aggressively for 3 seconds before standing with the bar still locked tightly overhead.

the transition.

The depth of the receiving position of a jerk will depend directly on the height the lifter has been able to elevate the bar, and therefore indirectly on the weight being lifted. When learning and training with light weights, such as those that can be easily pressed or push pressed, a reasonable depth should be achieved despite it being physically unnecessary to bring the bar overhead. Practicing the jerk with a particularly shallow receiving depth will typically result in trouble in the future when the athlete begins attempting to jerk with heavier loads and finds him- or herself unable to achieve an adequately deep receiving position.

In actual practice, of course, the lifter must receive the bar at whatever height necessary, just as he or she must do with a snatch or clean, to prevent the weight from crashing and becoming unstable, or having to press it up. That being the case, the actual depth of the receiving position will vary with every lift, even lifts of the same weight since it's unlikely an athlete will accelerate the bar to an identical degree with every attempt.

In this learning stage, and with very light weights, the lifter will need to intentionally reduce the amount of force generated in the drive in order to receive the bar at the desired depth. This reduction of force should not involve any change in the motion in terms of positions and amplitude, however; in other words, the lifter should still perform the same complete drive of the legs, but with less aggression to allow the desired receiving depth.

The lifter should hold the receiving position for 3 seconds, maintaining tension throughout the body and continuing to actively and forcefully lock the overhead position, before returning to a standing position with the bar still locked overhead. From these earliest stages, athletes need to be taught to remain active overhead during the recovery, as a reduction in aggressiveness overhead during the recovery is a common source of pressouts and dropped lifts later. Only once the lifter is standing fully again with the bar locked overhead is the lift complete.

Split Jerk Behind the Neck

With the athlete now capable of performing the jerk in its simplest form, the complexity of the split receiving position will be added. The split jerk behind the neck will make this introduction somewhat easier by simplifying the bar path and maintenance of balance; jerking from behind the neck also helps athletes feel the proper timing and rhythm of the dip and drive, as well as the final explosion, with the more secure and comfortable rack position.

With the bar beginning behind the neck, it is already in the same plane it will need to be in the overhead position. That is, rather than the lifter and bar having to move horizontally into their final positions as they do with the jerk from the front, the path of the bar and lifter are perfectly vertical.

The movement of the dip and drive in essence is unchanged, but with the bar racked behind the neck, the trunk will need to be inclined forward slightly, which means the posture diverges from what is needed in the jerk somewhat. This will mean a greater tendency for the lifter to push the hips back and lean the chest forward in the dip—this needs to be actively avoided with the lifter's effort to maintain the starting trunk angle throughout the dip and drive.

The athlete will stand in the drive position with the bar racked as it would be for a back squat—on the meat of the traps near the base of the neck—with the hands in the jerk grip. Many athletes will take a significantly wider grip unless monitored. The elbows should be under the bar as much as possible without sacrificing the bar's security to allow a vertical press, rather than lifted up and back behind the bar as will be natural for many athletes.

---

48 *Progression Summary*

Split Jerk Behind the Neck

Begin with the feet in the drive position and the bar secured behind the neck with the elbows down.

Pressurize and stabilize the trunk, settle the balance over the heels with full foot contact with the floor, and keep the knees straight but unlocked.

Dip at the knees only while maintaining connection with the bar, brake quickly, and drive straight up aggressively.

As the legs near complete extension, push against the bar with the arms to begin moving it into the overhead position.

As the arms push against the bar, lift and move the feet into the split receiving position quickly and aggressively, moving the hips and trunk straight down under the bar.

Lock the bar forcefully in the overhead position at the same time the feet reconnect with the platform.

Hold the receiving position aggressively for 3 seconds before recovering by stepping a third of the way back with the front foot, and then bringing the back foot forward to meet it, with the bar still locked tightly overhead.

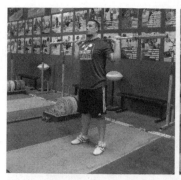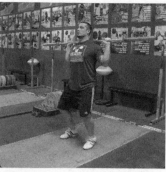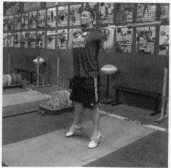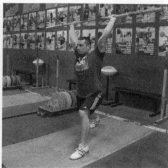

FIGURE 24.11 The split jerk behind the neck introduces the split receiving position to the jerk while simplifying the bar path and helping the lifter feel the proper rhythm and timing of the movement.

Following the same dip and drive practiced in the power jerk, the lifter will push vertically on the bar while lifting and reaching the feet into the proper split position determined previously. The inclination of the trunk should not change from the starting position, as it is already inclined forward slightly as it should be in the proper overhead position; likewise, the hips and trunk should move straight down from their beginning positions. The weight should be balanced evenly between the front and back feet immediately upon their reconnection with the floor, and legs set tight as the elbows lock out.

The movement of the feet into the split position should adhere to the same criteria outlined previously during the foot transition drill—the back foot remaining close to the floor and the front foot lifted to step out adequately. After holding the receiving position for 3 seconds—adjusting as needed first—the athlete will recover by stepping back a third of the way with the front foot, and the remaining distance forward with the back foot, actively pushing up against the bar and ensuring minimal horizontal movement.

Jerk Balance

The jerk balance is a drill that emphasizes the proper movement into the split position in the jerk. Typically used as more of a remediation exercise, it has great utility in a learning progression to prevent the bad habits it would otherwise be used to help correct—the diving of the head and chest forward during the

split and the excessive backward movement of the rear foot and hips that accompanies it.

While in the split jerk behind the neck, the path of the bar and lifter were perfectly vertical, during the jerk from the front, some horizontal movement of each needs to occur. With the forward movement of the foot in the split position, it's very easy to unintentionally dive or jump forward improperly during the split jerk from the front rack position. The jerk balance helps the athlete develop the feel for the proper movement under the bar.

With the bar in the jerk rack position, the athlete

49 Progression Summary
Jerk Balance

Begin with the feet in a partial split position approximately two-thirds the length of the full split position and the bar secured in the jerk rack position.

Dip straight down and drive straight back up to accelerate the bar upward.

As the bar leaves the shoulders, keep the back foot planted and lift the front foot to step out into the full split length.

Keep the trunk upright and land in the full split length with equal balance between the two feet.

Punch the bar up into the overhead position and lock it as the front foot reconnects with the floor.

Greg Everett

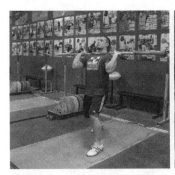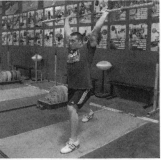

FIGURE 24.12 The jerk balance is an intermediate step that teaches the lifter how to properly move into the split position while maintaining proper balance and posture.

The key to this drill—and the reason it's helpful—is moving into the split position without leaning forward or shifting the weight excessively to the front leg. Focusing on a vertical trunk orientation and equal balance between the feet will help ensure the movement is correct.

Split Jerk

The final step in the jerk progression is the split jerk, which will be the chosen jerk style for the majority of weightlifters. All elements of the split jerk have been learned and practiced with the previous drills; the athlete simply needs to now become comfortable performing the lift.

will enter a partial split position—approximately a foot-length less than the athlete's full split length or slightly shorter. The easiest way to find this position is to step out into the full split position first, and then bring the front foot back about a foot-length or slightly more. In this partial split position, the lifter's trunk should be vertical and the weight balanced equally between the two feet.

From this partial split starting position, the athlete will dip straight down and drive straight back up just as he or she would in the dip and drive of any other jerk. Once the upward drive is complete, the athlete will lift the front foot, keeping the balls of the back foot planted on the floor, and step the front foot forward into the full split length, maintaining the properly upright trunk and equal balance between the feet, while punching the bar up into the overhead position. Like other drills, the athlete should attempt to lock the bar out overhead at the same time the front foot reconnects with the floor.

Possibly the most important point to understand with regard to the split jerk is that the dip and drive does not vary in any way from the power jerk. That is, it still needs to be performed with the same balance and drive up and slightly back; many athletes will naturally dip and drive forward in the split jerk even if they do not in the power jerk, confusing the forward movement of the front leg in the split for forward movement of the entire lift. This is the primary reason the power jerk is such a valuable training exercise even for split jerkers—it reinforces the proper balance and bar path in the dip and drive.

The athlete will begin with the feet in the drive position and weight balanced toward the heels but full foot contact with the floor, the trunk pressurized and tight, and the bar in the jerk rack position. The knees should be unlocked but straight, with tension

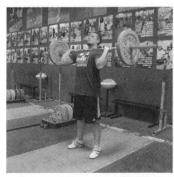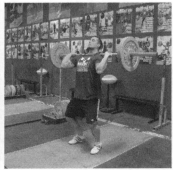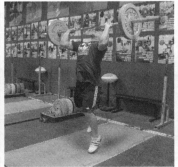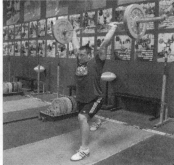

FIGURE 24.13 The split jerk is the final step in the jerk progression as the primary jerk style used by competitive lifters.

in the quads, to ensure a smooth dip without any separation of the bar from the shoulders.

Once balanced and stabilized in this position, he or she will dip smoothly, keeping the grip relatively loose, the rack position tight and unchanging, and the torso upright, braking abruptly at the bottom of the dip and driving straight back up violently with the legs. With a final upward explosion against the bar, the athlete will begin pushing against it with the arms and transitioning the feet into the split position.

As the bar leaves the shoulders, the head needs to be pulled back out of the way, and the elbows spread out and moved under the bar, directing it in a slightly backward line from its starting position.

The athlete will continue driving aggressively against the bar with the arms to move the body down into position underneath it. Again, it's important the athlete keep the trunk upright as he or she reaches the front foot forward rather than reaching with the chest and head. The slight forward inclination of trunk in the proper overhead position should actually occur after the feet have already reconnected with the floor, although this won't be visible in real time.

If the athlete reaches the chest forward, it will more than likely cause the back leg to reach too far back, and to actually pull the hips back out from under the bar, causing the lead foot to reconnect before the rear foot, and leaving the athlete behind the bar rather than directly under it, unable to create the necessary structure and balance to support the weight.

If the lifter's posture and balance are correct during the split, the replacement of the feet on the platform in the split position will be slightly staggered—the back foot should hit an instant before the front (This staggered reconnection should not be significant enough to be visible in real time, and it is not something the athlete will likely be able to feel.). This allows the athlete to drive off of the back foot, which helps keep the hips under instead of behind the bar. If the rear foot is disconnected and front foot connected while the athlete drives the torso forward, the backward shift of the hips out from under the bar described above is inevitable.

The locking of the elbows in the overhead position should be the signal to quickly tighten the lower body in the split position. If the elbow lockout is quick and aggressive, this should happen somewhat naturally, as the lockout and foot reconnection

50 Progression Summary

Split Jerk

Begin with the feet in the drive position and the bar secured in the jerk rack position.

Pressurize and stabilize the trunk, settle the balance over the heels with full foot contact with the floor, and keep the knees straight but unlocked.

Dip at the knees only while maintaining connection with the bar, brake quickly, and drive straight up aggressively.

As the legs near complete extension, push against the bar with the arms to begin moving it into the overhead position, moving the head back out of the way.

As the arms push against the bar, lift and move the feet into the split receiving position quickly and aggressively, moving the hips and trunk straight down under the bar.

Lock the bar forcefully in the overhead position at a quarter squat depth at the same time the feet reconnect with the platform.

Hold the receiving position aggressively for 3 seconds before recovering by stepping a third of the way back with the front foot, and then bringing the back foot forward to meet it, with the bar still locked tightly overhead.

will feel like they occur simultaneously. However, if the athlete instead develops the habit of timing the lockout of the lower body position with the connection of the feet to the floor, pressouts become more likely, as additional depth in the split may be needed following the feet landing to achieve complete lockout overhead.

If the back knee is locked and not allowed to flex along with the front, it will drive the lifter forward as he or she settles under the weight, pushing the bar forward as well. At best this will force the athlete to recover forward to maintain balance, and at worst it will cause a miss with the bar too far forward of the center of the base to be supported adequately.

Ensuring the back knee is unlocked and allowed to bend in concert with the front will allow the athlete to drive and settle vertically down under the load and maintain the necessary balance.

The jerk demands a certain aggressiveness and confidence. It will be the most weight the lifter ever places overhead—with the exception perhaps of exercises such as jerk supports in which a bar is lifted from a rack a short distance—and consequently it has the tendency to instill potentially debilitating fear in the lifter as the attempts near maximal. From the earliest stages of learning, a great degree of viciousness with every jerk needs to be encouraged.

Just as in the snatch, once the weight has been received overhead, the priority is stabilization before recovery. Settling into the split position will allow adjustments to be made to bring the barbell and lifter into balance; premature recovery attempts will magnify existing imbalance. Once the weight has been stabilized and the athlete feels secure, he or she will recover by stepping a third of the way back with the front foot and the remaining distance forward with the back foot, aggressively maintaining the locked out overhead position and pushing straight up against the bar to minimize its movement and prevent any softening of the elbows.

If an athlete cannot recover properly with the front foot first, it indicates a forward imbalance even if that imbalance is not significant enough to be otherwise observable.

Practice should consist of sets of 2-5 repetitions with weights that allow correct and safe execution. In the early stages of development, large volumes of very lightweight practice is appropriate and most effective; partial lifts and assistance exercises will be used to develop strength for the jerk. For practice of the jerk as part of the earliest training program, weights should be approximately 50-60% of bodyweight, or what the athlete and coach feel could be lifted without trouble for 5-6 repetitions (Medvedyev 1986/1995). Of course, lighter weights should be used if needed and the initial practice stage extended as much as needed for each athlete prior to beginning a more structured training program. This process is discussed in detail in the Program Design & Training section of the book.

Missing Jerks Safely

Generally speaking, missing jerks is not a particularly troublesome issue in terms of safety, but can become one with deeper receiving positions, so understanding how to miss safely is valuable. The fundamental idea is of course the same as the other two lifts—guide the bar away from the body and move the body out of the way as quickly as possible.

Like the snatch, jerks can be missed in front and in back, with misses in front far outnumbering misses in back. As is the case with the snatch, which direction the bar is dropped will depend on the bar's location relative to the lifter and its momentum, not

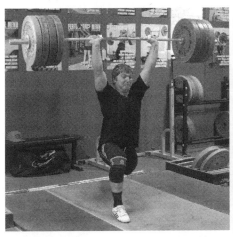 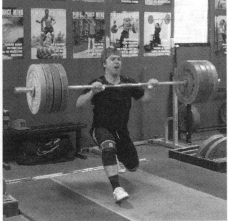 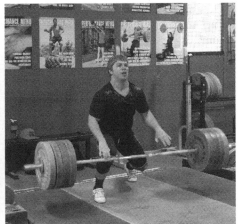

FIGURE 24.14 To miss a jerk in front, the athlete will push the bar forward and move backward, being particularly careful to step the front leg back out of the way.

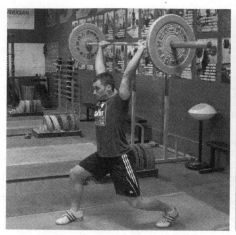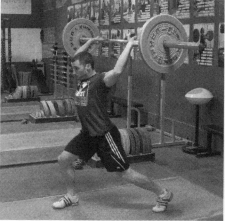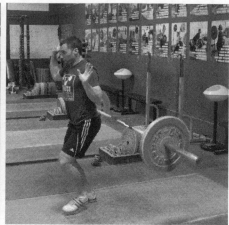

FIGURE 24.15 To miss a jerk in back, the athlete will guide the bar backward as much as possible while moving forward.

the lifter's preference.

With a miss in front, the bar is too far forward of the lifter's center of base to be supported, and may or may not be locked out. The most critical action to safely miss a jerk in front is quickly moving the lead split leg back out of the way so that the bar doesn't fall onto the thigh or knee.

If the lifter manages to bring the bar too far behind the center of the base, or the elbows break after a lock out and the bar has backward momentum on it, the bar will naturally drop behind the lifter's head. Lifters typically react naturally to this and quickly jump forward out from under the bar; in any case, the lifter needs to get his or her body out from under the bar as quickly as possible so it can drop safely to the platform.

The Squat Jerk

The squat jerk, as discussed briefly in the previous chapter, is a relatively uncommon jerk style due to its great demands primarily on mobility and precision, as well as squat strength. However, it does prove to be the best jerk style for certain athletes, and can have utility as a training exercise even for split or power jerkers.

Essentially the squat jerk is performed identically to the power or push jerk with the difference being the ultimate depth of the receiving position, which is a squat below parallel. However, the lift may also differ slightly in the magnitude of the upward drive on the bar and the ultimate height the bar reaches. The primary advantage of the squat jerk over the other styles is that it greatly reduces the necessary elevation of the bar because the lockout in the overhead position can be achieved through greater downward movement of the lifter. In addition to this, it allows the athlete to absorb the weight in a more stable position rather than in a low power position, which can be difficult in terms of both balance and the mechanics at that particular knee angle.

Lifting and moving the feet during the drive under can make the lift more difficult with regard to absorbing and stabilizing the weight overhead by making the receipt of the initial downward force of the weight somewhat more abrupt. Maintaining the feet's connection to the floor can help the lifter absorb the weight more smoothly. Obviously if the feet remain connected to the floor during the lift, the drive position needs to be altered to match the desired squat receiving stance.

The squat jerk is best suited for lifters with relatively short legs and long torsos, which is the reason for its more common use by Asian lifters in the

Greg Everett

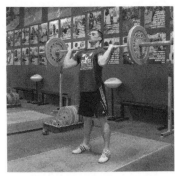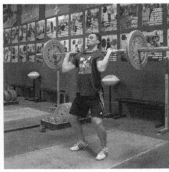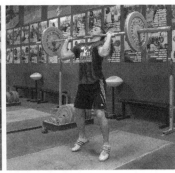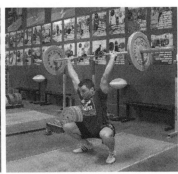

FIGURE 24.16 The squat jerk is a relatively uncommon jerk style in which the athlete receives the bar in a full squat position.

lighter weight classes who more frequently possess such builds. Shorter legs create stronger squatting mechanics, reduce the demand on squat mobility, and naturally produce a more upright squat posture, making it easier to stabilize in and recover from the bottom of the squat jerk.

For split jerkers, the squat jerk can be used as a training exercise at certain times. It can be used as a more advanced variation of a jerk-grip overhead squat, or in combination with jerk-grip overhead squats, to improve upper back mobility and strength in particular, and overhead mobility and strength in general (Jerk-grip overhead squats, however, are arguably more effective for this purpose because of the eccentric component and greater time in the position in question per rep.). Additionally, the squat jerk can be used simply for variety in a training program for the sake of both a physical and mental break from the typical monotony of weightlifting training, or as a variation during recovery periods when the lifter will not need to be lifting near maximal weights in the jerk.

Understanding the Jerk

While of course the identical phases of the snatch and clean can't be applied to the jerk, the lift can still be broken it into a series of phases that closely mirror their snatch and clean counterparts. Rather than the first pull, second pull and third pull, the jerk will be divided into the dip, the drive and the push under—in essence, accomplishing the same task of elevating and accelerating the barbell with the lower body, and then using the upper body to relocate the athlete under the bar to receive it.

Starting Position

The starting position of the jerk concerns two primary elements: the stance of the feet and the rack position. Each can have dramatic effects on the lift, and each will vary somewhat among lifters based on individual peculiarities. Additional but more minor elements will also contribute to the success or failure of the lift.

Drive Stance

The starting point for the position of the feet places the heels at hip-width or slightly wider to orient the legs approximately vertically and the toes turned out approximately 10-20 degrees relative to the centerline.

A vertical leg orientation in theory allows maximal force to be applied to the elevation of the bar, as the force generated by the leg extension will be directed straight down against the ground and straight back up against the barbell with none lost to horizontal displacement. Additionally, a vertical leg orientation will create the highest possible elevation of the bar-

bell when the body is in an extended position simply by virtue of the lifter's height.

However, other factors must be taken into consideration: primarily, the ability to brake in the bottom of the dip abruptly and powerfully. This is actually more important than the benefits of a perfectly vertical leg orientation, as this dictates the lifter's ability to generate the maximal elasticity, both of the barbell and the body, to create the most upward acceleration on the barbell in the drive of the jerk. The maximal height in the extended position and perfectly direct force application will not overcome an inability in that stance to execute a quick dip and an abrupt stop and change of direction.

Ultimately, just as is the case with the pulling stance of the snatch and clean, the drive stance of the jerk needs to be adjusted to best suit each athlete's build, strengths and weaknesses, which will require some experimentation. Generally speaking, athletes with weaker and/or longer legs will find a wider stance more effective.

Balance

The balance over the foot should be primarily over the heel while maintaining full foot contact with the floor. This means that there will remain pressure on the balls of the foot, but that it is minimal. Shifting the weight excessively to the heels will typically create subsequent forward shifting during the dip and or drive as the athlete rocks forward on the foot, creating a net forward imbalance from the initial rearward balance. Ensuring that the entire foot remains in contact with the floor is the simplest way to prevent excessive rearward balance on the heel.

As in the pulls of the snatch and clean, the goal is to maintain the balance over this same point throughout the dip and drive. The center of pressure on the foot, however, will shift forward as the balls of the feet push through the floor and the ankles extend as a natural part the legs' drive against the platform. Again, just as in the snatch and clean, this forward shifting of the center of pressure does not necessarily indicate—and should not be accompanied by—a forward shifting of the center of mass of the barbell-body system.

Rack Position

The details of the rack position were covered in great detail in the Learning the Jerk chapter. The most important points to understand are that the barbell must be connected directly and securely to the trunk rather than the arms, the hands must be around the barbell as much as is allowable by the athlete's proportions and mobility, and the elbows in as close to an optimal pressing position as the athlete's proportions and mobility allow with the previous criteria met.

The width of the jerk grip does not have to be the same used in the clean. If two different grip widths are used by a lifter, most commonly the jerk grip is wider than the clean grip. The adjustment between the two grips following the clean is discussed in the following chapter.

The effects of different grip widths in the jerk are in essence the same as in the snatch. Wider grips will require the lifter to elevate the bar and lower the body shorter distances and will allow greater overhead mobility; however, they will also make the rack position more awkward past a certain point, placing more strain on the shoulders and elbows, compromise pressing mechanics for the drive under the bar, and reduce the structural integrity of the overhead position.

Narrower grips will improve the structural integrity of the overhead position, allow for better pressing mechanics in the drive under the bar and, to a point, typically allow a more comfortable rack position; they will, however, require the lifter to elevate the barbell more and drive farther under it and increase the demand on overhead mobility.

In any case, the grip on the barbell while in the rack position should be relatively loose. An excessively tight grip on the bar will tend to cause the shoulders and elbows to drop, which reduces the security of the bar in the rack position, slow the elbow extension in the drive under, and somewhat limit the ultimate degree of elbow extension in the overhead position, which must be maximal for the optimal lockout. This does not mean the hands need to be open; they may be wrapped completely around the barbell as long as they are not gripping tightly. However, lifters may find through experimentation that they prefer leaving the hands somewhat open in the rack position, as this guarantees the grip will not be inadvertently tightened prematurely.

Occasionally lifters will also jerk with a thumbless grip—that is, the thumb is brought underneath the bar with the rest of the fingers rather than wrapped around it. This is generally done in cases of mobility restrictions, often as a result of previous injuries, that prevent the lifter from achieving an effective rack position with the thumb around the bar. In other cases, the lifter has simply found that he or she feels the drive and or push under the bar is stronger with this grip.

The thumbless grip is arguably slightly less stable overhead, but not dramatically so. While it should not be taught to new lifters or encouraged, if neces-

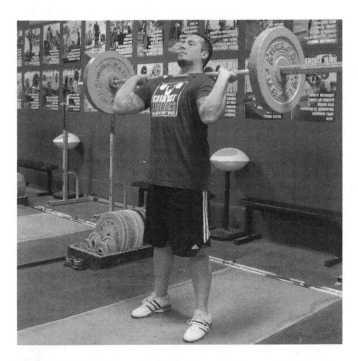

FIGURE 25.1 The starting position for the jerk creates the proper balance, posture and stability to optimize the lift.

sary for a given lifter because of a genuine inability to establish a solid rack position otherwise, it should be allowed.

Trunk Pressurization & Stabilization

The pressurization and stabilization of the trunk is critical in the jerk. The body must essentially act as a piston, moving vertically down and up to load the legs and then drive the barbell upward; any loss of rigidity in this process not only reduces the ultimate upward acceleration and elevation of the barbell due to the dissipation of force through the deformation of the body, but will also misdirect the force through the change in position of the barbell relative to the base of support.

The manner of taking in a stabilizing breath and activating the trunk musculature to lock it in and establish rigidity is discussed in detail in the Breathing & Trunk Rigidity chapter of the book. With regard to the jerk, timing is an important consideration. Generally speaking, it will be preferable for the lifter to take in the final pressurizing breath prior to initiating the dip of the jerk. This action will often naturally shift the lifter's balance forward slightly, so finalizing the breath and stabilization prior to the dip will allow the lifter to re-establish proper balance over the foot before beginning the jerk. Often lifters will naturally try to take in the final breath as they dip, which may work initially, but eventually, as lifts become heavier, will be increasingly more likely to create balance problems.

This breath needs to be complete, which, as discussed in the Breathing chapter, requires contraction of the diaphragm and expansion of the abdomen. This may require the lifter, at least above certain weights, to momentarily elevate the bar through a shrugging motion or a subtle push with the legs to reduce the pressure of the bar on the shoulders. In any case, this breath should cause an observable expansion of the abdomen, not just lifting of the ribs, prior to the final circumferential tightening of the trunk musculature.

An important element of trunk rigidity specific to the jerk is the activation of the lower abs. This is critical to stabilizing the orientation of the pelvis and its relationship with the spine during the dip. Without tension in the lower abs, the pelvis is more likely to anteriorly rotate prior to or during the dip, which will encourage the hips to move backward rather than straight down.

Dip

Like the starting position, elements of the dip will vary among lifters, such as depth, speed and acceleration, depending on each lifter's inherent abilities with regard to the relevant physical characteristics. Essentially, there is an idealized version of the jerk dip that then needs to be modified to the degree and nature that best suits each athlete and produces the most successful jerk. Some of this modification is predictable based on a lifter's performance metrics, and some will require experimentation.

Position & Balance

Maintaining the proper balance and producing the correct barbell trajectory in the dip demands a particular posture—the trunk must remain vertical throughout the movement. The barbell, hips and ankles should remain in approximately the same vertical plane as the lifter bends and extends the knees—this maintains the balance over the foot and prevents any unintended horizontal deviation in the bar path. Such a posture can only be maintained by the lifter if it is carefully reinforced and trained throughout his or her career, as it depends on very specific positional strength that is unnatural for most athletes.

Dip & Braking Speed

The ideal jerk dip is quick, although without accelerating more rapidly than what allows the barbell to remain connected solidly to the shoulders—that is, the rate of acceleration cannot be so great that the lifter's shoulders drop out from under the barbell and creates separation. Greater speed creates a greater stretch-shortening reflex, which then allows for a faster and more forceful subsequent contraction during the upward drive with the legs and allows for more upward whip of the barbell.

At least equally, and arguably more, important is how abruptly the dip is stopped and reversed; in fact, if this braking of the dip is not adequately abrupt, the speed of the dip will lose its potential effectiveness, and past a certain point, will actually become counterproductive. Faster braking of the dip creates greater tension in the muscles, which means greater potential force and speed in the drive; additionally, the more abruptly the dip is arrested, the more the barbell will flex down around the support area in the center (its connection to the lifter on the shoulders). This flexing of the barbell increases the tension in the leg muscles further, and can contribute directly to its own upward acceleration and elevation.

This elastic loading of the barbell creates a subsequent upward "whipping" as the downward bending reverses after reaching its maximal amplitude. As the loaded ends of the barbell accelerate upward with this action, the resistance of the barbell is reduced momentarily, allowing the athlete to accelerate to a greater extent in the leg drive. Although it will vary slightly among different barbells, this bar whip will typically become noticeable with approximately 120kg on a men's bar (Zhekov 1976/1992) and considerably less on a women's barbell.

The importance of this rapid braking motion to achieve maximal muscular tension and barbell oscillation dictates the depth of the dip to a large extent. That is, a given lifter's ability to arrest the dip will change as the depth of the dip increases, generally decreasing as depth increases. This requires the lifter to dip to a depth that allows adequate downward speed and amplitude of knee flexion for meaningful and effective knee extension, but does not exceed the ability to brake rapidly. This ideal depth will typically be arrived at by the lifter over time without explicit instruction, as the body will tend to shape its movement to optimize the action in question.

Strength vs. Elastic Jerkers

The pertinent abilities of lifters exist on a gradient, but jerk dips can be broadly categorized into two styles: elastic and strength. These categories describe a given lifter's most effective method of jerking based on his or her physical traits.

The elastic jerk is what is considered optimal, as discussed in the previous section. This method of jerking exploits the properties of the barbell and body to the greatest extent for maximal results. However, its effectiveness is predicated primarily on the lifter's ability to brake rapidly in the dip and secondarily on his or her capacity for explosive knee extension in the drive. Lifters for whom the elastic jerk will be ideal are those who exhibit above average explosiveness, particularly in countermovement jumps. Not all lifters possess the necessary capabilities in sufficient quantities for a successful elastic jerk; for those who do not, this approach to the jerk will actually be less effective.

These less explosive lifters will fall into the category of the strength jerk. This style of jerk will involve a somewhat slower dip and a greater dip depth. The slower dip will improve the lifter's ability to brake rapidly, as the downward force generated will remain within his or her ability to do so. The force experienced at the bottom of the dip can reach as much as 250% of the weight on the barbell (Zhekov 1976/1992); consequently, each lifter must control the downward speed to remain within his or her ability to withstand the commensurate force at the bottom of the dip, which is reduced along with downward speed.

Speeds beyond this threshold will result in a slow, soft braking in the bottom of the dip, often forcing unintended additional depth because of the inability to brake rapidly enough, which robs the muscles and barbell of much of the elastic energy that otherwise would have been generated, and typically will shift the lifter out of position forward. The greater dip depth provides a longer distance of drive travel, which means more time for the lifter to generate muscular force to reach the ultimate maximal speed of the drive.

In short, by modifying the style of the jerk appropriately for each lifter's individual physical characteristics, the effectiveness of the jerk can be maximized, while forcing a lifter to use the style that does not best suit him or her will result in poorer performance. Again, this is not a pair of categories with a rigid line of demarcation—lifters will fall along a gradient that spans the two extremes, and the actual execution of each lifter's jerk will accordingly reflect the position on that gradient.

Dip Depth

As discussed previously, the depth of the dip will vary among lifters based on what style of jerk is most appropriate. As a loose guideline, dip depth will typically be approximately 8-10% of the lifter's height. For example, a 5' 6" (168 cm) lifter will have a dip of approximately 5.3-6.6" (13.5-17 cm).

However, depth should be determined according to feel on the lifter's part and appearance (in terms of performance) on the coach's part. The lifter will typically, with some time and practice, gravitate to an appropriate depth, as the body will naturally attempt to optimize the movement. Adjustments will need to be made if a lifter obviously fails to find this ideal depth or is intentionally attempting to change it to ostensibly suit an inappropriate recommendation.

Arms & Rack Position

During the dip of the jerk, the rack position should remain static—the shoulders, arms and hands should remain unmoved from the position set in the start of the lift. The barbell's security in the rack position is critical for the transfer of force from the leg drive. Any movement of the barbell during the dip or drive will absorb force that should be going to either elastic loading of the bar and muscles (in the dip) or upward acceleration of the bar (in the drive). The lifter must actively and aggressively support the barbell and maintain the positions of the upper back and shoulders, combating the great force generated by arresting the downward motion of the barbell.

Dynamic Start

While completely different in appearance (and in specific effect) from the dynamic start of the snatch or clean, a dynamic start can be utilized in the jerk as well. The purpose of this action is to increase the downward force of the barbell in the bottom of the dip while still allowing the lifter to brake as rapidly, increasing the elastic loading of the barbell and leg muscles.

The basic action is to elevate the barbell slightly immediately prior to the initiation of the dip by lifting the shoulders quickly. This can be done, and is often done inadvertently, with a final inhalation that elevates the ribs and shoulder girdle. This motion creates a slight initial upward whip of the ends of the barbell, which then reduces the downward force of the bar as the lifter descends into the dip (because the dip is initiated as the weights are travelling upward), but increases the downward force as the weights reach the bottom of the barbell's downward whip at the bottom of the dip. However, because the athlete has by this point reached a static position, the increased force should still be within the isometric strength abilities of the lifter (Zhekov 1976/1992).

Just as with the dynamic start of the snatch and clean, a dynamic start in the jerk has the potential to improve performance, but also the potential to create problems in position and balance. If the movement of the barbell during the initial elevation diverges at all from vertical, the balance of the barbell-lifter system will be accordingly shifted—most probably forward—consequently misdirecting the dip and subsequent drive. Additionally, if the dip speed is excessive and the barbell and lifter become significantly discon-

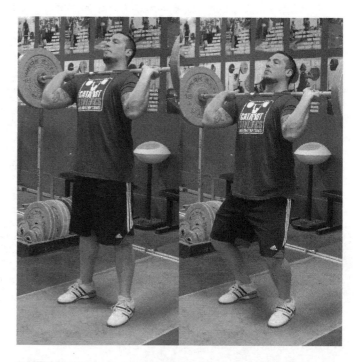

FIGURE 25.2 The depth and speed of the dip will vary among lifters based on their inherent athletic qualities, but will generally be 8-10% of the lifter's height and fast enough to elicit some degree of a stretch-shortening reflex.

nected, there will be a crashing effect as the barbell reconnects with the lifter in the bottom of the dip, again potentially shifting him or her out of position and balance. The dynamic start should be reserved for advanced lifters with consistent lift technique and well-developed postural strength and timing.

Drive

The drive of the jerk provides the necessary acceleration and elevation of the barbell to allow the athlete to move under it, similar to the first and second pull of the snatch and clean. As should be obvious from the previous section, the proper execution of the preceding dip will contribute significantly to the success of the drive; likewise, a poorly performed dip will dramatically reduce the effectiveness of even the best drive effort.

Speed & Timing

As was described with regard to the dip, as the athlete brakes and reaches the bottom of the dip, the barbell will bend around the support area (the lifter's shoulders) to allow the loaded ends to continue traveling down farther with their momentum. If the lifter reverses the dip and begins driving upward before the weights reach their lowest point, the legs will be working against force greater than the weight of the barbell and greater than what is necessary (remember from above that the force in the bottommost point of the dip can reach as much as 2.5 times the weight of the bar).

Instead, the drive should begin as the weights begin rebounding upward after reaching their lowest point. This will mean that the barbell already possesses some upward speed that will add to the speed generated by the lifter, and that the resistance to the drive will be reduced, allowing the generation of greater bar speed with a given magnitude of leg drive force.

This timing will change slightly with changing loads—the bending of the bar will last longer with heavier weights and take longer to reverse directions. Different barbells will also have slight variances in

elasticity even at a given weight. While these differences are subtle, they can have a significant effect on the lift. As a consequence, optimal timing of the drive is largely dependent on the lifter's rapid and accurate reaction to the feel of the bar. This is a skill that seems to have a significant inherent component, but also requires training experience to develop fully like everything else.

The barbell actually reaches its maximal upward speed prior to the full extension of the legs (Zhekov 1976/1992). This does not mean that the legs should not reach nearly maximal extension in the jerk, but that the lifter should begin initiating the push against the bar with the arms somewhat before that maximal extension is reached in order to capitalize on that speed, and to preserve as much of it as possible with the arms' push on the bar.

This changes slightly with strength jerkers, who must continue applying maximal force in the leg drive somewhat longer than their elastic jerker counterparts because of the need for more time and distance to generate maximal acceleration.

Even if the active leg extension is stopped prior to full knee extension, momentum will carry the lifter through further extension. However, like in the snatch and clean second pull, the knees will not reach anatomically maximal extension in the jerk drive.

Position, Balance & Direction

As weights in the jerk increase relative to the lifter's bodyweight, the ability of the lifter to correct the barbell's trajectory following the dip and drive decreases. That is, with a light weight, the lifter can correct for a somewhat misdirected drive with the active push of the barbell back into the overhead position because the inertia of his or her body is greater than that of the barbell. With heavy weights, however, this becomes impossible, and the importance of a properly balanced and directed dip and drive increases dramatically. Whatever direction the barbell is driven is the direction it will continue to travel despite any subsequent efforts of the lifter.

The balance over the foot should remain unchanged during the drive from its original point in the start and during the dip—behind the middle of the foot but not to an extreme. However, during the drive, the center of pressure will shift forward to the balls of the foot as the ankles naturally plantar flex with the effort of the legs to push against the ground. Just as in the pull of the snatch and clean, the line of gravity should remain in its original position, however, to maintain a static point of balance of the barbell-lifter system.

The same vertical-trunk posture from the dip must be maintained during the drive in order to ensure continued balance and a correct bar path. This is to a large extent dependent on a properly executed dip—the probability of a lifter being able to produce a vertically-oriented drive following a forward-shifting dip is essentially zero. However, even with a perfectly vertical dip, a vertical drive will still require active control of the movement by the lifter, as the natural tendency will be to shift the line of gravity to the balls of the foot and lean forward into the drive, both because this to most athletes naturally feels more powerful, and because athletes will often conflate the horizontal foot movement of the split with the movement of the drive.

Ideally, the upward trajectory of the barbell is actually directed slightly backward rather than perfectly vertically. This will assist in bringing the barbell into the proper relative position to the body overhead without forcing the lifter to lean or drive forward in the split movement. This backward path is produced by a combination of both the orientation of the leg drive and the motion of the arms' push under the barbell following the drive.

Arms & Rack Position

During the initial part of the drive, the rack position should remain static as it has prior to this point, with the barbell supported securely on the shoulders and the hands and arms inactive in any way other than their supporting roles in the rack position's integrity.

As the lifter nears the end of the productive leg drive—sooner for elastic jerkers and later for strength jerkers—the arms will begin pushing against the bar. The timing of this push is important for preserving as much of the existing bar speed as possible to create a fluid transition between the drive and push under, and to maximize the elevation of the barbell. This push with the arms should begin at the time the

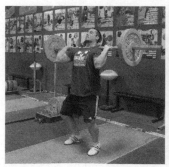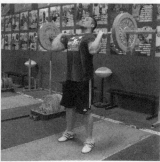

FIGURE 25.3 The drive of the jerk must be aggressive to impart maximal upward acceleration on the bar and oriented correctly to ensure the barbell and body reach the proper positions relative to each other.

barbell reaches its maximal upward speed (Zhekov 1976/1992), which again will vary in time and location depending on the lifter's jerk style. Like many technical elements, the proper timing requires practice and the ability to react quickly and properly to the feedback during the movement itself.

Push Under

The jerk is in principle identical to the snatch and clean—the barbell is first accelerated and elevated through the actions of the lower body, and then the lifter accelerates down and relocates his or her body into the receiving position under the bar with the upper body. In the case of the jerk, this downward relocation is achieved through a push against the bar rather than a pull, but like in the snatch and clean, it must also be as active and aggressive as the initial upward acceleration of the barbell. This action achieves three basic functions: driving the lifter down under the barbell into the receiving position, moving the body primarily and barbell secondarily into the correct horizontal positions relative to each other, and, very importantly, preserving as much of the existing upward speed of the barbell from the drive as possible. The heavier the barbell relative to the lifter, the less this action will continue elevating the barbell and the more it will push the lifter down, but any contribution to the barbell's elevation is helpful, and with proper timing and aggression, it can still be significant.

Timing

As was discussed in the previous section, the precise timing of this push under with the arms will vary slightly among lifters. The initiation of the push with the arms should coincide with the barbell's maximum upward speed—for elastic jerkers, this will be as soon as approximately halfway through the leg drive, and for strength jerkers, this will be nearer the end of the drive. To a degree, this timing can be observed and guided by the coach, but it will require primarily the lifter to feel the movement—with proper timing, the athlete will feel the least resistance against the bar, as it will already possess its greatest speed during the lift. There should be no observable hesitation between the drive and push under phases—it should appear to be a single, continuous action.

Direction

While the direction the barbell travels is determined overwhelmingly by the orientation of the drive (which is determined to some extent by the dip), the lifter can manipulate the position of the barbell and body to a degree with the action of the arms during the push under. This will be possible only if the barbell does not already possess antagonistic momentum—that is, if the bar is already traveling, as a product of the drive, in a direction opposite of what's desired, the upper body will not be capable of effecting any significant change.

Relative to its starting position, the barbell should travel slightly backward as the lifter's trunk inclines slightly forward, maintaining the same basic relationship between the barbell and the hips, achieving the proper overhead position for maximal structural integrity, and maintaining the same approximate line of gravity of the barbell-lifter system.

In order to achieve this slight backward direction, the lifter will need to intentionally push back as the bar leaves the shoulders rather than straight up. Obviously the head will need to be pulled back out of the way of the bar to clear the path and keep it as direct as possible. Ideally the head is pulled back without excessive backward tilting to allow the lifter to maintain a continuous focal point during the lift, but some lifters will find this impossible for various reasons; in such cases, a backward tilting of the head to allow the bar to pass is acceptable as long as the head and eyes are returned quickly to the neutral position.

Upper Body

The movement of the arms can influence the outcome of the lift considerably—like all other elements, its precision and timing are important components of a successful jerk. As mentioned previously, the initial motion of the barbell as it leaves the shoulders should have a slight backward orientation. This will assist in guiding the barbell and body into their prop-

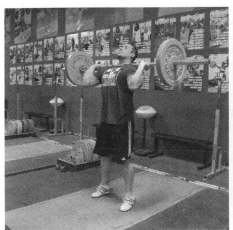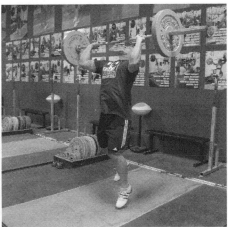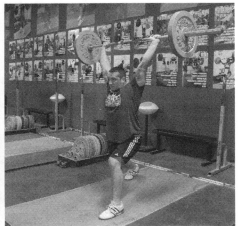

FIGURE 25.4 The push under the jerk preserves as much of the barbell's upward speed as possible, relocates the lifter under the barbell and positions the barbell and body correctly relative to each other. The feet will transition from the drive stance into the split position during the push under.

er respective positions, taking advantage of the barbell's existing momentum following a proper movement in the drive.

Because the arms have started, ideally, in a relatively advantageous pressing position, this should occur naturally to some extent; if a lifter is forced to begin the lift with a less than optimal rack position, even more care must be taken to ensure the proper movement of the arms during this phase of the lift.

Beginning with the elbows at least slightly in front of the bar helps with the backward inclination of the bar path initially. As the bar leaves the shoulders, the athlete should keep the elbows out to bring them under the bar as soon as possible; if the elbows are allowed to stay forward, or even move inward, the pressing mechanics are compromised and the push will be weakened as well as the direction of the barbell changed.

The grip should remain relatively loose around the bar during this push to allow maximal elbow extension speed. The action of this push under should be considered more of a punch than a press—that is, it must be quick, violent and complete. Never should this motion become a slow, hesitant press into the final lockout position. Like with the snatch, the lifter should attempt to lock the bar overhead by the time the feet reconnect with the platform to encourage maximal speed.

The bar should be supported in the palms of the hands to allow the most direct transfer of force. If a lifter must begin the jerk with the barbell in the fingers, part of the push under must include the immediate effort to shift the grip around the bar to the full hand and into the hand and wrist orientation desired for the overhead position.

The hips must move forward very slightly along with the chest and head, although not to the same extent, as the inclination of the trunk will be shifting from a very slight backward lean or, at the very least, vertical orientation, to a slight forward lean.

Lower Body

During the push under, the legs must transition from the drive stance into the split receiving position. Like in the snatch and clean, this transition must be timed precisely to prevent any loss of upward acceleration of the bar due to premature disconnection of the feet from the platform, and any failure to achieve adequate movement into the correct position due to a late or slow transition.

The timing of the leg transition will coincide with the lifter's initiation of the push under the bar, which again will be when the bar reaches its maximal upward speed—slightly different depending on the style of the jerk performed by each lifter. The rear leg will typically separate naturally slightly before the front—this is not something the lifter must concern him- or herself with. The rear foot should be kept relatively close to the floor as it moves back into position, while the front foot will need to be lifted more to allow the forward step into position to be completed before the push under drives the lifter back down onto the platform.

The rear foot, if moved properly (i.e. not lifted excessively and reached too far back), will reconnect with the platform a split second before the front foot. This momentary connection without the front foot creates an anchor for the lifter to push against that helps move the hips and trunk under the bar properly, which is slightly forward. If the rear foot is lifted too high, or the lifter reaches it too far back, it will pull the hips back out from under the bar and cause the front foot to reconnect with the platform prematurely and fail to reach far enough forward.

The rear foot should connect with the floor on the balls of the foot—not the toes. That is, there should be a decent amount of surface area in contact with the platform despite the heel being lifted. Additionally, the heel should be angled out away from the body slightly to keep the foot aligned with the lower leg. If the rear foot connects directed straight forward, there is a significant chance of the heel spinning inward and compromising the integrity of the split position.

The front foot should reconnect flat with the platform, either oriented straight forward or with the toes turned in slightly. In real-time observation, it should appear that the feet reconnect with the platform at the same time, and that the lifter locks the bar out overhead at the same time the feet hit.

Receiving the Bar

The jerk involves the difficult combination of heavy weights and a high center of mass. This requires that the receipt of the bar be as precise and aggressive as the rest of the lift.

The feet will reconnect with the platform before the elbows achieve the final locked out position, even though these actions will appear in real time to happen simultaneously. What this means is that the legs must absorb the lifter to some extent following the feet hitting the platform to allow the overhead lockout to be completed without hesitation; immediately locking the lower body upon the reconnection of the feet is likely to cause the lift to be pressed out overhead. This is not a dramatic movement—the lifter must simply time the lockout of the legs with the lockout of the elbows, rather than with the reconnection of the feet with the platform.

The balance should be approximately equal between the front and rear feet, although typically the lifter will feel slightly more pressure on the front foot. In any case, there should be no need to move forward or backward to establish a balanced position—if a jerk is properly performed and the receiving position properly balanced, the lifter will be capable of holding the position without adjustment.

The back knee must be soft and slightly bent—there is no need for a significant degree of knee flexion, and how much is used is largely a function of each lifter's build. However, a locked back knee will prevent the lifter from absorbing the lift with the legs to achieve lockout while maintaining balance—the stiff back leg will force any additional depth to be achieved by bending the front knee exclusively, which will shift the lifter forward without accompanying flexion of the rear knee.

The lead shin should be vertical or even slightly behind vertical to create the strongest possible position. Once the knee moves forward of the ankle, it becomes increasingly difficult to resist any forward momentum, and the lifter will typically fail to stop it. In a strong position, the lifter is able to push back off the front leg to secure the position and prevent any unwanted forward sliding.

Like in the snatch and clean, the lifter must stay connected to the bar and prevent it from crashing down into the receiving position. A push off the bar into an excessively deep split will allow the lifter to achieve a locked out overhead position, but will cause the bar to be unsupported initially, creating unnecessary and abrupt downward impact. This typically results in bending and re-extension of the elbows, illegal in competition, and unstable in practical terms. The depth of the split must be commensurate to the height the bar is driven; that is, the heavier the bar, the lower the split will need to be, and lighter weights must be received at somewhat higher levels to avoid separation between the lifter and the bar.

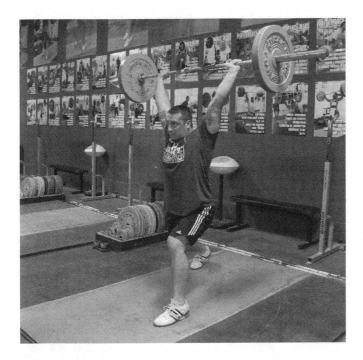

FIGURE 25.5 The receipt of the jerk must be precise and aggressive.

Recovery

With the highest center of mass and heaviest weight with which the lifter will contend, the jerk offers a lot of opportunity for instability in the receiving position, and the process of recovering to the standing position with the bar overhead to complete the lift creates even more potential for a loss of control. There are two primary concerns during the recovery of the jerk: maintaining the lockout of the overhead position and preserving stability.

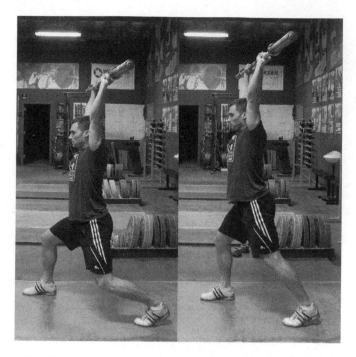

FIGURE 25.6 In the recovery from the split jerk, the lifter is attempting to "wedge" him- or herself up under the bar to keep it in approximately the same vertical plane. This minimizes movement of the bar and consequently maximizes the stability of the system.

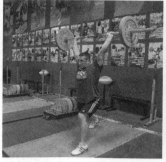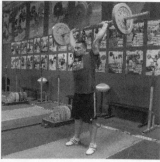

FIGURE 25.7 Recovering from the jerk must be active and aggressive to maintain stability and balance by minimizing barbell movement.

The first issue, maintaining the overhead lockout, requires continued effort to stabilize the shoulder blades and squeeze the elbows tightly in extension. It's frustratingly common to see the elbows soften and bend during a lifter's recovery simply because he or she fails to actively maintain what had been a perfectly locked out overhead position. The lifter has to keep in mind that the movement of the recovery introduces new forces to the system and without active, aggressive resistance, the lockout can very easily be compromised before the lifter has time to react and correct. Maximal effort to maintain the lockout position until the lift is complete and the athlete is intentionally dropping the bar should, from day one, be made a habit.

The second concern is the maintenance of the barbell's stability overhead. Upon successful receipt of the bar overhead in the split position, there will be little to no movement (the more movement, the poorer the execution of the lift was). However, the action of standing from the split introduces movement again and the attendant potential for instability. The goal must be to minimize the movement of the barbell to maximize its stability. This is managed through the proper recovery protocol described previously in the book: stepping approximately a third of the split length back with the front foot and then bringing the back foot forward to meet it. This in essence "wedges" the body up underneath the bar without requiring any significant horizontal movement of the weight, which is the larger percentage of the system's mass, and movement of which will consequently create greater instability than movement of the body.

Once the athlete is standing fully with the feet in line with the barbell and is demonstrating control, the bar can be dropped. Competitive lifters in particular should emphasize this establishment of complete control in a fully recovered position in preparation for competition in which the jerk may not be dropped until the judges have given a down signal. Training with incomplete recoveries and lazy overhead positions prevents the maximal development of overhead strength, stability and awareness, and creates unnecessary difficulty in competition.

Greg Everett

The Barbells' Path

Like in the snatch and clean, the precise bar path in the jerk will vary slightly among even elite weightlifters. However, all successful jerks will have elements in common. The most important element of the bar path of a successful jerk is that at no time does the barbell travel forward to any significant degree. It is possible to successfully make jerks with some very minimal forward movement of the barbell, but only because of the broad base and potential for moving that base the split receiving position provides. There is certainly, however, a limit to how much weight can be successfully jerked with such forward deviation, and consequently, the goal is to eliminate it.

The bar starts balanced over the lifter's base. In the dip, the barbell should travel down vertically to its lowest point, remaining in the same vertical plane in which it started. In the drive, the bar may travel approximately vertically, or ideally slightly backward. As the lifter initiates the push against the bar with the arms, there should be a continuation of the slight backward angle of the bar path, or the beginning of one. As the lifter reaches the overhead lockout position and settles into the final split depth, the bar will drop very slightly.

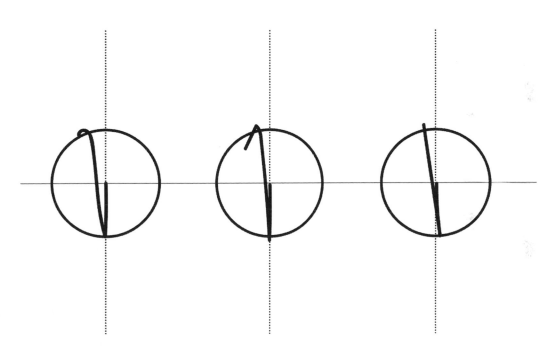

FIGURE 25.8 Pictured are the bar paths of successful jerks by three different technically proficient world-class lifters from three different weight classes. What should be immediately obvious is that, while they differ very slightly, they all conform to the same basic shape.

The Clean & Jerk

The athlete is now familiar with both the clean and the jerk in isolation. The clean & jerk as a single lift is considerably different than either lift performed individually. While the clean is quite taxing physically and psychologically, the clean & jerk presents even more of a challenge because of the need for both great strength and commitment for each, and the often remarkable fatigue that follows a heavy clean effort.

A few points need to be clarified with regard to performing the two lifts together as the clean & jerk. There will be two basic transitions between the clean and the jerk—the foot position and the rack position (including any change to grip width).

As has been mentioned previously, there may be minimal or no difference in the foot stance in the receiving position of the clean and the drive stance of the jerk for certain athletes. In these cases, this transition will not exist—the athlete will simply keep the feet in the same position. For most athletes, however, following the recovery from the clean, the feet will be moved back in to a narrower drive posi-

tion in preparation for the jerk. This can be done in whatever manner is most comfortable and stable for the athlete.

More dramatic, and more critical, will be the shift from the clean rack position to jerk rack position—sliding the hands in deeper under the bar and bringing the elbows down and out. This can be accomplished a few possible ways. Occasionally athletes will be able to reposition their hands in a standing position without any movement of the bar. This is unusual, however, with weight on the bar. Far more commonly, the athlete will need to unload the bar from the shoulders briefly in order to drive the hands farther under it.

Often athletes will stand from the clean, and then spend a great deal of time attempting to reposition the hands and arms in preparation for the jerk. This is an enormous expenditure of energy in an already fatigued state, and the more time spent in this position struggling with this adjustment, the less likely a successful jerk becomes due both to additional fa-

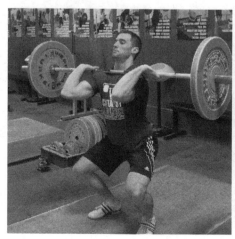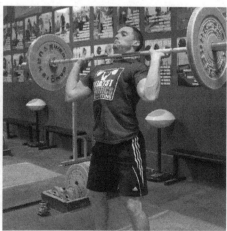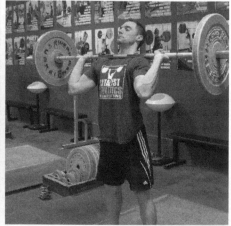

FIGURE 26.1 The rack position should be adjusted using the momentum from the clean recovery to unload the bar from the shoulders.

tigue and increasing discouragement. Heavy weights in the clean rack position are crushing both physically and psychologically, and the more time the athlete feels the weight of the bar pushing him or her into the floor, or has to struggle to achieve the desired position, the less confident he or she becomes in his or her ability to drive the bar overhead.

Once standing after a clean, the athlete can quickly dip and pop the legs to lift the bar slightly off the shoulders and create space to drive the hands in deeper under the bar (and possibly move the grip to a wider or narrow position) and bring the elbows into the desired down and out orientation. Once the bar settles back on the shoulders in the jerk rack position, the athlete is ready to jerk. This technique works, and will be the fallback if the better option fails or the difficulty of the clean recovery is such that the athlete simply wants to stand up without worrying yet about the jerk, but it's an unnecessary expenditure of energy and time.

Instead, the athlete can use the momentum already being generated from the recovery of the clean to pop the bar up as he or she reaches a standing position (Figure 26.1). This is much quicker and uses less energy than the previous method.

There will be times when one or both of the athlete's hands slip out from under the bar during the clean recovery. This is still a legal lift as long as the bar remains racked in the same position on the shoulders (i.e. it does not slide down the chest and have to be lifted back up onto the shoulders), and the athlete can make the attempt to re-grip the bar in preparation for the jerk. The method for doing so is the same for normally repositioning the hands—a quick pop with the legs to briefly unload the bar from the shoulders, although it may need to be more pronounced. In the case of both hands slipping from the bar, it's usually most prudent to re-grip one at a time to minimize the potential for dropping the bar. It's important that the athlete keep the arms raised high in this situation to ensure the bar remains securely racked deep on the shoulders—the bar cannot legally be allowed to slip down and then be readjusted back up.

Despite the desire to hold the bar for as little time as possible between the clean and the jerk, the athlete must be patient and adequately prepare for the jerk. This involves ensuring correct balance on the feet, the proper rack position, enough control of heavy breathing to bring in a sufficient breath to stabilize the torso, and the mental focus to perform the lift.

The necessity of mental preparation is often underestimated. Clean recoveries will generally be very taxing both physically and mentally. No other lift will place as much weight over the lifter's head as the jerk, and this demands a great deal of confidence and commitment. Far too often athletes miss jerks they're normally well capable of making because of a failure to adequately prepare mentally for the effort in the wake of a difficult and demoralizing clean.

The athlete can make only a single attempt at the jerk. Once initiating the dip, the athlete must commit to the attempt. It's important that efforts to adjust the grip or rack position are clearly such to prevent being mistaken as aborted jerk attempts.

Introduction to Error Correction

The correction of technical errors in the snatch, clean or jerk is a complex endeavor in many respects, and due to the inordinate number of possible errors, an overwhelming and frustrating subject for many. However, like many complex subjects, understanding a relatively small collection of principles will dramatically improve the coach's ability to manage error correction. This foundation of conceptual understanding will also allow coaches to effectively correct any possible error without having ever encountered it previously rather than relying on the memorization of predetermined approaches for specific mistakes. One of the characteristics that distinguishes great coaches from mediocre coaches is not only the ability to diagnose the causes of errors, but to simplify corrections for the lifter.

The primary component of the coach's ability to correct technical errors in the lifts is the genuine understanding of lift mechanics; this understanding is what allows the recognition, diagnosis and correction of errors. Without this knowledge, the only option for the coach is to implement others' instructions. Instead, the goal is for the coach to be capable of operating independently and devising corrective strategies for any conceivable error as it is encountered in the process of training weightlifters.

All of the information discussed previously in this book is part of this foundation of understanding. Additionally, the learning progressions for each lift provide a collection of potential remedial drills—these drills are used to teach specific elements of technical execution in specific segments of the lift, and consequently can be similarly valuable for correcting improper execution of those same elements and segments. These drills also provide a useful framework from which variations of given drills can be derived to most appropriately address a particular problem.

As a part of this process, it's important to recognize that the response of athletes to coaching cues and exercises can vary dramatically—methods that work well for some may be ineffective for others. The art of coaching lies in finding ways to improve *any* athlete's performance, and this can be accomplished only with smart experimentation based on a thorough understanding of technical principles of the lifts. It's the coach's responsibility to adjust the approach according to the needs of the athlete in question.

Technique correction should focus on the practical—that is, the coach should instruct the athlete regarding the performance of the given exercise without including superfluous information. Theory and extensive detail can be discussed with the athlete outside of the technique training sessions if the athlete is interested in understanding the rationale. Otherwise, the additional information overcomplicates the process and spreads the athlete's focus too thin, particularly when, as is true in many cases, the athlete does not genuinely understand and consequently arrives at incorrect and even contradictory interpretations.

Where to Start

It's unlikely an athlete will ever demonstrate a single technique flaw. While he or she may display a single error repeatedly and even consistently among attempts, it will invariably be accompanied by additional problems. This is due largely to the fact that errors in one part of the movement typically produce errors in other parts of the movement even with compensatory efforts (often other errors *are* compensatory efforts).

Early in an athlete's development, the list of errors

on each attempt will be extensive and may even vary considerably among attempts. Despite any variation, typically these athletes will repeatedly display a core set of errors, present irrespective of the changing peripheral errors. These core errors are the priority and must be addressed and corrected before any significant effort and time is invested in the peripheral errors. Often correction of these core errors will result in the attenuation if not elimination of the peripheral errors, which are generally products of the more fundamental errors. As the athlete progresses, the list of errors will diminish, as will the severity. However, the longer these errors have been performed, the more established they will be and consequently the more difficult to correct.

In addition to following the order of core to peripheral, efforts to correct technique errors should generally follow the order of their occurrence in the movement. Again, errors will nearly always produce subsequent errors; correction of the earlier faults often eliminates the cause of the later faults. For example, if an athlete's weight is too far forward on the feet at the initiation of the snatch or clean, it will typically cause the bar to swing forward away from the body. We can attempt to correct this bar path by encouraging the athlete to more actively pull the bar into the body, but this neglects the actual cause of the problem. That cause will continue to result in trouble with the lift even if the specific error of the barbell diverging from its intended proximity to the body is corrected through overcompensation. If we instead start with the earlier error—improper balance of weight immediately off the floor—we can correct it and in the process eliminate the second error as well.

Finally, it's critical to understand that an athlete has the ability to focus on and address a very limited number of errors at any given time. No matter how extensive the list of problems may be for a particular lift by a particular athlete, limit the focus to one or two at a time—this means both in a given rep or set, but also to a large extent, in a single training session. If errors have been properly prioritized, selecting which to focus on will present no problem. Ideally, additional errors aren't even discussed with the athlete to avoid distraction. Of course, if the athlete inquires about errors he or she suspects may be occurring, they can be addressed. But the more focused the

athlete can be kept on the highest priority problems, the more quickly they will be corrected. The longer the list of mistakes athletes are aware of, the more frustrated and overwhelmed they're likely to become, greatly reducing the effectiveness of corrective work.

Types of Errors

We can separate technical errors into two broad categories: conceptual and practical. A conceptual error is the result of the lifter not knowing how to do something (that is, having never been instructed on the element in question) or having learned incorrectly through improper instruction or misunderstanding. A practical error is the improper execution of an element of the lift despite the athlete's possession of the correct conceptual understanding of that element. As a lifter advances in skill, the bulk of errors will shift from conceptual to practical.

The protocol for correcting each type of error is different. For conceptual errors, the process is relatively simple: educate or re-educate and practice. Practical errors will require more work on the part of the coach and lifter. First the problem must be identified and the cause diagnosed—this is often the most difficult step, and it relies heavily on the coach's understanding of lift mechanics and proper technique. Next, the coach creates the means of correction—this will be the corrective exercises or drills determined to be most suitable for the lifter and error, and this decision will depend again on the coach's understanding of the lifts, but also on previous experience with implementation and experimentation. Finally will be the implementation of these exercises—the coach will determine when and how the exercises will be performed and the athlete will perform the work until achieving a satisfactory degree of improvement.

Observation

How the coach observes the athlete when attempting to evaluate a movement will depend on the movement and the element of the movement on which the coach is focusing. For general and initial observation of the movement as a whole, the coach is best positioned at an oblique angle and at a distance. This allows an easy view of the entire movement without shifting of the eyes to obtain a reliable picture of the whole lift in a general sense. This initial impression will provide the coach the information needed to adjust the observation position to more closely inspect the element(s) that stand out as the highest priorities.

For example, if the bar path appears to be problematic, the coach can stand at the lifter's side to more accurately assess it and also determine the source of the problem. In addition to this live observation, video can be helpful in diagnosing particularly troublesome errors with the use of slow motion or frame-by-frame analysis. However, while these tools can play a role, the coach should avoid becoming dependent on them.

When to Correct

If we're discussing correction of lifting technique, there is an assumption that all of the initial teaching has already taken place. In other words, the lifter has transitioned into a legitimate training program rather than a more introductory program focused primarily on lift instruction and the development of basic movements and work capacity.

If significant errors exist, it may be best to use focused technique training sessions in which only one or two lifts are trained with the appropriate remedial exercises. For example, a lifter may train five days a week, with two of those days being technique sessions in which the only work is remedial in nature, while the remaining three are of a more conventional composition. This training should be modified appropriately to avoid having the lifter continue practicing improper movements any more than necessary (That is, some amount of practice will always be done with less than perfect lifts until the athlete has reached technical mastery—the key is to ensure they represent the smallest possible fraction of the lifter's training possible.).

For less significant errors, corrective work should be added into the lifter's current training plan. How this is done can vary based on the training program, the errors in question, the time available and the nature of the corrective exercises. Technique primers are a very effective approach—select a corrective ex-

ercise to be performed immediately before the lift it's intended to correct. For example, to improve aggression and precision in the third pull of the snatch, a lifter can perform 3-5 sets of tall snatch triples before beginning his snatch training for that day. This not only provides the benefits of the corrective exercise itself, but will also improve the performance of the subsequent snatches, further reinforcing the corrections.

In all cases, corrective exercise of a technical nature should be performed at the beginning of the training session when the athlete is freshest and most focused. Remedial work of more of a strength nature can be placed toward the end of sessions as long as it will not be negatively affected by fatigue accumulated during the session.

In other cases, the program itself may be modified somewhat to address technical issues. For example, if we would normally have a training session with snatches from the floor, we may change this to snatch + overhead squat to include additional overhead strength and stability work without adding significant time to the workout; or we may change to a somewhat different exercise like snatch pull + hang snatch to address a specific need of the athlete without changing the fundamental effect of the exercise.

Again, limit the number of corrections a lifter has to focus on in a given training session or the effectiveness will be limited. That said, one of the benefits of using exercises to correct is that they require, in general, much less thought on the part of the lifter and consequently are less taxing in terms of nervous system fatigue and mental burnout because, as simplified segments of a lift, they are relatively simple to perform. These can be used in greater quantity and with more variety in a given session than technique work that involves more focused coaching and practice of a specific lift along with conceptual learning.

How to Correct

How corrections are made will depend somewhat on the coach's experience and preferences, but primarily on the circumstances—the nature and degree of the problem, the athlete's temperament, the available time and energy, the level of priority for the correction and the details of the training program into which it needs to be integrated.

As was explained previously, conceptual and practical errors will be corrected differently. Conceptual errors can be addressed with verbal instruction and demonstrations when the lift in question is being performed. Ideally, this is discussed immediately prior to the athlete beginning the exercise and one or two points of focus are determined for that session, and then reinforced by the coach during the session.

Practical errors will require more extensive intervention. This will involve various strategies mentioned above such as technique primers, standalone remedial exercises, modifications of lifts, and complexes. In any case, the first step is identifying the problem and diagnosing its source. This can be done only with experience and genuine understanding of lift mechanics and technique, although the specific errors discussed in this section of the book will help new coaches begin to learn to identify causes more quickly.

Next the problem needs to be isolated in some fashion to allow optimal focus on correction. For example, if an athlete is slow to punch up against the bar when finishing the turnover of the snatch, the least effective approach is to simply tell the athlete when snatching to punch up against the bar (although this should still be part of the total strategy). More effective is isolating the problem and providing an opportunity for the athlete to physically practice the movement with limited distractions. In this case, that could mean adding exercises like the snatch balance to the training program, and/or adding drop snatches or snatch balances as technique primers before snatch training sessions.

If needed or appropriate, we can then expand the isolated element to bring it closer to the complete lift. Staying with the above example, when the athlete has improved on the drop snatch or snatch balance adequately, we may progress to a tall snatch or dip snatch to allow the lifter to integrate this improved ability to punch up against the bar into the actual third pull, but still with an abbreviated movement that allows focus on the element in question.

Another step that can be taken after this, or instead of this, is combining corrective drills with the lift as a complex. For this example, that might be something like a dip or high-hang snatch + snatch.

The first rep allows more focus on the finish of the turnover, which then can be integrated into the full lift immediately after.

Another consideration with regard to practical errors is whether or not the cause is related to position-specific strength. A perfect example of this is the tendency for a lifter to begin extending the hips for the second pull prematurely. This may very well be a simple technique error that can be corrected with instruction, drills and practice, but it may also be due to a strength deficit in the necessary positions. That is, with heavier snatches or cleans, the lifter may be physically incapable of staying over the bar longer; in such cases, no amount of coaching or practice will correct the problem. In addition to this, it will be necessary to add strength work that addresses the position in question. For example, this athlete may use halting snatch deadlifts or segment snatch pulls rather than or in addition to snatch pulls.

Repetition Quality & Quantity

The quality of repetition during error correction is critical. Frequently athletes and coaches will concern themselves with the quantity of work at the expense of the quality, believing that the greater the volume of practice, the better the effect. The problem with this approach is two-fold. First, a lack of quality is the very element we're attempting to correct. Practicing a motor skill poorly will improve the athlete's ability to perform that motor skill in that same poor manner—never will it magically create correct motor patterns. Second, as a product of the first, that large volume of sub-optimal practice establishes motor patterns very similar to the ones we're attempting to create yet still incorrect. These patterns compete with the correct ones and make learning and establishing the correct ones far more difficult when compared to establishing those correct patterns in the absence of the similar incorrect ones. In other words, this approach to practice is not simply ineffective—it's counterproductive. A small number of precisely performed drills is far more effective than any number of inaccurately performed drills. Quality practice will produce quality performance.

Positive Instruction

Whether working with conceptual or practical technique faults, a final point needs to be considered with regard to the nature of cues or instruction: ensuring positive instruction. Positive instruction refers to three different elements: telling the athlete what to do instead of what not to do; aligning the cue with the action; and balancing critique and praise in a net positive quantity.

If an athlete is performing a lift incorrectly, it's a safe assumption that he or she doesn't know how to correct it. Consequently, simply telling athletes to not do what they're doing wrong is going to be unproductive—likely they know it's wrong, and even if they don't, simply learning that it's wrong doesn't give them any idea of how to approach correcting it

Instead, the coach needs to provide the athlete with an action to perform; something to do rather than *not* do. For example, if the bar is swinging away from the athlete's body during the snatch or clean, we can tell the athlete to not let the bar swing away, but this is a marginally useful instruction at best. The athlete needs to know what to do instead of allowing the bar to swing. In order to do this, we need to identify the source. Is the athlete locking the elbows? Is he or she allowing too much space between the bar and body and then banging the bar away with the hips? Is he or she not actively and correctly performing the upper body mechanics of the third pull?

Once we have the source identified, the appropriate instruction can be provided. If the problem is improper mechanics in the third pull, for example, rather than telling the lifter not to let the bar drift away, we can tell them to pull the elbows up and out in order to keep the bar close on the turnover. This provides the athlete with a very clear action to attempt and will more often than not produce better results than the negative counterpart. (This being said, there will be times when a vague cue like *keep it close* is effective—these times are when the coach and athlete have already established previously how exactly this is to be done. The cue, in this case, is simply a reminder rather than the actual instructions.)

Aligning the instructions or cues with the action means providing something for the lifter to do in harmony with the lift rather than in opposition to

it. An example of this would be an athlete who allows the hips to rise too quickly relative the shoulders during the first pull of the snatch or clean. Instead of instructing the athlete to keep the hips down, we can instruct him or her to keep the chest up. In this case, both cues gave the athlete an action to perform like we want, but the latter is better aligned with the movement being executed—that is, we gave a cue of upward lifting during an upward movement of the body.

Finally, it's important to always be cognizant of how critique is received by each athlete, and to balance that critique with recognition of the positives. For any given lift, even with several technical errors, the athlete is bound to have done something right. If all an athlete ever hears is what he or she is doing wrong, it can become discouraging, even when the coach is not intending it to be so. It's simple enough to add to any critique of a lift something that the athlete did well; for example, letting the athlete know that while the bar drifted away during the third pull, the second pull was executed with excellent aggression and timing. This helps keep the athlete motivated to continue correcting errors rather than giving up in frustration.

Coaches also need to keep in mind how each athlete hears critique and adjust his or her approach somewhat. Some athletes will be more sensitive than others, and often hear simple critique as a value judgment, believing, irrespective of the intent, that the coach is upset, disappointed or believes the athlete is hopeless. While coaches shouldn't coddle athletes and bend to their every irrational and unreasonable whim, there does need to be an effort made to ensure that the correct information is being communicated and received properly by each athlete.

Specific Corrections

The following three chapters provide corrective strategies for the most common technical errors in the snatch, clean and jerk. Descriptions of all exercises can be found in the Exercises section of the book. Again, these are guidelines and starting points. Experimentation and creativity are encouraged.

Each error has both cues to help with conceptual or more easily corrected errors, and more involved corrective methods such as drills, remedial exercises, technique primers and complexes, organized according to specific causes of the problem. Coaches will need to decide which is appropriate based on the circumstances.

The effectiveness of the corrective exercises listed with each error is dependent on their proper execution. For example, if we're attempting to correct the imbalance between leg and hip strength that can cause excessive leading with the hips in the first pull of the snatch, we may choose to perform segment snatch deadlifts. If the lifter loads the exercise excessively or rushes the movement and consequently performs it with the same unwanted hip leading, it not only won't help fix the problem, but will strengthen and reinforce it. Be sure to understand the purpose of each exercise in each case and enforce proper execution for that purpose.

Not surprisingly, in any given lift, errors and causes are often interrelated with others. I've attempted to avoid redundancy as much as possible without sacrificing the organization or clarity of the information and maximizing the section's usefulness as a quick reference tool.

Universal Errors

The following are errors that may occur in either the snatch or clean and have the same basic causes in both lifts, although there may be slight differences in how they appear and in what related errors they produce. For each error, possible causes and appropriate corrections for those causes are listed, including coaching cues when non-strength-related causes exist.

Leading with the Hips

Leading with the hips refers to the hips rising faster than the shoulders in the first pull to a degree larger than what is acceptable. That is, for most lifters we will expect to see a slight shift in the back angle during the pull from the floor, but too much creates a number of possible problems and can be indicative of imbalanced strength in the athlete.

Weak Legs Relative to Hips

If an athlete's hips are significantly stronger than his/her legs, the natural tendency, to an increasing degree with increasing weights, will be to extend the knees to a larger angle without moving the shoulders and bar to the same extent in order to shift more of the responsibility for lifting the weight to the hips. This is especially true for athletes with longer legs who already have a bigger leverage disadvantage at the knee. In order to prevent this natural shifting, the athlete's knee extension strength will need to be increased to allow him to extend the knees from the desired starting position with the full load.

Exercises to help correct this problem include anything that strengthens knee extension, and in particular, knee extension with the body in the posture we want the lifter to maintain during the first pull.

- Snatch/clean deadlift/pull on riser
- Snatch/clean deadlift/pull
- Snatch/clean segment deadlift/pull
- Halting snatch/clean deadlift
- Halting snatch/clean deadlift on riser
- Floating halting snatch/clean deadlift
- Snatch/clean lift-off
- Pause back squat
- Front squat

Rushing off the Floor

If an imbalance of strength is not the cause, the error is often the result of the lifter rushing the initial lift from the floor without being tight and controlled enough to maintain the correct posture. The body's natural tendency will be to unload the knees and shift more of the work to the hips with few exceptions (such as naturally very strong-legged athletes or athletes with relatively short legs and long torsos); consequently, if the movement is not controlled actively, we can expect the hips to rise faster than the shoulders.

Exercises to help correct this problem include anything that will force the athlete to control the posture off the floor correctly and help him or her feel the proper position and balance. These are largely the same as the exercises that will be helpful for correcting a strength imbalance. Additionally, complexes involving a partial pull that focuses on the correct first pull positions followed by a snatch or clean will be helpful.

- Slow-pull snatch/clean
- Segment snatch/clean (pause at knee)
- Segment snatch/clean pull/deadlift (pause at knee or at multiple points below, at and above knee)
- Snatch/clean lift-off
- Floating halting snatch/clean deadlift
- Snatch/clean segment deadlift/pull + snatch/clean
- Snatch/clean lift-off + snatch/clean
- Halting snatch/clean deadlift + snatch/clean

Cues that can be helpful, especially if used in combination with the above corrective exercises, include:

- Squeeze it off the floor
- Smooth off the floor
- Control off the floor
- Chest up off the floor
- Lead with the chest
- Tight off the floor

Jumping Forward

Jumping forward in the snatch or clean is always a symptom of a forward imbalance of the barbell-lifter system at some point during the lift. However, this imbalance can have a number of sources, and correction will vary depending on the cause. Often this error proves extremely difficult and frustrating to correct, but investing the time and effort is well worth it.

This is an error, however, that will sometimes respond to non-specific corrections. If the cause of the problem is proving difficult to diagnose or is not obvious, using this approach can be a smart way to begin resolving the problem sooner. First discussed are non-specific corrections that can be effective, followed by specific possible causes and suggested corrections for each.

Non-Specific Corrections

The first non-specific correction is the use of barriers to jumping forward by placing an object of some type in front of the lifter. While this can be very effective, it's critical to only use objects that don't create the potential for injuring athletes in the case they do still jump forward and contact the barrier.

The first choice is a scrap of thin rubber flooring or mat. Half-inch or thinner is ideal—this creates an adequate barrier but is low enough that the athlete will not have much of a problem finishing or bailing out of the lift if one or both toes land on the mat; it will also shift out of the way if the athlete kicks it with a toe. When introducing the mat, start it about as far in front of the lifter's toes as that lifter tends to jump and incrementally move it closer. Ultimately, it doesn't need to be actually touching the lifter's toes in the start, but it can be within an inch.

Another choice, which is better if part of the problem may be the bar swinging forward away from the lifter, is a vertical length of PVC pipe or wooden dowel placed in front of one or both ends of the bar (outside the plates). A brave coach can hold this pipe in place during the lift, but it needs to be held in a way that it can be released safely or allowed to move if the bar does contact it to prevent affecting the movement of the bar, and so that the bar will not hit the coach's hand. Another option to avoid these potential problems is to create a small base for the pipe (such as with a galvanized pipe flange added to one end of the pipe) that will allow it to stand vertically on its own, yet fall over out of the way if hit with the bar. This also allows the coach to view the lift from whatever position he or she prefers rather than be stuck right next to the athlete.

Virtual barriers can also be used, such as placing a length of tape or chalk line on the platform in front of the lifter's toes and providing the instruction to not jump over it. Despite the absence of a physical barrier and the attendant potential consequences, this can be surprisingly effective with some athletes.

We can also attempt over-correction through cueing alone or along with a physical or virtual barrier. That is, rather than instructing the athlete to not jump forward, we can instruct him or her to actually jump backward a small amount (such as half an inch) so that he or she somewhat exaggerates the effort to control the forward imbalance. Of course, if this results in a significant backward jump, it's not an appropriate strategy for that lifter.

The potential problem with all of the previous

strategies is that they may not correct the cause of the error but simply create some kind of compensatory effort that itself is a problem or leads to new problems. For example, the lifter may manage to avoid hitting a vertical pipe with the bar in the snatch, but does so by shifting his weight excessively far back over the foot in the pull, redirecting the lift backward. Or we may still see a poor bar path with excessive horizontal deviation, but the lifter leans farther back away from the bar to balance the system, resulting in excessive distance between the bar and body and the accordingly worse mechanics, and potentially preventing an adequately quick or proper movement into the receiving position.

Finally, performing the snatch or clean without lifting the feet from the platform is a non-specific approach to forcing the athlete to maintain balance over the same base throughout the lift. This can be successful for some lifters, but it also has the potential to cause other problems, such as confusing the lifter with regard to normal snatch and clean technique and forcing a pulling position with the feet in the receiving stance. If it is used, it should never replace standard snatches or cleans in the program, but be used in addition—employing the exercise as a technique primer for subsequent snatches or cleans, for example, is a good way to implement the exercise.

Failure to Shift Weight Back in First Pull

A part of the action of the first pull is to shift the center of mass of the barbell-lifter system slightly farther back over the foot into the balance we want maintained for the remainder of the lift. Needless to say, if this does not occur adequately or at all, the lifter's balance will be too far forward over the feet. If lifting with a proper upright posture, there will be very minimal effort to maintain the barbell's proximity to the body, as the bar will naturally hang approximately vertically below the shoulders. However, if the shoulders move or start excessively forward of the bar, the bar will swing forward unless actively controlled by the lifter.

Exercises that will help the athlete perform this backward weight shift and maintain both the proper posture and the bar's proximity to the body in the first pull include anything that allows controlled performance of and focus on this initial movement.

- Snatch/Clean segment deadlift/pull (pause at or below knee and/or immediately off the floor)
- Halting snatch/clean deadlift
- Segment snatch/clean (pause at knee)
- Slow-pull snatch/clean
- Halting snatch/clean deadlift + snatch/clean
- Snatch/clean pull + snatch/clean

Cues that may be helpful to encourage the athlete to perform the movement properly include:

- Back off the floor
- Bring it back
- Shift back right away
- Jump through the heels

Improper Starting Position

While some degree of adjustment can be accomplished early in the lift, it's limited, and an improper starting position can easily produce a forward imbalance during the snatch or clean. Starting with the weight too far forward over the feet is the most obvious mistake in this case, but starting with the weight too far back can actually produce a forward weight imbalance as well through the natural overcompensation that is typical in that case. The details of proper balance and posture in the starting position have been covered in detail previously—these criteria will need to be revisited.

Exercises that can help the lifter improve the starting position are the same as for the previous cause, as we are in essence trying to accomplish the same basic task. Of course, the focus will be primarily on the starting position. It will also be helpful to have athletes perform these exercises with a static start even if they employ a dynamic start in the snatch or clean and it's decided not to change this. If possible and reasonable, however, changing from a dynamic to static starting position itself is an effective way to correct problems in the starting position for newer lifters.

- Snatch/clean lift-off
- Segment snatch/clean deadlift/pull (pause

immediately off floor and/or knee)
- Floating snatch/clean deadlift/pull
- Floating segment snatch/clean deadlift/pull
- Snatch/clean deadlift/pull with slow eccentric (3-5 seconds) back into starting position
- Floating halting snatch/clean deadlift
- Slow-pull snatch/clean
- Snatch/clean without allowing weights to rattle as the bar leaves the floor

Cues in this case will be directed at helping the athlete establish the starting position itself correctly rather than with the movement of the first pull. These will of course vary depending on the nature of each athlete's deviation from the desired position and simply need to be instructions the athlete understands, along with possibly physically manipulating the athlete's position as needed.

Bar Moving Straight up Past Knees

A common mistake made by new lifters is lifting the bar straight up from the knees or lower thighs, continuing to lean forward over the bar and allow it to remain away from the body. The combined effort to keep the bar as close to the body as possible and initiate the explosion of the second pull should naturally bring the knees under the bar and the bar back into the hip (or upper thigh in the clean); however, new lifters will occasionally prevent this from occurring for various reasons, even simply having an unconscious aversion to allowing the bar to contact the body.

Exercises to help correct this problem should focus primarily on the movement between the knees and the power position or extension, the maintenance of maximal proximity of the bar to the body, and possibly the movement of the knees under the bar if necessary. Ideally the latter is not performed intentionally, but in some cases, remediation of that significant a degree is needed.

Note that it is actually possible to move the barbell too far back between the knee and hip, which will result in a snatch or clean in the lifter's weight shifting excessively forward or backward as the second pull is performed. Cues or practice to keep the bar back or push it back toward the hip should not

be misinterpreted to mean excessive backward movement past approximately the middle of the foot. See Pushing Bar Too Far Back Toward Hips below.

- Halting snatch/clean deadlift
- Hang snatch/clean (from the knee or mid-thigh)
- Segment snatch/clean (pause at knee and/or mid-thigh)
- Snatch/clean deadlift to power position
- Slow-pull snatch/clean
- Halting snatch/clean deadlift + snatch/clean
- Snatch/clean deadlift to power position + snatch/clean

Helpful cues will depend on what exactly the problem is, and include:

- Bring it in
- Bring it back to your hips
- Push it back into your hips
- Push it back into your lap
- Keep it close past the knees
- Bring it back past the knees

Bumping or Swinging Bar Forward in Second Pull

Any forward movement of the bar in the second pull has the potential to pull the lifter forward to a degree dependent on the bar's forward inertia and its weight relative to the lifter's. See more about and corrections for this error in its own section below.

Pushing Bar Too Far Back Toward Hips

Occasionally lifters will be so focused on bringing the bar back toward the hips that they move it too far back relative to the feet; that is, it moves behind approximately the middle of the foot. This shifts the line of gravity too far back over the foot, creating compensatory rocking forward on the feet, but also means that the bar is pushed forward a significant distance as the hips extend in the second pull, adding excessive horizontal force to the barbell. Lifters will need to be re-educated to understand that the backward movement of the bar is subtle and needs to be controlled properly—the purpose is to establish the proper balance and position for the second pull, not to push the bar back as far as possible. Exercises that can help the lifter practice the proper movement include:

- Halting clean/snatch deadlift (pause at mid-thigh or hip)
- Segment clean/snatch deadlift/pull (pauses at knee, mid-thigh and hip)
- Slow pull clean/snatch

Cues that may help the athlete maintain the proper barbell and body relative positions and balance over the feet include:

- Balance over the whole foot
- Keep the feet flat

Bar Swinging Forward in Third Pull

See more about this error and corrections in its own section below.

Bumping or Swinging Bar Forward in Second Pull

A forward-traveling barbell will cause forward movement of the lifter to a magnitude commensurate to the relative weights of the bar and lifter and the inertia of the bar in that direction; the heavier the barbell and the faster it's moving forward, the more it will pull the lifter forward (although, the heavier the bar relative to the lifter, the less it will travel forward under a given amount of contact force from the body). There can be a few different reasons the barbell moves forward away from the body at the finish of the second pull and each will have its own corrections.

Excessive or Improper Hip Extension

How and how much the hips are extended in the second pull will affect where the bar is directed to a large extent. While we want explosive and essentially maximal effort hip extension, it must be properly executed to be effective. We can imagine a vertical line running through a standing lifter's ankle, hip and shoulder when viewed from the side—essentially, the hip should never cross forward of this line at any point of the snatch or clean (the hip joint approximately, not the front of the body at hip level). Extending the hips through this line creates too much forward force on the bar that disrupts its upward movement and reduces its upward speed and elevation; additionally, it will cause the bar to gain excessive horizontal motion, either pulling the lifter forward or preventing a successful third pull. Part of preventing excessive hip extension is ensuring complete and adequately aggressive vertical leg drive; this is addressed specifically as its own error below.

Excessive hip extension in the finish of the second pull can be improved with a few different exercises:

- Dip snatch/clean
- Snatch/clean from power position
- Snatch/clean pull + snatch/clean

Helpful cues for preventing excessive hip extension include:

- Push hard with the legs
- Keep pushing with the legs
- Get tall
- Finish up
- Hips straight up
- Straight up

Inadequate or Incomplete Leg Drive

As mentioned above, one cause of the bar being pushed forward with the hips in the second pull is weak or incomplete leg drive against the floor—that is, the leg drive in the second pull is either not aggressive enough, or the lifter stops driving before the hips have finished extending. This leg drive creates the solid base for the hip extension and keeps the lifter's feet anchored to the floor and consequently, the hips in place; without that continued and forceful drive, the hips will slide forward too far through the bar. Not only will this move the bar forward, it will also reduce its elevation.

Conveniently enough, the exercises that will help correct this are largely the same as for the previous error, with a couple additions (the final three are to improve the power of the leg drive generally):

- Dip snatch/clean
- Snatch/clean from power position
- Snatch/clean pull + snatch/clean
- Back squat jump
- Quarter squat jump
- Jumping squat

Likewise, the cues are similar to the previous problem of excessive hip extension:

- Push hard with the legs
- Keep pushing with the legs
- Get tall
- Finish up
- Drive up at the top
- Push all the way up

Excessive Distance Between Bar & Body Before Contact

Failing to maintain proximity of the bar to the body prior to its contact with the hips in the snatch or upper thighs in the clean will make the bar being pushed forward more likely. The solution is not to reduce the power of the hip extension, but to improve the precision of the bar path to reduce the rebound of the bar off the hips.

If we face two cars bumper to bumper and have the drivers floor the gas, we may get a lot of burned rubber, but no collision to speak of, despite the cars creating maximal force against each other. However, if we back the cars up away from each other and repeat, we'll get a significant collision, resulting in both cars bouncing back away from each other. In the same way, the more distance between the bar and body prior to the bar contacting the hips in the final extension, the greater the collision, and the more the bar will want to bounce away from the body. Maintaining maximal proximity of the bar and body on the way up will allow maximal hip extension force with a minimal horizontal reaction of the bar.

Exercises to practice this proximity of the bar to the body include:

- Segment snatch/clean (pause at knee and/or mid-thigh)
- Halting snatch/clean deadlift + snatch clean
- Snatch/clean pull + snatch/clean
- Dip snatch/clean + snatch/clean
- Snatch/clean from power position + snatch/ clean
- Slow-pull snatch/clean
- Snatch/clean transition deadlift

Cues to help prevent excessive distance between the bar and body include:

- Keep it close
- Bar close
- Bring it into your lap
- Bring it into your hips
- Keep it close on the way up
- Smooth finish

Stiff Arms

Stiff arms (i.e. locked elbows) during the second pull can cause the bar to swing forward as the lifter finishes the extension—with upward momentum on the bar and the arms locked, the bar has nowhere to go, and it has to pivot around the shoulders and swing forward to continue moving. As was discussed in earlier chapters, we want the arms passively extended in the first and second pulls, allowing the weight of the bar to keep them extended rather than intentionally extending the elbows. This allows a quick transition between the passive arms in the second pull and the active arms in the third pull.

Exercises to help the lifter train passive extension of the arms in the second pull and transitioning to active arms in the third pull include:

- Snatch/clean high-pull
- Snatch/clean high-pull + snatch/clean
- Snatch/clean high-pull + hang snatch/clean
- Muscle snatch/clean
- Tall snatch/clean
- Hang snatch/clean

- Dip snatch/clean
- Snatch/clean from power position

Cues that may be helpful include:

- Long arms
- Loose arms
- Relax the arms
- Tight back, loose arms
- Let the bar stretch your arms long

Swinging Bar Forward in Third Pull

The bar may also swing forward during the third pull. This is often a continuation of forward swinging in the second pull, but it warrants its own section as it can be a problem specific to the third pull as well. Corrections for the latter will also help the former.

There are two basic causes of this problem: stiff arms and improper mechanics. They are combined here because the corrective strategies are the same.

Just like stiff arms will cause the bar to swing forward in the second pull, they will force the bar to swing forward in the third pull. If the elbows don't bend during the lifter's movement under the bar, the only possibility is the bar moving forward and the lifter moving backward to allow the bar to swing around the shoulders.

Likewise, failing to perform the mechanics of the third pull properly will cause the bar to either move or stay too far forward and either prevent a successful turnover or force the lifter to jump or lean forward to attempt to save the lift.

Exercises to correct the third pull and ensure maximal proximity include:

- Snatch/clean high-pull
- Snatch/clean high-pull + snatch/clean
- Snatch/clean high-pull + hang snatch/clean
- Muscle snatch/clean
- Tall snatch/clean
- Dip snatch/clean
- Snatch/clean from power position

Cues to help correct the problem and remind the lifter of the desired upper body movement include:

- Bar close
- Elbows high
- Elbows high and out
- Elbows high, bar close
- Pull the elbows up and out
- Elbows high before you turn it over
- Keep the bar so close you can smell it

Jumping Backward

Jumping backward during a snatch or clean is not necessarily problematic and therefore may not qualify as a technical error. However, it can become excessive and create problems in the receiving position, and can be unintentional and unwanted, in which case, it should be corrected.

Additionally, a distinction needs to be made between jumping backward and moving only the feet backward. Jumping backward here refers to the entire barbell-lifter system moving backward together. That is, the lifter's feet land farther back from their starting point, but the bar comes with the lifter and the receiving position is correct and balanced. If instead, only the lifter's feet move backward, but the rest of the body and bar remain in the original area of the base, this has the same basic effect as the bar going forward. This is a problem with different causes and different solutions and is addressed separately in the next section.

Weight Too Far Back in Pull

Any backward jump is caused by the lifter's balance being too far back over the feet at some point—in this case, it's too far back during the first and second pull or both. As was discussed earlier in the book, ideally we want the line of gravity to pass through the foot slightly behind the mid-point (around the front edge of the heel). Farther back than this, and the entire system will be directed too far backward. Exercises to help the athlete feel the proper balance over the feet and correct it in the pull include:

- Snatch/clean deadlift
- Segment snatch/clean deadlift

- Segment snatch/clean pull
- Snatch/clean pull
- Halting snatch/clean deadlift
- Segment snatch/clean
- Snatch/clean pull/deadlift + snatch/clean
- Segment snatch/clean pull/deadlift + snatch/clean

Cues to help encourage the lifter to maintain the proper balance during the lift include:

- Finish straight up
- Drive straight up with the legs
- Balance over the feet
- Balance across the whole foot
- Pull *up*

Excessive Hip Extension

Unlike the excessive hip extension discussed previously that causes the bar to swing forward, in this case, the excessive extension is occurring without the hips moving too far forward—in other words, the legs are still vertical or nearly so, and the shoulders are too far behind the hips and base.

Exercises to help the lifter feel the proper degree of extension will essentially simulate that finish position, and so must be done properly. For example, if the lifter is leaning back excessively in a snatch deadlift to fix excessive hip extension in the snatch, it will not be effective. All exercises for this must be done with the proper extended position described previously in the book.

- Snatch/clean deadlift with hold in simulated extension position
- Snatch/clean deadlift with hold in simulated extension position + snatch/clean
- Hang snatch/clean deadlift (knee) with hold in simulated extension position
- Hang snatch/clean deadlift with hold in simulated extension position + hang snatch/clean (knee)
- Snatch/clean pull
- Snatch/clean pull + snatch/clean
- Dip snatch/clean
- Snatch/clean from power position

Helpful cues may include:

- Finish straight up
- Drive straight up with the legs
- Get tall
- Finish tall
- Stretch out tall
- Pull straight up

Feet Sweeping Backward

Unlike in the backward jump discussed in the previous section, this error involves only the lifter's feet moving backward during the lift while the rest of the body and the bar remain over the same original area. The effect of this is essentially the same as the bar moving forward—in the receiving position, the center of mass is in front of the base and cannot be supported easily or at all depending on how significant the backward movement of the feet was.

Generally the reason for this error is the same in a basic sense as for actually jumping backward—the lifter's weight is too far back during the pull—but the timing may differ and likely the feet will move from the floor sooner in this case. Additionally, there is usually a weak, unaggressive or improper elevation of the feet in the third pull that causes them to drag rather than separate cleanly from the platform.

Incomplete Leg Drive

In this case, at least part of the problem is that the lifter has not continued driving with the legs against the ground long enough in the pull—the drive has stopped prior to the hips finishing their extension, which removes the pressure of the feet against the ground that is holding them in place against the backward imbalance, allowing them to slide backward in a natural reaction to the body's sense that it is falling over. The solution, of course, is to ensure the athlete continues pushing against the ground all the way through the pull. Exercises to help with this include:

- Dip snatch/clean
- Snatch/clean from power position

- Snatch/clean pull + snatch/clean
- Snatch/clean high-pull + snatch/clean
- Hang snatch/clean
- Power snatch/clean
- Power snatch/clean + hang snatch/clean
- Power snatch/clean + snatch/clean
- Snatch/clean with no jump
- Snatch/clean with no jump + snatch/clean

Cues to help encourage adequate and complete leg drive during the snatch or clean include:

- Keep driving
- Drive all the way up
- Keep the pressure against the floor
- Push hard through the floor

Improper Foot Movement in Third Pull

Backward sweeping of the feet can also occur without any significant imbalance in the pull due simply to poor mechanics in the relocation of the feet itself. This is usually due to a lift of the feet rather than of the knees—that is, the lifter picks up the feet by bending the knees rather than by essentially performing a squatting motion with the knees and hips together. A rubber mat can also be placed on the platform behind the lifter's heels during snatches or cleans or any of the related drills being used to correct the problem in the same way it's used to help correct jumping forward.

Exercises to help practice moving the feet correctly include the following. All need to be performed with a focus on completely lifting the feet from the floor and replacing them flat and in the correct location.

- Tall snatch/clean
- Snatch balance
- Drop snatch
- Dip snatch/clean
- Snatch/clean from power position
- Snatch/clean with no jump
- Snatch/clean with no jump + snatch/clean

Cues to help with proper foot movement include:

- Land flat-footed

- Land on the heels
- Feet right under the bar
- Heels right under the bar
- Lift the knees

Premature Arm Bend

Ideally during the first and second pulls of the snatch and clean, the lifter's arms are passively extended. This allows the maximal transfer of force into the bar from the legs and hips. The more hip-dominant the lifting style, the less of a negative effect premature arm bend will have, but it does not improve the snatch or clean in any significant way other than possibly improving the location of the barbell's contact with the body, and excessive bending can create new problems. The Understanding the Snatch chapter of the book discusses this topic in detail. Reasons for premature arm bend can vary widely, and strategies to correct them vary accordingly. As will become evident below, many of these problems are causes and effects of each other.

Non-Specific Correction

We can attempt some non-specific corrections for premature arm bending if the cause is not clear. Essentially these will simply allow the athlete to focus on maintaining relaxed arms and moving through the correct positions with the correct timing. Generally it's best to reduce the movement as much as possible and start with a snatch or clean pull from the hang at knee level. Ensure correct posture and balance in the starting position, and begin with a slow extension, focusing on maintaining relaxed arms. Gradually increase the speed and aggressiveness. Once the hang pulls are correct at full speed, a complex of 1-3 hang pulls followed by 1 hang snatch or clean is a good next step. Once these hang snatches or cleans are being done consistently correctly, the process can be repeated from the floor. It's especially important once the lifter has moved to the floor that, at least initially, the first pull is kept to a low speed to ensure correct posture and balance, as these things can be the source of the problem.

Forward Imbalance in Pull

If the athlete's weight is too far forward over the feet during the first and second pull and the bar is consequently pulling him or her forward, a natural reaction is to row the bar back and up toward the body to correct the imbalance quickly. Similarly, if the athlete is too far forward, often because the hips have started or ended up too high relative to the shoulders, he or she will have to rush to get under the bar to restore balance, and this often manifests as an early scoop coupled with early arm bend. In such cases, correcting the imbalance will correct the early arm bending.

Exercises to work on this include:

- Snatch/clean deadlift
- Snatch/clean segment deadlift
- Snatch/clean pull
- Snatch/clean segment pull
- Snatch/clean deadlift + snatch/clean
- Snatch/clean segment deadlift + snatch/clean
- Snatch/clean pull + snatch/clean
- Snatch/clean segment pull + snatch/clean
- Segment snatch/clean (pause at knee and/or mid-thigh)
- Dip snatch/clean
- Snatch/clean from power position
- Dip snatch/clean + snatch/clean
- Snatch/clean from power position + snatch/clean

Cues that may prove helpful include:

- Chest up
- Stay back in the finish
- Straight up with the legs
- Stay back
- Shift back off the floor

Too Far Over The Bar

While the shoulders should be at least slightly in front of the bar as the lifter enters the second pull, being too far over the bar can create a number of problems, including forward imbalance, a premature second pull, a forward jump, and premature bending of the arms. This posture needs to be corrected both

in terms of technique, but also through ensuring the lifter is strong enough to maintain the correct position over the bar.

- Halting snatch/clean deadlift (mid-thigh)
- Segment deadlift/pull (pause at mid-thigh and/ or knee)
- Segment snatch/clean (pause at mid-thigh and/ or knee)
- Halting snatch/clean deadlift (mid-thigh) + snatch/clean
- Slow-pull snatch/clean

Cues to help prevent the lifter from allowing the shoulders to move too far in front of the bar include:

- Chest up
- Stay back
- Shoulders above the bar

Premature Second Pull

Initiating the second pull early will mean that the bar is relatively low on the thighs when the knees begin to move forward, creating interference for the barbell's path and pushing it forward. In reaction to this (usually unconscious), the lifter will often bend the arms to bring the bar higher toward the hip to avoid being pushed away by the forward-moving thighs. Exercises to correct this problem will focus both on maintaining the proper posture and balance upon entering the second pull, and the timing of its initiation.

- Halting snatch/clean deadlift (mid-thigh)
- Halting snatch/clean deadlift (mid-thigh) + snatch/clean
- Segment snatch/clean (mid-thigh)
- Slow-pull snatch/clean

Cues to help the athlete maintain the correct position and time the second pull properly include:

- Hit high (thigh)
- Stay over it
- Be patient
- Get it to high thigh before you explode
- Wait on it

Grip Too Narrow

The simplest possible cause for premature arm bending is too narrow of a grip on the bar. This causes the bar to be too low on the thighs as the second pull begins, creating the same kind of interference described in the previous error. This causes the lifter to naturally bend the arms to bring the bar higher toward the hips to avoid this problematic contact with the thighs.

The grip width should be corrected to allow optimal contact with the body (crease of the hip for the snatch and high thigh for the clean) if possible. In some cases, this will not be possible, however. For example, a lifter with very long arms and a short torso will be unable to achieve the perfect grip width, usually because the angle of the arms is so extreme that it causes problems with the structure of the overhead position and with the grip in the pull. The grip should be moved to as close to the optimal width as allowable and then the lift technique adjusted as well as possible to accommodate it.

In order to allow the bar to contact higher toward the hip without bending the elbows, the lifter can shrug the shoulders back and slightly up—this can move the bar a significant amount and will have less of a negative effect on the lift than bent elbows.

Lack Of Confidence

A lack of confidence with the lift will often cause the lifter to bend the arms early, either in an attempt to lift it higher or to pull under early—neither will work if the weight is significant. The confidence in the ability of the legs and hips to adequately accelerate and elevate the bar is something that often needs to be learned over time with more experience, but to encourage the athlete to keep the arms relaxed, he or she can be instructed to think of lifting the shoulders (or the body as a whole) instead of the bar itself. If the athlete is focused on elevating the bar directly, its height will often become a concern irrespective of the current position of the body. If instead the athlete focuses on lifting the body, the bar is more likely to remain in the correct relative position and be better accelerated.

Exercises to help correct the problem include:

- More snatch/clean volume at threshold of problem
- Snatch/clean waves: work up to weight where problem occurs, reduce weight, work back up slightly higher, repeat 2-3 times.
- High hang/block snatch/clean
- Dip snatch/clean
- 3-position snatch/clean working from top to bottom

Cues to help remind the lifter to trust the legs and hips include:

- Trust the legs
- Jump it up
- Forget the bar and lift the body

Grip Too Tight

Premature arm bending may be the result of an excessively tight grip on the bar, which will create excessive tension in the elbow flexors. Gripping the bar too tightly may be a simple mistake or the result of a weak grip or poorly executed hook grip. To correct a weak grip, direct grip strength work should be incorporated into the program, and the use of straps for the snatch reduced if not eliminated. Snatches and cleans without the hook grip can also be used periodically to further strengthen the grip.

Using straps, however, may help a lifter whose grip strength isn't a problem get the feel for using only the necessary tension rather than over-gripping. This doesn't mean that all snatching should be done with straps; they can be used in occasional snatch workouts, during warm-up lifts, or for snatches being used as a technique primer.

Under-Extension

New lifters will often cut the second pull short in a rush to get under the bar—the hips will not open fully and the shoulders will remain above or even slightly in front of the bar rather than finishing behind the hips and bar. This transforms the lift to something resembling an upright row with considerable space between the bar and the body.

Exercises to help correct this include:

- Snatch/clean deadlift to simulated finish position
- Snatch/clean deadlift to simulated finish position + snatch/clean
- Hang snatch/clean deadlift to simulated finish position + hang snatch/clean
- Hang snatch/clean (knee or above)
- Dip snatch/clean
- Snatch/clean from power position

Cues to encourage complete extension in the pull include:

- Shoulders behind the hips at the top
- Open up
- Hips through the bar

Misunderstanding Maintenance of Proximity

Arm bending may be the product of simply misunderstanding how the bar is to be kept close to the body. In this case, the athlete can practice bringing and keeping the bar in properly using the back and shoulders rather than rowing it with the arms. Exercises to help include:

- Everett snatch/clean pull
- Stiff-legged deadlift
- Romanian deadlift

Cues that may help include:

- Tight back, loose arms
- Let the weight stretch your arms long

Early Scoop

An early scoop can be a symptom of another problem, as seen previously, and can be a problem itself by reducing speed, power and bar elevation, and shifting the lifter's balance forward.

Improper Timing of Second Pull

The athlete may simply be initiating the final upward explosion too early due to improper instruction, impatience or lack of confidence. Exercises to help train and practice better timing include:

- Halting snatch/clean deadlift (mid-thigh)
- Halting snatch/clean deadlift (mid-thigh) + snatch/clean
- Segment snatch/clean (mid-thigh)
- Slow-pull snatch/clean

Cues to help the athlete improve the timing of the second pull include:

- Hit high (thigh)
- Stay over it
- Be patient
- Get it to high thigh before you explode
- Wait on it

Intentional Double Knee Bend

As was discussed in the Double Knee Bend chapter of the book, the phenomenon is a natural reaction to the proper timing, positions and actions of the snatch and clean pull. Performing it intentionally will nearly always cause the knees to move forward too soon, resulting in poor balance over the feet, reduced bar speed, and less power in the final extension. The lifter will need to be re-educated regarding the double knee bend and encouraged to focus on positions and timing surrounding the movement of the knees rather than that movement itself.

Exercises to help the athlete learn to allow the double knee bend to occur naturally and at the correct time include:
- Halting snatch/clean deadlift (mid-thigh)
- Halting snatch/clean deadlift (mid-thigh) + snatch/clean
- Segment snatch/clean (mid-thigh)
- Slow-pull snatch/clean
- Snatch/clean pull + snatch/clean
- Hang snatch/clean (knee; initiate with a push of the legs against the ground)

Forward Imbalance in Pull

Forward imbalance in the pull will usually force the lifter to initiate the second pull (and the scoop as a part of it) prematurely in order to rebalance the system before it exceeds the threshold of possible correction. This includes the shoulders being too far in front of the bar, a poor starting position, failing to shift the weight back in the initial pull from the floor, and any other error that results in a forward imbalance. See the exercises and cues under the Jumping Forward section.

Postural Weakness

Finally, a premature scoop may simply be the result of the lifter being physically incapable of maintaining the proper position over the bar to a high enough point. No amount of cuing or technique work will correct this, although it will be helpful in combination with exercises to improve the postural strength to stay over the bar long enough.

- Halting snatch/clean deadlift (mid-thigh)
- Snatch/clean segment pull/deadlift (pauses at knee and/or mid-thigh)
- Segment snatch/clean (pause at mid-thigh)
- Floating halting snatch/clean deadlift
- Stiff-legged deadlift
- Romanian deadlift
- Good morning

Slow Third Pull

The third pull of the snatch or clean can be slow for a number of reasons, some of which are not directly related to the third pull itself—any error that creates distance between the bar and the athlete will slow the third pull. See previous sections for corrections of such errors.

Improper Mechanics

Like with any other segment of the lift, optimal mechanics will allow maximal speed with any given magnitude of effort. Improperly performed movements will always be slower. The third pull is often neglected and taken for granted rather than recognized as a segment of the lift that requires just as much active engagement as any other.

Exercises that can help teach, reinforce and train the proper mechanics of the third pull, as discussed in detail in previous sections of the book, include the following. In order to be effective, of course, all must be performed properly to meet the criteria outlined for a correct third pull.

- Tall snatch/clean
- Muscle snatch/clean
- Snatch/clean long pull
- Snatch/clean high-pull
- Dip snatch/clean
- Snatch/clean high-pull + snatch/clean

Cues that can help remind the athlete how to properly perform the third pull include:

- Elbows high before you turn it over
- Pull the elbows up
- Elbows up and out
- Bar close on the pull under

Poor Timing

Proper timing of the third pull will maximize its effectiveness, but often lifters don't understand conceptually what should be occurring, and naturally believe the turnover should be completed when they hit the bottom of the squat, which is, in fact, too late. The turnover should be completed as quickly and at as high a level as possible—the level at which it's actually completed will be reduced as the weights increase, but the effort to complete it as soon as possible will still produce the desired effect. Teaching lifters that the completion of the turnover—locking the bar overhead in the snatch and fixing the final rack position in the clean—should coincide with the feet reconnecting with the floor is a simple way to encourage maximal speed and ideal timing.

- Tall snatch/clean
- Dip snatch/clean
- Snatch/clean from power position
- Power snatch/clean
- Power snatch/clean + snatch/clean (attempting to finish turnover at same time/height for each)
- Hang/block snatch/clean from above knee height
- 2 and 3-position snatch/clean (low to high)

Cues that can help encourage better timing in the third pull include:

- Lock it overhead at the same time your feet hit (snatch)
- Elbows up at the same time your feet hit (clean)
- Snap it overhead (snatch)
- Elbows up right away (clean)
- Turn it over as high as possible
- Rack it high (clean)

Lack of Aggression

As with any movement, a lack of aggression will result in a lack of speed. Lifters typically have no trouble understanding that the upward extension of the snatch and clean must be extremely aggressive, but it's less intuitively obvious that the movement under the bar must be equally aggressive.

The exercises and cues that will help improve aggression in the third pull are the same as listed above for improving timing.

Hitching

Hitching is the momentary pause or reversal of the bar's upward movement during the transition from first to second pull—that is, the bar is pulled up to the thighs, then stops or drops slightly, and is then reaccelerated upward. This is illegal in competition and is an ineffective approach to lifting a bar outside of it—it can be likened to driving at 40 mph and coming to a stop so you can accelerate to 60 mph.

Hitching can have a number of sources, and more often than not, is a result of a conceptual misunderstanding or a lack of confidence. The abrupt re-acceleration feels explosive, and consequently the lifter will often believe they are creating more bar speed and elevation than they would otherwise.

For all causes, re-educating the lifter regarding the positioning and timing of the first and second pull is helpful, and then practicing and training the pull with a focus on constant pressure against the floor and never allowing the bar to slow down will aid in reinforcing this. Initially, the first pull can be kept fairly slow to help the lifter feel the basic rhythm, and then the speed progressively increased as competence is demonstrated. Exercises that can help accomplish this include:

- Snatch/clean pull
- Snatch/clean pull + snatch/clean
- Slow-pull snatch/clean
- Snatch/clean deadlift + snatch/clean pull + snatch/clean

Cues to help remind the athlete to pull properly include:

- Constant pressure against the floor
- Keep it moving through the middle
- Keep pushing with the legs
- Don't let up with the legs
- Smooth through the middle

Locking Knees in First Pull

This is an uncommon problem, but one that does occur, and that can be unusually difficult to correct. The athlete's knees will actually extend completely (or nearly so) before the scoop, arresting the smooth continuation of the lift, tipping the lifter too far over the bar, and placing excessive strain on the lower back. This arises usually because of conceptual misunderstanding (e.g. the lifter believes the knees must be "pushed back" in the first pull, and is doing this excessively) or in reaction to continually hitting the knees with the bar.

Exercises that can help the lifter work on maintaining the proper posture and degree of knee flexion leading into the beginning of the second pull include:

- Snatch/clean deadlift to power position
- Floating halting snatch/clean deadlift (shin to mid-thigh)
- Snatch/clean deadlift to power position + snatch/clean
- Snatch/clean transition deadlift

Cues that may help the lifter avoid locking the knees include:

- Keep your chest up past the knees
- Keep pushing up with the legs

Bar Scraping Shins or Knees

While we always want to keep the bar as close to the body as possible throughout the lift, contact at the shins or knees that causes scraping or any noticeable collision is problematic and indicative of an error in the position or movement.

Shoulders Behind the Bar

If the shoulders are behind the bar rather than above or slightly in front of it, the bar will naturally want to swing back against the legs to center itself under the shoulder joint. This can occur at any point, including in the starting position. The solution, of course, is to correct the lifter's posture and movement in the pull. Exercises that will help include:

- Snatch/clean deadlift
- Floating snatch/clean deadlift
- Halting snatch/clean deadlift
- Snatch/clean segment deadlift (pause 1 inch off floor, knee, mid-thigh)
- Snatch/clean deadlift + snatch/clean
- Floating snatch/clean deadlift + snatch/clean
- Halting snatch/clean deadlift + snatch/clean
- Slow-pull snatch/clean
- Segment snatch/clean (pause 1 inch and knee)

Cues to help encourage the proper position include:

- Shoulders over the bar
- Stay over it
- Hips higher (if appropriate)

Pushing Bar Back Excessively

The bar may still scrape the shins and/or hit the knees when the shoulders are positioned correctly relative to it if the athlete is attempting to push the bar too far back in the effort to maintain proximity at a given point of the lift. The lifter simply needs to adjust this effort and practice the movement properly. The same exercises listed above for the previous cause can be used here. Cues will consist simply of reminders for the athlete to avoid pushing the bar back excessively.

Premature Second Pull

This is essentially the same as the first cause above—that is, the shoulders move behind the bar before they should. See the corrections for this in its own section above.

Under-Pulling

Under-pulling refers to a failure to adequately extend the legs or hips, or both, when completing the second pull. Aside from failing to sufficiently accelerate and elevate the bar, this will usually also result in a forward imbalance. The proper position in the finish of the second pull has been discussed in detail previously—this will be the goal for the lifter during the remediation process.

Although it should be clear by this point, it's worth reiterating here that extending completely in the second pull in no way means prolonging the extended position. Prolonged extension is itself an error, and is addressed in the next section.

Conceptual Misunderstanding

Occasionally under-pulling is simply the product of the athlete not knowing what they should be feeling in the final position. This is likely the cause if the problem occurs at all weights; if it only begins occurring at near-maximal weights, the next cause below is more likely.

The simplest way to allow the athlete to feel the proper extension position is to simulate it in a controlled fashion. With a barbell loaded just enough to provide the feel of some weight, the athlete will simply stand flat-footed with the legs straight and vertical, and, keeping the abs and glutes tight, open the hips to bring the shoulders slightly behind them. This will place the lifter in an approximation of the desired position with the exception of the absence of plantar flexion.

The lifter can repeatedly deadlift (from the floor or hang) into this position and hold for a few seconds. When they're consistently able to achieve the proper position and have a reliable sense of where they need to be, they can progress to a complex of this deadlift into the simulated finish position + a snatch or clean from the hang, aiming to finish the lift in the same extended position they practiced with the deadlift. This complex can contain 1-3 reps of the deadlift plus 1 rep of the snatch or clean, and can be done from the floor or hang. Performing it initially from the hang at knee height will usually produce better results.

Cues that may help the athlete extend properly include:

- Open up all the way
- Shoulders behind your hips at the top
- Hips through the bar

Lack of Confidence, Aggression or Strength & Power

A lifter may fail to extend completely in the snatch or clean because of a lack of aggression, a lack of confidence at a given weight and the consequent rush to move under the bar, or inadequate strength and power to achieve complete extension at a given weight. While these are all distinct causes, they're similar in nature and have similar approaches to correction.

Strength can be addressed with basic exercises like pull and deadlift variations emphasizing complete extension, stiff-legged deadlifts, and good mornings. Exercises to help with explosiveness, aggression and confidence in the finish of the lifts include:

- High-hang snatch/clean
- Block snatch/clean (mid-thigh)
- Dip snatch/clean
- Hip snatch
- Segment snatch/clean (mid-thigh)
- Power snatch/clean
- Hang power snatch/clean

Cues that will encourage the lifter to be aggressive in the extension include (aside from the obvious such as *aggressive* and *explosive*):

- Explosive finish
- Attack the finish

Prolonged Extension

As has been discussed throughout the book, hesitating in the extended position at the end of the second pull limits the opportunity for the athlete to pull under the bar and with significant loads will prevent successful lifts. Despite being broken into segments for the sake of teaching, the snatch and clean should be in practice single, continuous actions without hesitation at any point. Hesitation in the top of the pull can have a few different causes.

Over-Pulling

In this case, the lifter is attempting to continue elevating the bar beyond the point of maximal productive extension. In other words, the maximal acceleration has been achieved but the athlete is continuing to try to pull the bar up rather than moving under it. This can be a conceptual misunderstanding, a lack of confidence at a given weight, or simply poor timing.

Exercises to help improve all three of these issues include:

- Dip snatch/clean
- Snatch/clean from power position
- High-hang snatch/clean
- Block snatch/clean (mid-thigh)
- Power snatch/clean
- Dip snatch/clean + snatch/clean
- Snatch/clean from power position + snatch/clean
- High-hang snatch/clean + snatch/clean
- Power snatch/clean + snatch/clean

Cues to help encourage the lifter to transition under the bar more quickly and at the proper time include:

- Quick change of direction at the top
- Up and down right away
- Get under it right away
- Quick up-down

Delayed or Slow Third Pull

If the lifter fails to initiate the third pull with adequate aggression, it can significantly delay the transition at the top of the pull. Training the third pull directly to be stronger and more aggressive will be helpful in addition to working on the timing at the top of the pull. Exercises include:

- Muscle snatch/clean
- Snatch/clean long pull
- Tall snatch/clean
- Dip snatch/clean
- Snatch/clean from power position
- High-hang snatch/clean
- Block snatch/clean (mid-thigh)
- Power snatch/clean
- Dip snatch/clean + snatch/clean
- Snatch/clean from power position + snatch/clean
- High-hang snatch/clean + snatch/clean
- Power snatch/clean + snatch/clean

Cues that may help include:

- Pull the elbows up as hard as you can
- Elbows up and out right away

- Accelerate down right away
- Aggressive under the bar
- Aggressive turnover
- Lock it overhead/turn it over at the same time your feet hit

Bar Dragging or Early Second Pull

A premature second pull resulting in an early scoop and the bar dragging up the thighs can greatly slow the entire lift, but also cause the lifter to over-pull and delay the movement under the bar because of the lack of speed. There is also the absence of the abrupt contact of the bar with the hips or high thigh that normally causes a reflexive reaction to pull under the bar. See the corrections described previously in the Early Scoop section.

Excessive Lifting of Feet in Third Pull

While lifting of the feet during the third pull is the recommended technique for most lifters, it is possible for this elevation to become excessive or improper. If the athlete is lifting the feet higher than is necessary to achieve adequate speed under the bar and the bar tends to crash down onto the lifter overhead in the snatch or in the rack position in the clean, it can be considered a problem. If the foot elevation is significant, but there is no problem with crashing and instability, it's not a significant concern and can be moved toward the bottom of the priority list for technical corrections.

Occasionally this excessive lifting takes the form of what is often called *donkey kicking*—this is not just excessive elevation, but a backward kick of the feet rather than a vertical elevation. In such a case, the same corrective exercises will be helpful, but the athlete needs to focus on lifting the knees rather than the feet. In other words, the movement is identical to a squat, but with the knees being lifted toward the body rather than the body being lowered toward the feet. This will help keep the feet level and landing flat, and maintain their proper position under the bar and body.

Abbreviating the lifts to focus on the third pull or end of the second pull and third pull will allow the athlete to focus on the proper movement of the feet. These lifts can also be combined with the full lifts as complexes, or started as abbreviated lifts (e.g. high-hang) and gradually extended until back at the full lift—for example, beginning with a dip snatch, then moving to high-hang, mid-thigh, knee, below knee, and floor as the athlete improves satisfactorily at each stage.

- Tall snatch/clean
- Drop snatch

- Snatch balance
- Snatch/clean with no jump
- Dip snatch/clean
- High-hang snatch/clean
- 3-position snatch/clean (top to bottom)

Cues to help remind the athlete to move the feet properly include:

- Quick feet
- Get the feet back down right away
- Land on flat feet
- Knees up on the way down
- Plant the feet right under the bar

Snatch Errors

The following technical errors are specific to the snatch. Some corrections will refer back to information in the previous chapter, Universal Errors.

Press-out or Soft Overhead

Having a solid, aggressive lockout position overhead is one of the most critical skills for a lifter. Not only is a completely locked out overhead position required to meet the rules of competition, it's necessary for supporting maximal loads and lifting safely.

There are a few different possible manifestations of this problem. The lifter may receive the bar with the elbows slightly bent and then press into the locked position; the lifter may receive with straight elbows that then bend and possibly re-extend; or the lifter may never achieve a fully locked out position. While these are different from each other, they can be addressed in similar manners by finding the cause.

Improper Timing or Slow Turnover

Timing of the third pull is critical, and if a lifter's timing is off, the lockout will not occur properly. See the Slow Third Pull error in the Universal Errors chapter for more information on this. Exercises to help improve the timing and speed of the turnover in the snatch include:

- Tall snatch
- Muscle snatch
- Dip snatch
- High-hang snatch
- Drop snatch
- Snatch balance

- Snatch high-pull + hang snatch (knee or higher)

Cues to help the lifter focus on better speed and timing include:

- Punch it up right away
- Lock it out the same time your feet hit
- Turn and punch
- Stay aggressive in the turnover
- Elbows up hard before you turn it over

Weak or Unaggressive Overhead Position

In some cases, a lifter may have a lack of overhead strength relative to his or her pulling strength and skill; in other words, they can lift more overhead than they're capable of holding there. In these cases, obviously the solution is to increase the relative amount of overhead strength work in the training program until the disparity is corrected.

Exercises to improve overhead strength include:

- Overhead squat
- Snatch push press
- Snatch press
- Press in snatch
- Push jerk in snatch
- Heaving snatch balance
- Hold all snatches and related exercises for 3 seconds in the bottom position

Exercises that will improve aggressiveness in the overhead position include:

- Drop snatch
- Snatch balance
- Tall snatch

Cues to help the lifter improve the overhead position include:

- Squeeze the shoulder blades tight
- Upper back locked in
- Elbows locked
- Push up
- Reach
- Squeeze the elbows locked

Limited Mobility

Mobility limitations in both the upper and lower body will significantly detract from a lifter's ability to successfully and securely lock out snatches overhead. Where the relevant limitation exists is important to determine so that effective mobility work can be prescribed. Generally speaking, if the lifter can achieve a solid lockout position overhead when standing with a slight forward inclination of the trunk, but not when squatting, the lower body is at least the primary source of the problem. See the Mobility & Flexibility section of the book for details on mobility work.

Exercises that can help with mobility for the overhead position include:

- Clean-grip overhead squat
- Press in snatch
- Push jerk in snatch
- Press behind the neck
- Push press behind the neck

Excessive Grip Tightness

As was discussed with regard to the overhead position in an earlier chapter, gripping the bar too tightly will limit the speed of elbow extension, and can reduce how completely the elbows will extend. The lifter will need to focus on gripping the bar only as tightly as needed to maintain control once punching up against it. This can be practiced with any snatch overhead exercise or snatch variation, but in particular the following:

- Drop snatch
- Snatch balance

- Tall snatch
- Dip snatch
- High-hang snatch

Missing Behind

It's not uncommon to hear lifters and coaches refer to a miss behind as a "good miss", the assumption being that a miss behind is closer to a make than a miss in front. While in certain cases this is true, it is not true universally. More importantly, no miss is good, and diagnosis of the cause of the miss is important for correcting it effectively.

There are quite a few possible causes of missing snatches behind, only one of which could be considered having "too much" power or pull (and even this is not really an accurate description—there is no such thing as too strong, too explosive, or too high when it comes to the pull of the snatch, only failure to accurately receive and control the bar).

Excessive Grip Width

One of the simplest reasons for frequent misses behind in the snatch that is commonly overlooked is an excessively wide grip. The wider the grip, the more easily the bar can continue moving past the proper position and point at which the lifter can still control it. A simple illustration of this idea is the shoulder dislocate—the wider the grip, the easier it is to move the bar behind the head. The narrower the grip, the tighter the movement becomes, eventually reaching a point at which the lifter cannot move behind the head with any effort. In the same way, a wider grip in the snatch means that if the bar has backward momentum on it during the turnover, it will be much harder to stop it from continuing backward past the point of no return.

Obviously fixing this problem is not necessarily as easy as narrowing the grip—presumably the grip width was chosen for a reason. The wider the grip, the quicker and easier the turnover tends to be, and this is a tough thing to argue with, especially for a lifter who is accustomed to lifting this way. However, if the lifter is missing frequently enough, it should be an easier case to make for a narrower grip.

If the grip is excessively wide to account for the lifter's proportions (short torso and/or long arms) and bring the bar higher into the hip, this can also be accomplished through some elevation and retraction of the shoulder blades during the second pull, and waiting longer to initiate the second pull (that is, staying over the bar longer with the shoulders—waiting until the bar is higher on the thigh to initiate the final upward explosion).

Make grip width changes incrementally. Making a dramatic change is a good way to create new problems and possibly earn some new wrist and elbow pain.

If for some reason the grip absolutely can't be narrowed, emphasis on strengthening the overhead position and the ability to maintain the position of the bar in the slot needs to be made. Exercises to help this include:

- Snatch push press
- Snatch press
- Overhead squat
- Push jerk in snatch
- Press in snatch
- Heaving snatch balance
- Snatch balance
- Holding bottom position of snatch and overhead exercises for 2-5 seconds

Poor Overhead Position

Failure to secure the bar in a proper overhead position will allow easier movement of the bar out of position, and if there is any imbalance backward, the bar will more easily fall behind the lifter. The proper overhead position has been covered in detail in earlier chapters—this position should be re-instructed, practiced, and monitored.

If the position is improper because limited mobility is preventing achieving it, mobility improvement must be made a priority. Don't neglect the lower body—limited ankle and hip mobility can prevent proper overhead position in the bottom of the squat. In fact, this specifically can contribute to a tendency to miss snatches behind because this limit on lower body mobility will result in the lifter's trunk being in-

clined forward to a greater degree, bringing the arms back to a greater angle, which maintains balance of the system over the feet, but destroys its structural integrity.

Exercises to help reinforce the proper overhead position include:

- Snatch push press
- Pressing snatch balance
- Heaving snatch balance
- Overhead squat
- Press in snatch
- Push jerk in snatch

Cues to help encourage the lifter to achieve and maintain the proper overhead position in the snatch or any of the previous exercises include:

- Squeeze the top inside edges of the shoulder blades together
- Lock in the upper back
- Bar behind your neck
- Squeeze the elbows locked
- Punch up on it

Diving the Head & Chest in the Turnover

The turnover of the snatch needs to bring the lifter into the correct overhead position immediately in order to allow the lifter to secure the structure and stabilize the bar. For this to be possible, there needs to be adequate space and time—that is, the bar must be lifted high enough before the lifter moves under it. Very common as snatch weights increase is diminishing confidence and the consequent premature pull under the bar. Because it's early, there either isn't adequate time and space or the lifter believes there isn't, and in response he or she will tend to try to sneak under the bar by diving under it—ducking the head and chest forward and down to be shorter and squeeze under the low bar. This results in the same poor overhead structure discussed in the previous section in which the trunk is inclined forward and arms backward excessively.

The most important correction is focusing on proper timing—completing the upward extension prior to pulling under the bar, but never hesitating before changing directions or pulling too far. The lifter should also focus on squatting straight down under the bar just as he or she would in a snatch balance, maintaining the proper upright posture and sitting the hips down instead of back. Finally, the upper body mechanics of the third pull need to be correct—the elbows moving up and to the sides to maintain the proximity of the bar and body.

Exercises to help correct this problem include:

- Tall snatch
- Dip snatch
- Snatch from power position
- Muscle snatch
- Snatch high-pull + hang snatch
- Snatch balance
- Drop snatch
- Heaving snatch balance

Cues to help encourage the athlete to avoid diving include:

- Head up in the turnover
- Chest up in the turnover
- Squat straight under it
- Straight up, straight down
- Chest/head up

Swinging the Bar Forward

This error was discussed in the Universal Errors chapter under the Bumping or Swinging Bar Forward in Second Pull and Swinging Bar Forward in Third Pull sections. Swinging the bar forward will create a bar path that loops back toward the lifter with excessive horizontal momentum and makes it difficult for the lifter to secure it in the overhead position. Read more about this error and find corrective exercises and cues in the Universal Error chapter.

Lifting the Feet Prematurely

Releasing the pressure against the floor by lifting the feet or ceasing to drive with the legs too early can cause the lifter's body to move forward under the bar.

Even if the path of the bar is correct, the net effect is that the weight is too far behind the lifter's base to be supported overhead, resulting in dropping of the weight backward.

Exercises to help train better leg drive and better timing of the movement of the feet include:

- Snatch pull + snatch
- Hang snatch
- Dip snatch
- Snatch from power position
- Power snatch from power position
- Power snatch

Cues to help the athlete driving with the legs adequately include:

- Keep the pressure against the floor
- Push hard with the legs
- Keep pushing with the legs
- Get tall
- Finish up
- Drive up at the top
- Push all the way up
- Keep driving against the floor all the way up

Missing in Front

The overwhelming majority of unsuccessful snatch attempts will be missed in front of the lifter with numerous possible causes—assuming here the weight is not simply more than the athlete can snatch. When trying to diagnose the source of the problem, always start at the beginning and work forward. Use the Universal Errors chapter to help determine the source of the problem and find corrective strategies.

Dropping Bar During Recovery

One of the most frustrating ways to miss a snatch is during the recovery after a seemingly good lift. This can be caused by an unrecognized imbalance during the lift; that is, despite the lift looking good, the bar or lifter was actually out of balance either too subtly to be visible, or simply not visible because of the coach's vantage point (likely in front of the lifter).

Rushing to Recover

Often a rush to stand after receiving a snatch overhead will result in a miss, or a near miss with the lifter taking a few quick steps forward to get back under the bar. This can be due to the lifter not actually being as balanced as he or she initially appeared, but more often it's a loss of balance due to a failure to maintain the proper position and structure in the hurry to stand up.

The solution to this is simply to have the lifter hold each snatch in the bottom position for 3 seconds before standing. Not only will this prevent a rush to stand, it will improve strength, position and confidence in the receiving position, and act as a diagnostic tool to recognize imbalances or improper positioning that is not otherwise obvious.

Improper Squat Mechanics

An improper squatting movement in the recovery from the snatch will shift the lifter out of the ideal structure to maintain the bar overhead. Lifting of the hips without commensurate movement of the shoulders and bar will mean an excessive forward inclination of the trunk. This can result in either a forward imbalance which causes the lifter to drop the bar in front, or can cause the body to attempt to maintain balance through compensation, shifting the arms and bar farther back, and reducing the structural integrity of the system, leading either directly to a drop of the bar backward, or a series of adjustments to try to re-establish structure and balance that exceed the

ability of the lifter to maintain control.

The athlete should always stand from the snatch by pushing up against the bar and following it with the body; this will encourage the lifter to lead with the bar and the chest and maintain not only the upright posture necessary for a stable structure, but also will help maintain focus on stabilizing the bar overhead. Exercises to help train the proper recovery position include:

- Overhead squat (especially with a pause in the bottom)
- 1¼ Overhead squat
- Overhead squat with slow eccentric

If a lifter is consciously attempting to recover properly but is physical incapable, this indicates a strength imbalance between the legs and hips, just as was discussed with regard to squatting and pulling from the floor in general. If the knee extensors are weaker than the hip extensors, the body will naturally shift more of the load to the hips by bringing the knees into a more extended angle without moving the weight significantly—the same forward leaning posture described above. Exercises to improve leg strength in order to avoid this tipping include:

- Front squat
- Pause front squat
- Pause back squat

Cues to help the lifter recover properly include:

- Push up on the bar and follow it with your body
- Push up
- Push up on the bar
- Head up
- Chest up
- Lead with the bar

Clean Errors

The following technical errors are specific to the clean. Some corrections will refer back to information in the previous Universal Errors chapter.

Bar Crashing into Rack Position

A smooth delivery of the bar to the shoulders is critical for successful cleans—failure to meet the bar well results in the load crashing onto the athlete, dramatically increasing the difficulty of maintaining the proper structure of the torso to support the bar, as well as reducing the ability of the lifter to stand from the bottom of the squat. The difference between meeting the bar well and allowing it to crash is analogous to performing a front squat from a rack compared to having the bar dropped onto the shoulders halfway down in the squat. It should be obvious which will be easier to recover from.

Any crashing of the bar onto the shoulders is the result of the bar and body not being actively brought together, but there are a few possible causes for this.

Indiscriminate Movement Under Bar

As was described in the Clean section of the book, the turnover must involve not simply an indiscriminate movement down into a squat, but a precise pull to relocate the athlete in the receiving position, wherever the bar may be. If the bar has been pulled high, the athlete needs to move into a relatively high squat position to meet it, just as if the bar is elevated less, the athlete needs to move into a deeper squat position. Successful cleans require precision, not just a launch of the bar upward and a careless drop into a deep squat. Part of the turnover should be the active

attempt to push the shoulders up into the bar as the elbows move up into the rack position.

Exercises that will help improve the mechanics and accuracy of the turnover and teach the athlete to meet the bar properly at any height include:

- Rack delivery drill
- Muscle clean
- Clean long pull
- Tall clean
- Dip clean
- Clean from power position
- Power clean + hang clean

Cues to encourage the lifter to accurately turn the bar over and meet it include:

- Meet the bar
- Shoulders up into the bar
- Tight under the bar
- Rack it high and tight

Inactive, Unaggressive or Slow Turnover

This error was address in detail in the Slow Third Pull section of the Universal Errors chapter. Exercises to specifically increase the speed and aggressiveness of the clean turnover include:

- Tall clean
- Dip clean
- High-hang clean
- Power clean
- Power clean + hang clean

Cues to encourage a faster and more aggressive turnover include:

- Aggressive turnover
- Turn it over hard
- Rack it high and tight
- Rack it right away
- Rack it at the same time your feet hit

Improper Mechanics

If the movement of the third pull is incorrect, it will be inaccurate, poorly timed, and too slow, all of which can easily result in the bar crashing onto the shoulders. Most common is the failure to initially pull the elbows up and to the sides, and instead to pull them back and down. Exercises to improve the mechanics of the clean turnover include:

- Rack delivery drill
- Tall clean
- Muscle clean
- Clean high-pull
- Dip clean
- Clean high-pull + hang clean

Cues that can help remind the athlete how to properly perform the third pull include:

- Elbows high before you turn it over
- Pull the elbows up
- Elbows up and out
- Bar close on the pull under

Bar Swinging Forward

Again, this error has been addressed in the Universal Errors chapter, which can be referred to for more information. Exercises to help correct this problem in the clean include:

- Clean high-pull + clean
- Clean pull + clean
- Dip clean
- Clean from power position
- Hang clean (knee or higher)

Cues to help the athlete focus on keeping the bar from swinging away include:

- Keep it close
- Push the bar in
- Keep pushing it in
- Keep it against your body all the way up
- Elbows up and out
- Elbows high

Premature Grip Release

Loosening the grip on the bar too early during the turnover can cause the lifter to lose the tight connection with the bar that is necessary for a smooth delivery to the shoulders. A full grip on the bar ideally is maintained throughout the turnover; however, if immobility or proportions prevent achieving a clean rack position with a full grip, the grip should be released only after the elbows have moved forward of the bar and are moving up—at this point the bar should already be connecting with the shoulders.

Exercises to help the lifter practice the maintenance of the grip on the bar or the properly timed opening of the grip into the rack position include:

- Muscle clean
- Clean long pull
- Tall clean

Cues to encourage the lifter to maintain the grip or release it properly include:

- Keep your grip
- Keep your grip as long as you can
- Stay connected to the bar

Over-Pulling

This is really only an issue with light weights, such as during warm-ups and lighter technique work. With such light weights, athletes will often put an inappropriately large force into the pull—it requires less upward force to lift 40kg than 140kg to a given height, so a lifter pulling maximally on light weights will find the bar flying up and crashing down.

Irrespective of weight and the amount of force put into the pull, the movement should never change in its essence—really the only difference between

40kg and 140kg should be the height at which the bar is secured in the rack position during the squat under. With all cleans, athletes should practice turning over the bar as quickly as possible and racking it as high as possible as they squat down. This will ensure that no matter the height of the bar, its delivery to the shoulders will be smooth.

Back Collapsing In Receiving Position

With the receipt of heavy loads in the clean, athletes will often find their backs collapsing and rounding forward. If not leading to a missed lift, this will result in unnecessarily difficult recoveries and exposes the athlete to potential flexion injuries of the back. Any flexion of the upper back lengthens the moment arm between the bar and the hips (and the remaining vertebral joints) and consequently makes it even more difficult to maintain the proper upright posture.

There are three potential elements of this problem: technique, strength and activation, and often all three are present to some degree. Technique involves the movement and positions of the lifter during the clean; strength involves the ability of the athlete's trunk musculature to support the desired posture under the bar; and activation involves the athlete's proper application of that strength.

Inadequate Trunk Strength

Both back and abdominal strength is critical for maintaining a rigid and properly oriented trunk in the clean. Exercises to improve back strength for receiving the clean include the following. The first three address the entire back, while the remaining exercises will help primarily with the upper back.

- Stiff-legged deadlift
- Good morning
- Weighted back extension
- Clean-grip overhead squat
- Press in clean (Sots press)
- Pause front squat

- Clean rack support
- Press behind the neck
- Push press behind the neck
- Bent row (arching upper back forcefully)
- Upper back extensions

Exercises to improve abdominal strength are numerous, but those that will be particularly effective for receiving the clean include:

- Hanging leg raise
- Weighted sit-up
- Weighted plank
- Roman chair/GHB sit-up
- Weighted planks

Failure to Activate Trunk Musculature

Even if the strength of the trunk musculature is adequate as evidenced by performance in the above exercises, it will be of no use if this musculature is not properly activated in the clean. First, the trunk needs to be locked in tightly from the beginning of the lift—there will not be time to achieve tightness during the third pull if it doesn't already exist, although certainly the athlete can brace further for the expected receipt of the weight on the shoulders.

Additionally, the attempt to aggressively establish and maintain posture is critical. An effort to lift the chest and drive the shoulders up into the bar as it's received will help strengthen the receiving position; further, the effort to drive the shoulders and elbows up during the receipt and recovery will help maintain the extension of the upper back, which will help keep the entire system stronger and help the maintenance of the upright posture, which itself is preventative of forward collapse.

Inadequate Trunk Pressurization

The final strength and activation related element is inadequate or unmaintained pressurization of the trunk. If the lifter fails to draw in an adequate breath to pressurize the trunk and maintain its rigidity throughout the lift, the back will more easily collapse under the weight of the bar on the shoulders, particularly if it isn't received smoothly. If the lifter fails to actively maintain the pressurization during the receipt and recovery of the clean, the effect will be similar—a crashing bar can force air out of the lungs if the athlete isn't actively fighting to maintain proper pressurization.

Bar Crashing

The barbell crashing down onto the shoulders in the turnover of the clean will for obvious reasons make the maintenance of proper posture and back extension more difficult. See the Bar Crashing into Rack Position section above for more information and corrections.

Hyperkyphotic Thoracic Spine

Excessive rounding of the upper back (hyperkyphosis) or immobility in the thoracic spine that prevents the lifter from flatting the natural thoracic curve to create the desired position will make the forward rounding and collapse of the back more likely in the clean. This places the bar farther forward relative to the hip and the rest of the spine, meaning the body must resist more force at any given weight to avoid collapsing forward.

Thoracic mobility is critical for all aspects of weightlifting and should be a priority for all lifters. More information on flexibility and mobility can be found in the Mobility & Flexibility section of the book.

Exercises that can help improve thoracic mobility and extension strength include:

- Clean-grip overhead squat
- Press in clean (Sots press)
- Press behind the neck
- Push press behind the neck
- Upper back extension
- Bent row (arching the upper back forcefully)

Sitting Back in Squat

The proper movement of the squat has been discussed in detail in previous sections of the book,

an emphasis of which is sitting as directly down as possible rather than reaching the hips back. The hips moving back in the squat forces the trunk to lean forward farther to counterbalance, and any increase of the torso's forward inclination increases the moment on the hip and spine, increasing the difficulty of maintaining spinal extension and an upright posture.

Exercises to help the athlete practice sitting down properly in the squat when receiving cleans include:

- Front squat
- Tall clean
- Dip clean
- Clean from power position
- Hang clean (knee or higher)
- Front squat + clean (front squat, drop the bar to the floor, clean, return to rack)

Cues to help remind the athlete to sit properly into the squat include:

- Sit straight down
- Head and chest up in the turnover
- Chest up into the bar
- Drive the chest up into it

Bar Too Far Forward

The effect of the bar being too far forward in the turnover and rack position is identical to the previous problem—the trunk must incline forward, making it more difficult to maintain back extension and proper upright posture. See the Bumping or Swinging Bar Forward in Second pull and Swinging Bar Forward in Third Pull sections in the Universal Errors about the bar moving away in the second and third pulls for more information and corrections.

Reaching with the Chest

A common mistake in the third pull of the clean is for the lifter to reach the chest forward to meet the bar rather than keeping the bar closer to the body and then pulling it back to the shoulders during the turnover. Again, this has the same effect of the previous two errors—forcing the trunk to incline forward excessively.

Exercises to help the athlete practice a proper turnover that brings the bar back into the shoulders include:

- Rack delivery drill
- Muscle clean
- Tall clean
- Dip clean
- Clean from power position

Cues to help the lifter avoid this problem include:

- Bring the bar back to your shoulders
- Bar close in the turnover
- Head and chest up in the turnover

Feet Sweeping Backward

Sweeping the feet backward out from under the bar and the rest of the body has the same effect as the bar being forward—the lifter's base is behind the center of mass, and likely the posture is not properly upright. See the Feet Sweeping Backward section of the Universal Errors chapter for more information and corrections.

Slow or Incomplete Turnover

The clean is largely dependent on the power of the third pull—because the greater weight can be elevated only a limited distance, the speed of the athlete under the bar is critical. The importance of this speed is paralleled by the importance of the security of the bar's placement in the rack position and the posture in the receiving position—these elements are connected by the timing and precision of the elbows' turnover. The Slow Third Pull error is addressed in detail in the Universal Errors chapter.

An incomplete turnover may or may not be slow, but the end result is a poor rack position that fails to secure the bar adequately.

Over-Gripping the Bar

While maintaining a full grip on the bar throughout the turnover is ideal for lifters possessed of the proper proportions and mobility, this doesn't mean a tight grip in the final portion of the movement and rack position. Gripping the bar too tightly in the final portion of the turnover can slow the elbows down and prevent the arms from reaching the final position entirely.

Exercises that can help the athlete practice the proper grip on the bar include:

- Rack delivery drill
- Muscle clean
- Tall clean
- Dip clean
- Clean from power position
- Power clean

Limited Mobility

Limited shoulder, wrist and thoracic spine mobility can greatly slow down the turnover and make settling into the rack position difficult. Even if a lifter can establish the proper rack position in isolation and in a front squat, mobility may be a problem—any drag created by limited mobility will slow the movement. Stretching specifics are covered in the Mobility & Flexibility section of the book.

Failure to Commit

Like with all aspects of the snatch, clean and jerk, commitment to the lift is imperative to success. Commitment is predicated on confidence and aggression, and these things are best developed over time with experience and a large volume of successful lifts. The accumulation of successful lifts is the product of smart programming, training and technique development. If an athlete misses 50% of his or her cleans above 85% by failing to rack the bar, expecting commitment to the turnover may be unreasonable because he or she has trained to expect misses and the fear of injury during a miss will prevent the necessary commitment to the movement.

However, athletes should be expressly taught that the most dangerous way to miss a clean is to not turn it over completely. Receiving a clean with the elbows down and the bar not secured on the shoulders properly opens the lifter up to hand, wrist, elbow and shoulder injuries. An inability to stand from the bottom of the squat is unlikely to cause injury unless the lifter is significantly out of position. Because of this, all lifters should be encouraged to commit to racking their cleans completely no matter what.

Exercises to help the athlete train aggression in the turnover and confidence without requiring the heavier weights that are problematic include:

- Tall clean
- Dip clean
- Clean from power position
- High-hang clean
- Block clean (knee or higher)

Block cleans are particularly helpful in this case because the blocks will support the bar in the case of a miss, meaning that, at least in theory, the fear of missing is eliminated (the athlete may require some convincing on this point initially). This elimination of consequences will help the athlete commit to the lift.

Cues to help remind the athlete to finish the turnover include:

- Elbows up all the way
- Elbows high right away
- Quick turnover
- Elbows up at the same time your feet hit
- Turn it over all the way

Bar Bouncing or Slipping Out of Rack

Occasionally athletes will find the bar bouncing or slipping out of the rack upon receipt of the clean. Although the bar crashing down onto the shoulders can exacerbate the problem, the underlying cause is poor positioning or inadequate effort. If the position

of the torso, shoulders and elbows is correct and aggressively maintained, the rack will be able to withstand significant crashing.

The bar bouncing or slipping forward out of the rack indicates that the torso is leaning too far forward, the upper back is not extended adequately, the shoulders are not pushed forward or elevated enough, the bar is too far forward in the rack position (i.e. on top of the shoulders rather than behind their peak), the elbows are not high enough, the grip is too tight, the athlete is giving up on the lift, or a combination of these things.

This problem will be most prevalent in athletes possessed of poor mobility because of its limitations on proper positioning at the bottom of the clean—either the position is unattainable, or the lifter's lack of mobility slows the movement into position, resulting in a failure to complete the turnover into a maximally secure position on heavier lifts. It may also be due to an inability of the athlete to maintain upper back extension under the load, which was addressed in a previous section.

While we want to encourage an immediate recovery from the clean in order to harness the power of the bounce, in cases of severe and frequent inability to secure the bar in the rack position, a pause in the bottom of the clean can be used temporarily. This should be limited as much as possible and a normal lift rhythm returned to as soon as the problem is resolved sufficiently. Another option is to use a complex of 1 clean with a pause in the bottom followed by 1 clean with a normal recovery.

If the issue is one of mobility, stretching will be necessary to improve the athlete's receiving position. See the Mobility & Flexibility section of the book for more information.

If instead the problem is technical, solutions can be found above in the Slow or Incomplete Turnover, Bar Crashing into Rack Position, or Back Collapsing in Receiving Position sections.

Failure to Recover

In the crowd at a world championships years ago, a coach leaned over and asked a former world-champion weightlifter why the lifter on the platform had just failed to succeed with his clean, presumably expecting a complex technical response. Instead, the lifter shrugged and said, "It was too heavy."

In the sport of weightlifting, sometimes the weight is just too heavy for the lifter, particularly in the clean. Of course, this should be re-framed in a way that helps us solve the problem: the lifter is not strong enough.

It isn't uncommon for a lifter to be capable of pulling and racking more weight than he or she is able to stand up with in the clean. No lifter will be perfectly balanced in the various physical abilities relevant to weightlifting, although the goal is always to bring up the weaknesses to the level of the strengths as much as possible. If a lifter is cleaning 95% of his or her best front squat, for example, that lifter is very technically sound, explosive and aggressive—but also has essentially no strength reserve. In such cases, an emphasis on improving squat strength is at least part of the solution to failed cleans.

That being said, there are also a few technical reasons for a failure to recover from a clean.

Imbalance

Possibly the most common reason for an athlete failing to recover from a clean is an imbalance in the receiving position—the body and bar not being adequately balanced over the lifter's feet. This prevents the optimal rhythm of the lift and shifts the body out of its strongest posture, and as a consequence, greatly increases the difficulty of standing from the squat.

See the Universal Errors chapter for information regarding diagnosis and correction of imbalances in the clean and snatch.

Receiving the Bar Too Low

Even the heaviest of cleans will be received at some height above the absolute bottom of a clean. In fact, most lifters are surprised when shown slow motion videos of their own cleans at how high they are when the bar first meets their shoulders. However, a slow turnover, poor timing, or a lack of aggression can result in a clean not being racked until the lifter is in or nearly in the bottom of the squat. This robs

the movement nearly entirely of the loaded eccentric movement that allows for a stretch reflex and the consequently more forceful concentric recovery. In other words, it turns what should feel more like a front squat into a pause front squat—and even worse, a pause front squat in which a bar was dropped roughly onto the lifter's shoulders.

In all cleans, regardless of weight, the lifter should attempt to turn the bar over and secure it in the rack position as soon as possible and in as high of a squat as possible. Even in the heaviest of cleans, this will usually be no lower than around parallel squat depth, even if it doesn't feel like it to the lifter and can't be seen in real time.

See the Slow Third Pull section in the Universal Errors chapter and the Slow or Incomplete Turnover section above for information and corrections for this problem.

Failure to Remain Rigid

The rigidity of the trunk in the receipt of the clean through pressurization and aggressive muscular activation is critical for success. Collapse of the trunk under the weight of the bar creates numerous problems that will limit the lifter's ability to recover, such as shifting the center of mass forward, preventing a maximal stretch reflex in the squat, and absorbing some of the legs' upward force in the attempt to stand.

See the Back Collapsing in Receiving Position section above for more information and corrections.

Improper Squat Mechanics

Security of the barbell in the rack position, and consequently, the lifter's ability to stand from the clean successfully relies heavily on the upright posture of the front squat. If this upright posture is lost during the recovery from the clean, the likelihood of success is significantly reduced. Excessive lifting of the hips without commensurate movement of the shoulders and bar will mean an excessive forward inclination of the trunk.

The athlete should always stand from the clean by driving the shoulders up against the bar, and reaching the elbows and head up; this will not only help maintain the upright posture necessary for a stable structure, but also will help maintain focus on keeping the bar securely racked. Exercises to help train the proper recovery movement include:

- Front squat
- Pause front squat
- 1¼ front squat
- Front squat with slow eccentric (forcing upright posture)

If a lifter is consciously attempting to recover properly but is physical incapable, this indicates a strength imbalance between the legs and hips, just as was discussed with regard to squatting and pulling from the floor in general. If the knee extensors are weaker than the hip extensors, the body will naturally shift more of the load to the hips by bringing the knees into a more extended angle without moving the weight significantly—the same forward leaning posture described above. Exercises to improve leg strength in order to avoid this tipping include:

- Front squat
- Pause back squat
- Pause front squat
- 1¼ front squat

Cues to help the lifter recover properly include:

- Shoulders up into the bar
- Head up
- Chest up
- Elbows up
- Drive up on the bar right away
- Hips in
- Lead with the elbows
- Shoulders and elbows up first

Poor Timing

Recovery from the clean is largely dependent on proper timing in order to take advantage of the stretch reflex in the squat. A failure to immediately and aggressively drive out of the bottom of the squat will prevent the lifter from exploiting the additional speed and force produced by a proper bounce, which, at heavier weights, can result in a complete failure to recover.

Exercises to help improve the timing in the clean recovery include (all focusing on the bounce and speed in the recovery):

- Front squat
- High-hang clean
- Block clean (mid-thigh or higher)
- Clean-jerk
- Front squat - jerk

Dizziness During Recovery

Dizziness or lightheadedness during the recovery of the clean can result from pressure from the bar occluding the carotid arteries, vagal stimulation from the combination of holding the breath and exerting forcefully, decreased cardiac output due to the intraabdominal pressure, or a combination of these elements. These things are discussed in detail in the Breathing & Trunk Rigidity chapter.

To avoid carotid artery compression, the clean rack position needs to include a degree of shoulder elevation, and may require additionally that the lifter pull the head back somewhat. Details of the proper rack position are discussed in the Clean section of the book.

A partial release of air during the recovery of the clean can help avoid dizziness from vagal stimulation and reduced cardiac output. This is also discussed in detail in the Breathing chapter.

Athletes should immediately bail out of a lift if dizziness or tunnel vision begins—blacking out under a clean, or any lift, is dangerous and the likelihood of reversing the process enough to complete the lift successfully is extremely small and not worth the risk.

Jerk Errors

The following technical errors are specific to the jerk. While there are a few problems and solutions similar to others for the snatch and clean, most are unique to this lift.

Poor Lockout or Pressout

As was discussed in regard to the snatch, a solid, aggressive lockout position overhead is one of the most important abilities a lifter can possess. A complete lockout is required to meet competition rules and maximizes the ability of the lifter to effectively support heavy loads overhead.

There are a few different possible variations of this problem. The lifter may receive the bar with the elbows slightly bent and then press into the locked position; the lifter may receive with straight elbows that then bend and possibly re-extend; or the lifter may never achieve a fully locked out position.

Improper Overhead Position

The first consideration when encountering a poor overhead lockout in the jerk is whether or not the overhead position is correct. If the athlete is not achieving the correct position, the structure will not be optimal to support the bar overhead, and the ability to lock out will be compromised. The overhead position is discussed in detail in the Jerk section of the book.

Exercises that will help teach and reinforce the proper jerk overhead position include:

- Press behind the neck
- Press behind the neck in split
- Push press behind the neck
- Push jerk behind the neck in split
- Power jerk behind the neck
- Split jerk behind the neck

Immobility

If athletes' overhead mobility is limited, they may either be unable to achieve a full lockout position overhead, or if they are capable of doing so, the additional "drag" on the system will often prevent them from achieving it quickly enough in heavier jerks, resulting in pressouts or re-bending.

Obviously the primary intervention in this case is to improve mobility as much and as quickly as possible. If the problem is severe enough and a temporary solution is needed to get by, widening the grip will reduce the demand on overhead mobility. Widening should be approached incrementally to find what works best, as extremely wide grips bring their own problems with them.

Exercises that will help as a part of the mobility work include:

- Press behind the neck
- Push press behind the neck
- Clean-grip overhead squat
- Push jerk behind the neck in split
- Press behind the neck in split

Poor Timing or Lack of Aggression

Like with all aspects of the jerk, timing and aggression are critical elements of a successful lockout overhead. While in fact the feet will reconnect with the floor before the elbows finish extending (just as with the snatch), in real-time, it should appear that these two things occur simultaneously, and the attempt by the lifter to lock out the bar overhead at the same time the feet hit the floor will encourage more speed and aggression. It's also necessary that the lifter not tighten the split position when the feet hit, but when the elbows lock to prevent stopping short before reaching adequate split depth.

Exercises that will help the athlete improve speed and timing of the overhead lockout include:

- Tall jerk
- Pause jerk
- Power jerk

Cues that will encourage better timing and speed in the lockout include:

- Lock the elbows at the same time the feet hit
- Punch
- Punch through the bar
- Quick elbows
- Quick hands
- Hands and feet together

Excessive Grip Tightness

As was discussed with regard to the snatch, an excessively tight grip on the bar in the jerk can slow and limit the extension of the elbows. A tight grip during the dip and drive can slow the bar down as it leaves the shoulders, and a tight grip during the drive under the bar can reduce the ability of the elbows to forcefully and rapidly extend.

During the dip and drive, a full grip on the bar is not problematic as long as the grip is no tighter than it needs to be. Likewise, the grip on the bar should remain as loose as possible as the lifter pushes under and only as tight as needed to maintain control of the bar and the position of the hand and wrist overhead.

Fear of Hyperextension

Some athletes, in particular those who have had previous elbow injuries, simply have a fear, conscious or not, of completely extending or hyperextending the elbows. The elbows should be kept strong with regular overhead strength work, primarily during preparatory mesocycles, and especially early in a new lifter's career, and elbow extension strength balanced as needed with elbow flexion work such as rowing movements, pull-up variations, and even curls. This work will improve the arms' strength and stability in the overhead position, reduce joint pain, and improve confidence, as will more and more training experience with the jerk.

Exercises that will help strengthen the arms overhead and improve confidence include:

- Jerk support
- Jerk recovery
- Push press
- Holding all jerks overhead for 3 seconds

Stiff Back Leg

A final possibility is a stiff back leg in the split position. As was discussed in the Jerk section of the book, if the back knee is locked or very stiff, it can push the athlete forward rather than allow him or her to move down under the bar to achieve the depth and position necessary for a solid lockout.

Exercises to help practice and strengthen a proper split position and a soft back knee include:

- Push jerk in split
- Push jerk in split behind the neck
- Press in split
- Jump to split
- Drop to split

Forward Imbalance

Easily the most common general error in the jerk is a forward imbalance. This is not surprising considering that essentially everything about the jerk creates a tendency for both the bar and lifter to shift forward if not carefully controlled. Following are the most likely underlying causes. Note that this is limited to actual forward movement of the bar and body; errors that create a similar result but involve the lifter moving backward are addressed in the next section.

Non-Specific Correction

Like with jumping forward in the snatch or clean, a non-specific correction may be effective for forward imbalance in the jerk if the cause cannot be diagnosed, or the imbalance is the product of more than one problem. The coach can stand with a vertical PVC pipe or forearm 1-3 inches in front of the sleeve of the barbell or the front edge of the plates to give the lifter an obstacle to avoid. The actual proximity is less important than the pipe or arm's presence—if either is in front of the end of the bar, the lifter can't see it anyway. The knowledge that it is there is usually adequate for the lifter to make the necessary corrections. The coach should immediately remove the PVC or arm once the jerk is overhead to prevent the bar from coming down onto either.

Dipping Forward

The dip and drive of the jerk feels awkward to most athletes new to weightlifting, as it is entirely dependent on the knees and excludes the hips. For some, this problem will be the result of simply being unfamiliar with such a position and knee-dominant movement; for others, there will be an actual strength limitation in the quads that prevents the movement from being possible with heavier weights. This results in the lifter either hinging forward at the hip along with the knee bend and/or shifting the weight too far forward over the foot.

Exercises that will help train the proper balance and movement in the dip include:

- Jerk dip squat
- Jerk dip
- Jerk drive
- Pause jerk
- Jerk dip squat + jerk
- Push press + jerk
- Power jerk + jerk

Exercises that will help strengthen the lifter to be more capable of the proper movement and posture include:

- Front squat
- Jerk dip squat (also with a pause in the bottom)

A forward dip may also be the result, at least in part, of the lifter's knees diving inward, which weakens the position and causes a forward shift of the weight over the feet. The knees should be actively pushed out to move in line with the feet, and creating tension in the quads and glutes prior to the initiation of the dip will help. Additionally, widening the drive stance may strengthen this position for such lifters.

Exercises that can help resolve the problem of the knees diving inward include (all performed with an effort to maintain the knees' alignment with the feet at all times):

- Jerk dip squat
- Push press
- Front squat

Cues that will help encourage the lifter to execute the dip in the proper position and balance include:

- Stay back
- Heels
- Keep your chest back
- Knees only
- Glutes and abs tight

Driving Forward

Even if the dip has been performed properly—that is, the balance and position in the bottom are correct—the athlete may shift forward in the drive. Often this is connected to the lifter being focused on the split movement, which then carries him or her forward prematurely. Other times, it is simply because most athletes will feel more powerful on the balls of the feet than on the heels. Like in the dip section above, this can be a technical or strength problem.

Exercises to help reinforce the proper position and balance in the drive include:

- Jerk drive
- Push press
- Power jerk

- Jerk drive + jerk
- Power jerk + jerk
- Push press + jerk

Cues to encourage the lifter to maintain the proper balance in the drive of the jerk include:

- Stay back
- Heels
- Keep your chest back
- Drive it back
- Get it back
- Behind your head

Pushing Bar Forward with the Arms

A proper dip and drive may still be coupled with a forward push of the bar with the arms. That is, the lifter has maintained the proper balance through the leg drive, but subsequently has failed to move the bar and body properly into the receiving position, resulting in the bar moving forward. This can be because of a misunderstanding of the proper upper body mechanics of this movement, which are described in detail in the jerk section of the book; a failure to be active and aggressive enough in executing this movement; or a lack of confidence that creates a fear of getting all the way under the bar.

Exercises to work on the proper upper body movement include:

- Press
- Push press
- Push press + jerk
- Power jerk + jerk
- Jerk behind the neck + jerk

Exercises to help with the lifter's confidence in the split position include:

- Jerk behind the neck
- Jump to split
- Drop to split
- Jerk recovery
- Jerk support
- Push jerk behind the neck in split
- Jerk balance

Cues to help the lifter push under the bar correctly include:

- Drive it back
- Get it back
- Behind your head
- Spread the elbows
- Push back right away

Short Split or Lifter Moving Backward

A short split position can be the result of failing to move the front foot far enough forward directly, or of the lifter moving backward out from under the bar. Possible causes and corrections for each follow.

Short-Stepping

If the athlete is performing the rest of the jerk correctly but failing to step the front foot forward adequately, it may simply be the result of a lack of effort or a misunderstanding of where the foot should be placed. Re-education regarding the proper split position is the first step, followed by encouraging the athlete to lift and reach the front foot more, and possibly to have more weight on the rear foot.

Drills to help work this foot movement include:

- Drop to split
- Jump to split
- Tall jerk
- Jerk balance

Cues to help encourage better front foot movement include:

- Step out
- Reach the front foot
- Kick the front foot

A more aggressive approach to forcing more aggressive elevation and reach of the front foot is to provide either an obstacle or a platform for the front foot while performing jerks or jerk-related exercises (not with considerably heavy jerks). An obstacle can be something like a small rolled or folded towel placed on the platform in front of the lead foot—something the athlete will have to lift the foot up and over, but won't result in disastrous consequences if the foot movement is inadequate. In other words, the lower, flatter and more stable the object, the better.

The platform approach is similar, but arguably safer. In this case, rather than having an obstacle to lift the foot above and then in front of, there is platform for the athlete to lift the foot up onto. A good option for this is a scrap of rubber matting. This can be as thin as half an inch, or multiple pieces can be stacked to increase the height; it can be as large as needed for more area for the foot to safely land; it is perfectly flat and stable; and it will not slide on the platform.

It should be kept in mind that using an obstacle or platform to train this footwork does carry risk with it, and it should be done judiciously.

Inadequate or Incomplete Leg Drive

In some cases, what appears to be a failure of the athlete to adequately lift and reach the front foot is actually the result of a failure to adequately accelerate and elevate the bar in the drive. Without sufficient upward drive on the bar, the lifter won't have the time or space to move the feet into the necessary split. This can be an inability to drive the weight adequately, a technical error of timing on the drive itself, or a premature movement of the feet into the split that causes a premature cessation of the upward drive.

Exercises to help improve the drive include:

- Power jerk
- Power jerk + jerk
- Push press
- Push press + jerk
- Jerk drive
- Back squat jump
- Jumping squat
- Quarter squat jump

Cues to encourage better leg drive include:

- Finish the drive
- Drive high
- Drive all the way up
- Drive high before you split
- Drive through it

Overreaching the Back Foot

A very common cause of a failure to step forward adequately, and for the lifter as a whole to move backward out from under the bar, is overreaching the back foot in the split. This excessive reach with the back foot will pull the hips backward and out of place under the bar, and prevent the front foot from moving forward adequately, as the rear foot will be the first to move after the drive. Lifters attempting to split longer will often mistakenly overemphasize the movement of the back foot and create this problem. This can be because of a misunderstanding of the split position or the movement into the split position. The lifter should be re-educated, and the position and movement drilled and strengthened.

Exercises that will help the lifter practice the proper split position and movement into it include:

- Jerk balance
- Tall jerk
- Push jerk behind the neck in split
- Split jerk behind the neck
- Drop to split
- Jump to split

Cues to encourage the lifter to move into the split without overreaching the rear foot include:

- Hips under the bar
- Back foot down, front foot forward
- Lift and reach the front foot
- Step forward
- Step through it
- Head and chest up in the split
- Back foot close to the floor

Diving the Head & Chest

Similar in effect to over-reaching the back leg, and usually connected, although each of the two can trade the cause and effect roles, is diving the head and chest forward under the bar. In other words, rather than splitting the legs and maintaining an upright position of the trunk, the lifter leans the trunk forward as part of the effort to move into the split. In reaction to the chest moving forward, the hips naturally move backward, shifting the entire base back rather than it remaining under the bar. In addition, this action will usually cause the front foot to reconnect with the platform early and before the back foot, pushing the hips and rear foot backward even more and exacerbating the problem.

Exercises to help the athlete train the proper upright posture in the split, strengthen the position, and reinforce the movement include:

- Push jerk behind the neck in split
- Jerk balance
- Tall jerk
- Drop to split
- Jump to split
- Step to split
- Walk to split

Cues to encourage the proper upright posture in the split include:

- Chest/head up in the split
- Chest/head up
- Hips right under the bar
- Vertical trunk
- Straight up, straight down
- Keep your chest back

Weak Split Position

A final consideration is inadequate strength and stability in a relatively deep split position, which can exist even in strong squatters. The ability to drive under a heavy jerk is predicated on the knowledge, both conscious and unconscious, that the athlete will be able to safely support the weight in the receiving position. Because the body will naturally avoid putting itself in a position it can't safely support, this will commonly prevent the lifter from splitting adequately.

Exercises to strengthen the position include:

- Lunge
- Walk to split
- Step to split
- Split squat
- Drop to split
- Jump to split
- Push jerk behind the neck in split

Inability to Brake in Dip

Much of the ability of the lifter to elevate and accelerate the bar in the jerk is dependent on the ability to abruptly brake the downward movement of the dip to maximize the use of elastic energy of both the barbell and body. This error will often appear as the lifter "bogging down" in the dip—a slow, sluggish change of direction, often accompanied with a forward shift in balance.

Some lifters will always naturally have a greater physical ability in this respect than others, but it can be improved in any athlete through training. The most important improvement to focus on is building a greater base of squat strength. Additional exercises to improve both strength to support the dip and the ability to brake and change direction include:

- Jerk dips
- Jerk dip squats
- Depth drops/jumps
- Quarter squat jumps

Back & Shoulders Collapsing in Dip

With the barbell on the shoulders in front of the neck as it is for the jerk, there is a tendency for the shoulders to drop and the upper back to round forward under the weight, particularly in the bottom of the dip when the athlete is braking and the downward force is much greater than the actual weight on the bar. Several factors increase the likelihood of the shoulders or upper back collapsing.

Poor Rack Position

The farther forward the bar is in the rack position, the longer the moment arm on the spine and hip, and consequently the greater the tendency for the shoulders and upper back to collapse. For this reason, the athlete should be sure to place the bar as far back toward the throat as possible and securely behind the peak of the shoulders, and support it directly with the trunk rather than with the arms.

A full grip on the bar rather than a rack position with just the fingers under the bar can help as well if adequate mobility exists. A full grip largely fixes the angle of the upper arm relative to the upper back; further effort to raise the elbows in the rack position will, rather than flexing the shoulder further and increasing that angle, cause the upper back to extend, securing its position further. The details of a proper rack position were discussed in the Jerk section of the book.

Weak or Immobile Upper Back

If an athlete's upper back is weak, or if immobility prevents it from being extended adequately, there will be a greater tendency for it to round forward under the force of the bar at the bottom of the dip. Mobility can be improved in ways addressed in the Mobility & Flexibility section of the book.

Exercises that can help with upper back strength and posture include:

- Clean-grip overhead squat
- Upper back extensions
- Jerk rack support
- Jerk dip
- Jerk dip squat

Tight Grip or Early Arms

Occasionally an athlete will begin with a solid rack position, but as he or she is dipping, drop the elbows, allow the shoulders to slide back and grip the bar tightly in premature preparation for driving the bar with the arms. This will cause the bar to slide forward and down, pulling the lifter forward and usually softening the upper back.

The lifter needs to maintain the jerk rack position for the duration of the dip and drive, and only bring the arms into play as the bar reaches maximum upward speed. This is often best encouraged by intentionally keeping the grip relaxed during the dip and drive and consciously pushing the shoulders up against the bar—not excessively elevating the shoulder blades, but thinking of supporting the bar by pushing the shoulders and trunk up into it.

Cues that may help the athlete perform this part of the lift properly include:

- Grip loose
- Keep your hands loose
- Shoulders up against the bar
- Patient arms
- Let the bar settle on your shoulders

Inadequate Trunk Rigidity

Another common cause of the upper back or shoulders collapsing forward is inadequate trunk rigidity due to inadequate pressurization. Again, the bar's placement forward of the spine creates a moment on the joints and a tendency to drop forward. As was discussed in detail in the Breathing & Trunk Rigidity section of the book, in order to create maximal rigidity of the trunk, it must be pressurized with air and all musculature around its circumference activated tightly. If the lifter fails to create or to maintain rigidity, the trunk is likely to collapse under the maximal downward force of the bar at the bottom of the dip.

The final pressurizing breath should be taken and held for a moment before the initiation of the dip to ensure the body has settled and is stable—often athletes will attempt to inhale as they dip, which produces very inconsistent results, and will often shift the lifter's weight forward over the feet.

Excessive Dip Speed

All things being equal, a faster dip will produce a better jerk by allowing the generation of greater elastic rebound. However, athletes differ in their braking strength in the bottom of the dip and the speed can exceed an athlete's ability to stop it abruptly and resist the force adequately while maintaining the correct posture and rigidity. Accordingly, dip speeds need to be adjusted to best suit each athlete's present braking ability.

The dip should also be initiated at a controlled enough speed to prevent any separation between the bar and the body. This control of dip initiation speed can be improved by tightening the quads and making sure the knees are not hyperextended prior to initiating the movement.

Exercises to both practice proper dip speed and improve the athlete's braking ability and elasticity in the dip include:

- Jerk dip
- Jerk drive
- Rebound jerk
- Power jerk
- Push press
- Jerk behind the neck

Narrow Split Stance

One of the primary advantages of the split receiving position for the jerk is the stability it provides in all directions. This stability can be reduced considerably, however, if the feet are too narrow—ideally the feet are approximately as wide as they would be in the squat stance or slightly wider. In any case of narrow foot placement, the athlete can be cued to drive the feet out from the center of the body as well as forward and backward. In particular, the athlete can push the back heel out at an angle, which will both keep the split stance wide enough and help align the back foot with the leg correctly.

Excessive Drive Stance Width

If an athlete has a particularly wide drive stance, it can occasionally result in a narrower split position. If this wide stance was not chosen intentionally to address another issue and is not considered necessary, the stance should be narrowed. If the wider stance is

being employed for good reason, other corrections will need to be made.

Excessive Split Length

Possibly the most common reason for a narrow split stance is the athlete's attempt to reach into an excessively long split. The farther forward and backward the feet reach, the narrower the stance must be to accommodate the distance until reaching hip width. The basic correction is more repetition with a shorter split to get the lifter accustomed to a default length and width.

Exercises to help reinforce and strengthen a more appropriate split length include:

- Push jerk behind the neck in split
- Jerk balance
- Drop to split
- Jump to split
- Walk to split
- Step to split

Cues that may help the lifter split at a better length include:

- Quick feet
- Tight split

Unfamiliarity, Weakness or Discomfort in Proper Split

A lifter may simply be unfamiliar with the proper split position, in which case re-education and practice is in order. Otherwise, it may be that the lifter is weak in the proper position, or has discomfort of some type in the proper position.

Exercises to help teach, practice and strengthen the proper split position include:

- Press in split
- Press behind the neck in split
- Push jerk in split
- Push jerk behind the neck in split
- Jerk balance

- Drop to split
- Jump to split
- Lunge
- Walk to split
- Step to split

Cues that may help the lifter achieve a wider split stance include:

- Push the back heel out
- Split out
- Split wide

Stepping Across

Finally, lifters will occasionally step the front foot across the midline toward the side of the rear leg. This not only produces a problematically narrow split stance, but creates additional imbalance or exacerbates the imbalance that caused the step in the first place. Most likely the source of the problem is a combination of being slightly out of balance to one side prior to initiating the dip—due to an off-center bar placement in the rack position, pain, injury or weakness on one side, or a particularly great strength imbalance—with a failure to establish and maintain adequate tightness in the dip and drive. Work related to creating and maintaining maximal trunk rigidity should be performed, and the lifter encouraged to take more time setting up for the jerk to establish that rigidity and balance between the two legs.

Separation of Bar From Shoulders in Dip

Separation between the bar and the shoulders during the dip of the jerk can make braking in the bottom of the dip and changing direction more difficult, disrupt the optimal rhythm of the dip and drive for exploiting elasticity to improve acceleration and elevation of the bar, and shift the lifter out of balance. Maintaining a tight and constant connection between the bar and lifter throughout the dip and drive will maximize the effectiveness of the upward lift of the bar. In general, this separation is caused by the lifter initiating the dip too abruptly. This is not an issue of the speed of the dip as a whole, but of the initial downward acceleration.

To avoid dropping out from under the bar, the lifter primarily needs to establish tension in the quads prior to initiating the jerk. Occasionally the athlete will be supporting the weight with a passive knee lock (in the same way that we naturally stand—relying on slight hyperextension of the joint to support most of the weight rather than significant muscular work).

Beginning the dip of the jerk from a passive knee lock will create slack in the system, leading to a brief moment of unsupported dropping as the dip is initiated before the quads tighten enough to catch up. By ensuring quad tension prior to unlocking the knees, the transition to movement will be much smoother and more controlled. Of course, the trunk should be pressurized and rigid, and some active tension in the glutes will help keep the dip smooth as well.

Additionally, this separation may be the result of an incorrect rack position. If the bar is not settled in securely on the shoulders and instead is heavy in the hands and arms, separation is likely, in addition to slipping. The bar should be settled completely in the rack position prior to the initiation of the dip to ensure a tight connection from the outset.

Exercises to practice maintaining a solid rack position and initiating the dip smoothly include:

- Jerk dip squat
- Jerk rack support
- Push press

Cues to remind the lifter to keep the rack position tight and initiate the dip smoothly include:

- Stay connected to the bar
- Settle tight
- Rack position tight
- Shoulders up against the bar
- Smooth dip
- Legs tight before you dip

Bar Sliding Down in Dip

Any movement of the bar in the rack position during the dip and drive of the jerk can disrupt the transfer of force from the body into the bar and likely create an unwanted shift in balance. There are a few possible causes, and often more than one is present for a given lifter.

Immobility

This problem is most common with athletes whose immobility prevents their establishing a proper jerk rack position, and who are as a consequence beginning their jerks with the bar at least partially supported by the arms rather than completely by the trunk directly. The obvious solution to this problem is continuing to increase mobility to improve the rack position, and these lifters may find that temporarily raising the elbows somewhat in the rack position will help.

Weak or Inactive Rack Position

For athletes who are capable of a correct jerk rack position, the problem is most likely the result of the athlete not actively maintaining a tight rack position throughout the dip and drive and/or not being strong enough in the rack position to withstand the downward force when it reaches its peak at the bottom of the dip.

Exercises to help strengthen the rack position and allow the lifter to practice maintaining it securely include:

- Jerk dip squat
- Jerk rack support
- Jerk dip
- Jerk drive
- Front squat
- Quarter front squat

Cues to remind the lifter to actively keep the rack position tight include:

- Shoulders up against the bar
- Rack position tight
- Keep your shoulders up

Inadequate Trunk Strength or Pressurization

Inadequate trunk rigidity in general will also contribute to the problem. Proper pressurization and aggressive circumferential muscular tension should be practiced and reinforced, and back and abdominal strength improved. See the Back Collapsing in Receiving Position section in the Clean Errors chapter for more information.

Premature Arm Drive

An early initiation of the push against the bar with the arms will naturally pull the shoulders back out from under the bar somewhat, reducing the security and stability of the rack position, and reducing the transfer of force from the leg drive into the elevation and acceleration of the bar.

Exercises to help the athlete practice better timing of the arms in the jerk include:

- Pause jerk
- Pause jerk + jerk
- Push press
- Push press + jerk
- Jerk drive

Cues to encourage better timing of the arms in the jerk include:

- Patient arms
- Drive high before you punch
- Finish your drive first
- Drive all the way up before you split
- Long drive
- Drive high

Pushing Bar Forward with Arms

If the bar is moving forward in the jerk, but the athlete's dip and drive is executed with proper balance and orientation, the lifter is pushing the bar forward with the arms. This can occur for a few basic reasons. This problem is also discussed as one of the causes of the Forward Imbalance error above.

Non-Specific Corrections

As a simple way to correct a forward push with the arms, the coach can stand with a vertical PVC pipe or forearm 1-3 inches in front of the sleeve of the barbell or the front edge of the plates to give the lifter an obstacle to avoid. The actual proximity is less important than the pipe or arm's presence—if either is in front of the end of the bar, the lifter can't see it anyway. The knowledge that it is there is usually adequate for the lifter to make the necessary corrections. The coach should immediately remove the PVC or arm once the jerk is overhead to prevent the bar from coming down onto either.

Improper Arm Mechanics

The problem may be as simple as the lifter not executing the motion of the upper body properly due to a lack of understanding or experience. The details of the movement are discussed in detail in the Jerk section of the book.

Exercises to help the lifter learn and practice the proper upper body mechanics include:

- Press
- Push press
- Press behind the neck
- Push press behind the neck
- Tall jerk
- Press to jerk

Cues that can help remind the lifter of proper upper body mechanics in the jerk include:

- Push it back right off the shoulders
- Spread the elbows
- Get it behind your head
- Get it back

Premature Push with Arms

If the athlete is beginning to push on the bar with the arms prematurely, there is a greater likelihood that it will be pushed forward.

Exercises to help the athlete practice better timing of the arms in the jerk include:

- Pause jerk
- Pause jerk + jerk
- Push press
- Push press + jerk
- Jerk drive
- Push press + jerk

Cues to encourage better timing of the arms in the jerk include:

- Patient arms
- Drive high before you punch
- Finish your drive first
- Drive all the way up before you split
- Long drive
- Drive high

Lack of Confidence

Finally, pushing the bar forward with the arms is a natural reaction to a lack of confidence or a fear of getting under a certain weight. This keeps the bar from moving directly over the lifter and makes bailing out easier.

Be sure to consider possible sources of this lack of confidence before prescribing remedial work. For example, if the lifter is weak in the split position, this may be causing him or her to unconsciously avoid it with heavy weights, and this will not be improved with the exercises listed below (see the Weak Split Position heading under the Short Split or Lifter Moving Backward error above for suggestions in this case).

Exercises to improve confidence with heavy weights overhead include:

- Jerk support
- Jerk recovery
- Jerk behind the neck
- Hold all jerks overhead for 3 seconds

Pushing Body Backward

Similar in effect to pushing the bar forward is the athlete pushing the body backward from the bar during the drive under. While the body is now what's moving out of position rather than the bar, the result is the same—the bar is too far forward of the lifter's center of balance and/or outside the range of structural integrity to be supported.

Non-Specific Corrections

Exercises that will help the lifter practice the proper movement of the body down into the split jerk receiving position include:

- Tall jerk
- Push jerk behind the neck in split
- Press in split
- Jerk balance

Backward Imbalance

If the lifter begins the jerk with the balance too far back over the heels, it's possible for it to remain too far back. The result will be the lifter traveling backward somewhat as he or she splits under the bar. While this is unusual, it is possible.

Exercises to help the lifter improve balance in the jerk include:

- Push press
- Power jerk
- Push press + jerk
- Power jerk + jerk
- Jerk dip squat
- Jerk drive

Lack of Confidence

The lifter moving backward in the jerk can actually be caused by essentially same action that causes a forward push of the bar with the arms—if the weight on the bar is significantly greater than the lifter's bodyweight and the feet move from the floor early, pushing forward on the bar will move the lifter backward to a greater degree. See the Lack of Confidence heading in the Pushing Bar Forward with Arms error above for suggested corrections.

Overreaching Back Foot

As was described above with regard to the Short-Stepping error, overreaching the back foot can pull the lifter backward when moving down into the split position.

Exercises that will help the lifter practice the proper split position and movement into it include:

- Jerk balance
- Tall jerk
- Push jerk behind the neck in split
- Split jerk behind the neck
- Drop to split
- Jump to split

Cues to encourage the lifter to move into the split without overreaching the rear foot include:

- Hips under the bar
- Back foot down, front foot forward
- Lift and reach the front foot
- Step forward
- Step through it
- Head and chest up in the split
- Back foot close to the floor

Missing Backward

Missing jerks backward is uncommon enough that it rarely requires any corrective work. Many lifters have never lost a single jerk behind themselves. Others will do it extremely rarely as a consequence of an odd isolated mistake that they've never performed previously and will likely never repeat. In short, it's generally acceptable to essentially ignore such misses with regard to corrective work.

However, if a lifter frequently misses jerks backward, there is an issue to resolve. Most commonly, this occurs with lifters who are naturally unusually strong and explosive in the jerk and are able to put a lot of upward force on the bar. Add to that a lifter who is also capable of a very long, deep split, and you have a recipe for backward misses in the jerk.

In any case, the solution is to reinforce and strengthen the receiving position—both the split position itself and the overhead position to prevent unwanted shifting of the bar in relation to the trunk and hips.

Exercises to accomplish this include:

- Lunge
- Walk to split
- Step to split
- Split squat
- Drop to split
- Jump to split
- Push jerk behind the neck in split
- Jerk recovery
- Jerk support
- Push press behind the neck
- Push press

Introduction to Program Design

The fundamental purpose of training program design is to exploit the body's biological ability and need to adapt to the stressors to which it's exposed. The stressors we intentionally apply to the body are the training exercises, modified by volume, intensity, frequency and other characteristics, chosen to elicit certain responses. In other words, the physical adaptation of the body is systematically manipulated to achieve the intended functional capabilities.

Training methodology is largely speculative and little can be considered irrefutable fact, although generations of coaches and athletes have certainly arrived at various dependable principles. It's for this reason—as well as the fact that responses to training vary widely among apparently similar athletes—that standard or formulaic approaches don't exist and there continues to be a great deal of contention regarding programming and training. Excellent results have been produced in many very different ways. In short, there is no correct approach to programming—there is effective and ineffective, and no single approach will be either for every athlete at all times.

The coach is left to rely overwhelmingly on practical evidence, logic and judgment. Experimentation is encouraged with the understanding that it's carried out with respect to the fundamental principles about which we're largely certain. Haphazard experimentation with no regard to common sense is a waste of the athlete's time.

This section of the book intends to present the underlying theoretical information and practical experience that guide program design, explanations of methods of implementation, and practical examples to provide coaches and athletes of all levels guidance of the nature and extent needed.

Program design and training results depend on the response of the athlete in question, and the potential variation among athletes is essentially infinite. While we can classify and categorize and generalize to create various systems and frameworks to guide program design, ultimately each athlete is unique in many relevant respects, and program design must be individualized for maximal effectiveness. It's the coach's responsibility to observe and adapt, and the lifter's responsibility to do everything in his or her power to maximize the effectiveness of training and restoration, including communicating clearly and regularly with the coach.

Progressive Overload & Variation of Stimuli

The most basic principle upon which all physical training is predicated is *progressive overload*. The body adapts to stress in order to survive—this is as basic a biological function as it gets. The key is that once the body has adapted to a given type and magnitude of stress, it will maintain that accommodation for as long as it remains regularly exposed to that stress. In other words, a stressor that once forced adaptation due to its novelty will eventually fail to stimulate further adaptation because it's no longer unfamiliar and the body has already biologically adjusted to manage it. In order to stimulate further progress, we need to expose the body to further unfamiliar stress. This describes the notion of progressive overload—the magnitude of a specific training stimulus must continually be increased, or its exact nature modified in certain respects, over the long term to produce gains.

While unfamiliarity of stress can be manifested in a number of ways such as exercise selection and even the speed of execution of a given exercise, the unfamiliarity with which we're primarily concerned in strength sports is, of course, increases in loading. In order to lift more weight, an athlete must continually lift more weight. This principle cannot be neglected. Fortunately biological adaptation involves a margin—that is, the body will adapt somewhat beyond the actual imposed demands. This is how an athlete is able to eventually lift a weight he or she has not actually lifted previously. Without this natural overcompensation, progress would be impossible.

Models of Adaptation

There are three models of physical adaptation in common use to conceptualize the response of the body to training: The General Adaptation Syndrome, the Fitness-Fatigue Model, and the Supercompensation Model. None defines the mechanisms in precise detail, but the principles they describe create general guidelines for the systematic manipulation of training load and restoration.

General Adaptation Syndrome

Although originally presented by Hans Selye merely as a general description of the body's response to stress of any type, the General Adaptation Syndrome has been adopted by coaches and exercise scientists as a vague guide for managing training stimuli and recovery. An exhaustive discussion of the GAS is unnecessary for our purposes here, but a clear picture of its essence can be helpful in guiding programming decisions in a general sense. Selye defined three stages of stress response: Alarm, Resistance, and Exhaustion.

Alarm: The alarm stage is the initial response to a stressor. In this context, this stressor would be an unfamiliar training stimulus. During this stage (immediately following a bout of training), performance will diminish to varying degrees depending on the type and dose of stress and the capabilities being measured. This stage includes muscle soreness, reduced speed and power, and reduced strength. Reductions in speed and power will be more pronounced than in absolute strength.

Resistance: The resistance stage can be considered the adaptation or recovery stage. During this stage, the body responds to the stress of the alarm stage with cellular, structural and neurological changes to prepare to better cope with similar stress in the future. This period will vary in duration based on the athlete's training history, the magnitude and nature of the stress, the athlete's genetic recovery abilities, and the athlete's restoration efforts.

Exhaustion: The exhaustion stage is what we're trying to avoid through planned training and monitoring of the athlete. At this point of the GAS, accumulated stress has exceeded the body's capability to cope with it in a positive fashion. This state of overtraining can be brought about not only by excessive training, but by inadequate restoration efforts or unusual outside stress. That is, an athlete may reach this stage with training volume and intensity no greater than what he or she has been able to manage historically because of factors such as lack of sleep, inadequate nutrition, or additional stress unrelated to training.

The key points to bear in mind are that training is stress and that it does not immediately or necessarily result in productive adaptation—adaptation requires time and recovery management. Additionally, there is a limit to how much stress an athlete can adapt to in a given period before reaching the point of overtraining.

Supercompensation Model

The Supercompensation Model in its most specific form describes the process of adaptation as a reduction in specific substances by training followed by their replenishment during recovery to a level greater than existed previously. While this precise notion of supercompensation has been dismissed as inaccurate because none of the substances have ever been identified (glycogen may be cited as one, but its depletion/replenishment can account for only one specific type of physical performance) (Zatsiorsky 1995), the elemental idea implied by the term *supercompensation* holds fast as a basic rule of training: an unfamiliar stress will encourage the body, given adequate time and resources, to prepare to better manage such stress in the future by adapting in a manner specific to that stress and to a degree beyond the demand of the stimulating stress. This is, of course, the underlying principle of progressive overload and the margin of adaptation mentioned previously.

Fitness-Fatigue Model

The Fitness-Fatigue Model avoids the detail that prevented the Supercompensation Model's acceptance by relying on more flexible terms. The important idea in this model is that training will simultaneously produce two basic responses: an improvement of physical capacity and fatigue (assuming the training is of an appropriate nature and magnitude). The nature of that physical capacity is specific to the training, as is the nature of the accompanying fatigue (e.g. heavy, low-rep strength training will produce much different fitness and fatigue responses than long distance running). This means that immediately following training, while the athlete's *potential* performance is improved, his or her actual performance is limited by fatigue.

Fortunately, and the reason training programs are effective, is that the improvements in physical capacity are more persistent than the fatigue (assuming appropriate training and restoration, and that the athlete is not in an overtrained state). In other words, the fatigue of training will abate adequately in time to allow the athlete to train again at necessary levels before the greater capacity developed by prior training returns to the previous level so that it can be built upon. By correctly manipulating training variables, including rest, the athlete is able to make net gains in physical performance—training and recovery must be coupled appropriately to allow the use of improved potential performance in the absence of the fatigue that initially accompanied it. Further, subsequent training must be undertaken before the newly developed capacity diminishes in order to create long-term progress.

It's estimated that for an average training load in a single workout, there is a 3:1 ratio of fitness to fatigue; that is, if the improved fitness lasts 3 days following the training session, the fatigue lasts 1 day (Zatsiorksy 1995). Of course, this is complicated greatly by the fact that training sessions are not undertaken in isolation, but in series and under varying degrees of accumulated fatigue and stress. The nature and magnitude of stress also varies dramatically among workouts. Accordingly, the precision of timing is far more complex than this ratio suggests.

Specificity of Adaption

As described by the SAID principle (Specific Adaptation to Imposed Demands), the nature of an athlete's adaptation to training will be specific to that training. This should to a great extent be quite obvious, and is glaringly so in the most general sense—for example, few individuals would expect considerable strength gains as a result of marathon running. However, the obviousness diminishes as specificity increases.

The snatch and clean & jerk are extremely nuanced combinations of strength, speed, explosiveness, precision, timing, focus and confidence; this combination cannot be replicated or developed completely by any other exercise. Consequently, the competition lifts themselves must represent a significant portion of the total training volume, although how much will vary among lifters, stages of development, and period of time relative to competition.

Specificity in training does not mean that no training other than maximal singles in the competition lifts should be employed; far from it. It does mean, however, that all elements of training must be selected specifically to develop the appropriate physical qualities and abilities necessary for optimal weightlifting performance. This ranges from exercise selection to exercise speed to posture to the number of repetitions per set.

This demand for specificity also applies to non-weightlifting physical activity. That is, weightlifting training must optimally drive physiological adaptation for weightlifting performance, but weightlifters must also limit or eliminate physical activity that does not support, directly or indirectly, weightlifting performance. Such non-specific activity has the potential to limit the desired adaptation in multiple fashions. For example, the performance of stamina- or endurance-oriented training or activity (outside of intentional GPP employed for specific reasons at specific times) will limit the ability of the body to optimally perform in the specific functional manner necessary. In addition to direct physiological competition for functional characteristics, non-specific training either limits the time available for specific training, or limits the athlete's capacity for recovery from specific training and consequently the desired adaptation.

It is not impossible to improve performance in weightlifting without complete specificity. However, the need for specificity increases along with the desired level of performance in a given activity, and program design must reflect this. The more advanced an athlete desires to be in the sport of weightlifting, the more specialized his or her training must become.

Genetic Potential

There is no scientific contention regarding the role of genetic potential in an athlete's success in weightlifting or any other sport, yet opinion on the subject varies considerably. This variation in opinion arises largely from genetically blessed athletes' common reluctance to accept the notion that they have natural advantages over other individuals. While the idea of genetics playing a significant role in one's athletic success can understandably be unappealing to those athletes, as the implication is that they do not or need not work as hard as others to achieve success, it should be understood that the recognition and acknowledgment of such genetic advantages is not intended to be insulting or belittling.

There is no argument that numerous physical traits (and their ultimate development) that allow excellent performance in a given sport are genetically determined. Such traits relevant to weightlifting include natural anabolic hormone levels, body segment proportions, joint structure, ratios of muscle fiber types, and number of muscle fibers in a given muscle. These characteristics control, at least to some extent, both the rate of improvement and the ultimate level of performance that can be attained through their influence or determination of characteristics like hypertrophy, strength, speed, recovery capacity, structure, mobility and leverage. Quite simply, this means that certain individuals are better suited than others for weightlifting, and will be capable of reaching levels of performance not attainable by those whose physical makeup diverges if the respective efforts and commitment to the sport are equal.

Clearly there are elements of performance that can be affected to various extents through training. Just because an athlete has extraordinary potential does not mean he or she will reach it without the proper training, motivation and discipline. Similarly, athletes with less than optimal potential can achieve considerable success with diligent training that exploits what strengths and advantages they do have and mitigates the limitations of their weaknesses. However, these individuals will still be working under a lower performance ceiling.

This of course does not mean that athletes not blessed with ideal genetic traits should give up on the pursuit of increasing weightlifting performance; it means simply that such individuals need to be realistic about both their potential rate of progress and their ultimate potential for development to ensure their training reflects their particular capacity and abilities, and consequently maximizes progress.

Strength & Power Principles

The development of strength and its related qualities is extremely complex from a physiological perspective. More often than not, training practices are developed in the gym independently of scientific understanding, at least at a significant level, and then evaluated much later by researchers to determine the underlying mechanisms. Generally speaking, a coach has little or no need to understand the higher level scientific underpinnings of training if he or she has a firm grasp of proven practical elements and their manipulation for intended effect. However, combining practical experience and ability with theoretical knowledge can only improve a coach's ability. The following are the principles most relevant to the development of weightlifters.

Strength Qualities

Strength can be divided into four basic qualities relevant to weightlifting, each of which is functional for given types of movements and activities, and must be trained specifically for maximal development.

Absolute Strength This is the ability of the muscles to produce maximal force; in other words, to lift as much weight as possible, irrespective of speed or acceleration.

Speed Strength This is the ability of the muscles to contract at high speed against resistance; in other words, to lift a weight at high speed.

Explosive Strength This is the ability of the muscles to generate maximal force in minimal time; in other words, to accelerate a weight as quickly as possible.

Strength Endurance This is typically defined as the ability to sustain repetitive efforts against resistance for an extended duration. In the context of weightlifting, it may alternatively be defined as the ability to continue to perform strength training over a long period of time, e.g. sustaining performance during a long training session, or work capacity, i.e. the athlete's ability to manage large training loads.

It should be apparent that while all four of these qualities are necessary to some degree for weightlifting, speed strength and explosive strength are of particular importance. What may be less apparent is the specificity of each quality. With regard to speed strength, one might assume that the higher an athlete's absolute strength, the higher his or her speed strength will be naturally. However, there is no correlation between the ability to produce maximal force and the ability to produce maximal velocity in the same movement with advanced athletes (Zatsiorksy 1995, Medvedyev 1986/1989). In practical terms, this means that in order to develop the speed strength so critical for weightlifting success, training must address, and even emphasize, this trait specifically rather than focusing exclusively or excessively on absolute strength.

Similarly, explosive strength is vital for success in weightlifting. The *explosive strength deficit* (ESD) represents the amount of an athlete's absolute strength that is inaccessible due to the high rate of contraction speed and consequent brevity of a given movement. It takes 0.3-0.4 seconds on average to achieve maximal force (or about 97-98% of it) (Zatsiorksy 1995); explosive movements can occur too quickly for maximal force to be generated, leaving the so-called deficit of strength—the remaining amount of strength the athlete is capable of generating but cannot apply to the explosive movement because of insufficient time to generate it.

Explosive strength can be improved by increasing absolute strength in athletes with relatively small explosive strength deficits in the movement in question (that is, their strength does not dramatically exceed the force they're able to put into the movement); however, this becomes far less effective as the ESD increases (that is, the athlete's strength far surpasses the force applied to the movement) (Zatsiorksy 1995). Consequently, in general terms, the more advanced the athlete and the greater his or her absolute strength, the more explosive strength must be trained directly rather than relying on increases of absolute strength to improve explosive strength.

Strength Development

There are two basic ways to increase strength: morphological and neurological adaptation. Morphological adaptations are alterations of the actual physical structures of the body. The primary change for strength is the accumulation of more contractile proteins within the muscle, also known as myofibrillar hypertrophy; in other words, the increase of the muscles' cross sectional area through an increase in functional tissue. Also included in morphological changes will be the strengthening of bones and connective tissue in response to increased loading.

The second is through neurological adaptation. This is the primary manner in which weightlifters improve strength and power over the long term, and the reason why a lifter can continue to gain strength over a long period of time without gaining weight or increasing in size. Neurological adaptations are changes to the following elements that control muscular action:

Recruitment The muscle fibers of a motor unit (collection of muscle fibers innervated by a single motor neuron) are either activated or not; there is no partial activation or contraction of an individual motor unit or muscle fiber. Higher magnitudes of force are generated when more motor units in the relevant muscles are activated simultaneously.

Rate Coding The frequency of a motor unit's repeated activation determines how much overall force is generated; higher frequency will produce higher tension.

Synchronization Typically motor units are activated in a given muscle during a given movement in a staggered fashion, or asynchronously. The more synchronized the activation of the motor units in a working muscle, the higher the total tension produced.

Golgi Tendon Organ Inhibition Golgi tendon organs (GTOs) are sensory organs near the transition of muscle to tendon that measure tension. When excessive muscle and tendon tension stimulates the GTO, force production of that muscle is inhibited. A reduction in GTO sensitivity reduces limitations on the muscle force that can be generated prior to this protective reflex being triggered.

Intermuscular Coordination The total force of a movement, as opposed to the force generation of a specific muscular contraction, is influenced through the precise coordination of many muscles via agonistic contraction and antagonistic relaxation. This coordination can be considered the skill of executing a given lift; the higher the athlete's skill of execution, the greater the strength of the movement because of the concerted work of the body as a whole.

Basic Strength Training Protocols

There are different approaches to training strength, each of which has benefits and drawbacks and must be implemented and emphasized appropriately for each athlete based on need, timing, and stage of development. In the broadest sense, these are maximal effort, maximal speed with limit weight, repeated effort (maximal or submaximal reps), and dynamic effort (Medvedyev 1986/1989, Zatsiorsky 1995).

Maximal Effort Maximal effort training is the use of the heaviest possible weights with consequently limited repetitions (1-3). This method is extremely effective for improving absolute strength and produces optimal improvements in intra- and intermuscular coordination. However, high frequency with such high intensity subjects the athlete to overtraining more than other methods, and it produces little if any hypertrophy because of the minimal amount of total work. Generally this is considered to be maximal effort without significant psychological arousal—that is, somewhat more weight could be lifted with maximal arousal, such as would be experienced in competition. Observing this rule in the gym will help reduce the tendency of this approach to lead to overtraining.

Maximal Speed Limit Weight This is the use of maximal movement speed with heavy weights (80-95%). Generally, maximal concentric speed should be used in all weightlifting training unless there is a specific reason not to in a given case, as this will better pace the development of the necessary speed strength with absolute strength.

Repeated Effort The repeated effort method can involve several repetitions to actual failure or short of failure. While this method is not as effective for improving absolute strength relative to maximal effort, it is more effective for stimulating hypertrophy, offers somewhat lower risk of injury, is less taxing physically and emotionally, and, if not taken to failure, allows for better preservation of optimal technical execution.

Greg Everett

Dynamic Effort This approach is the use of maximal speed with necessarily light weights. Dynamic effort does not increase absolute strength, but can help improve speed strength and explosive strength.

Periodization Structure

More advanced program design will typically involve periodization of some type. There are three primary levels of a training cycle that will be referred to in this book and commonly.

Macrocycle The macrocycle represents what could be considered the entire training program—that is, it's the complete training cycle that spans the time between subsequent meaningful events (usually competitions). A lifter may train on a single macrocycle beginning after every competition and leading to the next, or in cases of longer periods of time between competitions, may use more than one macrocycle between two meets, separated by some kind of max lift testing or other reason to split the time.

Mesocycle The mesocycle is the intermediate time period. Most commonly, this will be 4 weeks in duration, but generally can be anywhere from 3-6 weeks depending on the needs and content of the program and the competition calendar. This can be thought of as a training "month".

Microcycle The microcycle is a single week. Technically, a microcycle may be more or fewer than 7 days, but this is very rare because of the convenience of using the 7-day week.

Development Paradigms

In the US and other countries in which the sport of weightlifting exists in similar circumstances, generally the program design paradigm differs from countries with well-established systems of athlete development both practically and conceptually. In these latter countries, athletes are more often recruited and selected at the appropriate young age, and consequently they can be taught, trained and developed sequentially and systematically, exploiting the optimal periods of physical and mental development to appropriately time stages of training and achieving higher levels of mastery at younger ages to allow for longer careers at higher levels of performance.

In contrast, in the US athletes are more often arriving in the sport of weightlifting at later ages with broadly varying athletic backgrounds, including none at all. In consequence, the approach to instruction and program design often differs considerably because of the need to contend with older, less prepared athletes, and a broad spectrum of different backgrounds. The approach is more remedial in many respects, it often attempts to develop all qualities simultaneously rather than somewhat sequentially, and the development process overall is compressed to attempt to achieve maximal results prior to the athlete's more quickly approaching biological peak (or even to achieve them as quickly as possible to race waning capacity following that peak).

This book attempts to present the information necessary to deal with either situation and any in between to ensure the coach and athlete are able to implement the most effective system of training possible in their particular circumstances.

Progress & Expectations

Predicting the rate of progress and ultimate level of ability a lifter will attain is impossible with any legitimate precision. Generalizations can certainly be made, but the influencing factors—physical, mental, and circumstantial—are too numerous to allow a formulaic answer.

The most reliable fact with regard to the progress of a weightlifter is that the rate of progress will be maximal at the beginning of the athlete's career and will slow gradually over the course of that career. If the athlete remains in the sport long enough, the rate of progress will actually become negative as the aging athlete begins to regress. The actual rate of improvement will be greater the closer to the ideal age the athlete begins training.

The greatest rate of improvement will occur in the first year of training, with a relatively high rate of improvement (although decreasing over time) over the first 6-8 years of training, and progress continuing for 10-14 years in total. Athletes in larger bodyweight categories will typically maintain higher rates of improvement for a longer period of time than their lighter counterparts, and progress can be maintained longer if an athlete moves up a weight class near the end of the initial 6-8-year period of rela-tively rapid improvement (weight class increases will occur naturally when lifters begin at young ages—this natural progression should never be prevented). (Medvedyev 1986/1989)

In all cases, the rate of progress can be best preserved by the athlete continuing to dedicate more time, energy and focus to training, restoration and construction of the most conducive lifestyle to support sporting improvement. The more an athlete advances, the more his or her life will need to be shaped around the sport.

Assessment

When starting a new weightlifter, the coach must determine the present abilities and the potential of the athlete in order to plan his or her training. How formal such an assessment is will depend on the coach's preference and goals, and to some extent on the athlete. For example, a coach whose intention is to produce elite weightlifters will need a much more comprehensive assessment protocol than a coach who simply trains recreational lifters with no real aspirations of competitive success. If the former coach is actively recruiting new weightlifters, assessment will need to be thorough to discover appropriate talent with the potential for success. Similarly, a coach may choose to alter the thoroughness and formality of the assessment based on the basic profile of the athlete—a young athlete with obvious potential will likely earn a more in-depth evaluation than an older individual with no athletic background, for example.

Assessment may be split into two broad categories based on the type of individual being evaluated: youth or adult. Youth assessment will be predicated on the notion of long term, systematic development of a young athlete into a weightlifter; adult assessment will involve converting an existing or former athlete (or even an adult with no athletic background) into a weightlifter. Each will have somewhat different data available with somewhat different purposes.

The following points of assessment will help guide the coach in evaluating new lifters. Formal assessments should be undertaken prior to any training to determine the course and content of the subsequent training. Informal assessments may be made entirely or only partially prior to the initiating of training; in many cases, it will be expedient or even necessary for certain points of the assessment to occur during an initial stage of basic training.

With all of the collected information, the coach can build a training plan suitable for each athlete.

Formal assessments should be documented consistently by the coach; as these records accumulate, they will help reveal patterns to the coach and guide better decisions with regard to program design.

Physical Traits

Chronological & Biological Age

Chronological age—the number of years an individual has been alive—is a simple metric to get a basic idea of the athlete's status. This will also indicate what competitive classification a lifter falls into at present: youth, junior, senior or master.

More important to training is biological age—essentially the physical maturity of the athlete, which may not align perfectly with the expectations based on chronological age. With young athletes, the primary lines of demarcation are the onset of puberty and the completion of sexual maturation. Biological age in youth lifters will guide the training emphasis to exploit sequential periods of optimal potential adaptation. In all lifters, it will help guide decisions regarding elements such as training volume, average intensity and frequency.

Height & Bodyweight

The athlete's bodyweight initially will determine the weight class, but will also help guide decisions broadly regarding training volume. Generally larger athletes will recover more slowly and be capable of tolerating less volume than their smaller counterparts.

More important will be the athlete's height to

bodyweight ratio, as this will help determine the athlete's ideal bodyweight category to maximize competitiveness. The importance of appropriate bodyweight relative to height will increase with the lifter's progression and competitiveness. Beginning athletes will see natural changes in bodyweight in response to training in most cases, so no immediate decisions or actions will be necessary or truly possible. Recreational lifters will likely be unwilling to make modifications to bodyweight even if they were to be attended by considerable performance increases.

As lifters progress and likely begin to compete more seriously, the height to bodyweight ratio needs to be considered. Due to the disadvantages of height and long limbs described previously in the book, it's important to adjust bodyweight to move a lifter into a weight class in which they are competing with lifters of similar height.

Body composition and hormonal status will need to be taken into account when deciding on changing bodyweight categories. For example, if a lifter is already very lean, dropping bodyweight is very rarely a wise idea. If a lifter possesses higher body fat levels, dropping weight classes can be done more easily with much less of a negative impact on strength when done properly. Similarly, if a lifter has higher body fat levels, increasing a weight class may not be advisable unless body composition can be improved.

Body composition can be telling of a few things, such as an athlete's natural anabolic hormonal levels and his or her present and former training and nutrition practices. An athlete who comes into the gym muscular and lean will likely have an advantage over one who is not muscular and has a larger percentage of body fat, all other things being equal. This being said, body composition varies broadly among even the best weightlifters in the world; this is certainly not the ultimate indicator of either potential or present ability.

Tables 33.1 and 33.2 (adapted from Takano 2012) provide loose guidelines for optimal height to bodyweight ratios.

Proportions

An athlete's proportions, be they brachiomorphic, mesomorphic or dolicomorphic—will be to an ex-

Weight	Height	
56kg	149cm	4'11"
62kg	156cm	5'1"
69kg	162cm	5'4"
77kg	165cm	5'5"
85kg	169cm	5'7"
94kg	173cm	5'8"
105kg	176cm	5'9"
+105kg	186cm	6'1"

TABLE 33.1 Average male heights for weight classes (Pre-2018 classes)

Weight	Height	
48kg	148cm	4'10"
53kg	153cm	5'
58kg	154cm	5'1"
63kg	157cm	5'2"
69kg	158cm	5'2"
75kg	163cm	5'3"
+75kg	170cm	5'7"

TABLE 33.2 Average female heights for weight classes (Pre-2018 classes)

tent predictive of performance and training requirements and can help guide decisions on exercise selection to immediately begin shoring up weaknesses that result.

Mobility & Positions

The purpose of the mobility and position assessment is to determine how close the athlete is to being capable of achieving the necessary positions for the snatch, clean and jerk, and what, if any, are the limitations. This information will be used to determined mobility and sometimes exercise prescriptions (such as temporarily avoiding certain exercises until adequate ROM is achieved, or using certain exercises

Greg Everett

as part of the effort to improve that ROM).

Wrists Wrist mobility will need to be evaluated for the snatch overhead position and the clean rack position primarily. The best way to evaluate wrist ROM is to have the athlete perform these positions, taking into consideration potential interference from other areas, such as tight shoulders or internal arm rotators and adductors, that might prevent the display of the actual wrist ROM.

Elbows The elbows will need to be evaluated for their ability to fully extend (ideally into slight hyperextension). The best way to check this is by having the athlete hold the arm straight down at his or her side and extend the elbow maximally—this will prevent any interference from a tight shoulder girdle or thoracic spine, for example, limiting elbow extension in an overhead position. If an athlete is unable to fully extend the elbows, he or she is a candidate for extra overhead strength work to make up for the structural deficit.

Shoulders The ability of the shoulders to fully open to allow the lifter to establish the proper overhead position for the snatch and jerk needs to be evaluated. A simple method is for the athlete to lie on his or her back with the knees bent and feet flat on the floor, the lower back pressed flat against the floor, then lift straight arms up overhead and try to place them flat on the floor without arching the back. If this isn't possible, work needs to be done on the shoulders and possibly thoracic spine.

Thoracic Spine The thoracic spine needs to be mobile enough to flatten from its natural kyphotic curve, both to allow proper overhead positioning, and to contribute to a stronger back arch in the pull and squat. Thoracic spine immobility can usually be seen fairly easily as hyperkyphosis in the athlete's natural standing posture, or in a snatch or clean starting position as an inability to flatten the upper back. If the lifter can achieve a decent overhead position with a jerk grip, but is unable to press smoothly (or at all) with a jerk grip from behind the neck, thoracic spine mobility is likely limited.

Hips Hip mobility must be adequate to allow the lifter to sit into a full front and back squat with a properly arched spine, and set a proper back arch in the starting positions of the snatch and clean. It's simple enough to use these positions to evaluate hip mobility. In the squat, the contribution of the ankles to poor positioning must also be considered. If mobility seems limited, but the shin angle in the squat is relatively upright, or the athlete feels he or she is falling backward in the bottom position, the limitation is at least partially in the ankles.

Ankles Ankle mobility is critical for optimal lift performance; without it, the lifter will never be able to achieve the solid and balanced upright posture in the receiving positions of the snatch and clean that is necessary for maximal lifts. We're only concerned with the range of motion in a bent-knee position—any limitations due to gastrocnemius tightness will not affect the squat because the tension will be removed once the knee is bent unless it is severe. Again, we can simply evaluate the squat position—If an athlete is struggling to sit into the proper position and the elevation of the heels by ¼" or so makes a significant difference, ankle mobility needs to be improved. It will also usually be fairly obvious that an athlete is tipping or bouncing backward in the bottom of a squat if forced to hold it (unloaded), has a very upright shin angle, or feels it necessary to be actively attempting to dorsiflex the ankles to prevent falling backward.

Training & Performance

Training Age & Experience

An athlete's training experience in terms of duration and type will affect the training approach considerably. A youth with no athletic experience, an adult with extensive experience in a strength or power sport, and an adult with no training experience each requires a very different plan even if the ultimate goal for all is essentially identical.

Performance Traits

In order to be successful in weightlifting, athletes need to be strong, fast and explosive. These latter two traits in particular are largely genetically determined, but all three can be influenced by training to varying extents. The current status is an indicator of both natural ability and the nature of any previous training.

Formal assessments can be performed using tests such as vertical or broad jumps for explosiveness, short sprints for speed and basic barbell lifts for strength. The last is not possible with untrained youth candidates, but the first two will be useful.

Assessing these qualities can also be done informally during the earliest stage of training. For example, seeing an athlete squat in training will be a good indicator of strength even without actually testing a maximal lift; seeing an athlete perform a snatch, clean, jerk, or some variant during the learning stages will make it obvious if an athlete is naturally fast and explosive.

Technical Proficiency & Motor Learning Ability

The technical proficiency of current weightlifters can be determined with two basic criteria: the coach's visual observation of the competition lifts, and the ratio of the athlete's competition lifts to his or her squats and other basic strength lifts (See Table 33.3). The former is somewhat subjective, although not detrimentally so, and the latter is somewhat vague, as additional factors such as levels of explosiveness and mobility can influence this relationship independent of technical proficiency. In any case, this will provide a general sense of the athlete's abilities to help guide elements like exercise selection and the need for dedicated instructional training stages.

For athletes new to weightlifting, lift technique will not yet be established, meaning technical proficiency is not applicable. However, the coach will be able to evaluate a lifter's motor learning ability through the early stages of technical instruction. How well and quickly a new athlete learns and masters lift technique will guide the plan for the initial instruction stage and early training cycles.

Injury History & Related Limitations

Young athletes coming into the sport of weightlifting without athletic backgrounds should be devoid of significant injury history and consequently free of related limitations. This is one of the many benefits of starting lifters at the optimal age.

Athletes beginning weightlifting as adults will often have athletic and training experience and the injuries that accompany it. As a result of these injuries, they may have limitations on range of motion of certain joints, consistent pain during certain movements or in certain positions, or even performance limitations due entirely to fear.

It's necessary for the coach to design training to rehabilitate, strengthen, or accommodate such problems as much as possible. This can also be potential limitation on an athlete's ultimate lifting ability. For example, an athlete who has had a serious shoulder injury and now has limited range of motion that has not been correctable through rehabilitation may not be able to establish an ideal overhead position, and consequently will be unable to snatch or jerk as much as would otherwise be possible with their strength and technical abilities.

Competitiveness & Commitment

As with any competitive sport, success demands certain personality traits suitable to the particular demands of the sport on training and competition. How an athlete handles competition generally can be seen through previous performances in other sports, but this does not always translate perfectly into weightlifting. The nature of weightlifting competition is quite unique and an individual who does well in one sport mentally may not fare as well as a weightlifter. The coach will have to see the athlete in weightlifting competition to know how he or she will respond, although simulated competitions can be held in the gym to get an idea.

How competitive an athlete is will usually become fairly clear just through the observation of his or her daily training. Naturally competitive athletes will tend to keep an eye on what their teammates are doing and try to outdo them in the gym in one way or another, they will push themselves to beat their previous performances, and they will want to enter meets regularly.

An athlete's commitment to the sport and training is an important element of long term success. If an athlete is not enthusiastic about training, it will be obvious in his or her performance, and this will limit the effectiveness of the programming. Coaches need to be motivators, but to reach their true potential, athletes need to be driven, disciplined and goal-oriented on their own. If an athlete needs to be continually coerced into training and competing, it's very unlikely that athlete will be successful in reaching his or her physical potential.

Lift Performance & Ratios

Training lift performance can be used to gain a general sense of the athlete's experience and ability, absolute and relative strength, and strength imbalances. With experienced lifters, these will generally not require specific testing, but may be provided by the athlete. This can provide insight into what will require emphasis in the athlete's training program with regard to strength, technique or mobility (depending on what the rest of the assessment has determined

are limitations for given exercises).

The ratio of certain lifts to others will also describe an individual's relative strengths and weaknesses, which can guide program design emphasis and exercise selection, or indicate potential problems requiring direct correction. The ratios in Table 33.3 are descriptive of a balanced weightlifter. Reasonable divergence should not alone be considered to be indicative of a problem, as all athletes will possess natural strengths and weaknesses that can shift certain ratios without representing a problem needing to be addressed. Some ratios will also naturally diverge due to elements like body type and bodyweight category, and traits like explosiveness. For example, the lightest and heaviest weight classes tend to have higher squat to competition lift ratios (Laputin & Oleshko 1982/2007); a less explosive athlete will typically have a lower competition lift to squat ratio than a more explosive athlete; taller lifters will tend to snatch a higher percentage of their clean & jerk than shorter lifters. Such divergences will persist to a great extent regardless of training.

Circumstances

Before a training program can be designed, the coach needs to take into consideration the circumstances in which the lifter will be training. If the coach is fortunate enough to be working with a full-time weightlifter with no obligations outside the sport, this step doesn't exist and training can be planned optimally according to the athletic needs determined though the assessment.

However, this is unusual, particularly in the US. More likely, coaches will be working with weightlifters who have jobs, are in school and/or who have families, and these obligations and responsibilities will place restrictions on their training schedules as well as recovery abilities. These practical limitations will alter the ideal training program to some degree.

Facility & Equipment One of the possible limitations for coaches and athletes will be the facilities and equipment to which they have access. At best this may limit the number of athletes who can train at a single time, and at worst it will actually dic-

Lift	Of Lift	Percentage
Snatch	Back Squat	60-65%
Clean & Jerk	Back Squat	80-85%
Clean & Jerk	Front Squat	85-90%
Snatch	Clean & Jerk	80-85%
Front Squat	Back Squat	85-93%
Power Snatch	Snatch	80-85%
Power Clean	Clean	80-90%
Clean	Deadlift	70-75%
Press	Push Press	70-75%
Push Press	Jerk	75-85%
Overhead Squat	Back Squat	65-70%

TABLE 33.3 General lift ratio guidelines

tate exercise prescription irrespective of the determined needs of the athletes. For example, if a facility has only two platforms and two Olympic bars, but has twenty athletes and only two hours to train on a given day, there will certainly be a limit to how much work those athletes will be able to do with the competition lifts, and this will have to be taken into consideration when developing the training program. Here creativity in exercise selection and rotation among athletes will become critical.

Schedule It's rare for an athlete to have unlimited time available for training. Nearly all will have obligations such as work, school and family that, while clearly not as important as weightlifting, will be given priority in most instances. Programming may necessarily vary greatly among athletes based on how often they'll be in the gym and planning appropriately from the beginning of the process is simpler than attempting to modify the perfect program to fit into a conflicting schedule.

Financial To some extent, an athlete's financial means will dictate details of training and competition. For example, a lifter may not be able to afford to compete as frequently as a coach would otherwise prefer due to the cost of entry feels and travel, or to attend certain meets due to the related expenses. Similarly, an athlete's training schedule may be restricted if he or she cannot afford full-time gym fees. Many coaches and programs use various methods of fundraising to eliminate or mitigate these restrictions for promising competitive lifters.

Skill Classification

The Soviets developed a system of classification for weightlifters that allows the planning of appropriate training for lifters of increasing ability, guides the long term development process, and creates expectations and goals for performance. These classifications can be found in various sources and used instead of the following if the coach prefers.

The skill classifications in Table 33.4 (at the end of this chapter) are based on the Soviet idea, but have been created with the American weightlifter or those

in similar circumstances in mind—that is, more likely than not to be unable to train full time as a weightlifter and to arrive at the sport at a later age than ideal.

These classes were originally calculated based on three years of actual US and international competition results. As of July 2018, the IWF has adopted all new weight classes. Because at the time of this revised edition, there is no competition data from which to directly calculate these figures, they have been determined through extrapolation to predict figures for the new classes as well as possible. New figures will be calculated in a later edition when adequate competition data exists.

These classification levels will be used later to help guide elements of program design.

Recruiting Assessment

Recruiting athletes, particularly of the ideal age and ability, is very difficult in the US and countries with similar athletic landscapes. There is very little to offer to dissuade talent from accepting college scholarships, money and notoriety in the many other sports that provide such opportunities. Athletes must have a true love for weightlifting, which is not likely at the young age optimal for beginning the sport. While in some countries, access to talent of the appropriate age is far greater, alternative sport options are far fewer, and the recognition and appreciation of the sport of weightlifting is far more widespread, in the US, coaches are largely dependent on chance to find new athletes.

Recruiting in these circumstances, consequently, is more about persuading athletes to try the sport and continue in it long term rather than identifying the greatest talent and culling the group. However, recruiting assessment protocols can still be useful at least to identify the most promising athletes in a group for the sake of determining where to invest the most time, energy and possibly money, or to help stratify large groups of lifters according to talent and potential. Following is a testing protocol that will provide data to give the coach a sense of the athlete's suitability for weightlifting. Of course, these tests can and should be combined with the previously discussed assessments where they do not overlap.

Recruiting Assessment Protocol

The following should be measured and recorded by the coach. In most cases, rating will necessarily be somewhat subjective even if a numerical score is created to help clarify results. The coach will need to consider all data collectively.

Age The closer the athlete is to the optimal starting age range (11-13), the better.

Height:Bodyweight Ratio This will be more useful for senior athletes than youth and junior, as the latter group are likely still growing. However, typically it will be apparent if a young lifter will be relatively tall or short when fully grown; the stature of the athlete's parents can also be helpful to guide expectations for a lifter's ultimate height. The closer the senior athlete is to the height:bodyweight ratios supplied previously in Tables 33.1 and 33.2 at an appropriate body composition, the better.

Body Type Athletes with the mesomorphic or dolichomorphic body types will be more suitable than those with more brachiomorphic proportions.

Hand Size Larger hands confer a basic advantage in the ability to grasp the barbell, particularly in the snatch. This is of particular importance to male lifters in the lighter bodyweight categories.

Elbow Extension The ability to slightly hyperextend the elbows is ideal; somewhat greater hyperextension is preferable to an inability to achieve a perfectly straight arm.

Explosiveness Explosiveness is one of the most important physical traits a lifter can possess, and is largely an inherent quality. A simple test of explosiveness is the vertical jump, which conveniently tests the legs and hips specifically. Ideally the vertical jump is tested both with a standard two-legged countermovement jump and a jump from a still position in the bottom of a squat. High scores in both are desirable, as this indicates high levels of both elasticity and rate of force development. Keep in mind, this is a measure of actual vertical jump height, not the height of a box a lifter is able

Weight Class	Jump Height
56kg	67cm (26in)
69kg	68cm (27in)
85kg	70cm (28in)
105kg	66cm (26in)

TABLE 33.5 Vertical jump heights of experienced male weightlifters (Adapted from Laputin & Oleshko 1982/2007

to jump onto, which will be much higher.

Vertical jump heights will generally be greatest in the middle range of the weight classes (Laputin & Oleshko 1982/2007). Table 33.5 contains vertical jump heights from experienced male weightlifters as loose reference points. Of course the vertical jumps of untrained individuals will not reach these heights, but they can serve as a broad guidelines.

Mobility The simplest and most relevant test of mobility for weightlifting is for the athlete to perform a close-grip and narrow-stance overhead squat with a PVC pipe or wooden dowel. The closer the athlete is to being able to squat to full depth with flat feet and the arms extended completely straight overhead, the better his or her weightlifting-specific mobility. The width of the stance can be widened until reaching a natural squat stance and the width of the grip widened to a snatch-width if the athlete is not capable of the narrow stance and grip squat to verify at least the minimal required mobility.

Strength If the athlete is older and has training experience, basic strength lift numbers can be used to gauge the athlete's strength. For young new athletes, a grip dynamometer is a useful tool to measure basic strength levels, and grip strength itself is an important trait for lifters. The greater the grip strength, the better.

Some loose guidelines for experienced male weightlifters organized by weight class are shown in Table 33.6, and Table 33.7 shows average grip strength of the dominant hand according to age and gender. Notice that grip strength tends to peak in the mid-20s, and that the disparity in male:female strength is insignificant prior to sexual maturation.

Trunk Stability The athlete can be tested in holding a proper plank position to measure basic trunk stability. Athletes should be able to maintain the position for at least 1 minute.

Motivation The motivation to work hard is not an easy quality to measure without long term observation of an athlete. However, a sense of the athlete's will can be measured by testing his or her willingness to push him- or herself with a simple exercise not limited by the need for technical ability and that offers relatively low injury risk—two good choices are the bench press or press. A weight with which the athlete can do 8-12 reps should be used, and the athlete instructed to do as many reps as possible. The coach will then be able to observe how hard the athlete will push to complete reps.

Motor Ability A finger tapping test (also known as a finger oscillation test) can be used to get a basic sense of an athlete's motor ability. The higher the score, the better. This can be done on any computer with a sensitive keyboard (i.e. the keys must be depressed only a very short distance rather than deep keys). With a text editor program open, the athlete will set his or her dominant hand flat on a table with the index finger on a convenient key—any key that will record a letter, number or symbol. The athlete will then hit the key as many times as possible in 10 seconds, and the number of keystrokes can be counted by counting the number of letters, numbers or symbols recorded in the program. This should be repeated 5 times with breaks of 30-60 seconds between and the scores averaged. Scores will typically be between 70-100, but this can vary based on the setup used. It will be best to compare to other scores measured with the same method once enough have been collected.

Weight Class	Dominant Hand Strength
56kg	50kg (110lb)
69kg	56kg (123lb)
85kg	63kg (139lb)
105kg	73kg (161lb)

TABLE 33.6 Grip strength measurements for the dominant hand in experienced male weightlifters (Adapted from Laputin & Oleshko 1982/2007)

Age	Male	Female
10-11	18kg (40lb)	17kg (37lb)
12-13	25kg (55lb)	20kg (44lb)
14-15	36kg (79lb)	21kg (46lb)
16-17	43kg (95lb)	23kg (51lb)
18-19	46kg (101lb)	25kg (55lb)
20-24	47kg (104lb)	28kg (62lb)
25-29	48kg (106lb)	34kg (75lb)
30-34	46kg (101lb)	28kg (62lb)
35-39	46kg (101lb)	27kg (60lb)

TABLE 33.7 Average grip strength of the dominant hand by age and gender (Adapted from Zhongshan 2015)

Level 1 Men			
Bodyweight	Total	Snatch	Clean & Jerk
55	105	47	58
61	116	52	64
67	123	55	68
73	129	58	71
81	136	61	75
89	145	65	80
96	152	68	84
102	157	71	86
109	162	73	89
109+	167	75	92

Level 2 Men			
Bodyweight	Total	Snatch	Clean & Jerk
55	140	63	77
61	155	70	85
67	162	73	89
73	169	76	93
81	181	81	100
89	195	88	107
96	202	91	111
102	208	94	114
109	213	96	117
109+	221	99	122

Level 1 Women			
Bodyweight	Total	Snatch	Clean & Jerk
45	65	29	36
49	70	32	39
55	81	36	45
59	86	39	47
64	90	40	50
71	97	44	53
76	101	45	56
81	108	49	59
87	116	52	64
87+	120	54	66

Level 2 Women			
Bodyweight	Total	Snatch	Clean & Jerk
45	85	38	47
49	93	42	51
55	109	49	60
59	114	51	63
64	120	54	66
71	131	59	72
76	136	61	75
81	145	65	80
87	155	70	85
87+	160	72	88

Skill Level 1 The Level 1 classification will be the lowest level of beginning weightlifters who have established reasonable competition lift technique. Ideally these are young athletes, but in many instances, they may be adults. In the latter case, it's very likely that poor mobility may be the primary limiting factor in performance. In these cases in particular, there may also be a large disparity between basic strength levels and technical proficiency if the individual is coming from a previous sport in which strength was developed to a relatively high level.

Skill Level 2 The Level 2 classification will be higher level beginning to lower level intermediate lifters who have some weightlifting training experience, but are still in the relatively early stages of technical learning and development, and most likely in strength development. Ideally these are relatively young athletes, but in many cases they may be adults. In the latter instances, these athletes may have relatively high strength levels in basic movements in comparison to their competition lift performance due to previous athletic training. Such athletes are also likely to have mobility restrictions that limit competition lift performance.

TABLE 33.4 Skill Classification Levels

Level 3 Men			
Bodyweight	Total	Snatch	Clean & Jerk
55	157	71	86
61	180	81	99
67	194	87	107
73	205	92	113
81	222	100	122
89	238	107	131
96	245	110	135
102	252	113	139
109	257	116	141
109+	266	120	146

Level 4 Men			
Bodyweight	Total	Snatch	Clean & Jerk
55	174	78	96
61	204	92	112
67	225	101	124
73	240	108	132
81	262	118	144
89	280	126	154
96	288	130	158
102	295	133	162
109	300	135	165
109+	310	140	170

Level 3 Women			
Bodyweight	Total	Snatch	Clean & Jerk
45	102	46	56
49	109	49	60
55	125	56	69
59	135	61	74
64	140	63	77
71	151	68	83
76	156	70	86
81	163	73	90
87	170	77	94
87+	175	79	96

Level 4 Women			
Bodyweight	Total	Snatch	Clean & Jerk
45	118	53	65
49	128	58	78
55	140	63	77
59	155	70	85
64	160	72	88
71	170	76	94
76	176	79	97
81	180	81	99
87	185	83	102
87+	190	85	105

Skill Level 3 The Level 3 classification will be more advanced intermediate lifters who are bordering on the US national level of competition. They will still be refining their competition lift technique and developing a strength base, and likely have some remaining mobility limitations.

Skill Level 4 The Level 4 classification represents the lower tier of US national competition. These lifters will have a reasonable level of technical proficiency in the competition lifts, but may still have considerable work to do to refine it and develop consistency, especially at higher intensities. They will have decent levels of strength, and that strength will be fairly specific to weightlifting postures and movements. They will have reasonable mobility overall, but may still have limitations in specific local areas. These lifters will also have a reasonable amount of competition experience at the local level, and at least some experience at the national level.

TABLE 33.4 Skill Classification Levels (Cont.)

Greg Everett

Level 5 Men			
Bodyweight	Total	Snatch	Clean & Jerk
55	228	103	125
61	241	108	133
67	270	122	149
73	289	130	159
81	311	140	171
89	330	149	182
96	340	153	187
102	350	157	193
109	360	162	198
109+	376	169	207

Level 6 Men			
Bodyweight	Total	Snatch	Clean & Jerk
55	241	108	133
61	277	125	152
67	287	129	158
73	318	143	175
81	339	153	186
89	360	162	198
96	382	172	210
102	390	175	215
109	398	179	219
109+	414	186	228

Level 5 Women			
Bodyweight	Total	Snatch	Clean & Jerk
45	134	60	74
49	146	66	80
55	165	74	91
59	187	84	103
64	192	86	106
71	202	91	111
76	210	94	116
81	220	99	121
87	223	100	123
87+	240	108	132

Level 6 Women			
Bodyweight	Total	Snatch	Clean & Jerk
45	158	71	87
49	172	77	95
55	195	88	107
59	213	96	117
64	221	99	122
71	236	106	130
76	247	111	136
81	264	119	145
87	270	122	149
87+	278	125	153

Skill Level 5 The Level 5 classification represents the highest level of US national competition. These lifters have significant weightlifting training experience, have a fairly high level of technical proficiency and consistency, and optimal mobility overall. They will also be able to tolerate higher levels of volume, average intensity and training frequency, and will have a relatively large amount of competition experience, and may be competing at least at the lower international level, or at least be in range of making an international team.

Skill Level 6 The Level 6 classification represents lifters of mid-level world championships performance. These lifters have established consistent technique optimal for themselves and reached exceptional strength levels.

TABLE 33.4 Skill Classification Levels (Cont.)

Level 7 Men			
Bodyweight	Total	Snatch	Clean & Jerk
55	285	128	157
61	314	141	173
67	331	149	182
73	346	156	190
81	367	165	202
89	403	181	222
96	413	186	227
102	425	191	234
109	433	195	238
109+	451	203	248

Level 7 Women			
Bodyweight	Total	Snatch	Clean & Jerk
45	180	81	99
49	196	88	108
55	225	101	124
59	237	107	130
64	250	113	138
71	270	122	149
76	287	129	158
81	300	135	165
87	310	140	171
87+	319	144	175

Skill Level 7 The Level 7 classification represents the absolute best of the sport in all aspects of weightlifting performance.

TABLE 33.4 Skill Classification Levels (Cont.)

Training Variables

There are a number of training variables to be manipulated in order to produce desired adaptations, such as intensity, volume, repetitions, interset rest, and exercise selection. These elements will provide all of the necessary control to direct training stimulus and the consequent functional adaptations.

Intensity

Intensity is a measurement of the degree of effort. In the context of weightlifting, the term is very precise—the weight used in a given exercise. This can be represented as absolute intensity—the actual weight, measured in kilograms—or relative intensity—the percentage of the maximal weight of which the lifter is capable in the exercise. For example, an absolute intensity for a snatch might be 120kg, while the relative intensity would be 86% if that athlete's best snatch is 140kg (120/140). Each has its uses, and ideally both are documented in the coach's training records.

Objective Intensity: Objective intensity is an actual numerical value representing either absolute or relative intensity. Intensity prescriptions in a training program may be based on the athlete's best lifts in training, in competition, or even in that training session. What exactly relative intensity prescriptions are based on will of course need to be made clear by the coach.

Subjective Intensity: Subjective intensity is a valuable measurement when used in conjunction with its objective counterpart for evaluating progress, adjusting daily training, and even as a method of loading prescription. Instead of relying on the precision of numbers, subjective intensity describes the intended

loading more vaguely. Basic examples of subjective intensity would be *heavy* or *light*, or even *maximal*. In other cases, intensity may not be prescribed, but simply controlled during the session by the coach according to the intended goals.

This provides guidance regarding the desired loading for the exercise without assigning any actual weights or percentages and allows the athlete to adjust the training according to how he or she is feeling that day while still meeting the objective of the exercise.

Subjective intensity prescriptions are particularly useful with novice lifters who don't have established maximum lifts, or whose maximum lifts, because of the athletes' rapid improvements, are increasing quickly or otherwise unreliable. Similarly, for exercises like pulls, the intensity of which is typically based on the lifter's best snatch or clean, objective intensity may be inadequate because the new lifter's technical proficiency results in competition lift numbers that do not accurately reflect his or her strength. Subjective prescriptions are best accompanied by the observation and guidance of a coach during training.

Additionally, the coach and athlete can use subjective evaluations of intensity to gauge an athlete's recovery or the difficulty of a lift at a given percentage that has not been used previously.

Prescription Intensity can be either the cause or consequence of other training variables, such as the exercise itself and the set and repetition prescription. If the objective is a certain number of repetitions or volume, the reps and sets will be determined as the primary variables, and the intensity will need to be prescribed to accommodate them with respect to the exercise. If the objective is the use of a specific exercise, intensity will be determined according to what is possible and effective in that lift, and to meet the intended loading for that session and microcycle. If the objective is to test or train a maximal lift, the intensity will be the result of the lifter's performance in that session.

There will occasionally be instances with beginning lifters in which enough progress is made in a particular lift that the planned intensity prescriptions become inadequate. In these cases, the subjective intensity concept will allow the athlete and coach to make any alterations to the training plan deemed necessary. For example, if the athlete does not find a prescribed weight difficult when it's expected to be, this subjective evaluation of intensity indicates that the athlete's potential maximum lift has increased enough that the prescriptions based on the existing measured max are too low (In some cases, a cycle may be planned using max numbers that have not been tested recently and consequently may not be accurate.). The loading for the exercise can then be increased until the reps are appropriately difficult. The ability of athletes and coaches to function effectively in such a subjective manner will improve as experience is accumulated.

This problem, of course, is exactly why it's generally advisable to avoid objective intensity prescriptions with beginning lifters; however, they may be used as guidelines for progression, providing the lifter and coach a loose plan for how weights should be increasing or decreasing through a program, even if not followed directly.

Modulation Intensity needs to be varied during given training periods to allow both burdening and recovery. Generally a week of training will involve 2-3 genuinely heavy days and 2-3 somewhat lighter days. These days will alternate in some manner during the week (such as alternating daily, or 2 heavier days followed by 1 lighter day) to allow partial recovery between the heaviest training sessions. This does not mean that the lighter days are not challenging, and in the athlete's state of partial recovery following a heavy training day and with accumulated fatigue from the cycle as a whole, these reduced intensity days can actually be very challenging.

Trend While there will be a necessary fluctuation in intensity within each microcycle, intensity on average will increase over the course of a given macrocycle.

This is the most fundamental point of the training cycle, of course—to build to maximum intensity for single reps in the competition lifts for competition or testing. This increasing intensity is allowed by both the increase of the lifter's fitness in response to the training, and the accompanying decrease in training volume over the course of the cycle.

Average Intensity Average intensity is a figure of relative intensity (a percentage) representing some aggregate of sets. It may refer to all of the sets of a given exercise in a training session, all sets of the entire training session, or a given microcycle or mesocycle.

Adaptation & Purpose Training response will vary according to training intensity and the related repetition numbers and total volume. Consequently, intensity prescriptions reflect the purpose of the exercise at the given point in the training cycle (Table 34.1).

Maximal and Submaximal Intensity This top end range of intensity (90%+) offers unique training adaptation possibilities, but also potential problems. The highest threshold motor units in a muscle can only be recruited in this intensity range, and achieving maximal rate coding and synchronization are likewise only possible with such intensities (Zatsiorsky

Objective	Subjective	Application
50-70%	Light	Technique, speed, recuperative training, warm-up
70-80%	Moderate	Technique, speed-strength, explosive-strength, hypertrophy, absolute strength
80-85%	Moderate-Heavy	Absolute strength, speed-strength, explosive strength, hypertrophy
85-90%	Heavy	Absolute strength, competition lifts
90-95%	Submaximal	Absolute strength, competition lifts
95-100%	Maximal	Absolute strength, competition lifts, testing, competition

TABLE 34.1 General guidelines for intensity. The purpose and appropriateness of each intensity range will vary somewhat with the exercise, repetition range, total volume, lift tempo and interset rest.

Greg Everett

1995). This makes such intensity maximally effective for driving neurological strength adaptations.

However, the volume and frequency of maximal and submaximal intensity lifts needs to be regulated intelligently, as in excess they can produce incomplete recovery and low competition performance (Medvedyev 1986/1989). Interestingly, the Bulgarian method of training employs this intensity range exclusively. The key factors making this possible are high frequency, very low volume, and long term adaptation to this type of training. Additionally, competition lifts are typically similar to and even lower than training lifts. In short, this approach can be effective with proper implementation for improving competition lifts with appropriate athletes, but will not produce the increase in total in competition seen in more traditional training programs.

Technical Consistency Threshold This term refers to the intensity at which a given lifter's technical execution of the snatch, clean or jerk begins to break down and become unreliable. As lifters progress, the technical consistency threshold will increase in both absolute and relative terms as technical mastery improves and training shores up imbalances and weaknesses; that is, they will be consistent at heavier weights, but also at higher percentages of their best lifts.

Consistent Minimum The minimum weight an athlete is capable of lifting in a given lift in a given period of time when making appropriately heavy or maximal attempts. This is a baseline of ability that measures preparedness. For example, a lifter's maximum snatch may not measurably increase during a period of training, but he or she should have a higher consistent minimum relative to previous training cycles, indicating an improved baseline capacity.

Waves In some cases, intensity may be prescribed in repeated series of ascending weights. Rather than a uniform weight across the total number of sets, or ascending weights from the first to last sets, a series of 2-3 consecutive sets with ascending weights can be repeated. For example, a lifter might snatch singles at 80-83-86% and repeat the series 3 times for a total of 9 singles. Another variation is to increase the intensity for each repetition of the series—for exam-

ple, 80-83-86-82-85-88-84-87-90%. This variation is often an effective way to bring a lifter to a heavy lift he or she struggles to reach mentally. A final variation to either of the previous would also involve a change in repetitions during the wave—for example, 75% x 3, 80% x 2, 85% x 1. See the Waves heading below in the Repetitions section for more information.

Repetitions

Repetitions are the number of times a lift is performed in a single series, or set. Repetition prescription will be a primary determinant of training effect, but cannot function independently of intensity. A set of 3 reps doesn't necessarily encourage a particular adaptation—three reps of a given exercise at 80% will produce a very different effect than three reps at 50%, for instance. However, legitimate uses may exist for a certain number of repetitions across a spectrum of intensity even with a single exercise. For example, 3 reps at 50% can be used for dynamic work to train speed or as a warm-up set; at 70%, it can function as technical work, providing enough weight to require and allow proper movement, or to train explosive- and speed-strength; at 80% it can train explosive- and speed-strength and absolute strength; and at 90% plus, it can train absolute strength or serve as testing. In short, the effect of a given number of repetitions will depend primarily on intensity, lift tempo and the exercise.

Technical Complexity Generally speaking, the more technically complex a lift, the lower the repetitions that will, and should, be prescribed. The competition lifts, representing the highest technical complexity, will be employed nearly exclusively in the 1-3 repetition range; in contrast, squats may run the range from 1 to 10+ repetitions; lifts like snatch and clean pulls with intermediate technical complexity will generally reside in the 2-5 repetition range.

Repetition Ability Range The ability to perform repetitions at a given intensity in a given exercise varies among lifters. One lifter, for example, may be capable of squatting 90% for 4 reps, while another can only manage 2. This is primarily an issue of neurological efficiency—the higher a lifter's neurological efficiency, the fewer repetitions he or she will be capable of at a given intensity. This is not because the lifter has a low capacity for performing repetitions, but because he or she has a high capacity for lifting heavier weights through more advanced neurological adaptation; that is, he or she is able to generate more force with a given mass of muscle, making each repetition at a given intensity more difficult and taxing relative to the less efficient lifter.

Neurological efficiency increases with training experience. Beginning lifters will have low efficiency relative to advanced lifters, and consequently be capable of higher repetitions at a given intensity. Women also tend to have lower neurological efficiency than men due to the differences in testosterone levels; this difference is less pronounced in beginners as the efficiency across the board is so low. The nature of training will influence a lifter's neurological efficiency as well—the more time a lifter trains with higher intensities and lower repetitions, the higher his or her efficiency, and the better he or she will be at lifting high intensities with low repetitions; in contrast, a lifter who spends more time training with relatively high repetitions will have less neurological adaptation for maximal singles and be more capable of performing multiple repetitions at a given intensity.

Waves In some prescriptions, repetitions (and likely the associated intensity) will fluctuate among a series of sets, such as repeating sets of 3, 2 and 1 reps. The most common reason for doing this is to stimulate greater neurological activity with a higher intensity single (the single rep minimizes fatigue and maximizes neurological stimulation) and then follow it with a multiple-rep set (e.g. 3-6 reps). Following the stimulating single, the athlete will typically be capable of using more weight in the multiple-rep set. Using ascending waves, increasing the weight of both the single and subsequent multiple-rep set each time the pair is repeated, is a potentially effective way to allow the lifter to handle more weight in the multiple-rep sets that are the primary focus of the workout.

Back-Off Sets Also known as drop sets, if lower-intensity higher-rep sets follow high intensity singles, the lifter will typically be capable of handling more weight due to the neurological stimulation of the preceding heavy lifts as long as those sets are not of a volume sufficient to create too much fatigue.

Repetition Ranges

1-3 Reps Repetition numbers in the 1-3 range can generally be considered ideal for training absolute strength, speed-strength and explosive-strength. Strength gains are largely if not exclusively due to neurological adaptation (i.e. improved motor unit recruitment, rate coding, synchronization, and intermuscular coordination) due to the high intensity.

High intensity does not allow maximal speed or power (maximal power levels are generally seen in the 70-85% range). Speed-strength and explosive-strength are trained with more moderate intensity that would allow the performance of more than 1-3 repetitions; however, the lower repetitions in a set avoid the accumulation of fatigue that would prevent maximal speed and explosiveness.

While reps in the 1-3 range tend not to elicit significant muscular hypertrophy, this can be changed through manipulation of volume. 2-3 reps performed for 10-12 sets can in fact produce gains in functional muscle mass for some lifters.

This repetition range is ideal for the competition lifts and related exercises, the heaviest pulling variations, and heavy squatting.

4-6 Reps Repetition numbers in the 4-6 range will still encourage considerable strength gains—although not to the same degree as 1-3 reps—but will generally encourage more hypertrophy. This is the basis for the classic 5x5 and 6x6 strength programming—it's an attempt to balance strength and mass gains.

Reps	Application
1-3	Absolute strength, speed-strength, explosive-strength, speed, technique, competition lifts
4-6	Myofibrillar hypertrophy, absolute strength, youth/beginner strength
7-15	Sarcoplasmic hypertrophy, stamina, tendon strengthening, rehabilitation, youth strength

TABLE 34.2 General repetition guidelines

Greg Everett

There are two types of muscular hypertrophy—myofibrillar and sarcoplasmic. Myofibrillar hypertrophy is the result of aggregation of contractile proteins within the muscle fiber—that is, it's an increase in the quantity of functional structures in the muscle, which is accompanied by increased contractile capacity. Sarcoplasmic hypertrophy is instead an increase of intracellular fluid and aggregation of non-contractile protein structures—that is, the force-generation potential of the muscle fiber doesn't increase concomitantly with its volume. For certain activities, this type of adaptation is of value, but for the weightlifter is of relatively little use and counterproductive in the sense that it increases bodyweight without proportional increases in strength. Reps in the 4-6 range will encourage more myofibrillar than sarcoplasmic hypertrophy.

It's often stated that this rep range is ideal for power training because the loading allows the correct relationship between force and velocity. However, with technically complex lifts such as the snatch and clean & jerk, or any speed-based movement, neurological freshness diminishes quickly and despite the typically corresponding loading being ideal, speed and technique will suffer during the final few reps. For this reason, skilled power and speed training should generally be kept to the 1-3 rep range as noted previously, but with appropriate loading.

This range is appropriate for less technically complex strength-oriented exercises like squatting and pressing variations, and even pulling variations at times. It can also be appropriate for the earliest technique learning stage, especially with young lifters.

7-15 Reps Repetition numbers in the 7-15 range will most effectively produce local muscular stamina, sarcoplasmic hypertrophy and result in comparatively little strength gain, except in formerly sedentary individuals, who will respond positively to nearly any physical activity, and in young athletes.

However, this higher repetition range is effective for strengthening tendons, which do not progress as quickly as their associated muscles. This is a legitimate rationale for periods of higher repetitions in certain exercises like squatting and pressing variations.

This repetition range is appropriate for tendon strengthening, bodybuilding work, ab and back training, and youth training.

Sets

A set is a single series of repetitions performed without significant rest. The number of sets performed will be a product of the interrelated effects and demands of intensity, repetitions, volume, the type of the exercise, and the goal of the exercise at that time. The more advanced a lifter, generally the more sets will be performed, as the lifter will require higher volume to elicit adaptation. The lower the repetitions, the higher the number of sets to a point: once intensity reaches a high enough level, it will limit the possible number of sets. For example, a lifter may do 3 sets of 2 reps or 6 sets of 1 rep at 90%; but at 95%, he or she may be incapable of more than 2-3 sets of 1, and at 100%, it should be apparent that no more than a single set of a single rep is possible. If relatively low reps are being used for speed training, the intensity will be low, and consequently, many sets will be both possible and desirable. Finally, if hypertrophy is the goal, a higher number of sets, despite high repetition numbers, will be necessary to achieve a higher total of work, although with an appropriate intensity to accommodate this.

Prilepin's Table Soviet sports scientist A.S. Prilepin, using data from the training regimens of high-caliber weightlifters in the 60s and 70s, developed a table of intensity, rep and set relationships intended to describe what was assumed to represent optimal training (Table 34.3). The utility of this chart is limited, however, because of its broad ranges and the lack of specificity regarding the athlete and exercise; that is, it makes no distinction among skill level (although it can be assumed, based on its origin, to apply to advanced lifters), age, bodyweight, neurological efficiency, or any other factor that determines an in-

Intensity	Reps	Volume	Range
70%	3-6 reps	18 reps	12-24 reps
80%	2-4 reps	15 reps	10-20 reps
90%	1-2 reps	10 reps snatch / 7 CJ	4-10 reps

TABLE 34.3 Prilepin chart (Medvedyev 1986/1989)

dividual's need or capacity for volume, or between types of exercises, such as competition lifts, squats and pulls. Nevertheless, it can be consulted as a general check of the basic validity of certain training prescriptions or as a simple starting point for prescribing reps and sets for certain intensities.

Super Sets & Compound Sets Compound sets are sets of two or more different exercises performed in sequence rather than with the completion of all sets of one exercise before moving on to the next. For the weightlifter, this will generally be used only for accessory work like bodybuilding and trunk work, and often more as a way to keep this training efficient and minimize time requirements. A super set is simply a compound set in which no rest is taken between exercises in a given set.

Compound sets can be prescribed by organizing the exercises with letters and numbers indicating grouping and order—the letter indicates the group, while the number indicates the order in which each exercise is performed—and noting rest periods between each exercise within the set and between each set. For example:

A1. Weighted Back Extension – 3 x 10; 30 sec rest
A2. Hanging Leg Raise – 3 x 15; 1 min rest

would describe a compound set of back extensions and hanging leg raises. After the first set of back extensions, the athlete would rest 30 seconds, then perform the first set of hanging leg raises, and then rest 1 minute before repeating this compound set two more times. If the rest intervals are not important, rest times can be omitted and the athlete allowed to move between exercises freely, or they can be prescribed as a superset in which each group of sets of all exercises are performed without rest in between, but with rest after each group. If another compound set were to follow, we would restart the numbering with the letter *B* to describe the new group.

Volume

Volume & training load (sometimes called tonnage or workload) are figures that represent the quantity of training in a given period of time. Volume refers simply to the total number of reps performed (for a single exercise, in a training session, over the course of a week, or during a mesocycle, for example), while training load combines volume with intensity. Within this book, the term *volume* will mean the specific definition of total reps.

Volume is calculated by multiplying the number of reps by the number of sets; training load would then multiply that by the intensity. For example, volume and training load for a workout of 5 sets of 3 squats at 150 kg would be calculated as:

Volume: 5 x 3 = 15 reps
Training Load: 5 x 3 x 150kg = 2250kg

When calculating volume and training load, only working sets are included—that is, warm-up sets are ignored, as they have no significant effect on the athlete. This may mean a minimum intensity of 60-70% depending on the coach or source (in this book, 70% is the threshold with discretionary exceptions based on the demand and nature of the exercise). Accessory work like ab and back or bodybuilding is rarely if ever factored into this number, although its presence and approximate sense of volume needs to be considered in the overall planning and assessment of a program.

However, the coach will need to exercise discretion with each program because a certain lift may be prescribed in a way that results in a relative intensity below the threshold, but the volume should be accounted for. An example of this would be prescribing good morning or stiff-legged deadlift intensities based on the athlete's back squat—this will typically result in relative intensities in the 20-60% range, but the actual loading of the exercise warrants inclusion in volume calculations. In other cases, certain technical drills may employ relatively low intensity (50-70%), yet be taxing enough on the lifter that it's reasonable to consider them contributing to the total volume.

Relationship to Intensity The fundamental concept that needs to be kept in mind with regard to volume is that the higher the intensity, the lower the volume will necessarily be. This should be intuitively obvious to some extent, and will be reflected quite naturally in most programming efforts without conscious consideration. For example, few coaches or athletes would expect to be able to perform as many reps and sets at 90% as they would at 75%. An exception is the occasional "shock" microcycle, used very infrequently, that will employ both very high volume and high intensity.

Modulation Like intensity, volume needs to be modulated to some extent during a given microcycle to allow partial recovery and continued performance through a training cycle. Accordingly, we ensure that both intensity and volume fluctuate to an extent that allows adequate recovery from preceding higher volume workouts before the next. (Note that adequate recovery does not mean complete recovery; an athlete will not recover completely during a given training cycle, because that entire cycle is in a sense a single extended training stimulus.) Typically days of higher volume will alternate with days of lower volume, although like intensity, slightly different patterns like 2 days of higher volume and 1 day of lower volume may be used, or a series such as moderate-high-low in consecutive days.

Trend Over the course of a macrocycle, volume will decrease on average. However, it will not necessarily decrease weekly—volume may fluctuate week to week within a mesocycle, but with a trend of higher to lower overall, or may even remain approximately the same for 2-4 weeks before being reduced. How exactly volume changes within a mesocycle will depend on several factors, both of the program and the athlete.

Volume may also increase during certain periods of a training cycle. For example, if an athlete has just finished an extensive cycle emphasizing high intensity, low volume competition lifts, or has just completed a major competition and taken time off of training, it may take a few to several weeks to gradually increase weekly volume to the desired level for subsequent training.

Over the course of a weightlifter's career, training volume per cycle will increase gradually until reaching the optimal level. The optimal level for each lifter will vary depending on inherent qualities that determine the lifter's capacity and requirements, and on elements such as bodyweight, lifestyle and restoration factors, and the biological age of the lifter at the time of his or her peak is attained. As a lifter continues training past his or her physiological peak, training volume will decline from its peak to remain optimal for the time in question.

Progression Even with the nearly infinite possibilities regarding precise volume prescriptions, some loose guidelines can be used to steer planning. After determining the total volume for a particular mesocycle, it needs to be distributed into each microcycle according to the desired modulation and average reduction over the course of the mesocycle.

A loose rule with weekly volume reductions during a preparation mesocycle would be to reduce each week's volume approximately 10-15% per week relative to the previous week. For example, if week 1 contained 300 reps, week 2 would contain 255-270 reps.

However, if starting with a total volume for the preparation mesocycle, which is ideal, volume may be distributed into the microcycles with the following percentages of the total (Medvedyev 1986/1989), which will result in essentially the same numbers as above: Week 1 – 30%; Week 2 – 27%; Week 3 – 23% - Week 4 – 20%. In a mesocycle with 1000 total reps, for example, this would result in weekly volume of 300-270-230-200 reps.

The order of the middle week distributions may also be reversed: 30%-23%-27%-20%. This is advisable with very high volume mesocycles, as it provides somewhat more chance for recovery between the two weeks of highest volume, but still maintains the trend of reducing volume on average over the duration of the mesocycle.

Finally, it's possible in certain mesocycles to maintain the same or approximately the same microcycle volume for up to around 3-4 weeks before reducing significantly in the last week. An example distribution of volume with this approach is 27%-27%-27%-19% or 28%-28%-28%-16%. This can work well for simple intensity progressions in preparation mesocycles in which total volume is not extremely high.

Skill Level	Preparation Mesocycle	Weekly Average	Competition mesocycle	Weekly Average
1	630	158	n/a	n/a
2	822	206	n/a	n/a
3	1167	292	749	187
4	1511	378	964	241
5	1710	428	1196	299
6	1917	479	1273	318
7	2123	531	1350	338

TABLE 34.4 Volume guidelines based on skill level as described in Table 33.4

Competition mesocycles should typically contain approximately 65-75% of the volume of the preceding preparation mesocycle; however, the lower the total training volume in the macrocycle, the less dramatic the reduction will need to be. For a competition mesocycle, Medvedyev (1986/1989) recommends the weekly volume progression of 35%-28%-22%-15%.

In all cases, these percentages can be adjusted a few points in either direction as needed to still achieve the same basic effect. Similar progressions and distributions can be achieved with adjustments to shorter or longer mesocycles.

Recovery Generally speaking, training volume will be more taxing on a lifter's restorative abilities than intensity. That is, it's more common for a lifter to become overtrained with very high volume and moderate intensity than with very low volume and high intensity (an extreme piece of evidence of this is the Bulgarian style of training). If a lifter is unable to manage a certain training program, it's advisable to reduce volume rather than intensity (Medvedyev 1986/1989).

Missed Lifts Missed lifts in training should generally be considered in the calculations of the training volume. Despite being unsuccessful, the attempt at a lift requires essentially the same effort and consequently has the same effect on fatigue. Exceptions are attempts that are aborted before any significant

work has been performed (e.g. a clean that is stopped before the bar reaches the knees).

Volume Prescriptions Because of the incredible possible variation among athletes and circumstances, it's impossible to prescribe perfectly formulaic volume figures. It's important to reiterate that training volume, like most other elements, must be prescribed individually to maximize effectiveness. Table 34.4 provides guidelines that can be used as starting points based on the lifter's skill level, as described in Table 33.4 in the Assessment chapter. These figures consider only weights of 70% and heavier with the exception of exercises that according to the coach's discretion warrant inclusion (e.g. good mornings, presses and jumps).

Figures in the first two levels will not accurately reflect the total work, therefore, as much of the training in these stages is very light technique work, while despite constituting a significant number of repetitions, cannot be accounted for in the same way as heavier lifting (these figures do not include GPP training, such as repetitions of jumps). The Skill Level 1-2 sample programs will provide a sense of reasonable volume of all work.

Interset Rest Periods

Rest periods between sets should primarily reflect the intention of the exercise in that given training session, but can also be manipulated to somewhat alter the training effect of the same exercise, intensity, sets and reps.

For weightlifting, interset rest can typically be ad libitum—whatever the lifter feels is appropriate—as most will naturally rest according to need. If a certain lifter proves to exercise poor judgment with regard to rest periods (most commonly, resting too long), rest times can be prescribed.

Recuperation between sets involves two components: the replenishment of ATP (the molecule that directly provides energy for muscular contraction) in the muscles and the refreshing of the nervous system. Following a set, approximately 50-70% of ATP levels are restored within 20-30 seconds, and 100% in approximately 3 minutes (Bompa 1999). However,

CNS recovery can take considerably longer depending on the nature of the exercise and the intensity. When training primarily for neurological adaptations (absolute, speed and explosive strength, as well as technical mastery), as is done with weightlifting, neurological freshness for each set is typically desirable, requiring somewhat longer rest periods generally; this does not mean genuinely complete recovery between all sets, which is usually impossible in a practical sense, but maximizing freshness within the constraints of a given training session.

In general, the higher the technical complexity, higher the intensity, and lower the reps, the longer the rest period necessary for an exercise. For such lifts, rest times of 3-5 minutes are advisable. For lower intensity, lower complexity, higher-rep lifts, rest times of 2-3 minutes may be adequate. Moderately technical but very taxing lift sets (such as very difficult sets of 3-6 reps in the squat) will typically demand relatively long rest periods due to a combination of CNS and ATP restoration needs. Absolute maximum single-rep lifts can require as much as 10-15 minutes of rest for complete recovery (Zatsiorksy 1995); however, genuine maximal lifts will very rarely be performed in the gym, and when they are, they will likely not be followed by subsequent sets of the same exercise at the same intensity.

Beginning lifters will require less interset rest than advanced lifters with any combination of exercise, intensity and repetitions due to their lower neurological development and consequent inability to perform truly neuromuscularly demanding work.

Competition Preparation In competition mesocycles, it often makes sense to limit interset rest to 2 minutes between snatch and clean & jerk sets to condition lifters both physically and mentally for the sometimes quick pacing of competition. This may be done throughout the entire mesocycle, or limited to certain training days.

On The Minute Sets A notable exception to the rule of longer interset rest between high complexity lifts is the on-the-minute protocol for the snatch, clean, jerk and clean & jerk. This protocol was popularized in the US by coach Joe Mills with his 20/20 program.

The primary benefit to training the competition lifts on the minute is the technical consistency it nearly always creates. This is largely due to the inability of the lifter to think due to the brevity of rest between sets, and consequently to learn to rely on ingrained motor patterns rather than conscious thought to execute the lifts. A convenient collateral benefit is the ability to do a large number of sets without a proportionally large investment of time.

While this protocol contradicts the rule of longer rest for technically complex lifts, it seems to be possible and successful because intensities will be below maximal and submaximal, a more advanced lifter's competition lift technique is already established enough to require somewhat less CNS work, and the single repetition per set further minimizes the demand on the CNS. The high frequency itself seems to bolster the athlete's ability physically, and the consequent loss of adequate time and energy to think and worry about the upcoming lift contributes greatly to the success of each lift; this loss of conscious brain work also likely contributes to the overall lower CNS demand.

This approach is generally not appropriate for beginning lifters whose technique in the competition lifts is not adequately established. For superheavyweight lifters, rest may need to be increased to 90-120 seconds, particularly for cleans or clean & jerks, which will still provide similar results. Generally, using 1 minute rest for clean & jerks rather than performing them on the minute will allow the same basic effect but will be a more reasonable expectation with regard to conditioning.

Accessory Work For bodybuilding work and trunk strength and stability training, brief rest periods are appropriate. The complexity and intensity is very low, and limited rest will typically elicit a greater hypertro-

Shorter Rest	Longer Rest
Lower complexity	Higher complexity
Lower intensity	Higher intensity
Higher reps	Lower reps
Hypertrophy, conditioning	Strength, speed, explosiveness

TABLE 34.5 General interset rest guidelines

phic response. Additionally, it's often necessary or at least useful to maximize the efficiency of this kind of training to minimize the time demand.

Repetition Tempo

Prescription of tempos for lift execution is rare in weightlifting. As has been discussed elsewhere, maximal acceleration and speed in concentric movements should nearly always be employed by weightlifters to maximize development of speed-strength and explosive-strength. The less slow tempo training used in a program, the greater the development of speed-strength will be (Laputin & Oleshko 1982/2007). It should be noted that with high intensities, actual movement speed and acceleration will be limited unavoidably; however, the lifter must still attempt to apply maximal acceleration and speed, as this will still elicit the proper neurological adaptation.

In certain cases, it may be desirable to control the tempo of a lift to elicit certain responses. This will primarily apply to accessory work like back and abdominal training, or in some cases of weight gain and the like, to certain squatting, pressing and pulling variations. A simple way to reap the benefits of longer set time and greater work through reduced rep speed for the sake of hypertrophy without risking a loss of speed is to slow the eccentric movement, but perform the concentric movement with maximal acceleration and speed as usual.

Slow Eccentrics The most common use of repetition tempo prescriptions with primary training exercises is for slow eccentrics with lifts like pulls, deadlifts and squats. This can aid particularly in the development of postural strength in the specific positions necessary; in particular this can be helpful for improving back arch strength in the pull. Generally eccentric tempos for this purpose will be between 3-5 seconds, but may be as long as 10 seconds, with normal (i.e. fast) concentric speeds.

Compensatory Acceleration Compensatory acceleration is an approach to lift execution developed by Dr. Fred Hatfield. In any given lift, the leverage changes through the range of motion, resulting in different demands on force production by the muscles at different points—that is, one segment of the movement will be far more difficult than another. A simple example of this phenomenon is the squat—the same weight is much easier to move in the top of the squat than in the bottom, and particularly in the range around a horizontal thigh orientation. Compensatory acceleration is the application of maximal speed throughout a lift, which will mean greater speed through the ranges of better leverage, sustaining the maximal possible force production for better neurological adaptation; as resistance decreases due to better leverage, speed increases to maintain force levels (Hatfield 1989). This attempt to maintain maximal speed throughout the concentric segment of strength lifts should be employed by weightlifters at all times unless there is a specific and compelling reason not to.

Notation Australian strength coach Ian King developed a simple notation system for tempos that used three digits to describe the speed of the eccentric and concentric portions and time between the two. More recently this has evolved to include a fourth digit to describe the pause between the end of one rep and the beginning of the next. Each digit prescribes the number of seconds the segment is to take, with an X indicating maximal speed (most commonly used in the concentric phase position). The numbers prescribe the eccentric-pause-concentric-pause durations. For example, a tempo prescription of 30X0 would indicate a 3-second eccentric, no pause, a maximal speed concentric, and no pause before the next rep. If the pause between reps is not important, the fourth digit can be omitted. In cases in which only the eccentric speed needs to be prescribed, it can simply be noted alongside the exercise in the program (e.g. *5 second eccentric after last rep*).

Training Frequency

Training frequency refers to the number of training sessions in a given period of time—typically this will be weekly (microcycle). The frequency of training sessions will depend on several factors: the lifter's biological age, the lifter's level of development, the

Lower Frequency	Higher Frequency
Lower Skill Level	Higher Skill Level
Older/Younger	Ideal Age
Higher Volume	Lower Volume
Nearer Competition	Farther From Competition
Strength/hypertrophy emphasis	Competition lift/ technical emphasis

TABLE 34.6 Factors influencing training frequency

Skill Level	Frequency
Low	3-4 sessions/week
Moderate	5-6 sessions/week
High	Up to 12 session/week

TABLE 34.7 Training frequency guidelines (Medvedyev 1986/1989)

nature of the training cycle, the volume and average intensity of the training cycle, the proximity to competition, and the lifter's possible training schedule (Table 34.6). The higher the volume and average intensity in a microcycle and mesocycle, the greater the need for daily and weekly modulation of volume and intensity will become to maintain higher frequency training.

The training frequency that is possible will be largely dependent on the nature of the training. Heavy weightlifting can be performed very frequently with sufficiently low volume; higher volume training will force more recuperation time between sessions, greater modulation of volume and intensity among sessions, and greater exercise variety day to day.

Within a microcycle, a lifter will not achieve complete recovery between training sessions, but this is not the goal. An entire training cycle will involve the continual accumulation of training fatigue, although with periods of partial recovery between sessions, microcycles and mesocycles to prevent it from becoming overwhelming and counterproductive.

To maximize productivity with higher training frequency, some degree of variation in volume, intensity and movement patterns will be necessary among training sessions as was discussed previously with regard to volume and intensity. Because training fatigue is largely specific to movement patterns—both neurologically and physiologically—variations in exercises in consecutive days and training sessions will allow more productive training at high frequency. For example, a day that emphasizes pulling movements (competition lifts, pulls, deadlifts) is commonly followed by a day that emphasizes pushing movements (squats, jerks, overhead strength work).

In a Bulgarian-style training program, where the exercise variety is virtually non-existent and volume is very low, the primary variation will be of intensity. This is typically allowed to occur naturally rather than as a prescription, so that even if every training session is of maximal effort, the actual intensity fluctuates according to the lifter's present state of recovery. Generally with lifters trained over the long term with such an approach, this manifests as alternating days of higher and lower intensity, although the more specific training experience possessed by the lifter, the smaller the magnitude of fluctuation will be.

A loose guidline for training frequency can be seen in Table 34.7. Note that at the highest frequency levels, multiple training sessions per day will be necessary.

Workout Timing

The time of training sessions is a variable that can be manipulated for subtle changes in effect, although realistically athletes' training schedules will be dictated more by availability—theirs and those of the training facilities—than anything else. Physical capacity does fluctuate throughout the day, so ideally lifters can exploit this to some degree. Mobility will be worst in the morning and generally improve as the day proceeds. Strength is typically highest between 11:00am—2:00pm and 6:00pm—9:00pm (Laputin & Oleshko 1982/2007). Training during these windows is optimal.

It's important to maintain a buffer of 2-3 hours between heavy training and bedtime, as it will take a significant period of time for the athlete to relax following a significant workout.

Competition Preparation If a lifter's session in an upcoming competition will be at a time of day at which he or she is unaccustomed to training, it can be helpful to train at or near this time in the weeks leading into the competition. This applies for instances of time change as well in which the athlete will not be at the competition location to reasonably adjust to the time (usually 1 day per hour of time difference is needed to adapt). This can mean training at hours of the day that aren't possible or practical—in such cases, the lifter can get as close as possible and/or limit the practice to 1-2 days each week.

Exercise Selection

Exercises should be chosen primarily and overwhelmingly for their ability to most effectively deliver the necessary training responses. Exercise variety is a secondary concern, although it is an important consideration. For the weightlifter, very little divergence from the competition lifts, variations of the competition lifts (e.g. hang, block, complexes), and specific strength exercises (squatting, pulling, pressing) will exist.

Priority	Exercise	Presence
Primary	Competition lifts, significant variations (e.g. hang, block, power)	Always present
Secondary	Squats, pull variations; high priority technique work	Usually present; more in preparation mesocycles
Tertiary	Significant overhead work (e.g. push press, overhead squat, snatch balance); low priority technique work	More in preparation meso; reduces over duration of macrocycle

TABLE 34.8 Exercise priority classification

The core exercises for all weightlifters will always be the competition lifts. The next most common group includes squats, snatch and clean pulls and variations (e.g. partial pulls, segment pulls, pulls from risers, deadlifts, etc.). Finally on the periphery are less common competition and strength lift variations, overhead and pressing exercises (e.g. push press, press, snatch push press, overhead squat, snatch balance), and others that will be used by the fewest weightlifters and least frequently.

Accommodation & Variation Part of the underlying biology of training adaptation is the requirement for stimuli to remain unfamiliar to the body. Accommodation occurs when training stimulus does not change adequately to necessitate adaptation in response—at this point, such training will fail to stimulate progress.

Because the need for specificity in weightlifting is so great, relatively little of the variation required to stimulate adaptation will or can be derived from changes in exercise selection, at least in dramatic ways. Primarily the variety will come from changing volume and intensity—increasing volume over the course of a career until reaching the optimal level, and increasing average intensity indefinitely (until each must begin to be reduced for an aging athlete if a career lasts long enough).

Variations of basic lifts are possible without sacrificing the effectiveness, and if chosen intelligently, can increase effectiveness by addressing specific needs of the lifter. In fact, this is the only reason exercise selection should vary—to select exercises that will encourage the training responses most needed by the athlete in a given period of time. For example, a lifter who has a problem with improperly shifting his posture in the pull of the snatch off the floor may in a particular mesocycle use segment snatch pulls with a pause right off the floor and at the knee rather than classic snatch pulls. Overall the exercise achieves the same basic goal, but with lifter-specific benefits. In this way, some degree of variation is achieved to combat accommodation, and the training becomes more effective for the athlete.

Variation Among Mesocycles Generally the optimal approach to variation in exercise selection is to employ a somewhat different set of exercises among the mesocycles in a macrocycle. In the competition mesocycle, we will always have primarily if not exclusively the competition lifts, squats and possibly pulls. In preparation mesocycles, more variety is possible and useful. Each subsequent preparation mesocycle will typically use at least slightly different exercises from the previous. In this way, adequate variation can be achieved while also ensuring that each mesocycle properly addresses its goals.

Technique Work The most significantly and frequently varied exercises will often be the technique work performed. The technical remediation needs of the athlete and consequently the exercises selected to address them can change relatively frequently; additionally, it may take several different methods over a period of time to effect significant improvement.

Prioritization Exercises can be classified broadly according to their relative priority. Table 34.8 gives a simple outline of general prioritization. Exercises will need to be prioritized more specifically for each lifter in each macrocycle and mesocycle. If a particular quality in a lifter is lagging behind, it will need to be emphasized more than it usually would in a given mesocycle. For example, a lifter with a very weak squat will need to prioritize squat strength to reduce the disparity. While in a preparation mesocycle, strength lifts are already prioritized to some degree, it's possible to emphasize a specific lift to a greater degree. For example, work on pulling strength may be reduced somewhat in a given preparation mesocycle in order to allow greater volume and intensity in the squat.

Assistance & Accommodating Resistance

As discussed previously in the tempo section, the resistance against which the body is working will vary through the range of a movement as joint angles and leverage change. This results in a gradient of difficulty in any given lift.

One approach to addressing this variation—with the rationale that training effect is reduced because work is not equal throughout the range of motion—is to use accommodating resistance. This involves chains or elastic bands around the barbell to create variable resistance depending on the barbell's position. For example in a squat, bands may be attached to the floor and then around the bar so that as the lifter stands and the leverage of the position improves, the increasing tension of the bands increases the resistance. Similarly, chains may be hung from the bar so that in the bottom of the squat, more of the chain is on the floor and consequently not adding weight to the bar, and as the bar is elevated, more of the chains' weight is added to the bar.

Accommodating resistance is very rarely used in weightlifting, unlike in powerlifting. The primary issue is that every lift has a natural rhythm and tempo—part of successful weightlifting is mastering the nuances of the movement, which includes this natural rhythm based on the naturally changing leverage with different joint angles. Introducing accommodating resistance changes this natural rhythm and feel, and disrupts this neurological learning. It is best reserved for training absolute strength with lifts of limited technical complexity—hence its appropriateness for powerlifting.

More appropriate and effective for weightlifting to train the squat is the use of forced reps. A forced rep is a lift with weight somewhat above what the lifter is capable of that day, using assistance applied by the coach or training partner to help move the bar through the sticking point of the lift, usually around the middle of the range of motion. With this approach, the lifter is able to feel heavier weights, actually lift those heavier weights through the majority of the range of motion, receives the benefit to trunk and joint strength and stability of supporting heavier weights, gains the benefit mentally of improved confidence with heavier weights, and receives only exactly as much assistance as is needed for each rep and only in exactly the position necessary, which is often surprisingly little even for weights that exceed the lifter's best fairly significantly.

Jump Training

Jump training in the context of weightlifting serves three basic purposes: to improve explosiveness, speed and elasticity—the ability to convert the energy of an eccentric motion into subsequent concentric contraction with maximal speed and force. Virtually all movements in weightlifting benefit from improved explosiveness and speed, and elasticity plays a crucial role in the jerk in particular, but also in the clean recovery and in the start of the snatch and clean.

While novices will improve explosiveness and elasticity considerably simply by increasing absolute strength, more advanced lifters must train these qualities directly, as they are no longer even correlated with absolute strength (Zatsiorksy 1995). Weightlifting training, without jump training, naturally involves a significant volume of work that will address and improve these qualities, particularly when performed with proper speed and rhythm. For example, training all lifts with maximal concentric speed, training the squats and clean with a bounce in the bottom, and the dip and drive of the jerk all contribute to improving these traits. However, additional jump training will improve the results for any lifter.

In all jumping exercises, maximal speed is crucial for effectiveness. With loaded exercises like back squat jumps or quarter squat jumps, weights should never exceed what allows an explosive jump or the purpose of the exercise is defeated.

Introduction

All jump training should be introduced to athletes progressively and conservatively; the capacity to tolerate the work must be developed over time with gradually increasing volume, intensity and frequency. Ideally, this foundation is begun in the younger years with properly designed and implemented GPP. If

not, it's very important lifters not make the mistake of incorporating too much too quickly.

Less demanding jump variations should be introduced first, such as box jumps and back squat jumps, gradually increasing in frequency and intensity. Depth jumps should be used only by advanced lifters, and should also be introduced gradually with consideration of the other training being performed.

Programming

Jump training is deceptively taxing neurologically and can very easily be overdone, as it will not create a high perceived rate of exertion like other exercises and consequently lifters are less apt to recognize excessive volume and intensity at the time of performance. It is also considerably stressful to joints and connective tissue, which is why it should be done by lifters who have built the proper foundation with GPP and progressive development; if this has not been done, a gradual and conservative introduction and progression is even more critical.

Box jumps, back squat jumps, jumping squats and quarter squat jumps should generally be done with sets of 3-5 reps for a total of 10-20 reps per session, 1-3 days/week. The higher the intensity and less advanced the lifter, the lower the volume and frequency should be. These jump variations can be used throughout a macrocycle, with reduced volume and intensity as a competition nears.

Depth jumps are the most demanding jump variation and require the most care with regard to implementation. Less advanced lifters should use 2-3 sets of 3-8 reps at lower heights 1-2 days per week, and more advanced lifters can work to as many as 4 sets of 10 reps at greater heights 3 days per week. These jumps can be performed during any phase of training, but in greater volume and frequency in preparation mesocycles than competition mesocycles, and are generally best used in the latter half of the preparation period. During the competition mesocycle, the goal is to maintain explosiveness more than develop it; volume should be reduced, frequency should be reduced to once every 7-14 days, and depth jumps should not be performed within 10 days of competition (Laputin & Oleshko 1982/2007, Zatsiorsky 1995, Medvedyev 1986/1989).

Rest periods of 1-2 minutes between lower intensity jumps are adequate; 3-5 minutes of rest will be appropriate for depth jumps.

Jerk Elasticity Training

Aside from jumping exercises, there are a number of lifts that will train elasticity or components of it and have the added benefit of being entirely specific to the jerk. One that is overlooked, underused and even actively avoided is lowering the bar back to the shoulders between multiple reps of the jerk. This movement trains the legs to absorb the force and arrest the downward movement much as they will need to in the dip of the jerk; this movement involves considerably more force than is experienced in the dip itself with a given weight.

The jerk dip exercise is another that increases the downward acceleration of the dip to increase the force the legs must resist, and trains the ability to arrest the downward movement more abruptly. The more abruptly the dip can be stopped, the greater the potential stretch reflex will be.

Finally, the jerk drive exercise allows the dip and drive of the jerk to be loaded beyond the lifter's best jerk, and for the lifter to focus on this segment of the lift. The jerk drive is essentially a jumping exercise in the sense that downward force loads the legs, the legs arrest the movement, and then use the elastic energy to reverse the movement and contract more forcefully to drive upward.

Squat & Jump Complexes

An effective training protocol involves combining squats with jumps. Most commonly, this involves performing a set of box jumps or broad jumps immediately after a set of squats. However, the reverse order can also be used.

There are two possible reasons for the effectiveness of jumping after squatting. The first is *post-activation potentiation*—this is the phenomenon that allows muscles to contract more forcefully following a previous but non-fatiguing contraction (Lorenz 2011). In other words, this is more likely to occur following a heavy single in the squat; multiple heavy reps will more likely induce fatigue sufficient to reduce the forcefulness of subsequent contractions.

The other possibility is that, immediately following a fatiguing set of squats, performing a set of jumps forces the body to recruit higher-threshold motor units or units that have not yet been activated and fatigued; in addition, it may force better synchronization and rate coding in order to produce the voluntary forceful and explosive contraction with fewer fresh motor units available.

Reversing the order and performing a set of jumps, such as unloaded squat jumps, before a set of squats may induce a post-activation potentiation response that aids in contraction force for the squat.

At the very least, combining jumps with squats will teach the lifter to be consciously aggressive in a fatigued state, a critical ability for weightlifting, and make the training session somewhat more efficient.

Box Jump

Typically *box jump* refers to a simple countermovement jump onto a box. However, there are a few useful variations for weightlifting that can be specified in the program prescription.

Ideally all box jump variations are performed without a swing of the arms. While an arm swing will allow the athlete to jump higher, it does so independently of the leg and hip action the exercise is intended to train. By eliminating arm swing, the jump itself can be better emphasized. The hands can be held at the chest to keep them out of the way and not contributing to the jump effort, as well as keeping them immediately available to help in the case of a missed jump or stumble.

Countermovement Jump The countermovement jump is the traditional box jump variation (Figure 35.1). The athlete will stand with the feet in the pulling position or drive position, bend rapidly at the hip and knee, change directions abruptly, and drive maximally against the floor to jump up onto the box. This is a useful exercise for training both explosiveness and elasticity for the second pull of the snatch and clean, and the dip and drive of the jerk.

Non-Countermovement Jump To perform non-countermovement jumps, the athlete will dip into the starting position and pause for 2-3 seconds before initiating the drive against the ground. The athlete must drive from this position immediately and directly—it will be very tempting to sneak in a quick bounce of the legs as the jump begins, which simply creates a countermovement jump from a different starting position. This variation is useful for training explosiveness for the second pull of the snatch and clean, and the drive of the jerk.

Squat Jump In this variation, the athlete will perform a countermovement jump, but rather than a quick and shallow bend of the knees and hips, he or she will sit into a full squat (Figure 35.2). This exercise is useful for training explosiveness and elasticity in the squat, such as for the recovery of the clean.

Non-Countermovement Squat Jump Just like the conventional box jump, the squat jump can be performed without a countermovement to focus only

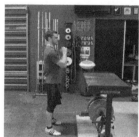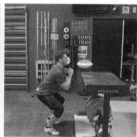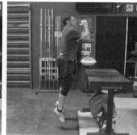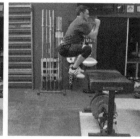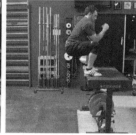

FIGURE 35.1 The conventional box jump is performed with a shallow countermovement, but can also be done from a shallow static starting position with no countermovement.

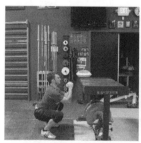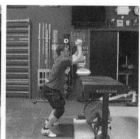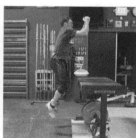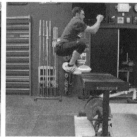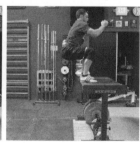

FIGURE 35.2 Box jumps can also be performed with a full squatting motion with and without a countermovement.

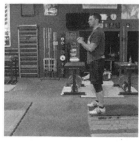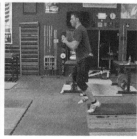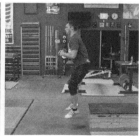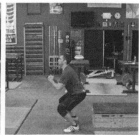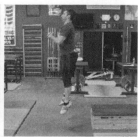

FIGURE 35.3 Depth jumps are the most effective jumping exercise for developing elasticity and explosiveness, but also must be used carefully due to their demanding nature.

on explosiveness without elasticity. The athlete will simply initiate the jump from a static position at the bottom of a squat. This is useful for training explosiveness in the squat, the pull off the floor of the snatch and clean, and the drive of the jerk.

For all box jump variations, box heights should be well within the athlete's ability. As heights approach maximal, athletes tend to cut the drive of the legs short in order to begin lifting the feet (much like as weights get heavier in the snatch and clean, athletes tend to rush into the pull under), which defeats the purpose of the exercise. A somewhat lower box should be used, and the complete and violent extension of the legs and hips emphasized over everything else. This should create a degree of floating onto the box rather than an aggressive reach up with the feet. Conveniently, this method also reduces the risk of injury due to a failed jump.

As much as is possible, the athlete should attempt to jump close to vertically and reach the feet forward onto the box instead of jumping directly forward onto it to prevent any bad habits from appearing in the lifts.

Dropping back to the ground following each jump to absorb the impact in a partial squat can serve conveniently as depth drops to train the legs' ability to absorb force. However, if this may be excessive, or the athlete for any reason needs to minimize impact, he or she should return to the floor after each jump by stepping down one leg at a time, or by planting the hands on the box and using the upper body to slow the drop.

Depth Jump

The depth jump (Figure 35.3) is the classic weightlifting jump exercise created and employed to maximize forceful muscular contraction—it creates more muscular activity in the jump phase following the drop than any other form of training stimulus (Medvedyev 1986/1989). This is also the reason the exercise must be implemented cautiously to avoid excessive volume and intensity.

The athlete will begin standing on a plyo box, step off to drop onto rubber matting on the floor, and as quickly as possible, absorb the drop and jump

vertically to maximal height. The arms should begin behind the body as if already in the back swing so that they may be immediately swung forward in the jump after the drop; the lifter should land on the balls of the feet but allow the heels to drop to the floor (Medvedyev 1986/1989). They can also be performed without an arm swing as described previously for box jumps.

The depth of the leg bend when absorbing the drop will vary among athletes, and will loosely correlate to the relative depth of that athlete's jerk dip; that is, more elastic athletes who employ a shallow dip in the jerk will also have a more shallow bend in the depth jump.

When first introducing depth jumps to an athlete, box heights should be no more than 30-40cm (12-16in) in height; over time, the box height can increase to 50-60cm (20-24in) for lifters over 94kg/69kg and as high as 70cm (28in) for lifters under 94kg/69kg. Reps and sets can be increased to the optimum of 4 sets of 10 reps for advanced lifters following a warm-up of lower effort vertical jumps and depth jumps. (Medvedyev 1986/1989)

Back Squat Jump

The back squat jump is a simple but effective jump exercise that improves general elasticity and explosiveness in the legs, and specifically for the squat and clean recovery. The lifter will hold a barbell behind the neck loaded with approximately 20% of his or her best back squat. The movement is simply a back squat with a rapid change of direction in the bottom and maximal concentric speed to allow the lifter to jump as high as possible. Subsequent repetitions should be performed continuously so that the lifter is utilizing the increased downward force in the eccentric motion due to the drop from the preceding jump. Sets of 3-5 reps are appropriate.

Quarter Squat Jump

The quarter squat jump is a shallow-depth countermovement jump with additional loading, useful for building elasticity and explosiveness for the second pull of the snatch and clean; it is less effective for

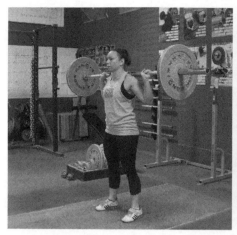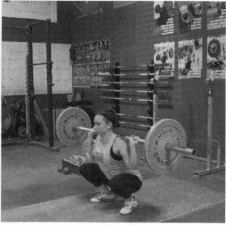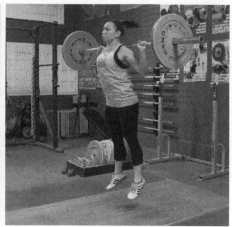

FIGURE 35.4 The back squat jump is a simple and effective exercise for general leg elasticity and explosiveness.

the dip and drive of the jerk because of the posture. With a loaded barbell held in back squat position, the athlete will perform a rapid quarter squat, change directions abruptly, and jump as high as possible. Each rep in a set can be performed from a still standing position rather than in a continuous series. The barbell should be held tightly against the traps to prevent it from moving or crashing onto the lifter when landing, and a belt can be worn to bolster trunk stability. Sets of 3-5 reps are appropriate, and the weight can range from 30-60% of the lifter's best back squat, and potentially heavier; however, the weight must be controlled to ensure relatively high speed in the jump.

Jumping Squat

The jumping squat is essentially a quarter squat jump in which the barbell begins supported on jerk blocks or a power rack. This means the movement is strictly concentric and all potential assistance in the concentric phase from a stretch reflex is eliminated; it also eliminates the need for the lifter to absorb the weight upon landing, which allows greater potential loading without injury risk, and allows somewhat different possible positioning, such as a more upright, knee-dominant posture that will transfer more to the drive of the jerk. The lifter will start the barbell on

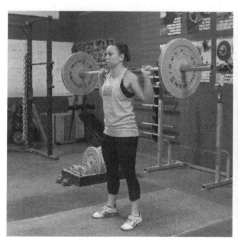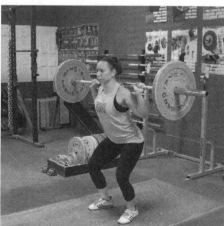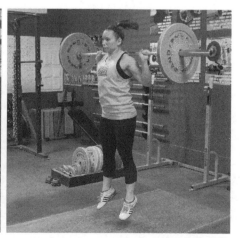

FIGURE 35.5 The quarter squat jump is effective for building elasticity and explosiveness for the second pull of the snatch and clean.

Greg Everett

jerk blocks or the pins of a power rack at a height that places him or her in quarter squat depth or jerk dip depth; the starting posture can be adjusted to resemble the second pull of the snatch and clean or the dip of the jerk depending on the need of the athlete. After pressurizing and stabilizing the trunk and generating some initial tension in the legs, the lifter will drive the bar up to perform a jump, the height of which will be minimal due to the weight, but the effort of which must be maximal. Upon landing, the lifter will drop out from under the bar to allow the jerk blocks or power rack to catch the weight.

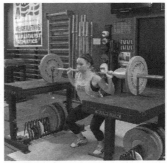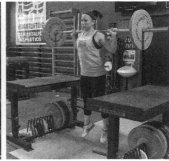

FIGURE 35.6 The jumping squat is a version of the quarter squat jump with only a concentric movement.

Accessory Work

Accessory work includes anything outside of weight-lifting specific training; this generally means trunk strength and stability (abs and back), bodybuilding, and any pre-hab exercises the lifter uses. Such training is not considered in the volume and average intensity calculations for the training cycle as its impact is minimal; this does not mean, however, that it is inconsequential and should not be factored in when considering the effect and demand of the program as a whole.

Trunk Strength & Stability

While the notion of trunk strength and stability typically conjures the abdominals in most athletes' minds, it includes all musculature surrounding the trunk, including the pelvic floor and diaphragm. These latter

Exercise	Activation	Movement	Demand
Good Morning	Isometric	Hip extension	Moderate-High
Stiff-Legged Deadlift	Isometric	Hip extension	High
Romanian Deadlift	Isometric	Hip extension	High
Back Extension	Dynamic	Back Extension	Low-Moderate
Reverse Hyper	Dynamic	Back Extension	Low-Moderate
Back Extension Hold	Isometric	Back Extension	Low
Kettlebell Swing	Isometric	Hip Extension	Moderate
Reverse Plank	Isometric	N/A	Low-Moderate

TABLE 36.1 Back exercises can be categorized according to the type of activation of the back musculature, the type of movement overall, and the degree of demand. Exercises like back extensions and reverse hypers can range from low to moderate demand depending on the presence of additional weight.

two, however, will be trained primarily though the pressurization of the trunk during structural lifting, leaving trunk strength and stability training to focus on the abdominals and back.

The competition lifts and common related exercises such as squatting, pulling and pressing variations inherently provide a considerable workload for the muscles of the trunk; however, additional direct training is necessary to maximize strength and stability. The ability of the lifter to establish and maintain maximal trunk rigidity during the lifts is one of the most critical factors in weightlifting success and injury prevention and its importance should not be underestimated.

Trunk work should be at maximal volume and intensity during preparation mesocycles, and at somewhat reduced volume and intensity during competition mesocycles. It should be minimal during the final week leading into a competition, and more focused on maintenance and activation than development.

Back Training

Back training is relatively straightforward with a limited number of useful exercises. Exercises can be categorized as involving spinal extension, hip extension, or combinations of the two, as well as combinations of isometric activation of one and dynamic activation of the other. They can also be loosely categorized in terms of demand—for example, unloaded back extensions are a very minimally taxing exercise, whereas stiff-legged deadlifts are a considerable training load. Table 36.1 contains a categorized list of the most beneficial back exercises for weightlifting.

Programming Low-demand back exercises can be performed as frequently as daily, while high-demand exercises will be performed less frequently—usually 2-3 days per week. The more demanding exercises are usually best included in training sessions emphasizing heavy pulling movements to allow more time for the lower back to recover before the next training session of this type. Lower-demand exercises will usually be performed with higher repetitions (8-15), and higher-demand exercises with lower repetitions (4-8) for 2-5 sets.

Abdominal Training

Like back exercises, ab exercises can be categorized according to activation and movement type, and intensity or demand to help with prescription. Movement types include spinal flexion, lateral spinal flexion, spinal rotation, hip flexion, and various combinations of these. Activation will either be isometric or dynamic. Demand will be dependent on intensity—generally speaking, the higher the repetitions or

longer the duration, the lower the demand or intensity.

Table 36.2 categorizes the most useful ab exercises for weightlifting, and provides guidelines for intensity and repetitions. Similar to back training, more demanding ab work should be performed in higher volume and intensity training sessions, while less demanding ab work should be performed with lower volume and intensity training sessions. This maximizes recovery and minimizes potential limiting of heavy lifting, and reduces the injury risk thereof, due to fatigued abdominal musculature.

Programming Ab work should be performed daily with the alternation of intensity, volume and movement and activation types. A simple but effective approach is to perform 3-5 sets of Category B followed by 3-4 sets of Category A on heavier training days, and 3-5 sets of Category C, D or E followed by 3-4 sets of Category A on lighter training days. Coaches can prescribe actual exercises if needed, or can sim-

Exercise	Rep Range	Intensity
A - Volume Trunk/Hip Flexion		
Crunch	15-30+	Unweighted
Reverse Crunch	15-30+	Unweighted
Sit-up	15-30+	Unweighted
V-up	15-30+	Unweighted
Jack Knife	15-30+	Unweighted
Knees to Elbows	15-30+	Unweighted
Glute-Ham Bench Sit-up	15-30+	Unweighted
Lying Leg Raise	15-30+	Unweighted
AbMat Sit-ups	15-30+	Unweighted
Ab Wheel	15-30+	Unweighted
Decline Sit-ups	15-30+	Unweighted
Roman Chair Sit-up	15-30+	Unweighted
Twisting Sit-up	15-30+	Unweighted
Hanging Leg Raise with Twist	15-30+	Unweighted

TABLE 36.2 The abdominal training matrix categorizes ab exercises and helps guide prescription.

ply prescribe categories and sets and allow the lifter to select exercises day to day. The latter is a good approach with more advanced lifters who are familiar with training and who make intelligent decisions to increase engagement with the program and allow them some control and variety for a generally unpleasant and tedious component of training.

Bodybuilding

Bodybuilding work may or may not be present in a lifter's program. The newer and younger the lifter, the more appropriate it will be to encourage balanced development around joints, help strengthen tendons

Knees to Elbows with Twist	15-30+	Unweighted
B - Intensity Trunk/Hip Flexion		
Sit-up	8-12	Weighted or difficult enough to limit to prescribed rep range
Hanging Leg Raise	8-15	Weighted or difficult enough to limit to prescribed rep range
Glute-Ham Bench Sit-up	10-15	Weighted or difficult enough to limit to prescribed rep range
Decline Sit-ups	10-15	Weighted or difficult enough to limit to prescribed rep range
Roman Chair Sit-up	10-15	Weighted or difficult enough to limit to prescribed rep range
Twisting Sit-up	10-15	Weighted or difficult enough to limit to prescribed rep range
C - Lateral Trunk Flexion & Isometric		
Side Bend	15-30	Unweighted
Windmill	10-15	Weighted or difficult enough to limit to prescribed rep range
Side plank	15-30 sec	Weight as needed to stay in duration range
Side plank lift	15-30	Weighted or difficult enough to limit to prescribed rep range
D - Trunk Rotation		
Standing Twist	10-30	Weighted
Russian Twist	10-30	Weighted
Windshield Wiper	10-30	Unweighted
Cross-Chop	10-30	Weighted
E - Isometric/Stability		
Plank	10-30 sec	Weight as needed to stay in duration range
Flutter kick	20-50 reps	Unweighted
L-sit	10-30 sec	Weight as needed to stay in duration range
Dead Bug	15-30	Unweighted
Ab Wheel	15-30	Unweighted
Roman Chair Sit-up Holds	10-30 sec	Weight as needed to stay in duration range
Turkish Get-up	3-8	Weight as needed to stay in rep range
Turkish Get-up Sit-up	8-15	Weight as needed to stay in rep range

TABLE 36.2 The abdominal training matrix (cont.)

with the higher-rep, lower-intensity lifting, and build a foundation of muscle mass. In lifters needing to gain weight, it will also be very valuable. It can be helpful, however, for all lifters during preparation mesocycles if dosed and timed appropriately so as to not interfere with the primary training. In the competition mesocycle, bodybuilding work should be reduced in volume relative to the preparation period and possibly eliminated, and eliminated in the last week before a competition.

Simple bodybuilding protocols can be used: 3-6 sets of 8-15 reps for 1-3 exercises per muscle group per session with interset rest periods of 1-2 minutes. More complex methods such as drop sets, supersets and rest-pause sets can be used if desired, and will introduce more variation for greater stimulus. Intensity will be low, although sets may be taken to failure to achieve a greater hypertrophic response. If multiple muscle groups are being trained in a given session, they can be completed in a circuit to minimize the time investment.

Bodybuilding work should be scheduled to match muscle groups to the emphasis of a given training session—generally this can be as simple as the broad categories of legs, upper body pushing, and upper body pulling. For example, a training session with a jerk emphasis is the appropriate time to incorporate bodybuilding pressing exercises. This will maximize the effect and the recovery of the muscles for the next similar training session.

One exception to conventional bodybuilding methods should be to always train through the full range of motion of the joint(s) in question. This will allow the training to contribute to tendon strengthening in addition to hypertrophy, and habitual limited range of motion lifting can set the athlete up for tendonitis and reduced mobility.

Pre-Hab & Activation Exercises

Weightlifting is very demanding on the range of motion and stability of the shoulders and hips in particular. While properly designed training and intelligent long term progression will develop the necessary stability and activation to a large degree, additional direct work can be beneficial. This training can be performed continuously throughout the entire macrocycle. Exercises and protocols can be found in resources dedicated to this subject.

Shoulder Pre-hab & Stability Using elastic bands and/or dumbbells, lifters can perform a number of exercises that train the many muscles involved in stabilizing the shoulder joint. These can be performed as part of the preparation work before a training session to contribute to the warm-up and activation, or along with post-workout accessory training.

Hip Activation Less commonly necessary than shoulder stabilization and pre-hab work, but not uncommon, is glute activation work to help stabilize the hip and allow optimal movement in the squat, pull and dip and drive of the jerk. This is typically performed pre-workout with various elastic band configurations to help the glutes fire properly in the subsequent training session.

Grip Training

For some athletes, grip will be or become a limiting factor in the snatch, and less frequently the clean. As with most other elements, the classic lifts themselves are generally the best exercise for training grip strength for the lifts. The athlete should also ensure he or she is gripping the bar correctly before worrying about additional grip work. However, supplemental grip work can be necessary and helpful at times if a lifter has not had the proper foundational development long term, or for other reasons, such as small hands, is limited in gripping ability relative to other capacities.

Strap use should be cut down as the first step to simply get more grip strength work out of the exercises already being performed. Warm-up snatches and cleans can also be done without the hook grip, and exercises like stiff-legged deadlifts and RDLs should be performed without straps or the hook grip.

If specific grip work is needed, grip exercises can be added to workouts 2-4 days per week.

Grippers

The quickest, easiest and often most effective additional grip work is the use of spring grippers (Figure 36.1). These can even be used in between sets of other non-grip-intensive exercises such as squats to save training time. The athlete should use a gripper weight that he or she is able to close completely for at least 5 reps and do 3-5 sets of maximal reps on each hand, starting with the weaker side. Once 3 sets of 10 reps at a given weight gripper can be done for a few workouts, the next heaviest gripper can be used as long as it can be closed completely for at least 3 reps. If the athlete is able to do only 3-5 reps with this heavier weight, he or she can do 3-4 sets there and then finish with 1-3 sets of up to 10 reps with the next lighter weight. If the transition between weights is too dramatic, the lifter can perform assisted reps on the heavier gauge gripper—that is, close it as much as possible and then use the other hand to help only as much as needed to close it the rest of the way for the desired number of reps. The athlete can alternate between simply performing the reps and doing some or all reps with a hold in the closed position.

Plate Pinching

Bumper plates can be used with a pinch grip in a few different ways (Figure 36.2). First is simply to pinch grip the plate and hold it for a pre-determined duration or as long as possible. Another is to perform farmer walks with a plate pinch gripped in each hand; this can be made more difficult by holding two plates in a single hand, especially metal plates that slide easily against each other. Walking will introduce some additional and uneven force the hands must resist.

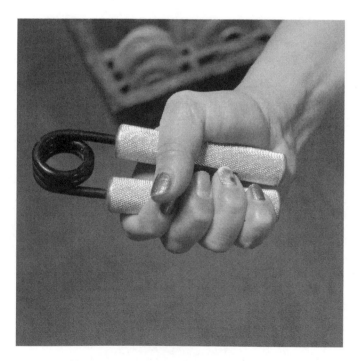

FIGURE 36.1 Spring grippers are a simple way to improve grip strength.

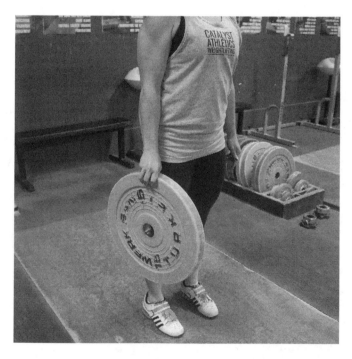

FIGURE 36.2 Plates can be pinch gripped for time, carried in a pinch grip during farmer walks, or tossed or flipped and caught.

Finally, a plate can be held in a pinch grip and tossed up slightly or flipped to be caught again in a pinch grip to add more downward force.

Snatch Grip Hangs

The classic hang from a pull-up bar for developing grip strength is a reasonable exercise, but is not specific enough for a couple of basic reasons. First, because of the possible durations for most athletes, it's far more of a stamina exercise than a strength exercise. More importantly, the primary issue is the increased force and weaker hand position in the snatch due to the wide grip. Using a snatch grip in the hang will improve the effectiveness of the exercise.

If the available pull-up bars are not similar enough in diameter to a barbell, or are not wide enough to accommodate a snatch-width grip, a barbell can be placed with each end in a squat rack so that the lifter can hang from the bar between the racks with a full snatch-width grip (the knees can be bent and lifted to bring the feet off the floor). (Figure 36.3)

An additional benefit of this exercise is that it provides decompression for the spine after heavy lifting.

Snatch Grip Holds & Shrugs

As an alternative to snatch grip hangs, and possibly preferable because of the more easily adjusted resistance, the lifter can perform standing snatch grip holds with a loaded barbell, or shrugs using slight leg drive to increase the force, both without straps or the hook grip (Figure 36.4). The bar should be started on high blocks to remove the need for it to be lifted from the floor each set.

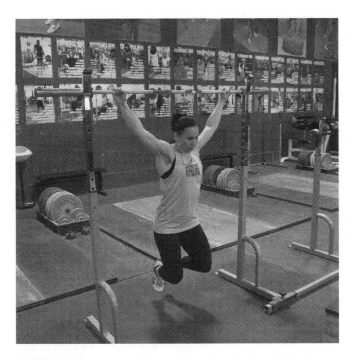

FIGURE 36.3 Hanging with a snatch grip from a barbell will provide specific positioning for grip strength work.

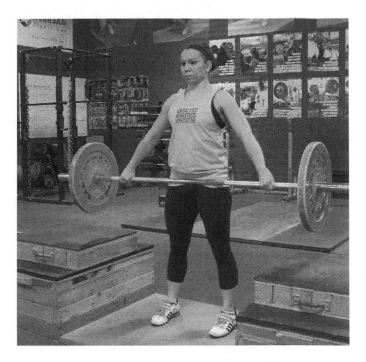

FIGURE 36.4 A loaded barbell can be held in the standing position with a snatch grip without straps or the hook grip, or the lifter can perform snatch shrugs with it to add more force.

The Bulgarian Method

The Bulgarian training method, created and practiced very successfully by former Bulgarian national coach Ivan Abadjiev, is a unique approach to weightlifting that appears to be extremely effective with proper implementation with the appropriate athletes at the proper time. In short, this type of training consists of frequent, heavy, low-volume training limited exclusively or nearly so to the competition lifts and the front and back squat. Ideally training is spread out among multiple sessions throughout the day, often each limited to only one or two exercises. This approach allows athletes to perform multiple times daily at very high average intensities. The philosophy emphasizes the unique ability of the competition lifts themselves, performed with competition parameters, to serve as the ideal training exercises.

To greatly simplify, Abadjiev explains that every lift signals genes to produce proteins in the muscles specific to that performance. For example, a snatch at 60% will create different gene signaling than a snatch at 95%. The athlete's training actually causes the body to reconstruct itself to be best suited for that exact nature and magnitude of performance. Abadjiev states that lifts above 95%, and especially 97%, are what's necessary to produce the adaptations required for optimal weightlifting performance (These are percentages of maximal effort at any given time, not percentages of a lifter's current best lifts). Further, the specificity of adaptation is critical, and for this reason all training must resemble competition as much as possible, from the exercises, the reps, the rest between sets, to the psychological arousal. In essence, this is an extreme application of the SAID principle.

In short, Abadjiev's training protocol involves only the snatch, clean, jerk and front and back squats, for singles and possibly doubles at times in the squat, for daily maximal efforts. He expects that each day following lifts that actually reach maximal, very near it, or over it, the lifter will have reduced results; although, with conditioning, these results will still remain very close to maximal (for example, he claims that in the period that Naim Suleymanoglu was clean & jerking 190kg, he never lifted less than 180kg in training). But despite the small and expected fluctuations in actual weights, every training day remains a maximal effort.

Weightlifting is very unique in the sense that the competition lifts are themselves the most effective training exercises in many respects—this allows a specificity of training not commonly possible. The snatch and clean & jerk develop the physical traits upon which the sport is based, and no other exercise provides more specific adaptation for these lifts than the lifts themselves. There are without a doubt traits, physical and psychological, that cannot be maximally developed and refined without training the competition lifts at very high intensity. A dominance of the total training volume by the competition lifts will also ensure that speed-strength and explosive-strength are developed very well, as the preponderance of all training reps will be performed with maximal speed and acceleration.

In addition to the obvious advantages of such an approach to training described above, this method has the additional benefit of greatly simplifying programming. As can be seen in this section of the book, programming of the more traditional nature entails expansive volumes of detail, which can be paralyzing for many, and often disruptive to progress. The Bulgarian method, and iterations thereof, reduce the involved planning to a remarkable degree.

Even if it were agreed that the Bulgarian method is the ideal approach for the training of weightlifters, it should be clarified that this method is very specifically intended for advanced weightlifters (on this point, Abadjiev agrees) who are technically proficient and have a solid foundation of strength and balanced development.

The effectiveness of this type of training is predicated on the ability of the athlete to snatch and clean & jerk at a level of skill and loading that makes the lifts demanding of the athlete's capacity. If an athlete is, due to technique deficiencies, unable to perform the lifts at such intensity, this approach will be ineffective.

Similarly, if an athlete is not possessed of a reasonable level of basic strength, the snatch and clean & jerk will be considerably limited in possible intensity, again failing to elicit adequate gains. In fact, it appears that the Bulgarian method may only be effective (and even possible in the long term) for lifters with excellent strength levels, i.e. very high squat numbers. In these cases, the athletes are snatching and clean & jerking weights that are not such large percentages of their absolute strength, despite being large percentages of their classic lift maxima, and consequently the training is not as taxing systemically. A lifter who clean & jerks 80% of his best back squat, for example, will have a very different experience from one who clean & jerks 70% of his best back squat.

Finally, it will often be beneficial for even more advanced lifters to spend at least occasional periods of time emphasizing strength lifts and volume over the classic lifts. For some, this variation will be necessary simply to combat mental stagnation and maintain motivation. More importantly, it's unusual for athletes to develop and improve in perfect balance. Invariably, athletes will develop relative weaknesses, which will begin to limit lift performance if not corrected. Minor weaknesses, particularly of a technical nature, can be addressed within a Bulgarian type program, but more significant weaknesses will require a more dramatic change in programming. Periodic higher-rep, lower-intensity training will help develop tendon strength to prevent tendonitis and injury during periods of Bulgarian style training.

Bulgarian Models

There are a number of ways to program in the spirit of the Bulgarian method without following Abadjiev's pure model. Following are a few examples to provide a sense of what is possible. No single approach is ideal for all athletes at all times, and the following is provided as description of what has worked rather than prescription of what will work. Shifting among iterations is a simple way to achieve variation in a system of limited variables. All of the following examples are presented as single daily training sessions because this is what will be most common. In any case, these training days may be broken up into multiple sessions without changing the total amount of work if the athlete desires and is able; if an athlete is able to train twice daily and would like to experiment with actually increasing the total workload by adding more training sessions to the week, a gradual progression should be used.

General Protocols

When working to the maximum lift of the day, the goal is to minimize volume by keeping warm-up sets to singles and doubles, and making relatively large weight increases set to set.

When lifting the daily maximum snatch or clean & jerk, the number of attempts at a given weight allowed should be determined with consideration of a few factors. First is the training experience and abilities of the athlete. The more advanced the athlete and the better conditioned to this type of training he or she is, the more maximal attempts he or she will be able to manage productively. However, less experienced athletes will also be able to manage a large number of maximal attempts because their lifts are limited more by technique than strength, and consequently the attempts are not as systemically taxing; the problem with these athletes performing multiple failed attempts is that because of their less established technical proficiency, there is a greater negative influence on lift technique and even confidence.

In any case, the decision to allow continued attempts at a given daily maximum requires confidence that a good lift is possible. This will mean that the lift is actually within the athlete's abilities in terms of strength and power, and that the preceding misses were a result of correctable technical imprecision or mistakes. If an athlete is attempting a maximal lift and it is clear the necessary strength and power are simply not there—either in terms of the athlete's absolute abilities or present abilities as limited by training fatigue—there is no benefit in repeating the lift, and there is risk of injury.

In general, 3-4 can be considered a maximum number of attempts to allow at a given weight. In some cases, it will be clear that the lift is not going to happen that day after a single attempt. In other cases, the attempts will get progressively better as the athlete continues—in such cases, further attempts can be allowed until the lift is made or this trend reverses.

Generally no deloading periods are used in such programming, although there may be periodic changes in exactly what protocols are used—for example, using different approaches for back-off sets following the daily maximum—and reductions in volume through such changes as the lifter nears a competition.

Daily Minimums

While the maximum of each lift is the most obvious and important metric for any weightlifter, a very important metric for Bulgarian style programming in particular is the daily minimum. This is the minimum snatch, clean & jerk or squat weight the athlete can lift any given day. The secondary goal behind increasing the maximum lifts is to increase the daily minimums. This represents an increasing base of ability and consistency, and is an indicator of how well the lifter is conditioned to this type of training.

Accessory Work

Accessory exercises may be used throughout the week to address trunk strength and stability in particular. Volume and intensity of trunk work should still be be varied to correspond with the rest of the day's training as discussed in the Accessory Work chapter.

Back work should be largely if not exclusively limited to low-demand exercises such as back extensions and isometric holds. Accessory work in general needs to be kept to an absolute minimum to not exceed the necessarily limited volume of this type of training.

Bulgarian Mesocycles

One approach for Bulgarian style training is to use it only in competition mesocycles with more traditional training in preparation mesocycles. While this can be effective for some lifters, it can also be problematic because the time is too limited for the athlete to become truly adapted to the training, reducing its effectiveness somewhat.

Competition

An important point to keep in mind with a Bulgarian style training approach is that competition lifts will often be lower than lifts in training, unlike with a more traditional program in which athletes will typically hit their biggest lifts in competition. The conventional tapering protocol does not produce the same results, and is largely impossible due to the already extremely low volume, although some degree of tapering can and should be done through the reduction of total training sessions and of squat volume in particular.

Americanized Bulgarian

When in the US for a few years and training American lifters, Abadjiev modified his program somewhat to be more suitable for the athletes he was working with. This was a simple program with a single daily training session in which all lifts were taken to maximal intensity, although Abadjiev would provide the lifters with expected weights. He would add jerks from the rack and snatch and clean pulls occasionally as well if deemed necessary for a given lifter.

- Front Squat – heavy single, 90% (of the heavy single) x 2 x 2
- Snatch – heavy single
- Clean & Jerk – heavy single
- Front Squat – heavy single, 90% (of the heavy single) x 2 x 2

Waves & Back-Off Sets

Another approach to increase the volume of lifts is to work to the daily maximum single, then perform a series of singles or doubles at a lighter weight, usually 80-95% of that day's maximum. These back-off sets may be at a single weight, or may increase set to set.

Another variation is to perform waves following the heavy single. This can be done in multiple ways. One is to reduce the weight following the maximal single to a certain percentage (usually 90%) and perform 1-2 series of sets of increasing weights—for example, 90-93-96%. Another is to use the same basic protocol, but to work back up to the original maximum lift. Finally, the lifter may actually lower the weight and try work back up heavier than the original maximum.

Prescribed Intensity

In some cases, it will make sense to prescribe intensity for some of the lifts. The two most common reasons for this would be to control squats to emphasize the competition lifts, or to force a greater degree of recovery on certain days.

Squat intensities can be capped to prevent the athlete from exceeding that threshold, or intensities can even be set uniformly every day as a way to maintain a high level of preparedness while minimizing the demand.

Intensities may be capped or prescribed below maximal on alternate days, such as 80-85%, to encourage somewhat more recovery between true maximal days. This may be done as a way to gradually condition a lifter to a Bulgarian style program, or to force a period of restoration. However, in the long term, the Bulgarian approach will be more effective with daily maxima by lifters adequately conditioned to the system.

Modification

Many variations of the basic program can be made to best suit a given athlete or emphasize certain lifts (usually the squat).

One example is a basic template often used by coach Steve Gough. Each lift would be taken to a maximum single for the day, possibly followed by back-off sets. This can be modified to a single training session on Monday, Wednesday and Friday with the same exercise order.

Monday/Wednesday/Friday
AM Session
• Front Squat
• Snatch
PM Session
• Clean & Jerk
• Back Squat

Tuesday/Thursday/Saturday
• Power Snatch
• Power Clean & Jerk
• Front Squat

A variation to emphasize squat strength may be the same basic template, but without back-off sets for the competition lifts, and up to 4-5 back-off sets for squats. Each day, these back-off sets can be different numbers of reps, and even different squat variations such as pause squats and parallel squats. Weights can be increased over the sets to a maximal or near-maximal effort by the final set.

Specific Populations

Youth

Starting weightlifters at a young age is ideal and argu-ably necessary for producing elite athletes in the long term. Such early starts are one element of the great success of many national sports programs. In the US, however, it's comparatively unusual to see legit-imate athletic training at young ages, particularly in the sport of weightlifting—in part because of the sport's obscurity, and in part because of the popu-lar notion that training with weights is dangerous for youths.

Young, new athletes will progress rapidly with any weightlifting training program; the goal, however, is building the proper foundation to support maximal long term progress and durability, not attempting to maximize short term improvements in the snatch and clean & jerk.

Health & Safety

The primary concerns with regard to the sport's safety are joint damage and limitations on ultimate bone growth. Damage to growth plates and relatively immature cartilage can in fact create problems, but such damage results from poor programming and improper training—neither is inherent to training with weights. In fact, proper training will improve bone density (among other characteristics like motor control, balance, mobility, etc.), and it's not difficult to find examples of athletes who began weightlifting at very young ages who now, as adults, have not only not had any joint development problems, but have grown to heights greater than either parent, often significantly.

Part of the myth that weightlifting stunts growth can be attributed to flawed logic, similar to that which persists with regard to gymnastics. Because elite gymnasts and weightlifters in lighter weight classes tend to be smaller in stature, many people assume that their training has limited their growth. This is a classic logical fallacy—*post hoc ergo propter hoc* (after this, therefore because of this). In other words, be-cause following sport training these athletes remain short, it is assumed (somewhat understandably) that this training was causative of the athletes' stature. This chronology, however, in no way demonstrates causation. Weightlifting has been show to not alter the physical maturation and development of youths age 12-14 (Medvedyev 1986/1989).

Quite simply, abilities in sports such as weightlift-ing and gymnastics are very dependent on leverage. Because shorter athletes have the advantage of better mechanics, they excel in these sports. In other words, the demands of the sports naturally select for short-er athletes. It's not that the sport has kept the ath-letes short, it's simply that taller athletes are unable to continue to elite levels because their mechanics don't allow for the necessary performance. (Interestingly enough, no one has ever argued that playing basket-ball causes athletes to grow to greater than average height, even though the reasoning is identical.)

While in gymnastics stature is always a factor both because the events are all based on movement of the body alone and there are no weight classes, in weight-lifting, heights vary dramatically because of the sepa-ration of athletes by their bodyweights. While short-er athletes lift less weight in absolute terms, they lift considerably more than their taller counterparts rel-ative to bodyweight because of the aforementioned leverage advantage. The heavier weight classes of weightlifting at the elite levels are certainly not lack-ing in men and women of above average height. While this does not prove weightlifting does not stunt growth, it does at least prove that any potential negative effects are not guaranteed, and certainly suggests that concerns are greatly exaggerated.

Training Stages

In order to reach elite levels, weightlifters are best started at age 10-14. However, it should be understood clearly that this does not mean the training program at this age will be identical to that of an older lifter with more training experience. It should, in fact, be considerably different, and managed in stages to both exploit the natural abilities of the athlete to learn and improve certain qualities in different stages of biological development, and to maximize safety. Following are age ranges and the qualities that training should emphasize in each.

In all of the following stages, GPP, mobility work, trunk strength, and grip strength should be emphasized. GPP should emphasize jumping, running and low-intensity, high-rep work to encourage tendon strengthening (Dvorkin 1982/1992)—muscle tissue is fully developed by age 15-16, but tendon strength is not equally developed (Medvedyev 1986/1989).

The primary goal for the earliest years of training is the learning and mastery of competition lift technique, not strength (Medvedyev 1986/1989). This not only takes advantage of the fact that athletes are best able to learn and perfect technique at young ages, but it also avoids potential problems of attempting to load strength lifts excessively heavily; additionally, strength training before sexual maturation will be largely ineffective in any event.

Any training program will result in improvements in the young athlete's abilities; however, the purpose of the earliest stages of training is not to elicit increases in snatch and clean & jerk weights, but to develop a strong foundation, physically and psychologically, that allows the greatest possible long term progress.

Age 10-14 The ability to improve speed, endurance, flexibility, and the ability to learn motor habits, is optimal at this age. Stretching, jumping, sprinting and games involving speed are important at this stage. (Dvorkin 1982/1992, Medvedyev 1986/1989)

Age 12-15 The ability to gain significant strength improves with the sexual maturation process. More strength work can be performed as biological age increases. However, most loading should be in the 70-75% intensity range, and the use of maximal effort lifts should be minimal (Dvorkin 1982/1992, Medvedyev 1986/1989).

Age 13-16 The ability to improve speed-strength is optimal at this stage (Medvedyev 1986/1995), so barbell lifts and jumping exercises are important. Average intensity in the competition lifts and strength lifts will be increasing during these years, and athletes need to develop the habit of training with maximal concentric speed and acceleration.

Competition Lift Learning

Young athletes can be taught the lifts with the progressions outlined in this book. One thing to keep in mind during the process, however, is that youth athletes will respond better to visual cues than spoken instruction (Medvedyev 1986/1989), so it's important to rely more on demonstrations of the movements than descriptions.

Very young athletes (under 13) can learn and practice the snatch and clean & jerk, as well as related exercises and drills, with empty technique barbells (5-10kg) or even lighter implements as needed. It's

Lift	Intensity	Reps	Sets
Snatch	40-50% of bodyweight	4-5	4-6
Clean & Jerk	10-15kg more than snatch	4-5	4-6
Snatch Pull	100% of or 10-15kg more than snatch	4-8	4-6
Clean Pull	100% of or 10-15kg more than clean	4-8	4-6
Front Squat	100% of or 10-20kg more than CJ	4-8	4-6
Back Squat	100% of or 10-20kg more than CJ	4-8	4-6

TABLE 38.1 Loading guidelines for the first month of training the full lifts (Medvedvey 1986/1995)

important for these athletes to accumulate a large volume of repetition.

Medvedvey (1986/1995) recommends the prescriptions in Table 38.1 for the initial month of training once the athletes are able to perform the full lifts. These weights would be used in all training sessions with no progressive increase.

Frequency

There is no reason that children of any age shouldn't engage in some manner of physical activity every day—in fact, they should be encouraged to. This doesn't necessarily mean high levels of exertion, but certainly legitimate durations of movement and play.

As young athletes begin transitioning into weightlifting specialization, barbell training may increase from 1-2 days to 3-4 days per week, with either rest or GPP activities on other days. The frequency and composition of training should be determined by the athlete's biological age and training experience. By their mid-late teens, there should be few athletes who cannot be training 3-5 days per week as weightlifting specialists, although this does not necessarily mean they are not still performing a significant quantity of GPP work.

Competition

While athletes may compete in weightlifting at very young ages, it should be kept minimal during the earliest stages of training. The inherent purpose of competition is contradictory to the goals of the early training stage.

If young new athletes do participate in competitions, the goals should be modified somewhat. Pressure to perform at any given level should be absent—the athletes should be able to enjoy the experience and learn from it, not be concerned about disappointing coaches or parents. The two goals should be to exhibit the best possible lift technique, and to make 6 out of 6 lifts. This will not only naturally keep the attempt weights from being excessively heavy, but will keep the athlete focused on the same goals of his or her program.

Women

The subject of women and weightlifting is one that attracts a considerable spectrum of opinions. Until this point, there has been no distinction within this book between men and women, and intentionally so. Overwhelmingly, the training of men and women need not differ, as both are in essence working with the same pertinent anatomy and physiology. In terms of psychology, there are arguably some general differences that can be effectively addressed with respect to coaching, but ultimately an athlete is an individual regardless of gender, and coaching and programming should be optimally suited for each individual.

The most significant difference between men and women is the respective levels of anabolic hormones. Men on average produce much higher levels of testosterone, allowing greater extents of hypertrophy and strength. There are of course exceptions to this, and some women possess hormonal levels that allow degrees of muscularity and strength beyond what are achievable by some men.

The neurological elements of strength, speed and explosiveness in women have a somewhat lower ceiling than in men due to relative testosterone levels, and this accounts for performance differences not attributable to disparities in actual muscle mass. This is also the source of the generally lower neurological efficiency of women and the resulting general ability for women to perform more repetitions of a lift at a given relative intensity.

Testosterone levels in women are elevated maximally two-three days following the onset of menses. For women using birth control, the pill schedule can be altered so that this testosterone peak coincides with major competitions. However, it is advisable to stagger the schedule so the competition date falls after menses and the cessation of any associated bloating and cramping; the performance-limiting effects of these elements can be more than enough to offset any benefits of elevated testosterone levels. Whether or not this kind of manipulation makes a noticeable difference will vary among athletes, and it is suggested that women experiment with it outside of competition first and only do so with a doctor's supervision.

These minor issues notwithstanding, men and women respond and adapt to training in the same elemental manner, and consequently no universal differences are required in program design. As is always the case, athletes must be trained as individuals, and their particular responses to training used as the ultimate guide to program design.

With regard to coaching specifically, it has been claimed (by female lifters; this author would never be so presumptuous) that the manner of communicating needs to differ somewhat between men and women. Because women tend to be more emotional where men tend to be more rational, the same kind of repetitive technical coaching that men seem to respond well to can sometimes become extremely frustrating to women because they may feel the coach is disappointed or upset, when in reality he or she is more likely simply emphasizing a certain technical element in need of improvement.

While this may be true in general, it is a great disservice to female athletes to assume they require any special treatment, and divergence from what is necessary to help improve their lifting is in a sense crippling them, both in terms of performance in the lifts, and in future coaching and performance situations. The coach simply needs to pay close attention—as he or she does with any athlete, male or female—to how a particular athlete responds to coaching of various manners, and adjust accordingly. Adjustment, however, does not mean coddling of fragile athletes—such athletes are responsible for doing their part to toughen up and meet the coach halfway in the effort.

Such adjustment for certain female lifters is often as simple as providing more encouragement and positive reinforcement along with any technical coaching. That is, where men are less likely to be upset by, or even notice, a lack of frequent outright praise and tend to be more receptive to continual technical correction without associating it with emotion, women tend to respond better to such technical correction when accompanied by consistent praise. There will never be a lift that is entirely wrong, no matter how many elements the coach may want to correct—it's not hard to find one good point to emphasize before making a correction. In reality, such an approach is reasonable for men as well.

Masters

Because the master categories in weightlifting begin at age 35, there is a very large range of ages falling into this classification, and consequently any discussion on training as a master lifter is necessarily vague. Masters age categories are broken into 5-year spans beginning at 35 (e.g. 35-39, 40-44, 45-49, etc.). Athletes vary dramatically even within a given 5-year age category, let alone among these categories, in terms of their performances and in their capacities to manage volume, frequency, average intensity and types of exercises (e.g. relative mix of competition and strength lifts) in training.

The single most important issue with regard to master lifters is a decreased (and decreasing) ability to recover from and adapt to training. Testosterone and growth hormone levels are significantly lower (often to the point of encouraging medical intervention; however, it should be noted that even with a doctor's prescription, it's still illegal for competitive lifters to use exogenous hormones) than during earlier training years, and this unavoidably limits strength, speed, explosiveness and the rate of recuperation from training.

In addition to less than optimal hormone levels, the master will often be dealing with decreased mobility due to past injuries and general wear, and increased time for recovery from inflammation and other aggravations. The treatment of injuries is best left to medical professionals with experience treating athletes. Mobility will need to become and remain an emphasis. While arguments exist regarding whether or not aged individuals can genuinely increase flexibility, there is no arguing that it's far easier to maintain flexibility than to re-establish it. Anecdotal evidence suggests compellingly that older athletes can certainly improve their flexibility, particularly if recovering former levels—in any case, stretching certainly can't hurt. The same approach to mobility discussed later in this book applies to the master; there may simply be a need for greater volume and frequency of stretching. In cases of extreme reductions of mobility, or particularly limiting injuries or joint conditions, athletes can consider the split variations of the snatch and clean, or employ only the power variations.

Arguably the most difficult element of training as a master is the psychological aspect of accepting a reduction in training and performance capacity for those who have trained and competed previously as senior lifters. Failure to accept it is often at the root of injury and regressing performance as athletes attempt to continue training with the same kind of intensity, volume and frequency they did as younger athletes.

Depending on age and experience, master athletes may find that they can only manage 1-2 relatively heavy training days each week, with 1-2 more light training days each week; some may find that they perform best training as little as 2 total days each week. In other cases, lifters may stay in the 80-85% range for the overwhelming majority of their "heavy" training, only exceeding this occasionally to prepare for a meet or test a max. Most will also find that it will be necessary or beneficial to place more emphasis on strength work than classic lift work to reduce the wear and tear on the joints.

In any event, volume will certainly need to be kept lower than for younger athletes. What works will vary greatly among athletes, so each will need to evaluate his or her own training and make adjustments as needed. The training journal is invaluable for such a process. Notes should not only include the details of each training session, but also comments regarding nutrition, sleep, bodyweight, fatigue, and enthusiasm for training. With this data, the athlete can make modifications to training appropriately to improve recovery and adaptation.

At a certain point, the goal of training will necessarily shift from increasing performance, to maintaining it, and eventually to simply trying to slow regression.

For more information on masters training and programming, see *Olympic Weightlifting for Masters: Training at Age 30-40-50 & Beyond* by Matt Foreman (Catalyst Athletics, 2014).

Greg Everett

The Program Design Process

Programming is a contentious subject even among coaches and athletes of similar caliber and experience, but based on performances, it's clear that no perfect method exists and that different approaches can all produce excellent results. What works for different athletes, and even for a given athlete at different times, can vary greatly, and much of program design is experimentation rather than simple implementation.

The purpose of program design is to manipulate training variables to elicit the desired response from the body—that is, to present the body with stressors specific to the desired physical qualities and provide the appropriate support for restoration and adaptation. How exactly this is done takes many forms, but all programming is predicated on this underlying principle.

The process can be organized into basic steps with loose guidelines applied, but it cannot be made entirely formulaic. The art of programming lies largely in predicting an athlete's response to training while having few absolute facts on which to rely—to this end, experience, particularly with the lifter in question, is easily the coach's most valuable resource. Proper record-keeping is a necessity to make this possible; these records allow the coach to create programming most effective for each athlete, and over time, to aggregate data to find general patterns and rules that can be applied to future athletes.

While the coach can predict on the gross level how athletes will respond to a given stressor, the finer details of response vary among athletes, sometimes dramatically, even within the broad categories to which general rules can be applied (for example, the skill level classifications in the Assessment chapter). For example, it can be trusted that an athlete who trains the squat regularly will become stronger in the squat, higher volume will take longer to recover from than lower volume, and training lifts with maximal speed and acceleration will improve an athlete's speed-strength and explosive-strength.

However, these rules provide no information regarding actual figures or measurements, and while individual athletes' responses to training will conform generally to certain expectations, they cannot be predicted with perfect accuracy. This variation will be manifested in tolerance to training variables like volume, average intensity, frequency, and exercise selection. And, of course, each athlete's response to these variables will not remain static throughout his or her career.

Perspectives & Timeframes

In the US, program design tends to be considered from the perspective of smaller timeframes than is common in other weightlifting countries. With more systematic athlete selection and education in many other countries, athletes with pre-determined potential as weightlifters begin training at appropriate young ages, and consequently, it's possible to plan training from the perspective of an entire career.

In the US and countries with similar circumstances, weightlifters are more likely to arrive in the sport somewhat older, and very often following considerable training time in other sports, or worse, with a poor or even absent athletic foundation. Related to this is the comparatively reduced likelihood that these athletes will remain in weightlifting for extended periods of time, both because that time is often not available due to late starting ages, and because opportunity to do so is limited.

These factors greatly limit the ability of coaches to take the long-term approach often possible in other countries' sports programs, and consequently, program design is often managed within smaller blocks of time in an effort to compress the process as much as possible. While this may produce quicker results within a given timeframe, it limits the ultimate possible progress. It still behooves both the athlete and coach to consider the training plan in the context of the long term as well as the short, irrespective of when and how the athlete arrives in the sport; the program can be altered as necessary to fit the less than ideal circumstances while preserving the original spirit as much as possible.

The Process

This chapter will provide a guide to the process of designing weightlifting programming. The intention is to describe the process in a way that arms the coach with the tools necessary to design training programs suitable for any lifter in any situation, not just the ideal athlete in the ideal circumstances, rather than simply provide formulaic prescriptions. Sample programs are provided in a following chapter to support this end, and to provide a starting point for coaches from which modifications can be made.

Planning Overview

The basic idea behind planning progress in a training cycle is for the athlete to begin relatively comfortably within his or her abilities and increase the burdening (a measure of the collective strain of intensity and volume) with increments consistent with factors such as the athlete's training experience, the nature of the exercise, and the demands of the rest of the training in the period in question. In a sense, the goal is to build momentum to push adaptation by the end of the cycle to a point beyond the athlete's present abilities. The more advanced the athlete, the more momentum must be gained and the smaller the ultimate increase will be. These increases do not necessarily refer to each exposure to an exercise—they may involve fluctuations of intensity and volume to create a trend of increase over a period of time.

Measurable Goals

Every training cycle planned should have a goal of measurable improvements—if the goal of a macrocycle is something other than increases in the snatch and clean & jerk in a competition, it must be an improvement in at least one specific exercise, such as the squat. Without such goals, evaluations of an athlete's progress and the effectiveness of a given cycle are impossible.

This does not mean that every training cycle will be completely successful with respect to such goals. In some cases, chosen goals may be unrealistic; in other cases, an untested training cycle may simply have not worked as expected. In both situations, the coach and athlete must reconsider the approach and correct as necessary, noting the mistakes to prevent repeating them.

Flexibility

All planning involves attempts at predicting an athlete's response to training, and by nature, predictions are fallible. Additionally, there exist no absolutes in regard to training—there are patterns whose accuracy invariably decreases as the focus narrows. The coach is left to rely on his or her own experience and that of others for guidance when designing programs, and to develop a continually greater degree of familiarity with his or her athletes in order to better predict their responses to various training stimuli.

For these reasons, programming may be considered equal parts science and art. Perfection is impossible, and no amount of care and calculation can change this or account for unexpected factors that disrupt recovery and possibly training. This being the case, flexibility in prescriptions is important to absorb not only misjudgments of an athlete's ability to progress, but also for unexpected factors that negatively influence recovery and limit adaptation. That is, while numbers will generally be prescribed, there will be times at which those numbers will need to be adjusted without prior notice based on an athlete's performance at the time in question. This kind of flexibility is critical for preserving progress in the long term—attempts at strict adherence to prescription irrespective of present circumstances will often result in stalled progress, injury or overtraining, resulting in retrograde performance.

Process Steps

Clearly there are a multitude of considerations to make when planning an athlete's training. In order to navigate this information, it will be helpful for the coach to have a simple protocol to guide program design. This process, while certainly involving chronologically distinguishable steps, is unavoidably nebulous to a degree. That is, each step cannot necessarily be completed before advancing to the next, and each new step may require adjustments to previous ones. It should be considered a progression from general to specific, with continual revision in light of graduating specificity. Over time, each coach will develop a better sense of how to begin and progress through program design. Additionally, he or she will accumulate training cycles that can be used as templates for future cycles, making the process far easier and quicker.

Following is a loose order of operations to for the process:

- Assessment
- Scheduling
- Goal Setting
- Exercise Selection
- Exercise Scheduling
- Final Details

Overall, the process will be working from the macro to micro scale in terms of time periods; that is, the details will be determined in order of the macrocycle, mesocycles, microcycles and finally individual workouts.

Assessment

While athlete assessment is in a sense continuous, it's important at the culmination of each training phase to perform a more formal, or at least more thorough, assessment of the athlete. This involves both objective and subjective measurements of performance.

We can use the athlete's actual lift numbers along with an evaluation of the athlete's strengths, weaknesses, and according needs. This evaluation should pertain to both strength and technique, and cover the spectrum of general to specific. For example, we may decide that the athlete is in need of improved leg strength; is in need of improvements in clean technique and strength; and specifically in need of correcting a sloppy turnover of the clean that allows the bar to crash onto his or her shoulders.

Schedule

Before we can build a training cycle, we of course need to know what its duration can be or needs to be. For competitive lifters, this will involve matching the training phases to the competition calendar (with the exception described below with regard to goal setting); for recreational lifters with no need to conform to outside schedules, this can be a product of other determinations like exercise selection and volume and intensity determinations. Generally we will be working with durations of 4-16 weeks.

Goal Setting

No planning can occur without goals in mind. Longer-term planning and related goals have been discussed previously; this goal setting is limited to shorter time frames. We need goals for the entire cycle as well as goals for periods of time within the cycle all the way down to single training sessions.

Exercise Selection

With the previous two steps completed, we will be able to make informed decisions regarding what exercises will be most beneficial for the training cycle. Again, this will involve both a general and specific perspective. Generally we need to consider the type of training phase—obviously a preparation phase will involve a greater proportion of strength exercises, while a competition phase will involve a greater proportion of competition lifts and their variants. Specifically we will need to address the athlete's needs as determined by the assessment and goal setting steps. This will involve both decisions regarding what lifts on which to focus, as well as what technical aspects of various lifts will be emphasized. To use the earlier athlete example, a preparation phase would need to involve a greater than usual emphasis on squatting and cleaning; more specifically, we would need to include exercises that address the turnover of the clean, such as clean high-pulls, tall cleans, muscle cleans, etc.

Part of exercise selection is prioritization. In order to know where to start when constructing the actual program, we need to know what will constitute the foundation. This will generally be squatting and/or pulling in preparation mesocycles, and obviously the classic lifts in competition mesocycles; in a broader sense, we will consider the most demanding exercises (such as squatting, pulling, snatching and clean & jerking) as foundational and build on and around them.

Exercise Scheduling

With these foundational exercises, we can lay down the framework of the cycle. This will simply involve the weekly schedule of these exercises—for example, we may back squat on Monday and Friday, and front squat on Wednesday. Around this, we may schedule clean pulls on Monday to coincide with the most demanding squat session and snatch pulls on Wednesday to coincide with a somewhat less demanding squat session. On Friday we might include snatch or clean deadlifts with a lighter squat session because we have a rest day following; or we might want to reduce the workload and drop the pulls entirely, or use partial pulls or shrugs instead. With these three days becoming our most demanding, we may add in a couple more strength-oriented exercises, determining the days in between to consist of more technique and/or classic lift related training.

In this manner, we can continue layering on exercises until we fill out the schedule appropriately with the exercises we've chosen. How many exercises are used each training day or session will depend on factors such as how much volume it's determined an athlete needs or can tolerate, the type of exercises selected, and the volume and intensity of each exercise.

A general rule of thumb is 3-6 exercises per training session, excluding less demanding supplementary exercises like core training. Of course, the weekly schedule won't remain the same for the duration of the cycle; it will change as the cycle progresses, at a minimum with each subsequent mesocycle.

Another detail that should be kept in mind when laying out the exercises in a program is how each flows with the following and preceding exercises with regard to time. For example, moving from snatches to snatch pulls will be quick because the lifter is already warm for that movement and will be able to start at a significant weight. In contrast, moving from jerks to squats will typically take longer because the dissimilar movements will require warming up for both. When trying to incorporate maximal training in a fixed period of time, taking this into account can allow much more effective planning.

Final Details

Finally, to the exercise schedule we need to assign volume and intensity prescriptions. This will be done according to the guidelines discussed previously in this chapter, creating a progression that will drive the adaptation we want, but that the athlete can tolerate.

Mesocycle Types

Mesocycles can be classified broadly in a few different categories based on their purpose, content and timing relative to competition. Generally speaking, the more advanced the athlete and the longer the macrocycle, the more pronounced the distinctions among mesocycles will be; with new lifters and short macrocycles, mesocycles will not necessarily be considerably different from each other, although certainly will contain the typical trends of volume and intensity. The two primary types are Preparation and Competition. Other types include GPP, Transition and Technique Education & Development.

It should be noted that program design does not necessarily need to conform to perfectly formal mesocycle structure in order to be successful. For example, weekly structure may transform gradually as the macrocycle progresses rather than being changed more significantly around clear demarcation points; duration of different training phases may be longer or shorter, and even be somewhat flexible and adjusted as the cycle progresses; some lifters will never use a distinct competition mesocycle in terms of intensity and repetitions, although volume will certainly decrease and intensity increase at the culmination of any macrocycle. In other words, it should be kept in mind that there are many ways to approach programming successfully; this chapter tries to present as much useful information as possible without prescribing how the work must be done with excessive rigidity.

Preparation
AKA Preparatory, Accumulation, Extensification, Strength & Power Development

The need for strength increases is in a sense infinite, as this is overwhelmingly what improvement in weightlifting will consist of once technical proficiency has been achieved. It's often said that there's no such thing as too strong. This statement does require qualification in this case, however. Greater strength and power are always needed, but disparity between general strength and specific application needs to be considered when planning an athlete's training. That is, a lifter with excellent absolute, explosive and speed strength but a relative inability to apply these qualities to the snatch and clean & jerk possesses a disparity in ability that needs to be addressed. In such a case, excessive emphasis on strength development with inadequate development of specific strength and power application is a misuse of training time.

The preparation mesocycle will be built primarily around strength exercises such as squats, pull variations, and press variations, as improving strength will be the primary purpose of this phase. The competition lifts will be performed, but in lower relative volume and frequency, and more variations will be employed rather than just the competition lifts from the floor, such as lifts from the hang or blocks and complexes. Speed- and explosive-strength work will also play an important role, including jumping variations.

It will typically involve exercises to address technical problems as well, or at least exercises that continue to improve the athlete's technical execution of the competition lifts.

During preparation mesocycles, the lifter's competition lift performance will decline with the accumulation of fatigue due to the high volume, and in particular, the high volume of strength work. However, the competition lifts will not be performed with maximal intensity during this phase, or if they are periodically, there should be no expectation of true maximal lifts.

Volume The volume in preparation mesocycles will be the highest of the macrocycle. This is due to the higher repetition numbers (in the competition lifts and variations, and the increase of strength exercises relative to competition lifts, which will generally employ higher reps), greater number of exercises, and possible higher training frequency.

Intensity The average intensity in the preparation mesocycle(s) will be lower relative to the competition mesocycle. This does not mean the training is not difficult; it's more a reflection of the volume and repetition numbers. That is, intensity is inherently lower when performing higher-rep sets relative to lower-rep sets, but a given set still may be very difficult and even maximal effort.

Frequency The training frequency in the preparation mesocycle(s) will be the highest of the macrocycle if there is a change in frequency in the macrocycle. That is, aside from the final week of a macrocycle in which frequency is nearly invariably reduced, frequency may remain constant for the entire macrocycle.

Specificity The similarity of training exercises, repetitions and intensity to competition conditions will be lowest in the earliest preparatory mesocycles. Specificity will increase with each preparatory mesocycle to some degree, although it will still remain more focused on strength exercises than the competition lifts in any case. The last preparation mesocycle in a macrocycle can be considered somewhat transitional in a sense, as it will bridge the least specific mesocycles with the most specific mesocycle.

Competition
AKA Pre-competition, Intensification,
Strength & Power Specification

The competition mesocycle is the final phase leading into competition, or for recreational lifters, testing of the snatch and clean & jerk. This phase has two basic purposes: to transfer the strength, speed and explosiveness developed in the preparation phase to the performance of the snatch and clean & jerk, and to begin reducing the fatigue accumulated during the preparation phase to prepare the lifter for optimal performance in competition.

The latter purpose will require more time the longer the preparation phase and the more preparatory training has been accumulated. This will typically be 2-6 weeks with an average of 4 (Zatsiorsky 1995).

The training focus will be on the competition lifts, primarily for single repetitions at relatively high intensity. Strength lifts will be reduced in number, volume and intensity and will remain primarily to maintain strength rather than increase it. Technique training will remain in volume and frequency appropriate for the needs of each athlete.

There are multiple approaches to the competition mesocycle, like any other phase.

Intensity The average intensity in the competition mesocycle will reach the highest of the macrocycle, as it will reflect the lower volume and repetition numbers, as well as the increasing focus on the competition lifts for primarily single reps. However, it will typically peak approximately two weeks from competition and then be reduced.

Volume The volume of the competition mesocycle will be considerably lower than the preparation mesocycle(s). This volume reduction serves the purpose of gradually reducing systemic fatigue accumulated during the preparation phase of the cycle in order to lead the lifter into competition, but it is also a natural reflection of the content of the mesocycle. That is, because the competition mesocycle is comprised of more competition lifts and fewer strength and accessory lifts, it inherently contains fewer reps.

Frequency The training frequency in the competition mesocycle will be the lowest of the macrocycle if there is a change in frequency in the macrocycle. That is, aside from the final week of a macrocycle in which frequency is nearly invariably reduced, frequency may remain constant for the entire macrocycle.

Peaking The final stage of the competition mesocycle is peaking for competition or testing. This is the final attempt to strip as much fatigue as possible while maintaining strength, speed and explosiveness, and maximizing the lifter's ability to snatch and clean & jerk when it matters. This period does not develop abilities further, but simply eliminates the factors preventing the athlete from fully accessing his or her present abilities.

Typically the lifter will have a final (or possibly the first and only for the macrocycle aside from the competition at its culmination) test of maximum snatch and clean & jerk 2-3 weeks before the competition date to test preparedness and allow planning for competition attempts. How far out from the competition this is done will depend on factors like the lifter's weight class (generally larger weight classes need more time), age (generally younger lifters need less time) and skill level (generally more advanced lifters need more time).

In the period between this test and the competition, average intensity and volume will be reduced. Intensity of squats and pulls in particular will need to be reduced. In some cases, pulls will be eliminated entirely.

Medvedyev (1986/1989) recommends that the last maximum snatch and clean & jerk be taken 10-14 days before the competition; the opening snatch weight be taken up to 4 days before the competition; and the opening clean & jerk weight be taken up to 8 days before the competition.

The final week leading into the competition will be extremely low volume and will taper in both volume and intensity as the week progresses. Generally the number of training days will be reduced as well. Exceptions to this will be less experienced lifters who will typically perform better by training each day but with extremely light weights on some (50-60%) to maintain technical preparedness.

General Physical Preparation

GPP training is non-specific work intended primarily to prepare the athlete for managing future training stress. This consists largely of basic strength and mobility work, joint preparation, work capacity development and coordination development. Such training might include basic barbell and dumbbell lifts, odd-object lifting, sprinting, jumping, throwing, carrying, basic gymnastic drills, and more play-oriented training and games.

The most important element will be jumping (Medvedyev 1986/1989). Grip strength is another critical element requiring focus and maximal development with new and young lifters.

GPP training is most commonly employed with young or new athletes without established training specialties; it serves to prepare the athlete for specialization by ensuring existing weaknesses are resolved and improving general work capacity. In particular, it's important to develop tendon strength, which develops more slowly than muscular strength, and in young athletes will lag behind the muscles in terms of natural physiological development. This is achieved primarily with low intensity, high volume, high amplitude work (Medvedyev 1986/1989).

The need and appropriateness for GPP decreases as the lifter advances in development. Rarely if ever will an established weightlifter employ a period of training genuinely dedicated to GPP. In some cases, these lifters may have a phase of training that contains more GPP-type training along with weightlifting-specific training after long lay-offs or when returning from an injury.

Technique Education & Development

The initial emphasis in terms of weightlifting-specific training with new weightlifters will be technique instruction and practice. This work will usually be combined with GPP training in the earliest stages of a young lifter's development.

Without a foundation of technical proficiency, further weightlifting specific training cannot proceed. This technique education involves primarily the competition lifts, but also the major supplemental strength and technique exercises.

With a long-term perspective, particularly with young athletes, it's wise to commit a significant period of time to technique instruction prior to using the competition lifts in particular in actual training. This will allow better ultimate proficiency and success. However, with the exception of young athletes, this will rarely be an option. Coaches will often have to shorten this instruction period dramatically with older athletes. In any case, no lift should be used in training without the proficiency to at least ensure safety. Guidelines for the early stages of training of young athletes are discussed in detail in the Specific Populations chapter.

How quickly an athlete develops technical mastery will depend on factors such as the quality of technique instruction, the athlete's natural learning abilities and athleticism, the athlete's commitment, the athlete's biological and training age, and the time and effort dedicated to training.

Athletes will be maximally capable of learning lift technique at younger ages (10-14); it's critical whenever possible to exploit this natural ability.

Transition

The transition mesocycle is a relatively infrequent and brief period that bridges consecutive macrocycles or the time between significant competitions and the subsequent macrocycle. This will typically be only 1-3 weeks.

Often after major competitions, lifters will take a short time off completely, or training will be very infrequent, light, low in volume and possibly even non-specific—more along the lines of active recovery—because of the extremely physically and psychologically taxing nature of such competitions. A layoff from training of more than 2 weeks will have measurable negative effects (Medvedyev 1986/1989).

Following time off from training, a period of transition back into full time training will be necessary. This will involve more GPP work, low intensity, and relatively low volume of the competition lifts, gradually shifting into the nature and volume of training that will comprise the beginning of the macrocycle to follow.

For short lay-offs such as a single week following a competition, this transition period will not need to be as long. One week is typically adequate, and it will be more specific to the following macrocycle from the start. The is the idea behind "Week 0"—this is the initial transition week of a macrocycle that prepares the lifter for the first genuine week of training. A simple way to compose Week 0 is to alter the first week of the macrocycle by reducing intensity by 10-15% and repetitions per set by 1-3.

Program Structure

The more advanced the athlete, the more complex the structure of the training program must become to continue driving positive adaptation. Initially, a very basic schedule of exercises, intensities, reps and sets with regular increases primarily in intensity will be adequate; as the athlete progresses, training cycles will increase in duration and their contents will require more extensive planning.

The term *periodization* refers to the partitioning of training into blocks of time. Within any given training block is the intentional modulation of training variables—in particular intensity, volume and exercise selection—during the period and among consecutive periods to maximize progress over the course of the entire training cycle.

Structure There are 3 primary levels of organization within a complete training program. The microcycle is a single week because of the convenience and practicality of this unit of time. The mesocycle is a

series of multiple microcycles—usually 3-6—with a common theme in terms of emphasis and variables like exercise selection, volume and reps. The macrocycle is the total duration of the program, comprised of 2 or more mesocycles.

Of course, training will also be contained within longer durations such as the entire year and even up to the quadrennium—the 4-year Olympic cycle. Such periods should always be considered at least in broad terms during the planning of individual macrocycles.

Schedule The schedule of the training program is primarily a concern for the competitive weightlifter, although it may become important in some instances even for recreational lifters. For the competitive lifter, all training programs must be designed according to the calendar of significant competitions primarily, and to less significant competitions secondarily, if at all. This is to ensure that the athlete achieves peak performance on the date of the most important competitions.

In the case of the recreational lifter, generally the training cycle can be constructed with the duration most appropriate for the lifter and the nature of the program. An exception to this will be foreseeable disruptions to the lifter's training, such as trips out of town in which the athlete will have limited or no ability to train. In these cases, programs should be designed around these dates, i.e. a training cycle ending before the athlete leaves, and a new one starting when he or she returns.

Duration Macrocycles will generally range in duration from 4-20 weeks. The more advanced the lifter, the longer the macrocycle will need to be until reaching a maximal productive duration, which will typically be 16-20 weeks, but may change dependent on the competition calendar. New lifters will generally work with durations of 4-8 weeks, while intermediate to advanced lifters will generally work with durations of 8-16 weeks.

The Year

The purpose of planning on the year scale is primarily to schedule macrocycles according to the competition schedule, and secondarily to create general goals

Period	Duration	Number
Microcycle	1 week	3-6 per mesocycle
Mesocycle	3-6 weeks	2-5 per macrocycle
Macrocycle	6-20 weeks	3-9 per year
Year	1 year	4 per quadrennium
Quadrennium	4 years	2-4 per career

TABLE 39.1 Periodization structure guidelines

Greg Everett

for each macrocycle and the year as a whole. The first step in scheduling is selecting the significant competitions for the year. These will vary among athletes depending on their level of competition.

For the beginning and intermediate lifter, competitions will be of the local and possibly regional level, meaning scheduling can be less predictable and may not be set as far out as a year, preventing a detailed plan for the year to be created early on. The coach will have to work with a more general plan until dates are set, at which time the plan can be adjusted and finalized as needed.

Additionally, all meets at the local level are essentially of equal importance, so it may not be necessary to prioritize. An exception is if a lifter wants to do several meets in a brief period of time, such as 3-4 weeks apart—in this case, it makes sense to select certain meets in that period to prioritize for more effective macrocycle durations. Another reason to prioritize a certain local meet might be that a lifter can earn prize money for a good performance.

Lifters at this level will generally be working with relatively short macrocycles and will be making relatively rapid progress, making it simple to peak for a greater number of competitions in a year. If such a plan doesn't interfere with the training program, the

lifter's year can be broken into as many macrocycles as there are competitions, and potentially more if there are unusually long periods without an available competition. For example, if a lifter competes in 6 meets in a year, there would be 6 macrocycles averaging 8-9 weeks each, although ranging in duration dependent on the actual competition calendar. If, however, there were a 3-month break between meets at some point, it may make sense, depending on the lifter, to break that into 2 6-week macrocycles rather than a single 12-week macrocycle.

For lifters competing at the national or international level, true competition peaking will need to be limited within a year. Typically these lifters will peak for no more than 2-3 meets in a year, and will train through other competitions (that is, simply compete in the course of a macrocycle without altering that cycle in any significant way to prepare for the meet) if any others are done. These insignificant meets will be used simply as competition experience—to help the athlete's composure, practice of the meet routine, or to experiment with higher openers or attempts in a risk-free situation.

These lifters will select the most significant competitions for the year—for the US national level lifter, for example, this will usually be the Nation-

CYCLE	MACROCYCLE 1: NATIONAL CHAMPIONSHIPS												REST	TRANSITION
MESO	MESO 1				MESO 2				MESO 3					
WEEK	1	2	3	4	5	6	7	8	9	10	11	12	0	0
EVENTS												NATIONALS		

CYCLE	MACROCYCLE 2: LEG STRENGTH EMPHASIS												TRANSITION
MESO	MESO 1				MESO 2				MESO 3				
WEEK	1	2	3	4	5	6	7	8	9	10	11	12	0
EVENTS								MEET				TESTING	

CYCLE	MACROCYCLE 3: AMERICAN OPEN												REST	TRANSITION
MESO	MESO 1				MESO 2									
WEEK	1	2	3	4	5	6	7	8	9	10	11	12	0	0
EVENTS												AO		

CYCLE	MACROCYCLE 4													
MESO	MESO 1						MESO 2				MESO 3			
WEEK	1	2	3	4	5	6	7	8	9	10	11	12	13	14
EVENTS						MEET								MEET

FIGURE 39.1 Example yearly plan for a national level lifter with 2 significant competitions (National Championships and American Open), 3 insignificant competitions, one macrocycle that ends in max testing in the gym, one macrocycle with a specific emphasis other than the competition lifts, and one macrocycle in which mesocycle duration is altered to suit the meet schedule.

al Championships and the American Open. For the international lifter, this would likely be the National Championships and the World Championships or continental championships (e.g. PanAm, European, Asian). The training in the year will then be scheduled around these dates so that the lifter will achieve peak performance for these competitions. Consideration will still be given to the insignificant competitions—small alterations may be made to the program prior to such meets if it will not negatively affect the macrocycle for the next significant competition, such as changing the timing of a back-off week to lead into a meet for better results, but any modifications will be minimal to ensure the training cycle is maximally effective for the competitions that matter. See Table 39.1 for a sample year plan.

The Macrocycle

Once the year schedule is determined, the macrocycles can be planned. The starting and ending dates of each will have been determined when planning the year around competitions unless, for a local-level lifter, all dates are not yet set. In this case, macrocycles can be planned based on the appropriate duration for the lifter, and then adjusted later when dates are finalized.

Goals The general goals of the macrocycle will need to be determined first. Of course the overarching goal for all lifters will be to increase the snatch and clean & jerk. However, certain aspects of training will often need to be emphasized at different times to support this goal. For example, a lifter may require a macrocycle that focuses on improving squat strength primarily, at least during the preparation period, rather than a more balanced approach. Such macrocycles are best used as far from significant competitions as possible, but may be used throughout the year as needed depending on the severity of the need—the sooner the problem is corrected, the faster the lifter will be able to progress in the long term, even if individual competition results in a given period are not as high as possible because of an emphasis on training other than specific preparation for snatch and clean & jerk in competition. Ideally, the competitions in

the year are prioritized so that macrocycles can be planned to maximize performance in the most important meet while still achieving the specific goals for the year overall.

For example, a national level lifter who will be competing in the American Open and National Championships will prioritize the National Championships, which is the more prestigious of the two. If the squat is lagging, this athlete may use an entire macrocycle that emphasizes the squat leading into the American Open, and then return to a more balanced macrocycle to maximize snatch and clean & jerk performance with this new squat strength for the National Championships.

Similar broad goals with regard to other disparities or technical problems should be enumerated for each macrocycle so that the coach can ensure the program will address these needs. This may include emphasis on the clean over the jerk if that is the weaker of the two, a focus on overhead strength and stability if that is a limiting factor in the snatch or jerk, more aggressive mobility work if needed, or any other specific problems that have been determined in the past year or macrocycle to be in need of resolving. With lifters who have started at the ideal age and have been developed properly, these issues will be less prevalent, as such lifters will possess better foundations and more balanced abilities.

Mesocycle Schedule Once goals have been created, the mesocycle schedule within the macrocycle should be determined. This will depend on a few factors. Any insignificant competitions, testing days or weeks, or other important dates within the macrocycle should be considered. If a competition falls very close (within a week) to a point in which there would be a transition between mesocycles, it may make sense to shift that break to coincide with the competition. For example, if a 12-week macrocycle is planned with 3 4-week mesocycles and a meet falls at the end of week 5, the coach may decide it's not disruptive to make the mesocycles 5 weeks, 3 weeks, and 4 weeks in duration, so that the meet will fall at the end of the back-off week at the end of the first mesocycle, and consequently the lifter will feel more restored for the competition. However, if this would require any adjustment beyond a week, the drawbacks will generally outweigh the benefits.

If a lifter will have to travel or for some other reason be unable to train in ideal circumstances at some point during the macrocycle, it will be ideal to schedule a back-off week during that period if possible to minimize disruption. The coach will have to consider the relative magnitude of the problem of trying to train in the suboptimal conditions and of rearranging the mesocycle schedule and choose the one with the least negative impact.

If no dates within the macrocycle will affect training, the mesocycle schedule should be determined based exclusively on the training content and goals—that is, the schedule that best suits the purposes of the mesocycles. The optimal length for the mesocycle is 4 weeks, with a reasonable range of 3-6. Employing the 4-week mesocycle unless there are compelling reasons to diverge is the recommended protocol. Reasons include the aforementioned scheduling conflicts or influences or the benefit of a change to the purpose of the mesocycle's content, such as extending the duration to accommodate more gradual intensity increases at uniform volume.

General Trends Over the course of a macrocycle, there will be consistent trends of certain key training variables such as volume, intensity, exercise selection, and frequency. The actual figures will vary among cycles and lifters, but the general changes of these variables will be reliable. These have been discussed in more detail in the Training Variables chapter. Figure 39.3 provides a simple graphical representation of these trends.

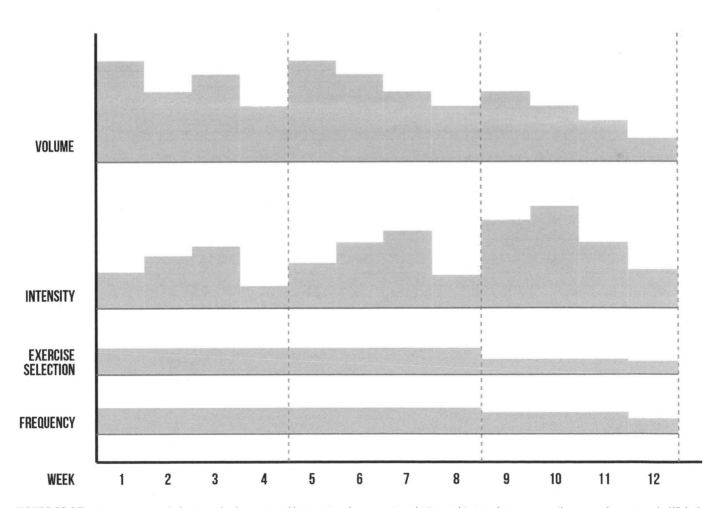

FIGURE 39.2 This figure represents the basic trends of average weekly intensity, volume, exercise selection, and training frequency over the course of a macrocycle. While the actual figures and order of loading & deloading microcycles may vary among effective macrocycles, the basic long-term trends will remain consistent.

The Mesocycle

The mesocycle is the level at which planning will be undertaken with the maximal level of detail. That is, while the year and macrocycle stages plan general elements like dates and broad goals, the mesocycle scale involves planning actual training variables such as exercise selection and volume.

When the details of each mesocycle are actually determined will vary among coaches. It is necessary to create the basic structure of the mesocycles, such as dates and volume prescriptions, and at least a general sense of exercise selection, prior to the beginning of the macrocycle. This provides a clear plan on which the coach can rely when prescribing the content of each mesocycle.

The final details of each mesocycle can then be determined as the previous cycle nears completion to allow for consideration of the athlete's present condition and most recent performances. Each mesocycle can even be prescribed in final detail one week at a time as long as a clear plan for the entire mesocycle and macrocycle exists. In this way the coach avoids having to invest a great deal of time into planning all details of an entire macrocycle at one time; additionally, finer details will likely need to be adjusted in the course of the macrocycle in reaction to the lifter's response to the training and the influence of outside factors, so finalizing such details upfront for the entire macrocycle is arguably creating unnecessary extra work, or locking the coach into a plan that may become less effective by preventing adequate flexibility.

Type As described previously, the content of the mesocycle will conform to the basic rules of its classification as preparation, competition, or transition. This will in the broadest terms dictate the details of volume, intensity, frequency and exercise selection.

Loading & Deloading Microcycles within each mesocycle can be loosely classified as loading (or burdening), maintenance, or deloading based primarily on the volume and intensity. Each mesocycle will require proper scheduling of such microcycles to allow the optimal loading, restoration, and potentially testing.

Typically deloading (also known as back-off or re-covery) weeks will be prescribed after 2-3 weeks of loading depending on the lifter, the type of mesocycle, and the magnitude of the loading. With certain training cycles, longer periods without deloading are possible, but usually no more than 5-6 weeks with a relatively low rate of weekly loading increase.

These deloading periods do not eliminate all fatigue produced by the mesocycle and macrocycle. Some level of fatigue will persist across the duration of the entire mesocycle and most of the macrocycle (the exception being the competition mesocycle during which this fatigue is systematically reduced). This is not necessarily problematic (only if not planned or managed properly to an extent that allows overtraining rather than progress), and in fact is the intention. That is, the entire macrocycle is one continuous stimulus to produce the intended increase in functional capacity.

Volume The longer a given mesocycle, the more fluctuation in loading and volume will need to be implemented. Unless dealing with rank novices with little or no training experience, volume cannot remain perfectly uniform for significant periods of time. Instead, volume must be modulated with a general trend of reduction, and possibly with fluctuation week to week that does not conform to consistent reduction, but achieves it overall on average. Graphical examples of how volume may be distributed in a mesocycle can be seen in Figure 39.2.

The total volume of the mesocycle should be calculated according to the need and tolerance of the athlete, and with respect to the nature of the mesocycle (i.e. preparation or competition, and more specifically, the precise exercises and intentions). Starting mesocycle volumes based on lifter skill development level can be found in the Training Variables chapter in Table 33.4. Manners of distributing the mesocycle volume among the microcycles is also covered in this chapter under the Volume heading. Eventually, the coach will also have data on each lifter from previous training cycles that should be used to guide appropriate volume prescriptions.

Intensity Generally through a mesocycle, the average intensity will increase from start to finish. However, it will fluctuate in some way dependent on how the loading of the microcycles is scheduled. Most commonly a mesocycle will increase in intensity over its duration until the final week, in which average intensity will be reduced. In other cases, the intensity of the mesocycle may increase until the penultimate week, in which it will be reduced, and then in the final week increased to the highest of that mesocycle.

In the former case, any maximal lifts or testing would occur in the second to last week and the final week serve as restorative in preparation for the subsequent mesocycle. In the latter case, the deloading week allows the athlete to restore to some degree for a maximal lifts or testing in the final week. The weekly increase in intensity will usually need to decrease in rate through progressive weeks; this is truer the longer the mesocycle and the period of increasing intensity is. For example, intensity may increase essentially linearly for 3 weeks, but if the mesocycle will increase intensity for 6 weeks, the rate of increase will diminish over the course of that 6 weeks, or fluctuation employed.

The rate of intensity increase will depend on the starting point—the lower the starting point, the higher the rate of increase can be (the closer to the athlete's maximal capacity it begins, the more difficult it will be to increase it). With all other elements remaining uniform (e.g. reps and sets), typically a 2-3% per week intensity increase is reasonable. This can be prescribed across all sets, or be the average increase. For example, the following starting and ending points can be achieved in two different ways while maintaining the same rate of average intensity increase (2-3% per week):

- Week 1: *5 sets of 3 reps at 75%*
- Week 2: *5 sets of 3 reps at 78%* Or *2 sets of 3 reps at 75%, 3 sets of 3 reps at 80%*
- Week 3: *5 sets of 3 reps at 80%* and/or *3RM*
- Week 4: *3-5 sets of 2-3 reps at 70%*

An example of an alternate 2-week increase, 1-week decrease, and 1-week increase would look something like:

- Week 1: *5 sets of 3 reps at 75%*
- Week 2: *4-5 sets of 3 reps at 80%*
- Week 3: *4-5 sets of 3 reps at 70%*
- Week 4: *3-4 sets of 3 reps at 85%* and/or *3RM*

Intensity may also be determined in each workout according to feel and observation with the goal of increasing the intensity on average over the course of a mesocycle. This does not necessarily require the lifter to perform an exercise with maximal intensity for the day; the coach may have an approximate level of effort he or she expects, and can help guide the athlete, with the athlete's feedback, to the proper intensity.

In other cases, exercises may actually be taken to maximal effort each day, and often followed by sets with reduced intensity for additional volume. The coach will need to differentiate between legitimate maximal effort, in which case there will likely be failed attempts in the workout, and near-maximal efforts, in which case the goal can typically be described as lifting as heavy as possible without missing or failed reps. With either of these approaches, volume will need to be monitored closely, as it can quickly far exceed what was planned with additional attempts.

This kind of approach may appear something like the following:

Snatch Pull + Snatch – 1+2RM, 90% x 1+2 x 2

This would require the lifter to take this snatch complex to a maximum, and then perform 2 subsequent sets at 90% of that maximum.

Exercise Selection Exercise selection will be based primarily on the type of mesocycle and secondarily on the assessed current needs of the lifter. That is, all preparation mesocycles will contain a relatively large number of exercises oriented more toward basic qualities like strength and technique, and all competition mesocycles will contain relatively large numbers of the competition lifts. However, based on the needs of the individual athletes, the ratios of each in a given mesocycle will vary, and the actual exercises selected will change to address the necessary physical qualities and technical abilities. Variation in exercise selection is discussed below under the Variation heading.

Prioritization The basic prioritization of exercises can be found in Table 34.8 in the Training Variables chapter. Exercises will need to be prioritized more specifically for each lifter in each macrocycle and mesocycle. If a particular quality in a lifter is lagging behind, it will need to be emphasized more than it usually would in a given mesocycle. For example, a lifter with a very weak squat will need to prioritize squat strength to reduce the disparity. While in a preparation mesocycle, strength lifts are already prioritized to some degree, it's possible to emphasize a specific lift to a greater degree. For example, work on pulling strength may be reduced somewhat in a given preparation mesocycle in order to allow greater volume and intensity in the squat.

When creating a program, the mesocycle should be built around the priority exercise(s). In the competition mesocycle, this is obviously the snatch and clean & jerk; those exercises are determined and scheduled first and foremost, and the remaining exercises then prescribed accordingly. In a preparation mesocycle that seeks to emphasize the squat, on the other hand, the squats would be scheduled and then the rest of the program built to accommodate them.

Variation Variation within a mesocycle and among subsequent mesocycles is accomplished primarily through changes in intensity and volume (including the changes to repetition numbers), and secondarily through exercise selection. Accommodation is easily avoided through the former as there will be an increase in intensity and decrease in volume over the course of a macrocycle and individual mesocycles.

Variation in exercise selection will be minor in some respects due to the need for specificity and the consequent limitation on variability; however, a significant degree of variation can still be achieved through the use of the many possible variations of the competition lifts, pulling exercises, squats and overhead work.

Generally, exercise selection can be kept uniform for the duration of a mesocycle, and in fact, this is typically the best approach, as the repeated exposure within the restraints of preventing accommodation allows progression. Exercises would then be altered at least to a minor degree in subsequent mesocycles to achieve some variation in stimulus along with the changing intensity and volume.

Variation should always serve a specific purpose rather than be assigned randomly for its own sake. Exercise selection should be based on the needs and goals of the macrocycle and mesocycle, as well as the assessed needs of the specific lifter. Several variations of an exercise may achieve the same basic goals appropriate for the mesocycle in question, but certain variations will also address the needs of the given athlete better than others. When selecting an overhead strength and stability exercise for the snatch, for example, a lifter who is strong overhead in the snatch but lacks aggressiveness and proper timing would benefit more from the snatch balance than the overhead squat; while both will achieve the basic goals of improving overhead strength and stability for the snatch receiving position, the snatch balance will also address the specific needs of the lifter to improve the timing and aggression of the lockout overhead.

Variation from mesocycle to mesocycle should also produce increasing specificity toward the competition lifts. That is, as the macrocycle progresses, the exercise selection shifts from more generally training basic qualities like strength and speed to training these qualities in manners more specific to the snatch, clean and jerk. Continuing with the example of overhead strength and stability for the snatch, subsequent mesocycles may employ the overhead squat, then heaving snatch balance, then snatch balance or drop snatch, incrementally progressing from a more basic strength emphasis to increasing demands on speed and precision. Similarly, squatting in early preparation mesocycles may employ more back squats than front squats and include variations like pause squats, parallel squats or slow eccentrics, and as the macrocycle progresses, squatting would eventually shift to using more front squats than back squats and being full speed with the use of the bounce out of the bottom to transfer maximally to the clean recovery.

Reps & Sets Repetition numbers will be assigned based on the exercise, the intensity, the type and schedule of the mesocycle. Details regarding proper rep and set numbers can be found in the Training Variables chapter. Repetition numbers and total volume will be highest near the beginning of the macrocycle and decrease as it progresses, and will together meet the volume requirements determined for the athlete for each phase of the macrocycle.

Testing While each macrocycle will culminate with a competition, a test of the snatch and clean & jerk, or at least the testing of some lift such as the squat, additional testing may be contained within individual mesocycles. This will generally take place in the final or penultimate week depending on the modulation of intensity and volume. For example, a 4-week mesocycle may build from week 1 to testing on week 3 and deload week 4; or it may build week 1-2, deload week 3, and test week 4.

This testing may be of a specific priority exercise or exercises in the mesocycle, or it may be of most if not nearly all exercises in the mesocycle. This will typically mean multiple-repetition maxima. For example, a mesocycle in which the lifter is back squatting for sets of 6 may build to a test of 6RM on the third week before backing off the final week.

Such testing is helpful to the coach by providing more frequent and diverse metrics to gauge progress and the needs of the athlete. While more advanced lifters will make records in the snatch and clean & jerk increasingly infrequently, they can and will make progress on other lifts more frequently. Seeing measurable progress more often is encouraging to athletes and helps maintain motivation that drives further progress; going months without seeing an objective improvement is disheartening to even the most motivated and dedicated lifter.

It's important to ensure that testing is scheduled appropriately and is supported by the training cycle. The only thing worse for an athlete's motivation than not being allowed opportunities for new records is failing to make new records that are expected.

The Microcycle

The microcycle, or week, will reflect the details determined for the mesocycle in which it's contained in terms of exercise selection, reps and sets, and total volume. As mentioned previously, the coach may elect to compose the final details of each microcycle as it approaches rather than prior to the initiation of the macrocycle. The two primary benefits to this approach are minimizing the time investment at the beginning of the cycle, and allowing more accurate prescriptions because of the accumulation of data from the preceding microcycles.

Volume The volume of the microcycle should be pre-determined based on the chosen distribution of the total volume of the mesocycle. This will be somewhat flexible and may be altered slightly as needed when the actual prescriptions are put in place—the total volume of the mesocycle and general trends of its distribution are most important.

Within the week, daily volume will need to be modulated rather than being distributed uniformly. Typically this is best done with daily fluctuation—that is, higher and lower volume days are alternated. In some cases, two consecutive days of higher volume may precede a day of low volume or rest if necessary to achieve some other purpose.

How much variation is necessary day to day is not formulaic, but dependent more on the needs of the lifter and the total volume of the microcycle. A lower volume day may contain 20-50% fewer reps than a higher volume day. Generally, the higher the total volume, the more dramatic the daily fluctuation will need to be. This is seen most clearly in training programs employing twice-daily workouts: the most common schedule employs two workouts on Monday-Wednesday-Friday and single workouts on Tuesday-Thursday-Saturday. Naturally, the double days have considerably greater volume than the single days.

This modulation of volume provides maximal restoration within the week to support the highest possible productive burdening of the athlete; reductions in volume will generally have a more pronounced effect on the athlete's recovery than reductions in intensity.

With a Bulgarian-style approach, daily modulation of volume is less of an issue, as the total training volume is extremely low already.

Graphical examples of daily volume modulation for weeks of 5 and 6 training days can be seen in Figure 39.3.

Intensity Like volume, intensity must be modulated within the microcycle to allow some degree of restoration to occur to support the highest possible average intensity for the week overall. Again like volume, how much variation is necessary is dependent somewhat on the athlete's tolerance and on the overall average intensity of the week—the higher the average intensity, the more dramatic the daily fluctuation will typically need to be. However, the modulation of intensity is considerably less than that of volume in any case.

There are two basic ways to create daily intensity modulation: direct prescription of intensity and exercise selection. The former is the obvious approach—the coach simply prescribes overall lower average intensity for one day than another. The latter relies on the inherent limitations of exercises to allow higher intensity or force lower intensity. For example, a program could prescribe maximal loading every day and still achieve this fluctuation simply by alternating the full competition lifts one day with power or hang variations another; these variations will naturally limit the possible loading relative to the competition lifts.

Note that with a Bulgarian-style approach, this daily modulation of intensity will occur naturally, forced by the limitations of the athlete's present state of restoration each day. However, the more conditioned the athlete is to this training system, the smaller the daily fluctuations will become.

Generally, days of higher intensity should coincide with days of higher volume in a microcycle to create an alternation of greater or lesser burdening overall.

Graphical examples of daily intensity modulation for weeks of 5 and 6 training days can be seen in Figure 39.3.

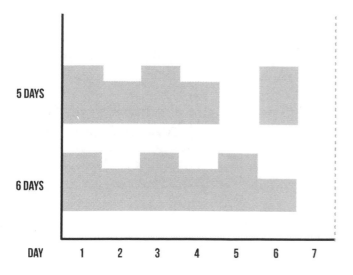

FIGURE 39.3 This figure represents the basic trends of volume and intensity in a microcycle; shown are examples of weeks with 5 and 6 training days.

Exercise Scheduling Exercise selection should have been completed for the entire mesocycle, and at this point exercises can be distributed among the training sessions of the week. The first consideration will be of the total number of exercises each day to ensure the necessary modulation of volume is achieved. Generally, a single training session will be comprised of 3-6 exercises, not including accessory work such as trunk strength or bodybuilding, or, in most cases, very lightweight technique work like technique primers. Obviously the higher the volume for the day, the more exercises will likely be scheduled.

Because the fatigue produced by training is specific to a large extent to the movements performed and muscles used (Zatsiorsky 1995), movement types should typically be alternated throughout the week. That is, identical movements as primary exercises should generally not be performed on consecutive days unless accompanied by significant variation of reps and intensity, and similar movement types are best alternated as well. Such alternation allows for higher training frequency, volume and average intensity overall in the week. This is the rationale for the common grouping of pulling-emphasis lifts and pushing-emphasis lifts on different days. For example, one day may contain a snatch or clean variation, pulling variation, and back strength work, and the following day a jerk variation, overhead strength work, and squatting. This is certainly not a hard and fast rule, but will be beneficial when allowed within all other parameters of the program design.

Some degree of daily variation of lift demand is important even if not totally necessary. This usually will mean alternating inherently higher demand lifts in one day, such as the competition lifts, pulls and squats, with lower demand lifts such as overhead lifts and power or hang variations of the competition lifts. It can also mean the alternation of days comprised primarily of high demand training exercises with days containing more technique-oriented exercises that are by their nature and loading less taxing. For example, one day may be cleans, clean pulls and back squats, and the next jerks, push presses and power snatches.

Finally, when possible, it's ideal to group exercises related to a single competition lift rather than mix exercises related to more than one competition lift

Greg Everett

in a single training session to maximize the proper development of the appropriate motor skills for each lift (Medvedyev 1986/1989, Laputin & Oleshko 1982/2007) —that is, snatch related exercises in one workout and clean or clean & jerk related exercises in another. These lift-specific sessions may be in the same day as long as they're separated by a significant rest period; for example, with double day training, it's common to have one session dedicated to the snatch and one to the clean or clean & jerk. This is most important for newer lifters with less technical proficiency (Medvedyev 1986/1995), but remains important indefinitely.

An exception to this rule is the periodic performance of the snatch and clean & jerk consecutively in a single session in order to prepare the lifter physically and psychologically for competition. Generally for preparation mesocycles, once weekly is adequate, and the frequency may be increased in the competition mesocycle. Performing the competition lifts back to back, particularly for singles at high intensity, is extremely different from performing each in isolation, and lifters who are not regularly exposed to the combination often struggle in competition. This strategy can be employed increasingly as the lifter advances and technical proficiency becomes better established, reducing the potential for problems, and its benefit increases due to the higher demands of competition of the advancing lifter.

The Workout

The final level of prescription is the individual training session. This includes all the finest details such as exercise order, repetitions, sets, intensity, tempo and interset rest, as well as any specific warm-up and cool down protocols requiring prescription.

Warm-up Warm-up practices should be established in the earliest stages of a new lifter's development and become routine over time. New lifters should be provided explicit instructions on warming up until they are capable of properly preparing for training on their own. General warm-up protocols are presented in the Warming Up chapter of the book.

Throughout a training cycle, the coach may as-sign certain warm-up elements on certain days that coincide with the training session's exercises or purpose, or to address observed needs for specific drills. In these cases, such specific warm-ups need to be prescribed.

Technique Primers As has been described previously, a technique primer is a lightweight technical drill that precedes the lift it's intended to improve. While it would be effective technique work in isolation, its effectiveness is magnified by its proximity to the primary lift. These primers should be prescribed based on the needs of the lifter as observed by the coach, and may change as frequently as each microcycle.

Exercise Order The order of exercises is an important element of the training session prescription, as it will influence both the effect of the exercises as well as the performance of each exercise in the session. The basic structure is to order exercises in descending degree of technical complexity and speed. That is, exercises that are faster and more complex (e.g. the competition lifts and their variations) will be performed first, and exercises that are less technically demanding and more strength-oriented (e.g. squats) will be performed last. Exercises like pulls, which are only moderately technical and speed-oriented will be performed in between. This ensures that the lifter's physical and mental resources are adequately available as needed. In the basic circumstances, if a lifter were performing snatches, snatch pulls and back squats, they should be performed in the order listed.

Order can diverge from this protocol to achieve certain objectives, however, such as when the necessary extent of prioritization of a certain exercise warrants overriding the normal order. If a lifter is emphasizing squat strength as much as possible during a preparation mesocycle, for instance, squats may be performed as the first exercise in the workout. This ensures the lifter performs the most important exercise of the session when he or she is freshest physically and mentally.

In other cases, such changes in order may be done to achieve a specific effect. Squatting before snatching, to continue with the example, may also be used occasionally to force the lifter to be more aggressive in the snatch due to being fatigued, and may, like jumping after squatting, force the body to recruit more and higher threshold motor units, and to improve rate coding and synchronization to achieve the necessary force, speed and explosiveness in a state of fatigue. Or, high intensity and very low rep (maximal stimulation of force production with minimal fatigue) squatting before snatching can improve the contraction force during the snatch. These kinds of changes should be used with experienced lifters, as they have the potential to interfere with optimal motor pattern development in lifters without established technical proficiency due to the performance of technical lifts in a more fatigued state.

Certain exercises may be ordered differently depending on their relative priority as well. For example, if a lifter is performing snatches, snatch pulls, snatch push presses and back squats in a workout, the order of the last two can be changed depending on the needs of the lifter. Generally the snatch push press would be best performed prior to the squat because of its greater need for precision, and because the leg drive for the push press will be reduced in power by the fatigue of preceding squats; however, if a lifter is strong overhead but relatively lacking in squat strength, it makes sense to perform the squats before the push presses. Another common example would be performing squats before rather than after pulls for a lifter whose squat strength lags considerably behind his or her pulling strength. While pulls are certainly more technical and speed-oriented than squats, they're not dramatically so, and the benefits of reversing the order for a lifter who needs it outweighs the drawbacks. In a session in which pulls are not particularly heavy, such reordering is unnecessary.

Exercises with similar movement patterns should generally be performed in series. As was discussed previously, generally a single training session should not combine lift variations of both snatch and clean due to the subtle differences in the rhythms and motions, so this ordering will naturally occur in most cases already due to the basic rules of order. For example, it's ideal to perform snatch pulls after snatches because of the similarity of the two movements rather than inserting another exercise in between.

A final consideration is how the order of exercises affects the timing and flow of a training session. When possible without interfering with more important criteria, exercises should be ordered to improve the efficiency of the session. For example, the transition time between snatches and snatch pulls is virtually none—simply the likely addition of weight and the donning of straps. If instead a lifter performs snatches, then overhead squats, and then snatch pulls, there is now the additional time of breaking the bar down, setting up the squat rack, reloading the bar, and then repeating that work in reverse to prepare for the pulls. If the overhead squats are instead performed after pulls, the change in the setup only needs to take place once rather than twice, saving considerable time. While it may seem like a minor detail, in a 3-hour training session, such fractions of time add up quickly. Additionally, the grouping of similar movements improves the development of motor patterns for the related competition lift.

Reps & Sets Typically, reps and sets will be determined, at least loosely, before intensity, although the two may be determined in different order or essentially simultaneously as needed. The repetitions will be determined according to the mesocycle type and timing (i.e. mesocycles nearer the start of the macrocycle will employ higher rep numbers than those nearer the end), the type of exercise, and the needs of the lifter (i.e. what they have historically responded to best). The sets will be determined based on the reps and intensities, and according to the calculated volume total needed for the day. More details on these determinations can be found in the Training Variables chapter.

Intensity Intensity for each set of each exercise will need to be determined according to the exercise, reps and sets, the purpose of the exercise in that training session, the lifter's capabilities and tolerance, and the type of microcycle (i.e. maintenance, loading or deloading). More details on these determinations can be found in the Training Variables chapter.

Rest, Tempo & Time As discussed in the Training Variables chapter, interset rest periods may or may not be prescribed. This will be at the coach's discretion depending on the need of the athlete or to achieve a specific purpose related to rest times. Tempos can be prescribed when appropriate to suit the purpose of a given exercise in a given training session. Generally the time of day the lifter trains will be determined more by availability rather than what the coach determines to be ideal, but when possible, the optimal training time can be prescribed; at the very least, multiple daily sessions can be assigned (e.g. morning and afternoon). Details on interset rest, tempo and training time can be found in the Training Variables chapter.

Accessory Work Accessory work like trunk strength and stability training and any bodybuilding work should generally be performed at the end of a training session. Relatively low intensity ab and back work can be performed at the start of the lifter's workout if it's determined the activation response is beneficial, but high-intensity and high-volume trunk work should be reserved for the end of the session to prevent the potential risk of injury due to excessive fatigue of the muscles stabilizing the spine. Details about each are provided in the Accessory Work chapter.

Additional Technique Work If additional technique work is deemed appropriate for a lifter, it's ideally performed first in the training session when the lifter is freshest and will have the greatest capacity for focus and concentration. Such work should not interfere with the most important elements of that training session, either in terms of time or fatigue. If drills are very simple and minor, such as footwork drills or basic empty barbell work, they can be performed at the end of a workout as time allows as long as the lifter is able to perform them properly.

Cooldown & Mobility Finally, any post-workout mobility work should follow the workout proper. Like the warm-up, lifters should be trained from the start of their careers to perform this work as routine, and changes, additions or omissions implemented periodically as necessary and appropriate. In these cases, certain work may need to be explicitly prescribed in the workout, or may be provided in a separate schedule to the lifter.

Medvedyev (1986/1989) and others also recommend a brief period of general cooling down (5-10 minutes) that includes hanging from a bar to decompress the spine in particular, but also the shoulders and hips, relaxation exercises, and concentration exercises. A simple and efficient way to include the latter is to perform visualization exercises during post-workout passive stretching.

Team & Individual Programs

Most weightlifting coaches will be working with more than one athlete, and some will have many in a team format. The question for this latter group is whether to write a single team program, or individual programs for each lifter.

In general, the need for individualization of the training program increases as the skill of the lifter increases. That is, the needs of newer lifters are more general and common than those of more advanced lifters.

There are certainly benefits to writing a single team program. One important one is that it creates an environment of supportive competition. It's easy for the lifters on the team to push each other and get competitive to push themselves harder when their teammates are doing the same lifts along with them. This can be informal competition—everyone is keeping an eye on what everyone else is doing and trying to stay ahead of them, whether in terms of absolute weight, or relative to bodyweight or current PRs. It can also be made more formal with prizes or money for the best performance of the day as a way to incentivize the lifters and garner a more competitive spirit.

The most obvious benefit of a single team program is convenience for the coach—writing one program demands far less time and effort than writing several.

The drawback of a single team program is of course the fact that a team is made up of individuals, and those individuals can be very different in terms of ability and needs. If the level of ability of all lifters on the team is essentially uniform, this problem is attenuated to an extent, but the likelihood of this is virtually zero. More often than not, any group of lifters is going to need to focus on different exercises or elements of technique, require and handle different levels of volume and intensity, possibly have slightly different training schedules, and even have different competition dates to which their training must conform.

Writing individual programs for a large team is very time-consuming and mentally demanding, and for some coaches, may not be entirely possible due simply to time constraints. In such cases, a reasonable solution is to stratify the team based on skill and competitive level. Lifters in the lower level or levels can train on a single program, as their needs will be more general and abilities similar. Minor alterations to this program can be made for individuals day to day if needed, such as using an alternative exercise that better addresses that lifter's needs, reducing volume or changing intensity, while maintaining the basic structure of the program.

Lifters at the higher levels will receive individual programs to provide the most appropriate and effective training for each. It's natural and entirely reasonable for the coach of a large team to invest the most time and energy in the best lifters on the team.

Intensity Prescriptions

There is unfortunately no simple formula to assist in determinations of intensity, and the interaction of a multitude of factors needs to be considered. Much prescription will be based on the coach's experience with his or her lifters, and particularly the specific lifter in question. There is certainly a considerable degree of estimation and experimentation, and therein lies the art of coaching that complements the science.

Skill Level Intensity prescriptions will vary depending on the lifter's skill level. The more advanced the lifter, the more established his or her abilities and tolerances will become, and the more familiar with them the coach will be, allowing programming to rely on historical performance for improved accuracy in prescription. The actual intensities will still vary somewhat among lifters based on factors like neurological efficiency, technical proficiency and age.

Accurate intensity prescriptions will be less possible for beginning and intermediate lifters. These lifters either have no established maxima on which to base relative intensities, or have inaccurate maxima due to their limited technical proficiency, mobility and similar factors.

Beginners generally should not be prescribed relative intensities for this reason. Instead, the coach and athlete together should determine appropriate weights for each session based on look and feel. As athletes progress in experience, percentage-based prescriptions will become possible and more valuable.

Exercises Intensity prescriptions will obviously vary among lifts even with the same number of repetitions. Generally, the higher the technical demand of the exercise, the fewer reps are possible at a given intensity, or from the other perspective, the lower the possible intensity for a given number of repetitions.

History Decisions regarding intensity prescriptions are best made based on experience rather than formula, and more experienced coaches will know off-hand approximately what kind of loading is not only ideal, but possible, in various cases, with consideration of not only the reps and sets for the exercise in question, but also of the surrounding training and its effects on fatigue, the athlete's current conditioning, and the unique abilities and tolerances of the athlete.

Coaches are encouraged to keep detailed notes of their athletes' performances with various exercises at given intensities and volumes. As these notes accumulate, they will become an invaluable reference for prescribing loading and volume when creating future programs.

Flexibility in Prescriptions

While all programs are intended to be as accurate as possible, no coach will be able to perfectly predict a lifter's state on any given day in the future. Factors in and out of the gym can affect a lifter's response to training dramatically and unexpectedly, and create situations in which prescriptions for a given training session are anything from inappropriately difficult for that day to physically impossible; in some cases, a prescription may even prove too easy.

In any event, the coach must always be willing and able to make adjustments to the training program as it progresses. Strict, unwavering adherence to prescriptions can transform a slightly imperfect program into a complete failure. With relatively minor adjustments as needed day to day and week to week, the spirit and basic structure of the program can be preserved and the effectiveness maximized.

This fairly predictable need for minor adjustment, of course, is the rationale behind not finalizing the details of prescription of the entire macrocycle up-front, but instead creating only the necessary details of the macrocycle and mesocycles, and then filling in the details of the microcycles as they arrive with the accumulated training data from the cycle in hand. This spares the coach the headache of more changes than necessary, and can save considerable time.

Modification for Injury

One of the unpredictable factors that can affect the training program, possibly dramatically, is injury. Depending on the nature and severity of the injury, training may need to cease entirely temporarily; in most cases, however, training can continue with appropriate modification to the program. This can require some serious imagination, but it's invariably possible if the coach and athlete are genuinely interested in finding a solution.

The first rule is to avoid aggravating the injury—the goal is to recover and return to normal training as quickly as possible, and this means ensuring the recovery period is not protracted by continual re-injury. Maintaining a long term perspective is critical—a short setback is preferable over a long one.

The initial steps are to determine what positions and movements need to be avoided completely, what positions and movements may be possible with limited loading and/or speed, and what the lifter's training priorities are that don't interfere with the injury (For example, if the injury is to the wrist and the lifter's first training priority is overhead strength, the next highest priority that doesn't interfere will need to be selected.)

Once these things have been determined, the program can be re-written accordingly. Essentially the process is to replace what was removed with the new work for the selected priorities—if work from the training program is omitted, space for other work is created. This opening should be exploited and filled with alternative training rather than self-pity. In the case of more severe injuries, the training program may need to be scrapped entirely and something new built from the ground up, but again using the same basic rules: not aggravating the injury further and focusing as much as possible on the needs of the lifter.

In the case of injury, not training isn't just a problem for the athlete's physical capacity—it's a psychological problem. Training in some way keeps the lifter focused and motivated and in the right mindset. Quitting and staying out the gym completely destroys the athlete's momentum and puts him or her in a position to have to get back up to speed from zero in *all* respects, not just the one or few that had to be modified. The athlete can be as upset as he or she wants, but needs to find some way to react productively instead of self-destructively.

Restoration & Recovery

Training cannot be effective in the absence of adequate restoration to provide the body time, resources and assistance to adapt to the imposed training stress. The foundation of training is the notion that by delivering the proper stimuli to the body, suitable adaptations can be achieved to improve the athlete's performance in the task in question. Such adaptation is neither immediate nor guaranteed—the body requires certain elements to allow the necessary physiological processes to occur.

Too many coaches and athletes invest inordinate amounts of time and energy planning and executing training programs while neglecting the issue of restoration and consequently make little progress. Interestingly enough, the recent increase in focus on recovery and restorative modalities has pushed some coaches and athletes too far in the other direction. Recovery is a critical element in any training program, but an athlete needs work from which to recover; no lifter is going to rest his or her way to success.

Rest Day Activity Days without training are intended primarily to provide the athlete time to rest and recover, both physically and mentally. This does not mean, however, that athletes should remain perfectly sedentary on their days off; sedentarism is not ideal, in fact, for restoration, even during a day of rest.

The goal is to allow the body to recover as much as possible by eliminating systemically and locally demanding activity, particularly of similar movement patterns to the athlete's training. Light movement, however, is helpful for promoting recovery by maintaining mobility physically and neurologically and improving blood flow and nutrient turnover to fatigued tissues.

Movement with resistance limited to the concentric phase such as rowing, cycling or swimming—at an extremely low level of effort—can be helpful if a lifter is particularly sore or stiff. Otherwise, dynamic range of motion exercise such as are used in the lifter's warm-up can be used once or twice throughout the day to keep the lifter moving and loose. Static stretching and SMR should also be performed, preferably when the lifter is somewhat warm, such as after some light activity or DROMs.

Mentally, it's important for lifters to take a break from their concerns regarding training and competition, and in fact to eliminate concern and stress over as much as possible. The mind needs time to relax, recover and reset as much, and possibly more at some times, than the body. Distractions like reading, television and socializing (in non-self-destructive ways, of course) will help the lifter's mind steer clear of the normal stresses of training. In this day and age of social media saturation, lifters should avoid viewing lifting photos and videos, especially of their competitors.

Finally, rest days should contain the largest volume and highest intensity of restorative modalities.

Sleep Sleep is the absolute first priority with regard to maximizing the ability of a lifter to train harder, train more, recover better and perform at a higher level. For baseline health and wellbeing, sleep is extremely important; add extremely demanding physical training with a serious psychological demand as well, and it becomes critical. As a period of genuine physical and mental recuperation, sleep has a profound effect on both individual training sessions and progress over the long term, as well as the athlete's general psychological state with regard to motivation, focus and discipline. The more physical and mental work performed, the more sleep is needed (Dvorkin 1982/1992).

Both quantity and quality are important. Unfortunately, neither can be achieved by a given athlete automatically. To improve quantity, the first step is structuring the day in such a way that a certain number of hours of sleep are possible. This scheduling should be of the same priority as the training schedule.

Possibly the most effective behavior for encouraging better sleep is maintaining a consistent schedule. If the body sleeps and rises at the same time every day, it will be more inclined to continue doing so. This of course can be very difficult with the obligations of work, family and friends, but some reasonable attempt should be made to at least minimize the variation.

The lifter's schedule should provide for a significant period of time prior to actual sleep in which he or she can wind down. Training should end more than 2 hours prior to bedtime. Light stretching and reading or other non-stressful, relaxing activities should always fill this period of time. Athletes should avoid television, computers, tablets or phones immediately before bed as well.

Developing a routine is key for consistent, high-quality sleep. For example, a lifter comes home after training, prepares and eats dinner, spends some time in the hot tub or contrasting, stretches and foam rolls, showers, brushes teeth and whatever other pre-bed hygienic activities are required, then gets in bed and reads until the pre-determined time to start sleeping. Such a routine will train the body and mind to be prepared for sleeping, and will gradually relax the body and mind.

Athletes require different amounts of sleep, but it's important to always err on the higher quantity side. Many individuals through years of habit have acclimated to reduced sleeping hours and may believe this short sleeping period is all they need. Invariably those who claim a need for extraordinarily little sleep have simply conditioned themselves over long periods of time to function adequately (or what appears to be adequately) on their limited hours. This is not necessarily indicative of a legitimate need for little sleep, but simply a demonstration of the remarkable ability of the body to adapt to the demands of life.

With a period of behavior modification, these individuals can successfully increase the duration of their nightly sleep, and with little exception will find they operate much better on more hours. If the lifter creates a regular bedtime and allows for an adequate number of hours of sleep, but he or she consistently wakes earlier than planned, there is no problem. However, if an athlete is forced to wake by an alarm each day, it's an indication that he or she is getting inadequate sleep. If a lifter blocks out more time for sleep than is needed, there will never be an issue.

There will always be, however, the occasional athlete who sincerely functions better with less sleep than seems necessary. In these cases it will be counterproductive to force unnatural patterns.

As much as possible, it's best to avoid sleep-inducing drugs, as they actually reduce the quality of sleep despite often making the athlete feel like he or she has slept longer or more deeply. That said, if a lifter has a genuine sleep disorder, this may be the only legitimate option at least temporarily—lower quality sleep is far better than no sleep. Supplements like holy basil that reduce cortisol or have systemic calming effects can be helpful.

The bedroom should be cool and as dark as possible—so dark a hand in front of the face can't be seen, if possible. This means blackout shades and covering or getting rid of any electronics with LEDs or similar lights that remain on all night. Research has demonstrated hormonal disruption during sleep with as little as a pinpoint of light on the skin.

Blue light should be avoided within the last hour or so before trying to sleep—this includes television and computers. This light spectrum encourages the hormonal process of waking up and can make falling asleep more difficult. Electronics, including cell phones, should be kept as far away as possible during sleep.

A notepad or journal can be kept alongside the bed in order to collect notes prior to sleep. Often this can help relieve the stress of a mind racing with necessary tasks and ideas and promote greater relaxation in less time.

Finally, it can be helpful to make notes on sleep in the training journal—over time this will likely demonstrate a clear association of the quality and quantity of sleep with subsequent training.

Youths require even more sleep than their adult counterparts—a minimum of 9.5 hours per night. Sleeping only 7.5-8 hours per night has been shown to result in a 30% reduction in work capacity (Dvorkin 1982/1992).

Nutrition The importance of nutrition's role in supporting recovery cannot be overstated. As direct support of physical activities and the processes in response, as well as indirect support through the maintenance of basic health and body function, nutrition is a critical component of all athletic training. Nutrition and supplementation are covered in detail in the Nutrition section of the book.

Outdoor Exposure Exposure to the outdoors can be very restorative (Medvedyev 1986/1989) for multiple reasons, ranging from exposure to sunlight, fresh air, reduced noise levels, and even simply pleasing views. This is particularly true for athletes who spend very little time outside in the course of daily life.

Caution should be exercised with the timing and dosage of sun exposure, however. Long durations of sun exposure can be physically draining, and consequently should not be allowed in the week prior to a competition or immediately before demanding training.

Stress Management All stress is essentially equivalent systemically in terms of how the body must cope with it, irrespective of its nature or additional local symptoms. That is, stress from work, relationships, traffic, or any other source is not substantially different from training stress, other than its potential to eventually result in positive functional adaptation. Interestingly, such non-training stressors can in fact result in physical adaptations, but not ones that will benefit the athlete.

In order to tolerate increased training stress (due to increased frequency of training, volume, frequency of intensity and average intensity), non-training stress needs to be reduced. Minimizing activities or approaches or mindsets that produce unnecessary stress will allow for greater recovery and training capacity.

Methods of stress reduction include better time management—such as creating a consistent, regular schedule that allows enough time for all necessary tasks—batching of tedious, small tasks into chunks of time rather than doing a lot of little things frequently throughout the day—and minimizing daily decision-making by planning ahead (meal-planning, scheduling, to-do lists with specific dates and times, etc.).

Reducing stressors is the ultimate goal, but the athlete will also need to find ways to minimize the damage from stressors that cannot be eliminated. Sleep is the primary method for this, but secondary is napping, meditating or some hybrid of the two. In practical terms, this can be something as simple as taking 15 minutes each afternoon to lie with the eyes closed in a dark, quiet room and not think about work, training, or any other source of concern or stress. This extremely minimal investment of time will go a long way in keeping systemic stress levels as low as possible.

Restorative Modalities

There are a number of active restorative modalities that need to be employed by lifters to maximize restoration and training capacity. Accessibility will vary among lifters, but efforts will need to be made to do as much as is possible financially and with the time available.

Lifters ideally alternate among available modalities to avoid any potential accommodation and consequent reduction in efficacy (Takano 2012).

Generally, more restorative work should be performed on rest days than on training days, and in the case of multiple daily training sessions, less intense modalities employed after early sessions and more intense modalities after the last session (Medvedyev 1986/1989).

Less intense modalities include stretching, napping, swimming and local cryotherapy; more intense modalities include massage, hydrotherapy (including cold plunge and hot tub), and dry and steam saunas.

Contrast Hydrotherapy This is arguably the most effective restorative modality available. Clinical research is somewhat ambiguous, and although some studies have shown significant improvements in recovery of strength and reduction of DOMS, results in the real world vary among athletes. Most support of this modality is anecdotal, but athletes with experience using it typically are adamant about its effectiveness. The contrasting temperatures improves circulation for improved blood and nutrient turnover in addition to the normal results of each, such as anti-inflammation and loosening and relaxing muscles and joints.

Not all athletes have regular access to hot tubs and cold plunges. If these are available, this modality can be used 3-5 days per week. If access to alternative modalities of similar intensity and nature like saunas to allow variation does not exist, contrast hydrotherapy can be employed as many days of the week as allowable by access.

5-10 minutes of hot alternated with 2-3 minutes of cold is a reasonable protocol. If significant soreness or joint pain is present, starting and ending in cold is recommended; if stiffness or tightness is the chief complaint, the athlete can start and end in heat.

Cold Plunge Cold plunges, or ice baths, are also very effective, at least anecdotally. Water temperature should be between 50-60 degrees F (10-15 degrees C). A bathtub filled to be just high enough to cover the athlete's legs will need about 20-40 lbs of ice. This plunge can be 10-15 minutes. Cold plunges are best after very heavy training sessions during particularly tough periods of training when athletes tend to be achy and inflamed.

Hot Tub Time in a hot tub can be a helpful way to keep muscles and joints loose and prevent stiffness from tough training. Hot tubs can also relax athletes in the evening and encourage better sleep as long as there is adequate time for body temperature to drop to comfortable levels before bedtime (the gradual reduction in body temperature itself is sleep-inducing to some degree).

Dry Sauna & Steam Sauna Typically in weightlifting, dry saunas are used primarily for cutting weight for competition, but they can also be used for restoration. For this use, it's important athletes stay hydrated while using the sauna. Ideally, sauna time is alternated with cold plunges or cold showers to induce effects similar to contrast hydrotherapy.

Massage Massage is a very effective restorative modality, but for most weightlifters is prohibitively expensive. However, even infrequent massage is better than none, although regularity even with infrequency will improve its effectiveness. Massage 1-3 times per week is ideal, but once monthly is still far better

than never.

Aggressive deep tissue work, except localized for a specific problem area to prevent injury, should be avoided within a week of an upcoming competition, as it can make the athlete feel slow and sluggish.

Stretching & SMR Stretching and foam rolling, even for already flexible athletes, will help keep muscles moving fluidly and reduce joint pain. It can reduce stiffness that accumulates between training sessions, making warming-up easier and training better. Passive stretching can also be helpful for recovery and preparation for future training sessions by preventing or reducing soreness (Zatsiorsky 1995).

Aside from the straightforward mechanical benefits to stretching and foam rolling, the practice can also serve as a calming, relaxing activity for athletes with benefits along the lines of napping or meditating, albeit to a lesser degree. Gentle passive stretching before bedtime can be helpful to settle the athlete down to prepare for sleep.

Swimming Light, easy swimming and treading water can be restorative through the anti-inflammatory response to the cool water, the decompression of the spine, and the ability of muscles and joints to move without the pull of gravity they typically have to work against. Keep in mind that this is not exercise—this is gentle swimming that elevates the heart rate minimally over baseline.

Napping As discussed with regard to stress management, napping—including no actual sleep, but simply lying with the eyes closed in a quiet, dark room—is incredibly beneficial both physically and mentally for restoration. It should be a goal for all weightlifters to schedule a nap of at least 20-30 minutes each afternoon. This is even more important for lifters training in multiple daily sessions.

Cryotherapy Cryotherapy, or icing, of locations of acute pain or chronic low-grade pain can both improve training and help prevent minor acute or chronic conditions from becoming more severe injuries when properly implemented. Cryotherapy is a contentious subject even among medical professionals, and recommendations vary considerably. In general, static icing should never exceed 10-15 minutes in duration no more frequently than hourly. Ice massage of a local area will only require 2-5 minutes, and can be punctuated on the minute with cross-friction massage.

Monitoring Recovery

With such an emphasis on recovery and the need to plan training around it, the question of how to monitor recovery status in some fashion naturally arises. The classic monitoring of resting heart rate and blood pressure are simple and convenient methods, but appear to have less value for the strength athlete than the endurance athlete. Heart rate variability (HRV) is becoming more prevalent and appears to be more accurate than orthostatic heart rate measurements. The practical objective measures that seem to have the best correlation with present condition are the athlete's vertical jump height and grip strength. That is, negative deviations from the athlete's baseline jump or grip strength appear to most accurately indicate under-recovery.

In any case, objective measurements, while being interesting, are typically unnecessary. Further, despite any level of accurate correlation between test results and the state of recovery, the actual implementation of the tests creates opportunity for inaccuracy. Jump testing, for example, requires some level of skill irrespective of how it's administered, and results can vary based on how well an athlete reaches a vane or how accurately he or she places a magnet, Velcro loop, or a chalk mark on a wall—all of which can vary day to day. Additionally, unmotivated athletes have been known to intentionally throw such tests in order to receive lighter training prescriptions; in other cases, this may not be entirely intentional, but due simply to a lack of psychological commitment to the activity.

In addition, an athlete's jumping ability will vary considerably during different phases of training emphasis. For example, jumps will tend to be much higher during lower-volume classic lift emphasis phases than during higher-volume strength-emphasis phases. This being the case, for jump testing to work, the baseline jump figure would need to be adjusted appropriately.

For objective metrics like resting heart rate or HRV that are not influenced by athlete performance, the challenge is determining how to appropriately adjust training in response to these measurements, as no formulaic strategy exists. It will be largely according to the coach's judgment.

A collection of subjective measures can be considered when trying to determine an athlete's condition. For most coaches, under-recovery will be quite obvious, often even before an athlete touches a barbell. Likewise, most athletes will not have trouble figuring out on what days they feel ready to train hard and heavy, and on what days they need to back off their planned training to some degree. Of course, there will be many days on which athletes would prefer not to train as hard as is planned, but need to push through it, and this is where the coach's observations and judgment play an important role. Depending on a particular athlete's disposition, he or she may be prone to undertraining without consistent pressure from the coach to work at full capacity. There are often times as well when an athlete appears and feels worn down, but has excellent and even record performance.

These subjective metrics will of course predictably fluctuate within training cycles, and even daily, so determinations will need to be based on a broader view of a given time period. That is, no athlete will be completely fresh every training day—if he or she is, the training is not demanding enough to elicit adaptation. However, under-recovery can only be maintained for so long before it crosses a threshold into overtraining and requires serious changes, often resulting in detraining, to bring the athlete back to a healthy baseline.

Overtraining is the result of continued training beyond the limits of restorative ability. In other words, it's the accumulation of stress at a rate or to a degree greater than what the body can respond to productively. Care must always be taken to balance training with recovery in order to maximize the adaptation potential of each athlete. Clearly it's more effective to improve recovery as much as possible rather than limit training unnecessarily. Much of a given athlete's recovery ability will be a product of genetics (e.g. natural hormonal levels and the ability to consistently attain adequate sleep quality and quantity); the remaining capacity can be improved and managed in the ways discussed previously in this chapter.

Typical signs of overtraining include:

- Chronic fatigue
- Insomnia or restless sleep
- Elevated resting heart rate and blood pressure
- Reduced speed of movement
- Reduced manual dexterity
- Increased joint soreness and stiffness
- Reduced enthusiasm for training
- Changes in personality or mood
- Irritability, frustration, anxiety
- Gastrointestinal distress, diarrhea
- Reduced grip strength
- Reduced vertical jump
- Retrograde performance (other than that expected as the result of normal training fatigue), including inability to perform prescribed training (assuming this training doesn't make unreasonable demands)

Diagnosing legitimate overtraining is not a simple task, as there is unfortunately no real measure of this condition, only a spectrum of physical states. Essentially indicators of overtraining need to be present consistently for a period of several days at least to consider it actually overtraining rather than simply a temporary bout of fatigue appropriate to the training, or that may simply be the result of work stress or similar non-training related elements.

If an athlete is determined to be legitimately in an overtrained state, the solution is significantly reducing intensity and volume in particular, and often forcing complete rest for a period of a week or more as needed. The deeper the state of overtraining and the longer the duration of this state, the more time it will take for the athlete to recover. After any complete rest that is taken, training can be resumed with very light weights (40-60%) and very low volume, and incrementally increased as tolerated, with closer daily monitoring of the athlete's recovery status.

Again, this is a delicate issue, as athletes should be expected to be fatigued, at times quite significantly, and challenged physically and emotionally by their training. Ultimately, much is left to the coach's and athlete's collective judgment.

Hand Care

Being covered in chalk and rubbing against knurled metal for hours every week will not exactly prepare hands for a modeling career—calluses will be commonplace, and blisters and tears will occur occasionally, or more often with inadequate preventative effort. As the connection of the body to the bar, the hands need to be taken care of well to prevent the disruption of training and competition. Seemingly minor wounds can prove painful and distracting enough to directly prevent a successful lift.

Hand care can be divided into two parts: prevention and correction. The greater and more consistent prevention efforts are, the less the need for correction will be, and the more consistent training can remain. Corrections are never perfect—the best strategy is to avoid needing them as much as possible.

Prevention The two keys of preventative hand care, which overlap considerably, are keeping the palms smooth and free of any hard, sharp edges, and keeping them adequately moisturized. Athletes will generally develop calluses near the bases of the fingers and possibly near the joints of the two smallest fingers depending on how the bar sits in the hands. If these

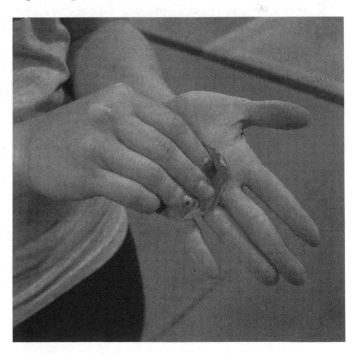

FIGURE 40.1 Calluses should be kept smooth with fine-grit sandpaper to prevent tearing.

calluses aren't maintained well, their edges can catch on the bar and be torn. If the tear is confined to the dead, callused skin, it will have no detrimental effect; but more likely, the tear will continue into the living skin and create a painful open wound that will be susceptible to further tearing and aggravation.

These calluses can be kept smooth by regularly sanding them down with fine-grit sandpaper (Figure 40.1). Small squares of sandpaper should be kept in the athlete's training bag for use during training if necessary. If this practice is consistent, rarely if ever will a callus develop to a degree that can cause problems. A simple way to make sure it's consistent is creating a habit of sanding the hands before each training session. Note that such sanding should not remove calluses completely, as they serve an im-

portant purpose, but simply keep them of reasonable thickness and remove any rough edges that may catch and initiate a tear.

If a callus is large enough or is beginning to separate from the hand, fingernail clippers can be used to trim any loose skin away, and the edge then sanded down to be smooth with the rest of the surrounding skin. Again, any palpable edges are potential locations for tears.

To keep the hands moisturized, they should be treated at night with a product like Cornhuskers Lotion. This is a non-greasy lotion created to help toughen the skin on the hands while keeping it healthy. A single application before going to bed each night should prove adequate for most athletes. For more severely damaged or more sensitive hands,

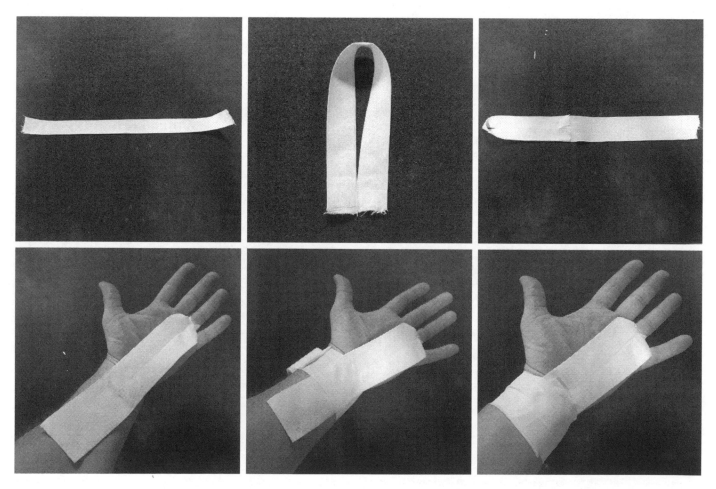

FIGURE 40.2 More extensive bandaging can be applied if needed to allow continued training. Fold one length of tape over down the middle of its length to make a long, thin strip with no exposed adhesive. Create a loop with this strip with the ends lying flat alongside each other. Apply another length of tape flat on the ends of the loop to hold them together and create a smooth, flat surface, leaving a long tail free, which will then be folded under and stuck to the other side of the loop ends. The loop is then slipped over the finger nearest the tear so it lies flat on the finger and hand, and tape is wrapped around the wrist to hold the end. The end can be folded back over the wrist tape and then wrapped over one more time to keep it more secure.

Greg Everett

it can be applied multiple times throughout the day, particularly following training and before bed. Additionally, larger quantities of lotion can be applied and then the hands covered in gloves to allow the hands to continue absorbing the lotion overnight. It's important as part of the moisturization effort to thoroughly wash chalk out of the hands after training.

Correction If prevention fails—or has not be duly performed—callus tears and blisters may appear. These will need to be managed properly in order to allow continued training.

Torn calluses should be trimmed with fingernail clippers and the rough edges smoothed with sandpaper. If the tear has left an open wound, the exposed area should be covered with a topical adhesive such as NexCare or Benzoin Tincture. A small piece of athletic tape can then be placed over the area, held better in place by the adhesive. This tape will likely not last an entire training session and may need to be replaced several times.

More extensive bandaging can be applied if needed to allow continued training (Figure 40.2). Fold one length of tape over down the middle of its length to make a long, thin strip with no exposed adhesive. Create a loop with this strip with the ends lying flat alongside each other. Apply another length of tape flat on the ends of the loop to hold them together and create a smooth, flat surface, leaving a long tail free, which will then be folded under and stuck to the other side of the loop ends. The loop is then slipped over the finger nearest the tear so it lies flat

on the finger and hand, and tape is wrapped around the wrist to hold the end. The end can be folded back over the wrist tape and then wrapped over one more time to keep it more secure.

If a blister occurs, it should be taken care of before it rips on its own—this will allow more control of the outcome (Figure 40.3). Once a tear occurs, the athlete is at the mercy of chance. The blister should first be lanced and drained—this can be done by clipping its edge with fingernail clippers or using the sharp point to puncture it. In either case, the hole should be placed on the edge of the blister nearest to the fingers—this will reduce the likelihood of the bar's movement in the hands from tearing the skin away.

Once the fluid is squeezed out and cleaned away, liquid adhesive such as NexCare can be injected into the empty blister through the hole. This will allow the dead skin to serve as a protective layer while the wound heals from the inside out. The blister should be smoothed out as much as possible as the adhesive is drying. Once dry, sandpaper should be used to further smooth out any rough edges and help prevent any further tearing. Athletic tape can be used to cover the area with the added adhesive of Benzoin or similar if desired. If a blister has already torn open, the remaining dead skin should be removed and the underlying skin treated in the same way described for a torn callus above.

If necessary or desired, topical lidocaine gel can be applied to any hand wounds to reduce the pain, although the effects are inconveniently short-lasting.

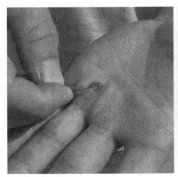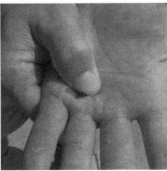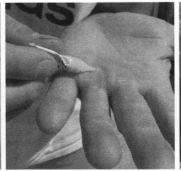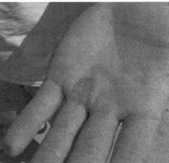

FIGURE 40.3 Repairing a blister: Blister prior to tearing; Lancing blister at edge nearest fingers; Draining fluid; Injecting adhesive; Finished.

Injuries

Despite the generally unrecognized low incidence of injury in weightlifting competition, as with all sports and training modalities, injuries are inevitable, particularly as the level of competition increases. Most can be avoided through intelligent training, programming and restorative methods, but once an injury does occur, its treatment is critical for the athlete's timely and full recovery and return to training.

The first issue is that of recognition. Competitive athletes are accustomed to training with pain and discomfort and often pride themselves on their abnormally high tolerances. However admirable in general this may be, there is in fact a threshold after which continued training is no longer respectable, but simply stupid. Many times an athlete's refusal to back off at appropriate times transforms minor problems into potentially career-ending injuries.

The distinction between the type and degree of pain the athlete can train through and a legitimate injury that requires treatment and rest is critical. Most athletes' first reaction is to deny the severity of an injury. Equally problematic is the genuine ignorance of the condition in question. Unfortunately, the recognition of a legitimate injury is often not straightforward. That being the case, it's wise to err on the side of caution, and if any doubt exists, seek the opinion of a professional familiar with the treatment of athletes.

It's important to always keep in mind the big picture when considering responses to an injury. Most athletes have a sense of urgency and a consequent refusal to miss any training. However, this failure to back off when appropriate often leads to exacerbation of the condition to a point at which rest is forced. If left to this, invariably a minor injury that may have required a brief time off will demand far more time off and more involved treatment. In other words, caring for an injury sooner will nearly always reduce the total amount of missed training.

Ultimately the most intelligent course of action is to consult with a medical professional experienced working with competitive athletes who understands both the demands of the sport and the urgency of achieving a complete recovery and return to training. This will allow the most accurate diagnosis, which in turn will allow the most appropriate course of treatment and modification of training.

Training Practices

One of the many important elements of training with an established coach, and even more ideally, in a team environment, is the natural acquisition of information regarding the myriad details of weightlifting training practices, etiquette and culture. Some of these things can be taught and learned in other manners, such as being presented in this chapter, but nothing can replace the daily experience of the weightlifting gym atmosphere. Sadly, this is one of the most commonly missing experiences of new weightlifters in the US with the sudden explosion of interest and relative dearth of established weightlifting gyms and coaches.

The 1 Kilo Rule

Weightlifting is a sport in which the rate of progress declines predictably over time. That is, the longer an athlete trains, the more slowly he or she will make progress. When a lifter reaches the more advanced stages in which progress is measured in small numbers over large spans of time, sound programming and strategy is even more important, and part of that strategy is doing everything possible to provide opportunities to measure that progress.

There's an almost irresistible compulsion to always try to make big PRs—a 5kg PR is a lot more exciting than a 1kg PR. Unfortunately, many lifters get greedy for large increases when not adequately prepared, and miss the attempts, repeatedly, sometimes for months. A 5kg PR is a lot more exciting than a 1kg PR, but a 1kg PR is a lot more exciting than continually failing to make any measurable progress at all.

Even worse, often to set up these big PR attempts, these lifters will actually lift their current PR as the last set before the PR weight. As it's already known that weight is possible, its repetition makes little sense; further, if the lifter is physically capable of lifting his or her current PR on a given day, there is a very good chance 1kg more is possible. Making incremental records at a higher rate will produce the same ultimate progress, but the more frequent measurable progress not only demonstrates the effectiveness of the training, but keeps the athlete more motivated to continue.

With this in mind, in most cases lifters should strategize in a way that sets them up to make the 1kg record first. If more is possible, it can be performed following this. Often in a training cycle leading into a testing day, the athlete's performances will be such that it's nearly guaranteed he or she will hit a big PR. In these cases, more aggressive numbers can be attempted. If the lifter can't honestly tell the coach he or she has 99% or more confidence in making a certain weight, a more conservative weight should be selected. If that degree of confidence doesn't exist, it's unlikely the lifter will be successful even if ready physically.

The PR attempt itself should be reached in a rational manner. Lifters typically take the same warm-up weights for certain exercises habitually. These weights should be adjusted as needed to set up the PR attempt with reasonable weight increases that both allow adequate physical and mental preparation and minimize unnecessary fatigue.

For example in the snatch, a lifter's best is 125kg, and he always take 5kg jumps past 100kg: 100-105-110-115-120. But the lifter is aiming for a 126kg PR. If the lifter takes his normal jumps, he will get to 120 and find that his normal 5kg jump matches his current PR, and to make 126kg, he either needs to take an odd, and excessively large, 6kg jump, or figure out a better way.

This better way is to adjust the attempt weights to provide for rational, decreasing increments as the PR weight is approached. In the above example, this could be something like 100-105-110-114-118-122-126 or 100-105-110-115-119-123-126, depending on the lifter's historical consistency and confidence. In the first approach, the final jumps are all kept to 4 kg (3%), and in the second, the lifter begins with 4kg jumps and then takes a smaller and less demanding, physically and mentally, 3kg jump to the PR attempt. With smaller maximal weights, this final jump can be reduced to 2kg—the final attempts being a weight 1kg under the current PR followed by a weight 1kg over the current PR.

This plan needs to be in place before the athlete begins the exercise. The coach should play an active role, either providing the lifter with the appropriate plan, or at the minimum, consulting with the lifter to verify that his or her plan is acceptable. Establishing a plan at the beginning improves the lifter's confidence and keeps him or her on pace to lift rather than leaving the lifter scratching his or her head and over-thinking the process between each set.

Repeating Cycles

It's fairly common for a lifter to repeat the same macrocycle if it's been deemed effective. However, in some cases, the maxima on which the relative intensity prescriptions of certain exercises are based have not been measurably improved. This does not necessarily mean that the athlete's ability in these exercises hasn't improved, but at the least, it means they weren't tested and consequently, recent updates to the figures are not available. This is most common with strength lifts like squats, pressing variations, and other overhead strength lifts.

In other cases, the lifter failed to accomplish new records in competition lifts themselves. While initially this may seem to indicate the macrocycle failed and shouldn't be reused, it can simply be the product of an unrelated problem and not a reflection of the cycle's efficacy. For example, if the only snatch and clean & jerk testing of the macrocycle was in its culmination in a competition, the lifter may have simply had a bad competition performance due to nerves,

poor meet conditions, or other complications not related to his or her physical ability. In these instances, the observation of the lifter and other metrics collected throughout the course of the macrocycle may satisfactorily indicate that the program was in fact effective.

In either case, when a program is repeated, it's important that the absolute intensities be increased regardless of the lack of change in the exercises' maxima. This may mean extremely minor increases over the previous cycle—such as a single kilogram—or more significant increases in exercises such as squats when the coach is confident, based on multiple-rep performance in the preceding cycle, that the lifter's squat has improved considerably. Repetition of an identical training cycle with identical intensities is a nearly perfect way to guarantee no improvement of the lifter's performance. However, if the lifter is able to repeat the training cycle with the same reps, sets, interset rest and volume with higher intensities, it should be obvious this will both drive and indicate improvement.

More commonly, an effective macrocycle may be repeated in essence but certain details changed. Generally this will be variation of certain exercises, such as different variants of the competition lifts to address the changing needs of the developing lifter, or adjusted volume or intensity based on determined need from the previous run through. This method allows the coach to be confident in the effectiveness of the training cycle, but also to continually ensure it remains maximally suitable for the athlete each time it's used.

Warm-up Reps

There are two kinds of weightlifters in the world: those who do the number of reps prescribed for their working sets in all warm-up sets, and those who do as few reps as possible as they warm up to the working sets. More advanced lifters can generally be allowed to employ the approach they find best, but in most cases, the coach should dictate the protocol based on what's most suitable for the lifter and the program.

The less experienced the lifter, the more important it is that they perform the full number of prescribed reps on all warm-up sets. These lifters have not yet established technical proficiency, and every rep they perform is an important motor learning opportunity. Reducing repetition numbers simply reduces their volume of repetition and protracts the technical learning process. Additionally, it's important for developing lifters to continually improve their work capacity; performing full warm-up reps is a very simple way to allow more training volume without extending the duration of training sessions.

The other consideration is the purpose of the exercise that session. There are two possibilities: training or testing. If the purpose is training, all reps should be performed—the goal is for the athlete to benefit from these repetitions as much as possible. If the purpose is testing a maximal effort, partial-rep sets may be used to warm-up in order to conserve energy. For example, if a lifter is going to test a 5RM squat, he or she may perform sets of 5 on the lightest warm-up sets, and then use triples and doubles the rest of the way up until reaching the first 5RM attempt weight. In a final case, the lifter may be working to a repetition maximum, but doing so more for the sake of training effect than testing. In this case, it's appropriate to perform full rep numbers on warm-up sets.

Barbell Loading Protocol

How the barbell is loaded can affect the feel of the barbell and even the outcome of a lift at times. Generally, however, the issue is more one of taking care of equipment. First, bumper plates of different brands or models should not be mixed on different sides of the bar—that is, a plate of one type on one end, and a different type on the other. Each plate will have somewhat different compositions and consequently bounce differently when dropped. Uneven bouncing causes unnecessary wear on the plates and the barbell. Different plates can be mixed on the same bar as long as they are balanced side to side, although this is still not ideal, as different plates can vary slightly in diameter, and this will mean more weight being supported by the larger plates.

Once 5kg in addition to the last bumper plate needs to be added, the next largest bumper plate should be used when possible. That is, if a lifter has a 15kg bumper plate and needs 20kg of weight on the side, a 20kg bumper plate should be used to replace the 15 rather than 5kg of change plates. This minimizes the abuse to the bumper plates by spreading the total weight out over a larger surface area (heavier bumpers are wider than lighter bumpers). This is particularly important with 10kg bumper plates, which tend to be very thin and more easily damaged. Of course, once a 25kg bumper is on the bar, this rule changes to 10kg worth of change, at which point a 10kg bumper plate can be added.

Multiple smaller bumper plates can be used in training, e.g. a 15kg and 10kg rather than a 25kg, and most commonly are, often out of convenience in loading, and sometimes out of necessity due to a lack of plates. This actually has the benefit of spreading the total weight over a larger surface area when dropped, which will reduce wear on the equipment. The downside is that it changes the behavior and feel of the barbell slightly. That is, the degree to which a bar bends and therefore whips depends not just on the total weight, but on the distribution of that weight. If a given weight reaches farther toward the ends of the bar due to multiple plate loading, it will produce somewhat more elastic rebound during a lift. This can be problematic for a competitive lifter who must be capable of lifting that weight properly loaded in competition.

Plates should also be loaded heaviest to lightest from inside to outside—that is, the heaviest plates closest to the center of the barbell. Weight markings, if only on one side of the plate (like on most change plates), should face outward. If using friction plates (change plates covered in rubber to limit sliding on the bar), weights less than 2.5kg can be placed outside of the collars.

Collars are relatively rarely used in training, again more because of inconvenience than anything. Competition style collars are also very expensive, and as a consequence, many gyms don't have enough collars for lifters to use regularly anyway. Spring collars can be used instead when collars are needed and the budget doesn't allow an adequate number of competition collars.

Collars should be used any time there is the potential for plates sliding on the bar during a lift. This can be due to a combination of a very slick bar and loose-fitting plates, or simply a lifter with poor control. In any case, plates sliding on the bar can be extremely dangerous for the lifter, and at the very least, can cause unnecessary damage to equipment due to bars dropping unevenly.

Competition style collars should be used at minimum when lifters are approaching a meet to prepare them for the different feel and sound of the bar. With such collars, the plates will spin slightly less easily (only the bearings of the barbell will spin rather than both the bearings and the plates on the bar themselves), and the bar will whip slightly more—without collars, the plates can move slightly and absorb some of the energy that would otherwise go into bending the bar.

More information on barbell loading with regard to competition preparation can be found in the Competition section of the book.

Record Keeping

The importance of a training journal cannot be exaggerated. Irrespective of what shape it takes, this reference allows the athlete and coach access to invaluable information to help guide programming and recovery efforts, as well as simply to evaluate progress over the long term. Memory is limited and unreliable and in no way adequate. A simple spiral-bound notebook from the drugstore is all that's necessary. Inside the athlete can, under each date, record the performed exercises, sets, reps and loading, as well as notes regarding how specific parts of the training felt, the status of injuries or other pain, energy levels, bodyweight, the previous night's sleep, and other relevant data.

As a coach, tracking the training data for a team of lifters gets more complicated. In this case, keeping electronic records like Excel documents or similar will make tracking each athlete's training and subsequent planning far easier. Each cycle should at minimum show the actual training (exercises, reps and sets) along with weights and percentages when appropriate. It's helpful to also note each athlete's relevant metrics at the start and end of each cycle, e.g. best lifts and any other markers the coach is interest-ed in (vertical jump, mobility metrics, skill level are a few examples). Some coaches prefer to note lifts as they occur in training for each athlete; others prefer to collect athlete's records periodically to update their own records. In any case, the coach cannot create maximally effective programming without having access to all of the data from preceding training.

Missing Lifts

Misses count as practice just as much as makes. Not only are missed lifts practice in the physical, technical sense, i.e. practicing the movement that produces a miss, but, more importantly, it's practicing mentally to miss. In any training cycle, lifts will be missed. In fact, if no lifts are missed in a cycle, it's an indication that the training is too easy. This doesn't mean cycles should produce a high number of misses, but simply that some should be expected.

Missing can become a habit like anything else a lifter practices. If an athlete becomes accustomed to missing lifts, it becomes routine and suddenly it's not a big deal anymore. The lifter may find him- or herself perfectly content to simply miss and try to repeat the set to make up for it. Repeating a set is acceptable in some cases, but making this a habit is training to not be prepared and focused when necessary. The coach needs to decide beforehand in a workout what will be accepted as misses and what will warrant repeating.

The number of misses should be a very small number relative to the total training repetitions in a given workout or time period. If a lifter is constantly missing prescribed lifts, the prescription is off. This may mean the intensity is too high, the repetition numbers are too high, or even that the choice of exercise is unsuitable for that athlete at that time.

Volume Calculations The volume of training is one of the metrics used to determine the burdening load on the athlete. The organism can't distinguish in these terms a difference between a failed lift and a successful lift—the only distinction is in the amount of work and effort. Consequently, genuine attempts at a lift should all be included in volume calculations whether completed or missed. The only case in which a failed lift can be ignored with regard to volume is if the attempt was aborted immediately—for example, the lifter gave up on a snatch or clean before the bar even reached the knees. If the lifter completed the pull and only failed to move under the bar, it should be consider, in terms of volume, a complete rep, just as a snatch pull or clean pull would be.

Response to Missed Lifts

There are times in a lifter's life when lifts aren't made. These times are, of course, the absolute worst, and in those moments following a missed lift, athletes can generally find indisputable proof that they'll never again succeed, that their abilities have already peaked and they're finally and terminally on the decline, and can explain in detail why, being in such a stage of life, they no longer have any value to the world.

There are two basic responses following a missed lift: To accept it and move on, or to refuse to fail and fight back. Neither is always the best choice, and it isn't always easy to know how to proceed after a missed lift. Unfortunately, prescribing a totally rigid protocol isn't possible. There will be many times in which the decision will need to be made based more on intuition than protocol. The following will provide some basic guidance, but there will certainly be times when diverging from these recommendations is reasonable and preferable.

Mistake or Failure The first consideration to make when trying to decide how to proceed after a missed lift is to determine if the miss was a mistake or failure. That is, did the lifter make a technical error that he or she can correct with some coaching input, or did he or she physically fail to lift the weight? The two are completely different experiences, and they warrant different responses.

If the lift was missed because it was genuinely beyond the athlete's physical capability, the obvious decision is to stop. If the lifter makes a technical mistake and both he or she and the coach are confident it can be corrected in a subsequent attempt, generally it's acceptable to repeat the set and make the correction. If the lifter misses again, the coach needs to consider the possibility that he or she and the lifter didn't actually know what the problem was, or that

it's not entirely technical.

If the lifter is tired, has a considerable amount of work left in the training session, or his or her confidence in making the lift has dropped considerably, the lifter should move on. If instead the lifter is feeling good, doesn't have much if any subsequent training to worry about, and the last miss was closer than the first one, the lifter can give it another ride.

Understand the Program A very important consideration when deciding whether or not to take a missed lift again is how that additional attempt will affect fatigue and as a consequence the rest of the training program. Training programs are (or should be) constructed carefully with volume and intensity within desired parameters; if a number of additional reps are added, makes or not, the stress of the program is increased and effects that were not intended or foreseen are created. This can be a significant enough difference to cause problems in subsequent workout or workouts, and if it's something that happens frequently, to seriously disrupt the entire training cycle. If this is happening frequently, the program needs to be re-evaluated.

It's also important to understand what the intention for the lift in question is. For example, is the goal to use the exercise to get stronger? Is it to improve a certain aspect of technique? Understanding this will help the decisions. If strength is the goal, and the missed lift was a strength exercise like a squat or press, assuming the athlete didn't make some kind of correctable mistake (much less likely with a basic strength exercise), the weight is too heavy.

If the missed lift is a more technical exercise, such as a competition lift or variant, there are more possible causes of a miss. The weight may be too heavy, but the athlete may also just be doing something wrong technically, or may not be focused or as aggressive as needed. If the goal is technical improvement, the priority is proper execution. If the weight the athlete is attempting to use is preventing him or her from performing the lift correctly, it's too heavy, whether the lift is actually made or not. If the goal is speed or explosiveness, a miss may mean that the athlete needs to make a technical adjustment or improve focus.

Reducing Weights When an exercise is intended to work primarily on lift technique, again the priority is proper execution. If a weight is preventing this, generally the best course of action is simply reducing the weight to a point at which the lift can be properly performed for the intended reps and sets. Decisions on what weight to use can usually be made using warm-up lifts or previous sets as guides. If any uncertainty exists, erring on the conservative side and dropping more is advisable; the weight can easily be increased on subsequent sets if the lifting is adequately improved (sometimes moving down and coming back up will even allow the lifter to make a weight he or she missed previously).

With strength exercises, the decision on what to do after a miss will depend a lot on what the rest of the program looks like, and whether the program at that point is more focused on intensity or volume. For example, if the lifter is back squatting heavy singles and doubles, the goal is obviously trying to achieve a certain level of intensity; a miss would indicate that the level of intensity desired is more than what the lifter can handle at that time. If the volume of the program is low, which it more than likely is with such a rep prescription, it's often wise to stop with the miss rather than accumulate more volume by reducing the weight and performing more reps.

In the case that the goal is accumulating a certain amount of volume, the weight can be reduced as needed to allow the lifter to finish out the prescribed sets and reps.

When possible, finish an exercise on a make even if it requires reducing the weight considerably.

Remainder Sets In some instances, there may be a certain number of sets and reps of an exercise that is somewhat technical in nature, but is also intended to build some strength and power, and the coach deems the intensity to be the most important factor. As an example, 5 sets of 3 reps snatching from high blocks. The first 2 sets are done successfully, but the third rep of the third set is missed. The first 2 reps looked fine, but the last one wasn't even close. Sometimes it makes sense, rather than reducing the weight to finish the remaining sets, to complete the remaining sets as doubles instead of triples, and to add one more set to make up for the missed reps in the abbreviated sets. In this way, the same amount of volume at the same intensity is being completed.

Gym Etiquette & Atmosphere

Most gym etiquette is simply common sense and courtesy. However, since both seem disappointingly rare, some of the basics are addressed here in addition to more weightlifting specific practices.

Respect of other athletes should be exercised during training at all times. Athletes should always be given an uninterrupted view forward while lifting, direct eye contact with a lifting athlete should be avoided, and noise should be kept to an absolute minimum during heavy attempts to allow the athlete to focus. In the team environment, team members should be at least moderately aware of what the other lifters are doing in order to ensure the suitable quiet and encouragement is provided when appropriate.

Lifters need to remember that their primary purpose is training. That is, socializing is secondary, and needs to be set aside to ensure not only the athlete's training, but the training of all team members, can be done properly without distraction or disruption. This doesn't mean the gym needs to be a silent vacuum of fun, but it does mean all behavior needs to support training first and foremost. If athletes don't want to come to the gym if they can't fool around or their favorite music isn't playing, they don't have the constitution to be successful weightlifters.

The culture of the gym is created originally by the coach, and reinforced by the coach and lifters. Lifters will model the coach's behavior, consciously or not, and consequently, the coach needs to be constantly aware of how he or she acts in the gym and in competition. Each lifter on a team or in the gym is a model for other lifters, especially the newer ones, who learn the gym's culture from the more experienced members. It's a collective responsibility for the team to create and maintain the proper environment and to ensure new lifters learn what's expected of them. While the coach is ultimately responsible for enforcing expectations, the team must share the responsibility.

Safety & Equipment

Care of equipment and the facility should be a priority for all athletes. Gear should be used appropriately and abuse should be limited to the expected stress of normal training use. Athletes should help keep the facility clean and orderly as much as is reasonable. This means primarily not leaving behind empty water bottles, used tape, or other trash, and controlling chalk use to prevent unnecessary spilling. More specific rules include the following:

Back Away from the Squat Rack If you're doing an exercise using a squat rack, whether it's squatting, jerking, or anything else, take more than half a step back from the squat rack. It's not a lot of effort, and if you miss a lift, you won't drop the bar on the base of the rack. When bumper plates land on racks, it will often chip pieces of the rubber away and the rack can be dented or certain plastic parts broken completely (for some perspective, bumper plates start at around $200/pair for 10kg to $400/pair for 25kg and squat racks are $400-600 each). You also won't have a near-death experience getting yourself tangled up with the bar and rack.

If You're Sketchy, Use Collars Weightlifters often train without collars on their bars because they lift them straight up and put them straight down, so there's no sliding of plates on the bar. If you're new, unsure, or otherwise sketchy when you lift, use collars. Weights sliding on your bar can be disastrous—the shift in weight magnifies whatever imbalance caused it, and your attempts to correct are usually too little, too much, or too late. Spare us all the fear of seeing you almost die and protect the rest of us and the equipment by keeping your weights secured safely on your bar with collars. If you don't know whether or not you're a sketchy lifter, you're a sketchy lifter.

Contain Yourself in Your Lifting Area This is usually a platform, but it may also just be a designated space on rubber flooring. If you're fighting a bad lift, and the only way you think you can save it is to chase the bar off your platform or outside of your lifting area, it's already over—drop the bar (under your control) inside your lifting area. Not only are you putting yourself at risk, but you're putting the people around you at risk. If you want to do irresponsible things that risk injury to your person that don't threaten the safety of others, knock yourself out. Do not do those things in a public place where you're around people who don't share your lack of regard for personal physical wellbeing. If you're not sure you can contain yourself in your designated lifting area, you shouldn't be doing whatever you're doing. Just because someone or something wasn't somewhere before your lift went sideways doesn't mean that remains true afterward—someone may have wandered into the space you think is clear, and may very well not be paying attention to you, operating under the assumption that you know what you're doing and you're not going to be running around the gym throwing barbells.

Keep Your Lifting Area Clear Whatever your lifting area is, whether a platform or an area on the floor, keep it clear. Don't leave change plates, collars, bumper plates, clothing, training journals, or *anything* on the floor in that lifting area. Hard, solid objects are things that a dropped bar can bounce unpredictably off of, causing a loaded bar to collide with you or someone near, or go crashing into other equipment. Soft items (clothing, towels, journals) are trip hazards, whether during a lift or not.

Don't Use The Best Bars in the Rack Quality weightlifting barbells are expensive, and they need to perform very well and safely. In order to do that, they need to be taken care of (like everything else, but especially these). Using barbells in squat or power racks, even when lifters are careful, over time results in the knurling being worn down where the bar rests in the rack. This means less secure grips on the bar during any exercise with a snatch-width grip, and this is not a problem that can be fixed. Use less expensive bars when doing rack work—especially squats—whenever possible.

Don't Spin or Slide Bars in Racks Related to the previous rule, when using a bar in a rack—whether it's the best or worst bar in the gym—don't spin it or slide it side to side in the cradles. If the bar is off center in the rack, it's your own fault for putting it back that way after your last set (see the next rule). If you got it in there that way, you can get it out from the same place—there's no way the bar is so off-center that you can't possibly lift it out of the rack. If you spin the bar in the rack when setting your rack position for jerks or pressing exercises, get your grip set loosely and let your hands spin around the bar as needed to get into position instead. You don't need to be choking the bar to death before you're even in position to lift it out of the rack. This sliding and spinning wears down the knurling and ruins the barbell, and adding insult to injury, is completely unnecessary.

Set Your Bar Down in the Rack When using a barbell from a squat rack, replace it under control when you're finished with your set. Don't throw the bar back into the rack, or slam it down into the cradles. This is either a sign of laziness, a lack of respect for the gym, or attention-seeking. If your set was so incredibly difficult that you can't possibly set the barbell down into the rack the way you should, you shouldn't be putting it into the rack—drop it on the platform like you would a snatch or clean & jerk. Even after the most difficult set of squats, it's not hard to lower a bar a few inches down into a rack until you feel it supported and can move out from under it. Aside from taking care of the equipment (both the bar and the rack), this is also an issue of safety. When dropping or throwing a bar into a rack, it's easy to miss the cradles, especially on one side only, resulting in a potentially injurious explosion of bar, rack and plates. (As an extension of this, move out from under the bar cautiously at first until you're sure it's actually in the rack completely.)

Don't Drop Empty Bars on the Floor Bars are meant to be dropped on the floor when loaded with bumper plates—dropping an empty bar directly onto a platform is unnecessary stress on an expensive piece of equipment that already has to survive a great deal of stress day to day. If you're not strong enough to set an empty bar down when you're done with it, you're not a weightlifter and you have zero chance of ever becoming one.

Place Racks Properly If jerking from a rack, position the rack along the front edge of the platform rather than significantly back from the front edge. This maximizes the available space on the platform for both the lift and a potential safe miss.

Keep Chalk Where it Belongs You're not flocking Christmas trees—you're lifting weights. Chalk all over the floor and elsewhere in the gym is not helping you hold onto your bar. Stick your hands in the chalk bucket and keep them in there while you rub the chalk in. Don't grab a handful of powder or a chunk and then proceed to rub it in outside the bucket, and don't slap your freshly-chalked hands together like an emotional slow-motion montage in a Lifetime original gymnastics movie. Yes, some chalk is going to end up on the floor in lifting areas—let it get there in unavoidable manners. Not only is it extra work for someone to clean up, it clogs HVAC filters and forces more frequent replacement, and it's a slipping hazard for lifters on the platform.

Control Your Bar When You Drop It After a snatch, clean or jerk, return the bar under control to the platform. This doesn't mean you can't drop it—it means keep your hands connected to it until it's fairly close to the floor, and pay attention to it until it's done moving. Don't let go of the bar from overhead and walk away, letting it bounce across the platform into another lifter, off of something back into your own legs, or into other equipment.

Don't Stand on Bumper Plates Bumper plates may seem indestructible because you drop them when you lift, but they're meant to be durable for exactly one thing—being dropped on an evenly loaded barbell on a proper lifting surface. Many times a bumper will be lying partially on top of something (a change plate, another bumper plate, or the edge of a platform, for example), and by standing on it, you're stressing the plate in a way it's not meant to be stressed—like being folded in half. Which leads nicely into the next rule:

Lay Bumpers Flat on the Floor or Stand Them Up If you need to lay a bumper plate on the floor, lay it flat so it's evenly supported by the floor in case someone isn't paying attention and breaks the previous rule or drops more weights on top of it. You can also lean them up against something if they're close enough to vertical to not be stepped on or end up on the bottom of a stack. Otherwise, put them away where they belong.

Barbell Rules Barbells should never been stood on, sat on, kicked, or spun with a foot. The former are abuses barbells are not intended to cope with, and the latter is both disrespectful on a fundamental level, and unhygienic.

Load/Unload One Plate Per Side When you're loading or unloading a barbell in a rack, do it one plate on one side, then one plate on the other side, and alternate in this way until all of the plates are on or off. Don't take multiple plates off the same side first, as this leaves the bar unbalanced and creates the potential for tipping out of the rack. Even if you're a world class physicist and are convinced that the relative weights and the positions of the rack supporting the bar prohibit such tipping, it's still possible when, for example, you bump the unloaded or less-loaded end with your shoulder or a plate, and suddenly your safely balanced system is flying through the air. The whipping end of a 6-7-foot long barbell will do very serious damage to whatever it comes into contact with, especially human tissue. Eyes have nearly been lost to this mistake.

Don't Throw Plates into Plate Racks Set your plates into the racks they belong in—don't throw them or drop them. Even if those racks are made of metal and you think they're the toughest things on Earth, it's just being lazy and will likely bounce the rack around on the floor, shifting it from where it's supposed to be and adding unnecessary wear to joints. If you're too weak or tired to lower a plate to the ground under control, roll it in from the side.

Don't Drop Bars into Vertical Racks If your gym stores barbells in vertical storage racks, slide them in gently. Don't stick the end of the bar into the top of the hole and then drop it—slamming a bar on its end damages the snap rings, which can lead to their eventual breaking, causing the bar sleeve to lock up during a lift, or even slide off of the bar—either is dangerous for the lifter.

Clean up Your Blood Sharing can be great, but not when it comes to blood borne pathogens. If you bleed on a bar from a torn callus, accidentally hooking your shin, or in any other way get your private internal fluids on any other public surface, clean it up properly, such as with Clorox, Lysol or a similar cleaning agent. If it's a bar or another metal surface, dry it off immediately after using any cleaning solution to help prevent it from oxidizing.

Clean up Your Spills Accidentally kicked your wa-ter or coffee or favorite pre-workout muscle-swelling beverage? Clean it up—this isn't astrophysics. If you don't know how to clean it up or what to clean it up with, find a responsible adult and ask. Don't pretend it didn't happen and leave it for that responsible adult to find later when it's sticky, nasty and staining.

Put Away Whatever You Use This is the easiest of all rules—put away everything you use where it belongs. If the person before you didn't put it away where it belongs, be the better person and do it right because it's the right thing to do, then tell the offender to do it right next time when you get the chance.

Lowering the Bar between Reps

Lowering the barbell between consecutive reps of a set in the snatch, clean or jerk can be difficult, but the difficulty can be greatly reduced with proper technique. Just as raising the weights requires a concerted effort of the entire body, so does lowering them.

Snatch & Clean When lowering the bar from overhead after a snatch, the athlete will begin by slowly bending the arms under control to bring the bar down as low as can be managed in this position, while simultaneously bending the knees. This brings the bar to a lower starting point. At the lowest position, he or she will quickly flip the elbows from under to over the bar, keeping it as close to the body as possible as it drops. The clean will begin with this flipping of the elbows from under to over the bar.

As the elbows flip over and the bar begins to drop, he or she will straighten the legs and pop up onto the toes to meet the dropping bar with the thighs, absorbing the force by dropping back to flat feet and bending the knees. The thighs will also create somewhat of a shelf to catch the weight and reduce the strain on the grip. From here, the weight can be lowered in the same manner as a deadlift.

In some cases of multiple-rep snatches from the floor when using straps, the lifter may choose to lower the bar before standing until the final rep. This can be done by, from the bottom of the squat, guiding the bar forward and down as the athlete begins standing in order to bring the hips and bar together. From this point, the rest of the movement is like lowering the bar from overhead; that is, the athlete will absorb the bar with a bend of the knees, and then drop the bar to the floor under control. This should only be done if explicitly allowed by the coach, and only by athletes with no problems stabilizing and recovering from the snatch.

Jerk With the jerk, the bar will be brought back to the rack position on the shoulders by the athlete first lowering it by bending the arms and legs to bring the bar to a lower starting position, then straightening the legs and popping up onto the toes to bring the shoulders up to meet the falling bar, and absorbing the load by dropping to flat feet and bending the knees as he or she would when lowering a snatch or clean, keeping the torso upright. From here the bar can be lowered to the floor as the clean is, or it can be replaced in a rack.

Overhead lifts can also be lowered to the shoulders behind the neck. This will be most common with snatch push presses, overhead squats or snatch balances, but may also be the preferred location for athletes after finishing a set of jerks, push presses or presses. The process is the same as for bringing the bar down in the front—the athlete simply needs to keep the head out of the way, keep the shoulders shrugged up to ensure a muscular landing pad rather than a bony one, and to prevent dropping the chest excessively as the weight of the bar is absorbed.

Dropping the Bar Dropping the bar after a successful lift should not be a careless action. The lifter should maintain contact with the bar until it passes his or her waist, guiding it down safely away from him- or herself. Failing to do so in competition is a technical rules violation and can result in a no-lift call (The new IWF rule requires contact with the bar only to shoulder height; continuing contact to waist height ensures no doubt in competition, and maximal safety in training); in the gym, the practice is an effort to maintain safety and prepare for competi-

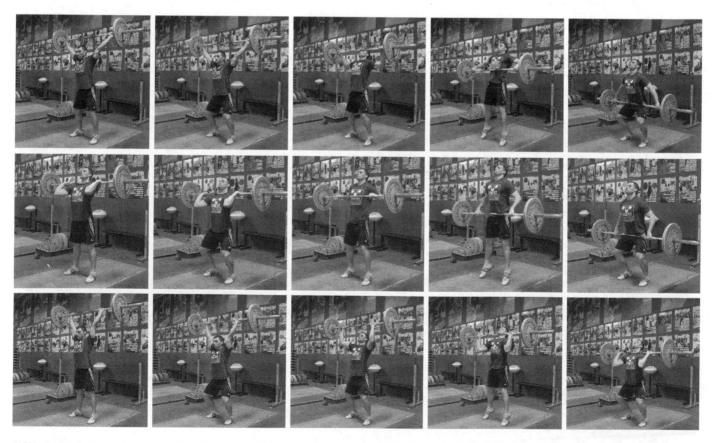

FIGURE 41.1 The bar can be lowered safely and under control after the snatch, clean or jerk by bending the knees and arms to first bring the bar to a lower starting point, then letting the bar fall while standing on the toes to meet the bar smoothly and absorbing it by bending the legs again.

Greg Everett

tion. Different types of bumper plates will bounce to varying heights when dropped—some quite high, particularly in combination with the springier rubber tiles of some platforms—so the lifter should be careful to continue watching the bar as it drops and bounces and to keep his or her hands clear to avoid jamming fingers or a wrist against a rebounding bar. It's important as well to make sure the platform is clear of any spare plates off of which the bar could bounce in an unexpected direction and collide with the lifter or another nearby. Along the same lines, before the athlete drops the bar, he or she should make sure no other lifter has wandered into the area and inadvertently placed him or herself in the path of the bar.

The Mental Game

As has been mentioned in passing a number of times throughout the book, weightlifting is a sport that demands a great deal of mental fortitude and skilled control of the mind in order to achieve the necessary physical tasks in training and competition consistently. Some athletes naturally possess exceptional mental control, focus and intrinsic motivation, while others must work over time to develop their abilities. In either case, athletes will benefit from actively improving these abilities further.

Much of this is very individual, and each athlete will need to find his or her own methods with experimentation and practice. The following provides guidelines for developing and organizing effective mental habits for athletes, and recommendations for how coaches can help their athletes with these tasks. More advanced visualization and other mental techniques can be found in resources by experts in the field.

Positivity for Productivity

Positivity is not just a general state of mind—it can be a very deliberate approach to considering and responding to events and circumstances with specific purpose. With regard to weightlifting, it's the intentional mastery of psychological reaction and fram-

ing of training, competition and all the many related elements in a way that constantly drives motivation, progress and focus, and reduces discouragement and distraction.

This type of positivity does not involve the alteration of one's fundamental personality—rather, it's a framework for managing day-to-day difficulties and demands for maximal productivity. It's the ability to replace the passive and useless hoping and wishing on which new athletes so often rely with mindful action and proactive strategy to accomplish clear tasks and achieve rational goals.

Athletes

The athlete's job as a weightlifter is to do everything in his or her power to improve in all aspects of the sport. Like most sports, weightlifting success requires the mastery of a multitude of elements, only some of which are actually related to the gym. The coach can write an incredible training program, properly dose praise and critique, and provide all of the structure and support the athlete needs, but ultimately, the lifter has to do the work, remain committed, and believe in what he or she is doing if he or she intends to get anywhere. Weightlifters cannot sit around hoping and waiting for their coaches to give them that one magical cue, exercise or inspirational speech that finally makes them great weightlifters. Each athlete must *be* a great weightlifter by creating the habits, work ethic and mindset of a great weightlifter before he or she becomes one in terms of actual lifting performance—if the athlete fails to do that, he or she will never actually achieve greatness.

Prepare for Workouts Weightlifters should always know the contents of their next workouts—not knowing is a perfect indicator of a lifter's lack of commitment and interest in weightlifting—if he or she can't even be bothered to have a quick look at the upcoming workout, it's obviously not even on the priority list, let alone at the top where it needs to be if becoming a great weightlifter is the goal.

Not only should the athlete know what the next workout is, he or she should be spending time thinking about it before reaching the gym, making goals and plans, and visualizing successful lifts. Athletes should study their next workouts at least several hours before they're going to happen. If he or she trains in the afternoon or evening, this should be done in the morning; if he or she trains in the morning, this should be done the night before. A lifter should be able to get through a workout without even having to look at the program because he or she is so familiar with it. Athletes should have specific goals to reach before they even tie their shoes. They should have the next workout in the backs of their minds all day leading up to it.

Further, athletes should be performing at least basic visualization of the most important parts of the upcoming workouts in preparation. Visualization is discussed in more detail below.

Reframe the Negative Positively When things go wrong in training, the lifter has two basic options: wallow in his or her misery and get worse, or reframe the situation in a way that allows improvement. Understand this is not a suggestion the athlete act like all the bad things are good, or to pretend the workout went well when it didn't; rather, it's the intentional reconsidering of the problems in a way that allows the athlete to improve going forward. The first part of this is using failures or mistakes as motivation rather than as fodder for self-flagellation. The second part is using these negative things to create clear and specific goals and plans to fix the problem.

For example, if the lifter had a terrible day snatching because he or she was allowing the bar to swing around into place overhead rather than actively moving it into position properly, he or she can indulge in anger briefly, but then move on quickly to motivation to improve; the lifter should create a task list of actions to fix the problem, and literally write this list in the training journal both as a method to internalize it, and to have a reference for the next training session with that exercise. In this case, the lifter might write that he or she needs to focus on pulling the elbows up and out aggressively on every single snatch next time, or write down a simple one-word cue he or she finds effective to tell him- or herself on each snatch attempt.

Whatever it is, it needs to be a simple, objective item—it can't be something vague like *Next time I need to snatch better*. Such a note is not only useless, it keeps the negative negative by focusing on what was done wrong instead of what the athlete is going to do right in the future.

Finally, the athlete should be sure the tasks are positive—that is, they are actions to do, not actions to *not* do. Using the same example as above, it's not productive to plan to not allow the bar to swing forward—the question is *how* is the lifter going to do that? That must be the focus. What is the athlete going to do? What is the proactive response? If the athlete can answer that concisely and specifically, he or she will have a valuable solution to the problem.

Journal Notes First, if a lifter doesn't keep a training journal, there are serious fundamental problems to address. A journal is a critical part of training and should be considered an absolute necessity for any serious athlete. The training journal should be used not just to track the numbers from workouts, but subjective information like how the athlete slept, how he or she felt in the workout, the level of enthusiasm for training that day, and other little things that help make sense of what's happening over the long term when the journal is referred to in the future.

There are also three things every lifter should be writing after each workout: What am I proud of from today's workout? What do I need to work harder on next time? What are my goals for my next workout? These questions must all be answered specifically and clearly.

Celebrate Success Weightlifting involves a lot of hard work over long periods of time with few significant successes. It's important, in consequence, to celebrate the successes that do occur and be aware of their existence rather than allowing the negative to consume the mind. However, celebration should never be excessive or serve to reduce a lifter's motivation to continue improving. It's imperative to distinguish between being happy or proud of a certain achievement, and being satisfied or content with current abilities. The former is important; the latter is detrimental to progress.

Appreciate the Process The process of training is an experience of every hour of every day for years; the results are few, irregular and infrequent. If a lifter can only be happy with results, that lifter will very rarely be happy, and as a consequence, is likely to lose motivation and even quit the sport. If instead the lifter learns to appreciate and enjoy the process itself, motivation will remain more constant and reliable. The athlete needs to appreciate the satisfaction of hard work and consistency and recognize such things as accomplishments themselves, not just as a means to accomplish more objective performance goals. Habitual emphasis on the kind of positivity described here will help make this appreciation of the process natural.

Coaches

The coach's attitude and behavior will both determine the kind of athletes he or she attracts and who remain in the program, and will also serve as the model his or her athletes emulate. A coach may have a charming vision in his or her mind of a dictatorial master being the ultimate coaching paradigm, but very few people can actually pull it off in a productive way—the most important element to making this approach viable is actually being a true master of the craft, and again, very few coaches genuinely are. Far more likely, a coach's success is going to rely overwhelmingly on his or her ability to develop meaningful relationships with athletes, be a model for them to emulate, and provide support—in other words, to make lifters *want* to be the best they can be, rather than trying to frighten or shame them into improving.

Balance Critique & Praise No matter how tough an athlete is, hearing nothing other than a list of what he or she did wrong is going to wear on someone. This is the easiest thing to do as a coach. Even a coach's best lifter is going to produce a long list of things that need to be corrected or improved. In reality, decent lifters usually know a lot of them and even most of them without needing them pointed out by their coaches. What's more difficult is properly triaging and knowing what the lifter needs to hear at any given time. A lifter can only manage so many things at once anyway, so coaches need to learn to prioritize the problems and focus on the most critical first.

In addition to this, a few pats on the back go a long way in general, but also in balancing the critique that is absolutely necessary for all lifters. This is not a suggestion to be dishonest or exaggerate—being

genuine with praise is imperative for it to be effective—nor is it a suggestion that coaches coddle their athletes like fragile, sensitive children. It's simply a recommendation that the coach provide a balance of drawing attention to what each athlete does right and does wrong.

No matter how bad a lift or training session was, the lifter had to have done at least one thing well. For example, maybe a lifter missed every jerk over 85% in a training session, but she was showing a lot of aggression with her attempts, which is one of the goals she and the coach have created for her. It's not hard to pick out at least one positive to include with the priority critiques provided. This keeps the lifter motivated to improve rather than just being discouraged from a continual barrage of negatives.

Positive Cues Technical cues should be positive in two different ways. First, they should align with the lift or part of the lift when possible rather than being contrary. For example, for a lifter who tends to yank the bar off the floor and shoot the hips up too quickly relative to the shoulders, a cue to keep the chest up is more effective than one to keep the hips down—lifting the chest aligns with the action of moving upward.

Cues should be positive also in the sense that they provide the lifter with an action to perform, rather than just being a reminder of something to *not* do. If the lifter is doing something incorrectly, there's a good chance he or she doesn't know how to fix it—if he or she knew how to stop, it probably wouldn't be happening. In that case, telling him or her to stop doing it is useless. Using our same example, rather than telling a lifter not to let the hips shoot up, telling him or her to stay tighter off the floor and keep the chest up will provide the lifter a clear and simple action to perform that will help correct the problem. The coach cannot simply point out what the lifter did wrong and hope he or she figures out how to fix it next time.

Support Finally, the coach's job is to provide the support necessary for his or her lifters to do what they need to do. This means helping them learn and practice the habits they need to develop; giving them ideas on how to implement changes; going to them and checking in regularly rather than always waiting for them to come to the coach; and being available for them when they need to talk. Every athlete will require a different nature and magnitude of support, and these things can change over time with a given athlete.

Again, athletes should never be coddled. Part of the support job is to helping athletes become more self-reliant, personally accountable and intrinsically motivated. The coach must steer them in this direction while providing the net they need in the process.

Attentiveness & Intention

Attentiveness is a constant attention to detail; intention is a clear plan with purpose. These two things are critical for becoming a great weightlifter. Too often, lifters are content to coast through the majority of their training by doing the minimal work required—simply going through the motions without any genuine thought about what they're doing or why, and without sincere intent. Suddenly they reach weights unachievable with such an approach and are unable to make the adjustment.

Habits are created by repeated actions; if the lifter most commonly performs lifts and training in general without attentiveness and intention, this will be the way he or she approaches all lifts to some extent even when trying consciously to change this for specific lifts. At this point, it's too late. True success requires doing nothing haphazardly or without clear understanding and purpose.

Awareness The lifter must always be aware of what he or she is doing. It may seem impossible for a lifter to do anything without knowing he or she is doing it, but it's entirely possible for lifters to perform many actions without conscious thought through routine. While routine and not overanalyzing are beneficial in many respects, they must be utilized properly. This is simply a matter of paying attention to the present action.

The lifter must next be aware of why he or she is doing what he or she is doing. This doesn't mean every lifter needs to have comprehensive knowledge and understanding of program design and biomechanics; it means that he or she must understand the purpose of the exercise or action. For example, the purpose may be improving aggression in the turnover of the snatch, or improving the stability of the overhead position in the jerk.

Next, the athlete must be aware of how he or she is doing whatever is being done. That is, it cannot simply be done automatically without thought. The lifter should have points of focus for every rep of every exercise he or she ever does. As has been explained throughout the book, this cannot be a list of points, but 1-2 per rep. Proper execution of every single repetition performed, particularly focusing on the specific needs of each athlete, is what creates the foundation for performance at higher levels. This is what builds the necessary habits that carry over into near-maximal and maximal lifts without requiring the lifter to think his or her way through the lift, which is impossible. Even the most seemingly unimportant exercise has at least one specific purpose—attention to that purpose and mindful execution is what makes it effective.

The athlete additionally needs to pay attention to whether or not what he or she is doing is effective. This is not always possible to know with a single occurrence of an exercise or action, but may require the evaluation of a series over time. However, the idea of evaluating effectiveness, both objectively and subjectively, should be on the athlete's mind. This can be communicated with the coach to help guide him or her in decisions on future training.

Finally, the athlete needs to remain cognizant of his or her mental and emotional responses to training. In this way, the lifter will know whether responses are positive and productive, or negative and counterproductive, and make the necessary changes.

Intent The athlete needs to have clear intentions for every exercise and the program as a whole. Of course, this is primarily the realm of the coach, but the athlete will be more successful by being engaged with the process.

The athlete and coach together should define realistic but ambitious goals at every scale—from an entire macrocycle down to a single exercise—and continually ensure the programming and daily training serves these goals.

Execution Proper execution of all reps in the program will build consistency and confidence in maximal lifts. There are general rules of proper execution, such as those described throughout the book with regard to posture, positions, tempo and the like for each lift. There are also occasionally rules specific to each athlete that may differ somewhat from the general rules—this is usually the result of using a certain exercise for a purpose specific to the lifter that is not its traditional purpose.

Consistency Again, athletes should attempt to perform every single repetition in every single workout with maximal precision and consistency. This is the only way the necessary habit of quality lifting can be developed.

Evaluate The success of every training cycle needs to be evaluated, both in objective and subjective terms. Objective measurements include the obvious, such as the weights lifted, the training volume of specific periods, and the lifter's bodyweight and body composition.

Subjective measures include the lifter's enthusiasm for training and how much they enjoy the process, his or her outlook on future training and performances, and his or her contributions to the training atmosphere through attitude and support.

Control Finally, the athlete needs to actively control his or her mental response to training, the program and goals. This involves the actions discussed previously with regard to positivity and productivity.

Visualization

Visualization is a skill, and like any skill, it requires practice. It's imperative that lifters learn to effectively visualize successful training and competition. Belief and confidence have very real effects on performance. Obviously there is a limit to its power, but it can be surprisingly effective. Keep in mind that the athlete has to genuinely believe what is being visualized (which is the ultimate purpose of visualization)—a lifter can't visualize snatching 400kg and expect it to happen no matter how realistic his or her visualization.

Lifters should practice visualization with a single lift initially to work on focus and details before trying to expand into more extensive processes. The first key is the level of detail—nothing should be left out, even the most seemingly irrelevant. Every single thing the athlete would do, see, hear, smell, and feel needs to be included. The second key is feeling confident throughout the visualization—that is, the athlete *knowing*, not just thinking, that he or she will be successful.

The athlete should start the process with the very first thing related to the lift he or she is visualizing. For example, loading the weight on the bar or writing the exercise and weight in the training journal—whatever it is that the lifter would do that could be considered the very beginning of that set depending on how he or she normally does things. From this point, the lifter must see, hear, feel, smell and do in his or her mind every single thing through the process of taking that lift until the bar is back on the platform and he or she is sitting and marking a successful lift in the training journal.

This means rubbing chalk into your hands and noticing how it feels, adjusting your wrist wraps and the sound the Velcro or leather makes, the smell of ammonia or the taste of your pre-workout beverage of choice, paying attention to the sensation of first grasping the barbell and how the knurling feels in your hands, your exact movements while you prepare and set up with the bar before lifting, the noise the plates make as the bar breaks from the platform and the feeling of the weight hanging from your arms, the shifting of the pressure over the soles of your feet and the sound of your knee sleeves creaking, the sound of the barbell and the feel of its contact on your hips or upper thighs as you extend and the sensation of aggression and exertion, noticing the speed with which you move under the barbell, hearing the sharp clap of your shoes reconnecting with the platform and the pressure returning to your feet as the weight settles overhead or on your shoulders, the sound of your expulsion of air and the strain of your legs and back to recover from the bottom of the squat and that thought in your mind of driving hard and fast and not letting up, the feeling of relief and satisfaction of making it up and the sounds of your teammates yelling for you, the feeling of the weight suddenly disappearing as you drop the bar, the deep sound of the heavy weight hitting the floor, and finally returning to wherever you started to rest for the next set and make a note in your journal.

Bill Starr made an important point many years ago in his book *Defying Gravity* with regard to visualization, and that is to work on it until the athlete feels no physical arousal from even the biggest lifts in the mind. The goal is to be able to mentally work through a PR lift in the biggest competition ever without feeling the heart or breathing rates increase. This will let the athlete know he or she has mastered that lift and made it routine and truly believable.

Over time, the lifter can progress to visualizing an entire competition or training session. Athletes can begin using this to prepare for upcoming training sessions and meets to build confidence.

Sample Training Programs

The following macrocycles are included to provide examples of program design for athletes at different stages of development and with different needs. Additionally, they should provide further clarification of the principles of program design discussed in preceding chapters.

These programs can all be used as-is by coaches and lifters, but their primary utility will be as templates on which to build programs modified appropriately for the athlete based on his or her particular strengths and weaknesses and the other factors that determine the various parameters of the training program. In other words, while they will be effective out of the box, their effectiveness will be considerably improved by appropriate tailoring for specific lifters.

Such alteration will primarily involve changes to volume, intensity and possibly frequency, but may also include changes to exercise selection. Exercises can be replaced by other similar lifts that better address the particular needs of the lifter but still address the same basic purpose. For example, a hang position may be changed, or a hang lift may be taken instead from the blocks; pulling exercises may be changed to different variations such as segment or partial pulls, floating or on a riser; and squats changed to emphasize the priority for the lifter, such as more front squats than back squats, or pauses added.

Most of these programs can be found in web, text, Kindle, Excel spreadsheet, and phone app formats on the Catalyst Athletics website for ease of use.

Notation

Exercises are followed by the prescribed loading, reps and sets in that order. For example, *Snatch – 75% x 2 x 5* indicates snatching 75% of the athlete's 1RM for 2 reps for 5 sets. If a loading prescription is absent, the sets and reps will be in the reverse order. For example, *Box jumps – 4 x 5* indicates 4 sets of 5 reps.

Complexes of more than one lift per set will contain rep prescriptions for each exercise in their order of execution. *Clean & Jerk – 80% x 2+1 x 3* indicates 3 sets at 80% of 2 cleans followed by 1 jerk, for example. *Snatch pull + snatch – 75% x 2(1+1) x 5* indicates 5 sets at 75% of 1 snatch pull, 1 snatch, 1 snatch pull, and 1 snatch.

Unless otherwise indicated, relative intensity prescriptions are of the athlete's 1RM of that exercise. One consistent exception is for pulling exercises—percentages for snatch and clean pull and deadlift variations refer to the associated competition lift maximum. For example, *Snatch Pull – 90% x 3 x 3* would mean 90% of the athlete's best snatch.

Percentages that follow a maximum refer to that max rather than the athlete's all-time best. For example, *Back Squat – 5RM, 90% x 5* indicates the athlete works to a 5RM, then performs 90% of that weight for a set of 5.

HS (Heavy Single) *HS* or *heavy single* indicates taking the exercise to the heaviest weight for a single rep that can be managed in that training session. This is determined simply by gradually increasing the weight until that criterion is met without any failed attempts. If an attempt does fail, but the reason for failure is obviously technical in nature, the athlete can make another attempt. Otherwise the loading increase should stop when the athlete completes a rep he or she is confident is approximately the best possible at that time. In other words, it's the heaviest weight reasonably possible that day rather than a true maximal test. Similar to the heavy single would be multiple reps with the "heavy" notation, e.g. *heavy 3 or heavy triple*. This simply means taking the exercise up to the heaviest set of 3 reps the athlete is able to do that day.

Max *Max* is a genuine test of a maximal effort. In this case, the athlete can give him- or herself up to 3 attempts at a given weight. An exception would be an athlete who is missing based on minor and known technical errors, and who is able to continue making attempts that are at least as close or better than previous attempts at that weight. In such cases, continued attempts are recommended until this trend reverses.

RM *RM* stands for *repetition maximum*, meaning the athlete will attempt the set with the heaviest weight possible for the prescribed number of reps, e.g. 3RM, 5RM, 1RM. If percentages follow an RM prescription, they are of that day's RM, not of the athlete's current 1RM. For example, *3RM, 90% x 3 x 2* would indicate taking the exercise up to a maximum weight for 3 reps, then doing 2 more sets of 3 at 90% of that maximum weight.

No Weight Prescription If a loading prescription is absent for a particular exercise, the athlete should choose the loading according to feel, knowing that at the beginning of a training cycle, these weights should be conservative to allow gradual progression in the coming weeks.

Accessory Work

Abdominal and lower back work should be included regularly in all of the following programs. Other training such as light bodybuilding-type work can be included as needed or desired. See the Accessory Work chapter for more information on its implementation.

Skill Classification Sample Programs

The following programs provide examples of macrocycles appropriate for the associated skill classification level as described in Table 33.4 in the Assessment chapter. These can be used as-is, but ideally are used as templates to be modified to optimally suit the individual athlete with exercises that address specific technical needs, strength disparities, mobility issues, volume and frequency tolerance and requirements, and competition schedule.

These programs are kept relatively simple in terms of exercise selection to allow easier modification for specific athletes through the substitution of simple competition lifts with more appropriate variations or complexes.

Programs for the highest skill levels have not been included because such programming demands an extremely high degree of individualization and, more importantly, coaches and athletes at that level have no need for help from this book.

- Level 0
- Level 1
- Level 2
- Level 3
- Level 4
- Level 5

Additional Sample Programs

The following programs are additional examples of different program structures and training ideas. All are programs that have been used successfully by many lifters. These can be used as-is, or may serve as templates to which modifications can be made to better suit specific lifters' needs and competition schedules.

- Beginner Template
- Simple 3-Day Template
- Masters Program
- Weight Gain Program
- Bulgarian Program
- Five-Week Front Squat Cycle
- Ten-Week Volume Squat Cycle
- On-The-Minute Cycle
- Risers, Waves & Positions
- Double Day Squats & Heavy Weights

Program **Skill Level 0**

This stage is the athlete's initial engagement in weightlifting. It involves two basic phases: the initial learning of technique, and then the initial development to graduate them to the next level. Ideally these are young athletes, but in many instances, they may be adults. In the latter case, it's very likely that poor mobility may be the primary limiting factor in performance. In these cases, there may also be a large disparity between basic strength levels and technical proficiency if the individual is coming from a previous sport in which strength was developed to a relatively high level. In such instances, training will need to be modified appropriately to allow the preservation and improvement of existing strength alongside the development of lift technique, mobility and work capacity.

The learning phase will involve the initial teaching of the lifts using the progressions outlined in this book, and the continued practice of the whole lifts and partial variations as needed and appropriate. The goal is for the athlete to develop a baseline of technique that will allow him or her to begin training in earnest. This does not mean they will be technically proficient, and in fact they will be far from it. Practice and remediation will continue for some time, but the lifter will possess enough skill that a systematic training program involving the competition lifts will be effective.

GPP Training Along with the following workouts, these athletes should be performing GPP training regularly. This work can be spread across the week according to time and availability, and should be dosed appropriately for each athlete—the younger the athlete or the less of an athletic background the athlete has, the more GPP will be appropriate. The volume of work should be increased gradually until reaching maximal, and should be reduced every fourth week. The suggested exercises are based on recommendations by Medvedyev (1986/1995) and can be modified based on available facilities and equipment.

Following are the GPP exercises and dosages. A minimum of one exercise from each category should be performed each week, with the emphasis on the sprints, jumps and throws. GPP can be consolidated into 2-3 workouts each week, or can be spread out over several days in the week.

Sprints
- High-Knees - 25m x 2-4
- 30m Walking Start - 50m x 1-3
- Standing Start - 50m x 1-4, 100m x 1-4

Jumps
- Standing Long Jump 2-leg Takeoff – 10-20
- Standing Long Jump 1-leg Takeoff – 10-20
- Standing Vertical Jump – 5-10
- Running Long Jump (5-7 steps) – 3-5

Throws
- Medicine Ball Hip Hinge Forward – 25-50
- Medicine Ball Hip Hinge Backward – 25-50
- Shot Put (3-5kg) – 15-25 (Substitute: Medicine Ball)
- Discus (Standing Start) – 15-25 (Substitute: Light Medicine Ball)

Carries
- Farmer's walk (1 and 2-arm)
- Overhead carry (1 and 2-arm, barbell and dumbbell/kettlebell)

Cross Country
- Run 1-2km or 10-15 minutes (Substitute: rowing, cycling, jumping rope)

Games
- Sports or athletic games – 15-20 minutes

Learning Phase

This phase is comprised of three distinct steps: learning basic barbell movements, learning the competition lifts, and then practicing all of the lifts in a systematic fashion to lay a foundation of technique that will allow the lifter to then progress to continually graduated weightlifting training programs. The duration of each step will depend on a number of factors—primarily, the speed at which the athlete learns at each step. Additional factors include the athlete's mobility, age, training schedule, and commitment. The coach will need to exercise his or her judgment when determining the athlete's readiness to proceed to the next step. Mobility work and GPP should be performed throughout this phase.

Step 1 The first step involves teaching and practicing basic positions and movements with the barbell: the back squat, front squat and press. This will create a simple foundation for the competition lifts and give the coach and athlete an opportunity to get an early assessment of the athlete's mobility and body control.

The progressions for these exercises presented in the book can be used for this purpose, taking as much time as is required by each athlete to gain a reasonable mastery. This may be as little as a single training session.

Step 2 The next step in the process is comprised of learning the competition lifts themselves using the progressions described in the book. Again, the duration of this process will vary considerably among individuals. Prior to moving on to the next step, athletes need to be able to consistently demonstrate reasonable technique in the full competition lifts and squats.

Step 3 The final step in this first phase of the process is a training program in which the athlete practices the competition lifts, squats, pulls and basic accessory lifts along with some basic GPP. This step ideally will last 12 weeks, but may be abbreviated or extended as appropriate for each athlete.

Each workout will focus on a single competition lift (snatch, clean or jerk) to improve learning, and each will include assistance exercises, GPP and mobility work. The goal is for the athlete, at the end of this period, to be prepared to begin a training program that will begin the development of the array of necessary physical traits such as strength, speed and explosiveness along with continuing the pursuit of technical mastery.

The initial loading recommendations (Table 42.1) are based on prescriptions by Medvedyev (1986/1995); these are simply loose guidelines that can be adjusted as needed and appropriate for each athlete. The principle, however, is the use of a uniform weight for an extended duration rather than an attempt to increase loading from the start; the purpose is technique learning and assimilation, not the development of strength. To this end, it's imperative that the chosen loading allows the athlete to perform the exercise properly. If after each 4-week period, the loading is obviously extremely easy for the athlete, it may be increased as appropriate, again with the understanding of the purpose of these exercises at this stage.

Every workout should begin with a full warm-up as described in this book and 5 minutes of practice of the snatch, clean or jerk with the empty barbell for sets of 5-10 reps, and conclude with ab work, back extensions and mobility work. Each workout should alternate between front and back squats. Additional skill work for the lift on which the workout is focused can be performed after the warm-up as well.

In the final (twelfth) week of this period, the lifter will test the snatch and clean & jerk to gauge his or her capabilities. These should not be considered absolute maximal effort lifts, but rather a reasonable

Lift	Intensity	Reps	Sets
Snatch Exercises	40-50% of bodyweight	4-5	4-6
Snatch Pulls	Snatch weight or 10-15kg more	4-5	4-6
Clean Exercises	10-15kg more than snatch exercises	4-5	4-6
Clean Pulls	Clean weight or 10-15kg more	4-5	4-6
Jerk	10-15kg more than snatch exercises	4-5	4-6
Squats	Clean weight or 10-20kg more	4-8	4-6
Pressing Exercises	Snatch weight or 10-15kg more	4-10	4-6
Back Extensions	Unweighted	6-10	4-6

TABLE 42.1 Initial intensities for the learning phase (Medvedvey 1986/1995)

test of the lifter's abilities before beginning the next stage of training. Proper execution of the lifts and the athlete's safety should be the top priorities.

Weeks 1-4

For the first 4 weeks, the lifter will repeat the following series of 3 workouts. On the final day of this block, the lifter will perform the Final Workout.

Day 1
- Hang Power Snatch (knee)
- Hang Snatch (knee)
- Segment Snatch Deadlift (1", knee, mid-thigh)
- Squat

Day 2
- Power Jerk
- Press
- Snatch Press + Overhead Squat
- Squat

Day 3
- Hang Power Clean (knee)
- Hang Clean (knee) + Power Jerk
- Segment Clean Deadlift (1", knee, mid-thigh)
- Squat

Final Workout
- Hang Snatch (knee)
- Hang Clean (knee)
- Power Jerk
- Front Squat

Weeks 5-8

For the next 4 weeks, the lifter will repeat the following series of 3 workouts. On the final day of this block, the lifter will perform the Final Workout.

Day 1
- Power Snatch
- Hang Snatch (knee)
- Segment Snatch Pull (knee) + Snatch Pull
- Squat

Day 2
- Split Jerk
- Push Press
- Snatch Push Press + Overhead Squat
- Squat

Day 3
- Power Clean
- Hang Clean (knee) + Power Jerk
- Segment Clean Pull (knee) + Clean Pull
- Squat

Final Workout
- Power Snatch
- Power Clean
- Split Jerk
- Front Squat

Weeks 9-11

For the first 3 weeks of the final block, the lifter will repeat the following series of 3 workouts.

Day 1
- Power Snatch
- Snatch
- Snatch Pull
- Squat

Day 2
- Power Clean
- Split Jerk
- Push Press
- Squat

Day 3
- Clean & Jerk
- Clean Pull
- Snatch Push Press + Overhead Squat
- Squat

Week 12

The final week of this phase will lead into a test of the snatch and clean & jerk to gauge the lifter's preparedness. The lifter should be evaluated not just on the weights of the lifts, but also on technique and mobility.

Day 1
- Snatch
- Snatch Pull
- Snatch Push Press + Overhead Squat
- Front Squat

Day 2
- Clean & Jerk
- Clean Pull
- Push Press
- Back Squat

Day 3
- Snatch
- Snatch Pull
- Front Squat

Day 4
- Snatch
- Clean & Jerk

Development Phase

Once the athlete has completed the learning phase and has developed a solid enough foundation of lift technique and mobility to begin working to increase the actual loading of the lifts, the development phase can begin. This phase will last until the athlete achieves the Level 1 standards in Table 33.4 (Chapter 33). Again, how long this takes will vary considerably among athletes. The actual program will vary as well depending on the specific needs of each athlete, which will vary primarily due to age and athletic background.

All workouts should begin with a complete warm-up and practice of the full snatch, clean or jerk with an empty bar for 5 minutes, and end with ab work, back extensions, and mobility work. GPP workouts should continue in the same manner as during the Learning Phase. Additional skill work for the lift on which the session focuses can be performed after the warm-up as time, energy and focus allow.

General principles of the Level 0 program include focusing on either the snatch, clean, jerk or clean & jerk in a single session in most cases rather than mixing elements of the two competition lifts, performing a variation of each competition lift at least twice weekly, and performing squat and pull variations at least three times weekly.

Training will be controlled primarily by feel and the coach's observation with guidance of the basic plan, an example of which follows. Weights should be selected to provide a challenge to the lifter while allowing proper execution, with the goal being gradual increase over time as tolerated, which at this stage, should be possible fairly consistently for extended periods of time. Every several weeks, weights and volume should be reduced considerably for 1-2 weeks to allow the athlete some restorative time both physically and mentally.

Exercises should remain uniform for 3-4 weeks at a time to allow the athlete continued practice and a chance to increase loading. Exercises can then be changed to somewhat different variations for another 3-4 weeks to provide variety while continuing to push long term progress in the same basic movements. For example, pulling variations may move from segment deadlifts, to deadlifts without pauses, to segment pulls, to pulls without pauses. Pulls may be done from a riser or from blocks of different heights as well. In all cases, correct movement and starting postures must be reinforced to allow such variety to contribute to technical improvement rather than limit it.

Following are two simple examples of training schedules for 4-week blocks that use the same basic structure with variations to exercises and reps.

Sample 4-Week Block 1

Day 1
- Hang Snatch (below knee) – 6 x 3
- Segment Snatch Deadlift (1", knee) – 5 x 3
- Overhead Squat – 5 x 3
- Back Squat – 4 x 8

Day 2
- Power Clean + Front Squat – 6 x 2+1
- Clean High-Pull – 5 x 5
- Power Jerk – 6 x 3
- Press – 5 x 6

Day 3
- Hang Clean (knee) & Jerk – 6 x 3(1+1)
- Segment Clean Deadlift (1", knee) – 5 x 3
- Back Squat – 5 x 5

Day 4
- Power Snatch + Overhead Squat – 6 x 2+1
- Snatch High-Pull – 5 x 5
- Front Squat – 5 x 4
- Snatch Press – 5 x 6

Sample 4-Week Block 2

Day 1
- Snatch – 6 x 2
- Snatch Pull – 5 x 4
- Overhead Squat – 5 x 3
- Back Squat – 4 x 6

Day 2
- Power Clean + Front Squat – 6 x 2(1+1)
- Clean High-Pull – 5 x 3
- Power Jerk – 6 x 3
- Press – 5 x 4

Day 3
- Clean & Jerk – 6 x 2(1+1)
- Clean Pull – 5 x 4
- Back Squat – 5 x 3

Day 4
- Power Snatch + Overhead Squat – 6 x 2(1+1)
- Snatch High-Pull – 5 x 3
- Front Squat – 5 x 3
- Snatch Press – 5 x 4

Program Skill Level 1

The Level 1 classification will be the lowest level of beginning weightlifters who have established reasonable competition lift technique. Ideally these are young athletes, but in many instances, they may be adults. In the latter case, it's very likely that poor mobility may be the primary limiting factor in performance. In these cases, there may also be a large disparity between basic strength levels and technical proficiency if the individual is coming from a previous sport in which strength was developed to a relatively high level.

These athletes will be training 3-4 days per week in macrocycles of 4-6 weeks in duration with relatively low volume and average intensity and a fairly high volume of GPP. There will be a significant volume of learning and remedial drills, and intensities will be prescribed subjectively and controlled by the coach during the workouts. Volume figures will be very loose, as much of the volume will be comprised of light exercises that do not have considerable systemic fatigue effects.

There will be significant possible variation with regard to the types and ages of athletes in this stage. Consequently, the recommendations for this level are somewhat vague. Generally speaking, more GPP work will be employed earlier in the period of time in which the lifter remains in this classification level, and the younger the athlete, the more GPP training will be done. Coaches will need to use their discretion to prescribe appropriate training for each athlete.

All training phases will be preparatory in nature. Youth at this stage in particular will be competing little, and when competing, should be attempting to make all 6 lifts with optimal technique rather than aiming for maximal weights. Adults in this stage will more likely compete similarly to more advanced lifters with regard to attempts and goals, but training leading into competition will still not require significant modification—moderate reductions in volume and intensity in the week prior to competition will be adequate.

The sample Level 1 program provides a simple example of how a program for this level of athlete can be constructed. Working in 4-week blocks, the coach or athlete can change the exercise selection each block both for variety and to best address the current technical or strength needs, using different lift variations or complexes. Intensities can be increased as tolerated essentially continually until no longer possible, at which time a 1-2-week break can be undertaken with reduced volume and intensity and limited barbell work before beginning the next 4-week block.

GPP Workouts

Example GPP sessions are included with the sample program to provide a general idea of what can be done. Again, the quantity and exact nature of the GPP training will vary depending on the athlete—more extensive for younger athletes or older athletes with little or no athletic backgrounds, and pared down appropriately for older athletes with a solid athletic foundation. Each workout lists the categories of GPP to be done that day. Following are descriptions of the work for each category. The dosage will need to be adjusted appropriately for each athlete and in consideration of the rest of the training program at the time—this means doing from only a single exercise to all in the category, and adjusting the total number of repetitions performed. GPP should be introduced gradually and increased in volume over time, and reduced in volume and intensity periodically, such as every 4-5 weeks, to coincide with the fluctuations in the barbell training.

Sprints
- High-Knees - 50m x 2-4
- 30m Walking Start - 50m x 2-3
- Standing Start - 50m x 2-4, 100m x 2-4

Jumps
- Standing Long Jump 2-leg Takeoff – 20-40
- Standing Long Jump 1-leg Takeoff – 20-40
- Standing Vertical Jump – 10-20
- Running Long Jump (5-7 steps) – 5-10

Throws
- Medicine Ball Hip Hinge Forward – 25-50
- Medicine Ball Hip Hinge Backward – 25-50
- Shot Put (3-5kg) – 15-25 (Substitute: Medicine Ball)
- Discus (Standing Start) – 15-25 (Substitute: Light Medicine Ball)

Carries
- Farmer's walk (1 and 2-arm)
- Overhead carry (1 and 2-arm, barbell and dumbbell/kettlebell)

Cross Country
- Run 2-2.5km or 15 minutes minimum (Substitute: rowing, cycling, jumping rope)

Games
- Sports or athletic games – 20 minutes

Week 1

Monday
- Snatch Skill Work
- Snatch – 5 x 3
- Snatch Pull – 3 x 5
- Back Squat – 3 x 8
- Back Extensions
- Abs

Tuesday
- Clean Skill Work
- Clean & Jerk – 5 x 3+1
- Clean Pull – 3 x 5
- Push Press – 3 x 5
- Back Extensions
- Abs
- GPP
  - Sprints
  - Jumps
  - Carries

Thursday
- Snatch Skill Work
- Power Snatch – 5 x 3
- Snatch Push Press + Overhead Squat – 4 x 5+1
- Front Squat – 3 x 5
- Back Extensions
- Abs

Saturday
- Jerk Skill Work
- Power Clean & Power Jerk – 5 x 3+1
- Clean Pull – 3 x 5
- Back Squat – 4 x 5
- Back Extensions
- Abs
- GPP
  - Throws
  - Jumps
  - Cross Country

Week 2

Monday
- Snatch Skill Work
- Power Snatch + Hang Snatch (knee) – 5 x 1+1
- Halting Snatch Deadlift (mid-thigh) – 3 x 3
- Back Squat – 4 x 5
- Back Extensions
- Abs

Tuesday
- Snatch Skill Work
- Power Snatch – 5 x 2
- Snatch Push Press + Overhead Squat – 3 x 5+1
- Front Squat – 3 x 5
- Back Extensions
- Abs
- GPP
  - Sprints
  - Jumps
  - Games

Thursday
- Clean Skill Work
- Power Clean + Hang Clean (knee) – 5 x 1+1
- Halting Clean Deadlift (mid-thigh) – 3 x 3
- Push Press – 3 x 5
- Back Extensions
- Abs

Saturday
- Jerk Skill Work
- Power Clean & Power Jerk – 5 x 1+3
- Snatch Pull – 3 x 4
- Back Squat – 4 x 5
- Back Extensions
- Abs
- GPP
  - Throws
  - Jumps
  - Cross Country

Week 3

Monday
- Snatch Skill Work
- Snatch – 5 x 3
- Snatch Pull – 3 x 5
- Back Squat – 3 x 8
- Back Extensions
- Abs

Tuesday
- Clean Skill Work
- Clean & Jerk – 5 x 1+3
- Clean Pull – 3 x 5
- Push Press – 3 x 5
- Back Extensions
- Abs
- GPP
  - Sprints
  - Jumps
  - Carries

Thursday
- Snatch Skill Work
- Power Snatch – 5 x 3
- Snatch Push Press + Overhead Squat – 4 x 5+1
- Front Squat – 3 x 5
- Back Extensions
- Abs

Saturday
- Jerk Skill Work
- Power Clean & Power Jerk – 5 x 3+1
- Clean Pull – 3 x 5
- Back Squat – 4 x 5
- Back Extensions
- Abs

- GPP
  - Throws
  - Jumps
  - Cross Country

Week 4

Monday
- Snatch Skill Work
- Power Snatch + Hang Snatch (knee) – 5 x 1+1
- Halting Snatch Deadlift (mid-thigh) – 3 x 3
- Back Squat – 4 x 5
- Back Extensions
- Abs

Tuesday
- Snatch Skill Work
- Power Snatch – 5 x 2
- Snatch Push Press + Overhead Squat – 3 x 5+1
- Front Squat – 3 x 5
- Back Extensions
- Abs
- GPP
  - Sprints
  - Jumps
  - Games

Thursday
- Clean Skill Work
- Power Clean + Hang Clean (knee) – 5 x 1+1
- Halting Clean Deadlift (mid-thigh) – 3 x 3
- Push Press – 3 x 5
- Back Extensions
- Abs

Saturday
- Jerk Skill Work
- Power Clean & Power Jerk – 5 x 1+3
- Snatch Pull – 3 x 4
- Back Squat – 4 x 5
- Back Extensions
- Abs
- GPP
  - Throws
  - Jumps
  - Cross Country

Program **Skill Level 2**

The Level 2 classification will be higher level beginning to lower level intermediate lifters who have some weightlifting training experience, but are still in the relatively early stages of technical learning and development, and most likely in strength development. Ideally these are relatively young athletes, but in many cases they may be adults. In the latter instances, these athletes may have relatively high strength levels in basic movements in comparison to their competition lift performance due to previous athletic training. Such athletes are also likely to have mobility restrictions that limit competition lift performance.

These athletes will be training 4 days per week in macrocycles lasting 6-8 weeks still with relatively low volume and average intensity, and a considerable amount of GPP and technical and remedial drills. In the same program, volume will remain approximately uniform for the first 3 weeks of each mesocycle and then be reduced on the final week for restoration.

Intensity prescriptions will remain primarily subjective and controlled by the coach during the workouts. All mesocycles will be essentially preparatory, as this stage of development will not require entirely specific competition preparation aside from some relatively minor reductions in volume and intensity in the final 1-2 weeks preceding competition.

As in previous levels, the exact amount and nature of GPP training will vary dependent on the age and athletic experience of each athlete.

Mesocycle 1

Weeks 1-3

Monday
- Snatch Skill Work
- Snatch – 5 x 3
- Snatch Pull on Riser – 3 x 4
- Snatch Push Press + Overhead Squat – 3 x 5+1
- Back Squat – 3 x 8

Tuesday
- Jerk Skill Work
- Power Snatch – 5 x 3
- Jerk – 5 x 3
- Power Clean – 5 x 3
- SLDL – 3 x 5
- Upper Body Push Bodybuilding

Thursday
- Clean Skill Work
- Clean – 5 x 3
- Clean Pull on Riser – 3 x 4
- Front Squat – 3 x 5
- Good Morning – 3 x 5
- Upper Body Pull Bodybuilding

Saturday
- Skill Work of Choice
- Snatch – 6 x 1
- Clean & Jerk – 6 x 1+1
- Push Press – 3 x 5
- Back Squat – 3 x 5
- Push/Pull Bodybuilding

Week 4

Monday
- Snatch Skill Work
- Snatch – 5 x 1
- Snatch Pull – 3 x 3
- Back Squat – 3 x 5

Tuesday
- Jerk Skill Work
- Power Snatch – 5 x 1
- Power Clean & Jerk – 5 x 1+1
- Snatch Push Press + Overhead Squat – 4 x 3+1
- Upper Body Push Bodybuilding

Thursday
- Clean Skill Work
- Clean – 5 x 1
- Clean Pull– 3 x 3
- Front Squat – 3 x 4
- Upper Body Pull Bodybuilding

Saturday
- Skill Work of Choice
- Snatch – 6 x 1
- Clean & Jerk – 6 x 1+1
- Push Press – 4 x 3
- Back Squat – 4 x 3
- Push/Pull Bodybuilding

Mesocycle 2

Weeks 5-7

Monday
- Snatch Skill Work
- Snatch – 6 x 2
- Snatch Pull – 4 x 3
- Snatch Push Press + Overhead Squat – 5 x 3+1
- Back Squat – 4 x 6

Tuesday
- Jerk Skill Work
- Power Snatch – 6 x 2
- Jerk – 6 x 2
- Power Clean – 6 x 2
- SLDL – 3 x 5

Thursday
- Clean Skill Work
- Clean – 6 x 2
- Clean Pull – 4 x 3
- Front Squat – 3 x 4
- Good Morning – 3 x 5
- Upper Body Pull Bodybuilding

Saturday
- Skill Work of Choice
- Snatch – 6 x 1
- Clean & Jerk – 6 x 1+1
- Push Press – 5 x 3
- Back Squat – 5 x 4
- Push/Pull Bodybuilding

Week 8

Monday
- Snatch Skill Work
- Snatch – 5 x 1
- Snatch Pull – 3 x 3
- Back Squat – 3 x 5

Tuesday
- Jerk Skill Work
- Power Snatch – 5 x 1
- Power Clean & Jerk – 5 x 1+1
- Snatch Push Press + Overhead Squat – 4 x 3+1
- Upper Body Push Bodybuilding

Thursday
- Clean Skill Work
- Clean – 5 x 1
- Clean Pull – 3 x 3
- Front Squat – 3 x 4
- Upper Body Pull Bodybuilding

Saturday
- Skill Work of Choice
- Snatch – 6 x 1
- Clean & Jerk – 6 x 1+1
- Push Press – 4 x 3
- Back Squat – 4 x 3
- Push/Pull Bodybuilding

Program **Skill Level 3**

The Level 3 classification will be more advanced intermediate lifters who are bordering on the US national level of competition. They will still be refining their competition lift technique and developing a strength base, and likely have some remaining mobility limitations.

These lifters will typically be training 5 days per week with minimal GPP work, mostly consisting of jump training and bodybuilding work, but adjusted appropriately for the athlete's age and athletic experience. Macrocycles will typically be approximately 12 weeks in duration, varying as needed based on the competition schedule. They will be able to rely on objective relative intensity prescriptions based on accurate maxima. Bear in mind that the percentages in the sample program may need to be adjusted for certain athletes.

These training programs will have distinct preparation and competition mesocycles, the latter of which may emphasize frequent, heavy single competition lifts, as these lifters should be at a level of technical proficiency that allows such training to be effective.

On Saturday workouts in the preparation phase, the lifter will perform clean & jerks with a double of his or her weaker lift; that is, if the lifter's clean is weaker than his or her jerk, he or she will perform 2 cleans + 1 jerk for this exercise.

Mesocycle 1: Preparation

Week 1

Monday
- Snatch Technique Primer
- Snatch – 70% x 3, 75% x 3 x 5
- Snatch Pull on Riser – 90% x 5 x 4
- Back Squat – 60% x 8, 70% x 8 x 4
- SLDL – 3 x 5
- Back Squat Jump – 20% (of Back Squat) x 5 x 4

Tuesday
- Snatch or Jerk Technique Primer
- Power Snatch – 70% x 3, 75% x 3 x 5
- Power Jerk – 70% x 3, 75% x 3 x 5
- Snatch Push Press + Overhead Squat – 70% (of Snatch) x 5+1 x 5
- Upper Body Pull Bodybuilding

Wednesday
- Clean Technique Primer
- Clean – 70% x 3, 75% x 3 x 5
- Clean Pull on Riser – 90% x 5 x 4
- Front Squat – 70% x 5 x 4
- Good Morning – 3 x 5
- Box Jump – 4 x 5

Thursday
- Jerk Technique Primer
- Jerk – 70% x 3, 75% x 3 x 5
- Power Clean – 70% x 3, 75% x 3 x 5
- Snatch Balance – 70% x 2, 75% x 2 x 5
- Push Press – 70% x 5 x 5
- Upper Body Push Bodybuilding

Saturday
- Snatch, Clean or Jerk Technique Primer
- Snatch + Overhead Squat – 1+1RM
- Clean & Jerk – 2+1 or 1+2RM
- Back Squat – 70% x 5, 75% x 5, 80% x 5 x 2
- Squat Box Jump – 4 x 5
- Barbell Lunge – 3 x 5
- Upper Body Push & Pull Bodybuilding

Week 2

Monday
- Snatch Technique Primer
- Snatch – 70% x 3, 75% x 3, 80% x 3 x 3
- Snatch Pull on Riser – 90% x 5, 95% x 5 x 3
- Back Squat – 65% x 8, 75% x 8 x 3
- SLDL – 3 x 5
- Back Squat Jump – 20% (of Back Squat) x 5 x 3

Tuesday
- Snatch or Jerk Technique Primer
- Power Snatch – 70% x 3, 75% x 3, 80% x 3 x 3
- Power Jerk – 70% x 3, 75% x 3, 80% x 3 x 3
- Snatch Push Press + Overhead Squat – 70% (of Snatch) x 5+1, 75% x 5+1 x 4
- Upper Body Pull Bodybuilding

Wednesday
- Clean Technique Primer
- Clean – 70% x 3, 75% x 3, 80% x 3 x 3
- Clean Pull on Riser – 90% x 5, 95% x 5 x 3
- Front Squat – 70% x 5 x 2, 75% x 5 x 2
- Good Morning – 3 x 5
- Box Jump – 4 x 5

Thursday
- Jerk Technique Primer
- Jerk – 70% x 3, 75% x 3, 80% x 3 x 3
- Power Clean – 70% x 3, 75% x 3, 80% x 3 x 3
- Snatch Balance – 70% x 3, 75% x 2, 80% x 3 x 2
- Push Press – 70% x 5 x 2, 75% x 5 x 3
- Upper Body Push Bodybuilding

Saturday
- Snatch, Clean or Jerk Technique Primer
- Snatch + Overhead Squat – 1+1RM
- Clean & Jerk – 2+1 or 1+2RM
- Back Squat – 73% x 5, 78% x 5, 83% x 5
- Squat Box Jump – 3 x 5
- Barbell Lunge – 3 x 5
- Upper Body Push & Pull Bodybuilding

Week 3

Monday
- Snatch Technique Primer
- Snatch – 70% x 3, 75% x 3, 80% x 3, 3RM
- Snatch Pull on Riser – 90% x 5, 95% x 5, 100% x 5 x 2
- Back Squat – 65% x 8, 75% x 8, 8RM
- SLDL – 3 x 5
- Back Squat Jump – 20% (of Back Squat) x 4 x 3

Tuesday
- Snatch or Jerk Technique Primer
- Power Snatch – 70% x 3, 75% x 3, 80% x 3, 3RM
- Power Jerk – 70% x 3, 75% x 3, 80% x 3, 3RM
- Snatch Push Press + Overhead Squat – 70% (of Snatch) x 5+1, 75% x 5+1, 5+1RM
- Upper Body Pull Bodybuilding

Wednesday
- Clean Technique Primer
- Clean – 70% x 3, 75% x 3, 80% x 3, 3RM
- Clean Pull on Riser – 90% x 5, 95% x 5, 100% x 5 x 2
- Front Squat – 70% x 5, 75% x 5 x 4
- Good Morning – 3 x 5
- Box Jump – 4 x 4

Thursday
- Jerk Technique Primer
- Jerk – 70% x 3, 75% x 3, 80% x 3, 3RM
- Power Clean – 70% x 3, 75% x 3, 80% x 3, 3RM
- Push Press – 70% x 5 x 2, 75% x 5, 5RM
- Upper Body Push Bodybuilding

Saturday
- Snatch, Clean or Jerk Technique Primer
- Snatch + Overhead Squat – 1+1RM
- Clean & Jerk – 2+1 or 1+2RM
- Back Squat – 70% x 5, 75% x 5, 80% x 5, 5RM
- Squat Box Jump – 3 x 4
- Barbell Lunge – 3 x 5
- Upper Body Push & Pull Bodybuilding

Week 4

Monday
- Snatch Technique Primer
- Snatch – 70% x 2 x 5
- Snatch Pull on Riser – 80% x 3 x 3
- Back Squat – 70% x 5 x 4
- SLDL – 3 x 5
- Back Squat Jump – 20% (of Back Squat) x 4 x 3

Tuesday
- Power Clean – 70% x 2 x 5
- Jerk Technique Primer
- Jerk – 70% x 2 x 4
- Push Press – 70% x 3 x 3

Wednesday
- Clean Technique Primer
- Clean – 70% x 2 x 5
- Clean Pull on Riser – 80% x 3 x 3
- Front Squat – 70% x 3 x 4
- Good Morning – 3 x 5

Thursday
- Snatch Technique Primer
- Power Snatch – 70% x 2 x 5
- Power Jerk – 70% x 2 x 5
- Snatch Push Press + Overhead Squat – 70% (of Snatch) x 3+1 x 5

Saturday
- Snatch, Clean or Jerk Technique Primer
- Snatch – 70% x 1, 75% x 1, 80% x 1, 85% x 1 x 3
- Clean & Jerk – 70% x 1+1, 75% x 1+1, 80% x 1+1, 85% x 1+1 x 3
- Back Squat – 70% x 5 x 2, 75% x 5 x 2
- Barbell Lunge – 3 x 5

Mesocycle 2: Preparation

Week 5

Monday
- Snatch Technique Primer
- Snatch – 70% x 2, 75% x 2, 80% x 2 x 5
- Snatch Pull – 100% x 3 x 4
- Back Squat – 70% x 5, 75% x 5 x 4
- SLDL – 3 x 5
- Back Squat Jump – 20% (of Back Squat) x 5 x 3

Tuesday
- Jerk Technique Primer
- Jerk – 70% x 2, 75% x 2, 80% x 2 x 5
- Power Clean – 70% x 2, 75% x 2, 80% x 2 x 5
- Push Press – 70% x 5, 75% x 4, 80% x 3 x 5
- Upper Body Push Bodybuilding

Wednesday
- Clean Technique Primer
- Clean – 70% x 2, 75% x 2, 80% x 2 x 5
- Clean Pull – 100% x 3 x 4
- Front Squat – 70% x 3, 75% x 3 x 4
- Good Morning – 3 x 5
- Box Jump – 4 x 5

Thursday
- Snatch or Jerk Technique Primer
- Power Snatch – 70% x 2, 75% x 2, 80% x 2 x 5
- Power Jerk – 70% x 2, 75% x 2, 80% x 2 x 5
- Overhead Squat – 70% x 2, 75% x 2, 80% x 2 x 5
- Snatch Push Press – 70% (of Snatch) x 5, 75% x 5 x 5
- Upper Body Pull Bodybuilding

Saturday
- Snatch, Clean or Jerk Technique Primer
- Snatch + Overhead Squat – 1+1RM
- Clean & Jerk – 2+1 or 1+2RM
- Back Squat – 70% x 3, 75% x 3, 80% x 3, 85% x 3
- Squat Box Jump – 4 x 5
- Barbell Lunge – 3 x 5
- Upper Body Push & Pull Bodybuilding

Week 6

Monday
- Snatch Technique Primer
- Snatch – 70% x 2, 75% x 2, 80% x 2, 85% x 2 x 4
- Snatch Pull – 100% x 3, 105% x 3 x 3
- Back Squat – 70% x 5, 75% x 5 x 2, 80% x 5 x 2
- SLDL – 3 x 5
- Back Squat Jump – 20% (of Back Squat) x 5 x 3

Tuesday
- Jerk Technique Primer
- Jerk – 70% x 2, 75% x 2, 80% x 2, 85% x 2 x 4
- Power Clean – 70% x 2, 75% x 2, 80% x 2, 85% x 2 x 4
- Push Press – 70% x 5, 75% x 4, 80% x 3, 85% x 3 x 4
- Upper Body Push Bodybuilding

Wednesday
- Clean Technique Primer
- Clean – 70% x 2, 75% x 2, 80% x 2, 85% x 2 x 4
- Clean Pull – 100% x 3, 105% x 3 x 3
- Front Squat – 70% x 3, 75% x 3 x 2, 80% x 3 x 2
- Good Morning – 3 x 5
- Box Jump – 3 x 3

Thursday
- Snatch or Jerk Technique Primer
- Power Snatch – 70% x 2, 75% x 2, 80% x 2, 85% x 2 x 4
- Power Jerk – 70% x 2, 75% x 2, 80% x 2, 85% x 2 x 4
- Overhead Squat – 70% x 2, 75% x 2, 80% x 2, 85% x 2 x 4
- Snatch Push Press – 70% (of Snatch) x 5, 75% x 5, 80% x 4 x 4
- Upper Body Pull Bodybuilding

Saturday
- Snatch, Clean or Jerk Technique Primer
- Snatch + Overhead Squat – 1+1RM
- Clean & Jerk – 2+1 or 1+2RM
- Back Squat – 70% x 3, 80% x 3, 85% x 3, 90% x 3
- Squat Box Jump – 3 x 3
- Barbell Lunge – 3 x 5
- Upper Body Push & Pull Bodybuilding

Week 7

Monday
- Snatch Technique Primer
- Snatch – 70% x 2, 75% x 2, 80% x 2, 85% x 2, 2RM
- Snatch Pull – 100% x 3, 105% x 3, 110% x 3 x 2
- Back Squat – 70% x 5, 75% x 5 x 2, 80% x 5, 5RM
- SLDL – 3 x 5
- Back Squat Jump – 20% (of Back Squat) x 3 x 3

Tuesday
- Jerk Technique Primer
- Jerk – 70% x 2, 75% x 2, 80% x 2, 85% x 2, 2RM
- Power Clean – 70% x 2, 75% x 2, 80% x 2, 85% x 2, 2RM
- Push Press – 70% x 5, 75% x 4, 80% x 3, 85% x 3, 3RM
- Upper Body Push Bodybuilding

Wednesday
- Clean Technique Primer
- Clean – 70% x 2, 75% x 2, 80% x 2, 85% x 2, 2RM
- Clean Pull – 100% x 3, 105% x 3, 110% x 3 x 2
- Front Squat – 70% x 3, 75% x 3 x 2, 80% x 3, 85% x 3
- Good Morning – 3 x 5
- Box Jump – 3 x 3

Thursday
- Snatch or Jerk Technique Primer
- Power Snatch – 70% x 2, 75% x 2, 80% x 2, 85% x 2, 2RM
- Power Jerk – 70% x 2, 75% x 2, 80% x 2, 85% x 2, 2RM
- Overhead Squat – 70% x 2, 75% x 2, 80% x 2, 85% x 2, 2RM
- Snatch Push Press – 70% (of Snatch) x 5, 75% x 5, 80% x 4, 85% x 4 x 3
- Upper Body Pull Bodybuilding

Saturday
- Snatch, Clean or Jerk Technique Primer
- Snatch + Overhead Squat – 1+1RM
- Clean & Jerk – 2+1 or 1+2RM
- Back Squat – 70% x 3, 80% x 3, 85% x 3, 90% x 3, 3RM
- Squat Box Jump – 3 x 3
- Barbell Lunge – 3 x 5
- Upper Body Push & Pull Bodybuilding

Week 8

Monday
- Snatch Technique Primer
- Snatch – (70% x 2, 75% x 1, 80% x 1) x 2
- Clean & Jerk – (70% x 1+1, 75% x 1+1, 80% x 1+1) x 2
- Front Squat – 70% x 3, 75% x 3 x 3
- Back Squat Jump – 20% (of Back Squat) x 3 x 3

Tuesday
- Jerk Technique Primer
- Power Snatch – (70% x 2, 75% x 1, 80% x 1) x 2
- Power Clean & Power Jerk – (70% x 1+1, 75% x 1+1, 80% x 1+1) x 2
- Clean Pull – 90% x 2, 95% x 2, 100% x 2 x 2, 90% x 2

Wednesday
- Snatch – (70% x 2, 75% x 1, 80% x 1) x 2
- Clean Technique Primer
- Clean & Jerk – (70% x 1+1, 75% x 1+1, 80% x 1+1) x 2
- Back Squat – 70% x 3 x 4
- Good Morning – 3 x 5
- Box Jump – 4 x 3

Thursday
- Snatch or Jerk Technique Primer
- Power Snatch – (70% x 2, 75% x 1, 80% x 1) x 2
- Power Clean & Power Jerk – (70% x 1+1, 75% x 1+1, 80% x 1+1) x 2
- Snatch Pull – 90% x 2, 95% x 2, 100% x 2 x 2, 90% x 2

Saturday
- Snatch, Clean or Jerk Technique Primer
- Snatch – 70% x 2, 75% x 1, 80% x 1, 85% x 1 x 3
- Clean & Jerk – 70% x 1+1, 75% x 1+1, 80% x 1+1, 85% x 1+1 x 3
- Snatch Pull – 90% x 2, 95% x 2, 100% x 2, 80% x 2
- Front Squat – 70% x 3, 75% x 3, 80% x 3, 70% x 3
- Squat Box Jump – 3 x 3

Mesocycle 3: Competition

Week 9

Monday
- Snatch Technique Primer
- Snatch – HS; (85% (of HS) x 1, 90% x 1, 95% x 1) x 2
- Clean & Jerk – 70% x 1+1, 75% x 1+1, 80% x 1+1, 85% x 1+1 x 3
- Front Squat – 70% x 3, 80% x 3, 85% x 3 x 3
- Good Morning – 3 x 5
- Back Squat Jump – 20% (of Back Squat) x 3 x 3

Tuesday
- Jerk Technique Primer
- Power Snatch – 70% x 1, 75% x 1, 80% x 1, 85% x 1 x 5
- Power Clean & Power Jerk – HS; 85% (of HS) x 1+1, 90% x 1+1, 95% x 1+1
- Clean Pull – 100% x 2, 105% x 2, 110% x 2 x 2, 90% x 2

Wednesday
- Snatch – 70% x 1, 75% x 1, 80% x 1, 85% x 1 x 3
- Clean Technique Primer
- Clean & Jerk – HS; (85% (of HS) x 1+1, 90% x 1+1, 95% x 1+1) x 2
- Back Squat – 70% x 3, 75% x 3 x 4
- Good Morning – 3 x 5
- Box Jump – 4 x 3

Thursday
- Snatch or Jerk Technique Primer
- Power Snatch – HS; 85% (of HS) x 1, 90% x 1, 95% x 1
- Power Clean & Power Jerk – 70% x 1+1, 75% x 1+1, 80% x 1+1, 85% x 1+1 x 3
- Snatch Pull – 100% x 2, 105% x 2, 110% x 2 x 2, 90% x 2
- Good Morning – 3 x 5

Saturday
- Snatch, Clean or Jerk Technique Primer
- Snatch – HS; (90% (of HS) x 1, 95% x 1, HS) x 2
- Clean & Jerk – HS; (90% (of HS) x 1+1, 95% x 1+1, HS) x 2
- Clean Pull – 90% x 2, 100% x 2, 105% x 2, 80% x 2
- Front Squat – 70% x 3, 80% x 3, 8085 x 3, 90% x 3 x 2
- Squat Box Jump – 4 x 3

Week 10

Monday
- Snatch Technique Primer
- Snatch – HS; (85% (of HS) x 1, 90% x 1, 95% x 1) x 2
- Clean & Jerk – 70% x 1+1, 75% x 1+1, 80% x 1+1, 85% x 1+1, 90% x 1+1
- Front Squat – 70% x 3, 80% x 3, 85% x 3, 90% x 2 x 3
- Back Squat Jump – 20% (of Back Squat) x 3 x 3

Tuesday
- Jerk Technique Primer
- Power Snatch – 70% x 1, 75% x 1, 80% x 1, 85% x 1, 90% x 1
- Power Clean & Power Jerk – HS; 85% (of HS) x 1+1, 90% x 1+1, 95% x 1+1
- Clean Pull – 100% x 2, 110% x 2, 115% x 2, 90% x 2

Wednesday
- Snatch – 70% x 1, 75% x 1, 80% x 1, 85% x 1, 90% x 1
- Clean Technique Primer
- Clean & Jerk – HS; (85% (of HS) x 1+1, 90% x 1+1, 95% x 1+1) x 2
- Back Squat – 70% x 3, 75% x 3, 80% x 3 x 3
- Box Jump – 3 x 3

Thursday
- Snatch or Jerk Technique Primer
- Power Snatch – HS; 85% (of HS) x 1, 90% x 1, 95% x 1
- Power Clean & Power Jerk – 70% x 1+1, 75% x 1+1, 80% x 1+1, 85% x 1+1, 90% x 1+1
- Snatch Pull – 100% x 2, 110% x 2, 115% x 2, 90% x 2
- Good Morning – 3 x 5

Saturday
- Snatch, Clean or Jerk Technique Primer
- Snatch – HS; (90% (of HS) x 1, 95% x 1, HS) x 2
- Clean & Jerk – HS; (90% (of HS) x 1+1, 95% x 1+1, HS) x 2
- Snatch Pull – 90% x 2, 100% x 2, 105% x 2
- Front Squat – HS; 85% (of HS) x 1, 90% x 1, 95% x 1
- Squat Box Jump – 3 x 3

Week 11

Monday
- Snatch Technique Primer
- Snatch – HS; 85% (of HS) x 1, 90% x 1, 95% x 1
- Clean & Jerk – 70% x 1+1, 75% x 1+1, 80% x 1+1, 85% x 1+1, 90% x 1+1
- Front Squat – 70% x 2, 80% x 2, 85% x 2 x 3
- Back Squat Jump – 20% (of Back Squat) x 3 x 3

Tuesday
- Jerk Technique Primer
- Power Snatch – 70% x 1, 75% x 1, 80% x 1, 85% x 1, 90% x 1 x 2
- Power Clean & Power Jerk – 70% x 1+1, 75% x 1+1, 80% x 1+1, 85% x 1+1, 90% x 1+1 x 2
- Clean Pull – 90% x 2, 95% x 2, 100% x 2, 90% x 2

Wednesday
- Snatch – 70% x 1, 75% x 1, 80% x 1, 85% x 1 x 3
- Clean Technique Primer
- Clean & Jerk – 70% x 1+1, 75% x 1+1, 80% x 1+1, 85% x 1+1 x 3
- Back Squat – 70% x 3, 75% x 3 x 3
- Box Jump – 3 x 3

Thursday
- Snatch or Jerk Technique Primer
- Power Snatch – 70% x 1, 75% x 1, 80% x 1, 85% x 1 x 3
- Power Clean & Power Jerk – 70% x 1+1, 75% x 1+1, 80% x 1+1, 85% x 1+1 x 3
- Snatch Pull – 90% x 2, 95% x 2, 100% x 2, 90% x 2

Saturday
- Snatch, Clean or Jerk Technique Primer
- Snatch – HS; 90% (of HS) x 1, 95% x 1
- Clean & Jerk – To Opener
- Clean Pull – 85% x 2, 90% x 2, 95% x 2, 100% x 2
- Front Squat – 70% x 2, 80% x 2, 85% x 2 x 2
- Squat Box Jump – 3 x 3

Week 12

Monday
- Snatch Technique Primer
- Snatch – 70% x 1, 75% x 1, 80% x 1, 85% x 1, 90% x 1 x 3
- Clean & Jerk – 70% x 1+1, 75% x 1+1, 80% x 1+1, 85% x 1+1 x 3
- Clean Pull – 90% x 2 x 3
- Back Squat – 75% x 3 x 3

Wednesday
- Snatch – 70% x 1, 75% x 1, 80% x 1, 85% x 1 x 3
- Clean Technique Primer
- Clean & Jerk – 70% x 1+1, 75% x 1+1, 80% x 1+1 x 3
- Snatch Pull – 85% x 2 x 3
- Front Squat – 75% x 2 x 3

Thursday
- Snatch – 70% x 1 x 5
- Power Clean & Jerk – 70% x 1+1 x 5

Saturday
- Competition

Program **Skill Level 4**

The Level 4 classification represents the lower tier of US national competition. These lifters will have a reasonable level of technical proficiency in the competition lifts, but may still have considerable work to do to refine it and develop consistency, especially at higher intensities. They will have decent levels of strength, and that strength will be fairly specific to weightlifting postures and movements. They will have reasonable mobility overall, but may still have limitations in specific local areas. These lifters will also have a reasonable amount of competition experience at the local level, and at least some experience at the national level.

These lifters will typically be training 5 days per week with minimal GPP work, mostly consisting of jump training and bodybuilding work. Macrocycles will typically be approximately 12 weeks in duration, varying as needed based on the competition schedule. They will be able to rely on objective relative intensity prescriptions based on accurate maxima. Bear in mind that the percentages in the sample program may need to be adjusted for certain athletes.

These training programs will have distinct preparation and competition mesocycles, the latter of which may emphasize frequent, heavy single competition lifts, as these lifters should be at a level of technical proficiency that allows such training to be effective. This is the first level in which depth jumps are introduced with the included jump training.

On Saturday workouts in the preparation phase, the lifter will perform clean & jerks with a double of his or her weaker lift; that is, if the lifter's clean is weaker than his or her jerk, he or she will perform 2 cleans + 1 jerk for this exercise.

Mesocycle 1: Preparation

Week 1

Monday
- Snatch Technique Primer
- Snatch – 70% x 3, 75% x 3 x 5
- Snatch Pull on Riser – 90% x 5 x 4
- Snatch Segment Deadlift (1", knee) – 80% x 3 x 3
- Back Squat – 60% x 8, 70% x 8 x 4
- SLDL – 3 x 5
- Back Squat Jump – 20% (of Back Squat) x 5 x 4

Tuesday
- Jerk Technique Primer
- Jerk – 70% x 3, 75% x 3 x 5
- Power Clean – 70% x 3, 75% x 3 x 5
- Push Press – 70% x 5 x 5
- Upper Body Push Bodybuilding

Wednesday
- Clean Technique Primer
- Clean – 70% x 3, 75% x 3 x 5
- Clean Pull on Riser – 90% x 5 x 4
- Clean Segment Deadlift (1", knee) – 80% x 3 x 3
- Front Squat – 70% x 5 x 4
- Good Morning – 3 x 5
- Depth Jump – 4 x 8

Thursday
- Snatch or Jerk Technique Primer
- Power Snatch – 70% x 3, 75% x 3 x 5
- Power Jerk – 70% x 3, 75% x 3 x 5
- Overhead Squat – 70% x 3 x 5
- Snatch Push Press – 70% (of Snatch) x 5 x 5
- Upper Body Pull Bodybuilding

Saturday
- Snatch, Clean or Jerk Technique Primer
- Snatch + Overhead Squat – 1+1RM
- Clean & Jerk – 2+1 or 1+2RM
- Floating Snatch Pull – 80% x 5 x 4
- Back Squat – 70% x 5, 75% x 5, 80% x 5 x 2

- Depth Jump – 3 x 5
- Upper Body Push & Pull Bodybuilding

Week 2

Monday
- Snatch Technique Primer
- Snatch – 70% x 3, 75% x 3, 80% x 3 x 3
- Snatch Pull on Riser – 95% x 5 x 3
- Snatch Segment Deadlift (1", knee) – 85% x 3 x 3
- Back Squat – 60% x 8, 70% x 8, 75% x 8 x 2
- SLDL – 3 x 5
- Back Squat Jump – 20% (of Back Squat) x 5 x 4

Tuesday
- Jerk Technique Primer
- Jerk – 70% x 3, 75% x 3, 80% x 3 x 3
- Power Clean – 70% x 3, 75% x 3, 80% x 3 x 3
- Push Press – 70% x 5 x 2, 75% x 5 x 3
- Upper Body Push Bodybuilding

Wednesday
- Clean Technique Primer
- Clean – 70% x 3, 75% x 3, 80% x 3 x 3
- Clean Pull on Riser – 95% x 5 x 3
- Clean Segment Deadlift (1", knee) – 85% x 3 x 3
- Front Squat – 70% x 5 x 2, 75% x 5 x 2
- Good Morning – 3 x 5
- Depth Jump – 4 x 8

Thursday
- Snatch or Jerk Technique Primer
- Power Snatch – 70% x 3, 75% x 3, 80% x 3 x 3
- Power Jerk – 70% x 3, 75% x 3, 80% x 3 x 3
- Overhead Squat – 70% x 3, 75% x 3 x 3
- Snatch Push Press – 70% (of Snatch) x 5, 75% x 5 x 3
- Upper Body Pull Bodybuilding

Saturday
- Snatch, Clean or Jerk Technique Primer
- Snatch + Overhead Squat – 1+1RM
- Clean & Jerk – 2+1 or 1+2RM
- Floating Clean Pull – 80% x 5 x 2, 85% x 5 x 2
- Back Squat – 70% x 5, 75% x 5, 80% x 5, 85% x 5
- Depth Jump – 3 x 5
- Upper Body Push & Pull Bodybuilding

Week 3

Monday
- Snatch Technique Primer
- Snatch – 70% x 3, 75% x 3, 80% x 3, 3RM
- Snatch Pull on Riser – 100% x 4 x 3
- Snatch Segment Deadlift (1", knee) – 85% x 3, 90% x 3 x 2
- Back Squat – 60% x 8, 70% x 8, 8RM
- SLDL – 3 x 5
- Back Squat Jump – 20% (of Back Squat) x 3 x 4

Tuesday
- Jerk Technique Primer
- Jerk – 70% x 3, 75% x 3, 80% x 3, 3RM
- Power Clean – 70% x 3, 75% x 3, 80% x 3, 3RM
- Push Press – 70% x 5 x 2, 75% x 5, 5RM
- Upper Body Push Bodybuilding

Wednesday
- Clean Technique Primer
- Clean – 70% x 3, 75% x 3, 80% x 3, 3RM
- Clean Pull on Riser – 100% x 4 x 3
- Clean Segment Deadlift (1", knee) – 85% x 3, 90% x 3 x 2
- Front Squat – 70% x 5, 75% x 5 x 3
- Good Morning – 3 x 5
- Depth Jump – 3 x 6

Thursday
- Snatch or Jerk Technique Primer
- Power Snatch – 70% x 3, 75% x 3, 80% x 3, 3RM
- Power Jerk – 70% x 3, 75% x 3, 80% x 3, 3RM
- Overhead Squat – 70% x 3, 75% x 3, 3RM
- Snatch Push Press – 70% (of Snatch) x 5, 75% x 5, 80% x 5 x 2
- Upper Body Pull Bodybuilding

Saturday
- Snatch, Clean or Jerk Technique Primer
- Snatch + Overhead Squat – 1+1RM
- Clean & Jerk – 2+1 or 1+2RM
- Floating Snatch Pull – 80% x 5 x 2, 85% x 5, 90% x 5 x 2
- Back Squat – 70% x 5, 75% x 5, 80% x 5, 85% x 5, 5RM
- Depth Jump – 3 x 3
- Upper Body Push & Pull Bodybuilding

Week 4

Monday
- Snatch Technique Primer
- Snatch – 70% x 3 x 4
- Snatch Pull on Riser – 85% x 3 x 3
- Snatch Segment Deadlift (1", knee) – 80% x 3 x 3
- Back Squat – 60% x 6, 65% x 6 x 3
- SLDL – 2 x 5
- Back Squat Jump – 20% (of Back Squat) x 5 x 3

Tuesday
- Jerk Technique Primer
- Jerk – 70% x 3 x 4
- Power Clean – 70% x 3 x 4
- Push Press – 70% x 5 x 3
- Upper Body Push Bodybuilding

Wednesday
- Clean Technique Primer
- Clean – 70% x 3 x 4
- Clean Pull on Riser – 85% x 3 x 3
- Clean Segment Deadlift (1", knee) – 80% x 3 x 3
- Front Squat – 70% x 3 x 4
- Good Morning – 2 x 5
- Depth Jump – 3 x 8

Thursday
- Snatch or Jerk Technique Primer
- Power Snatch – 70% x 3 x 4
- Power Jerk – 70% x 3 x 4
- Overhead Squat – 70% x 2 x 3
- Snatch Push Press – 70% (of Snatch) x 5 x 3
- Upper Body Pull Bodybuilding

Saturday
- Snatch, Clean or Jerk Technique Primer
- Snatch + Overhead Squat – 1+1RM
- Clean & Jerk – 2+1 or 1+2RM
- Floating Clean Pull – 80% x 3 x 3
- Back Squat – 70% x 5 x 3
- Squat Box Jump – 3 x 5
- Upper Body Push & Pull Bodybuilding

Mesocycle 2: Preparation

Week 5

Monday
- Snatch Technique Primer
- Snatch – 70% x 2, 75% x 2, 80% x 2 x 4
- Snatch Pull on Riser – 100% x 3 x 4
- Halting Snatch Deadlift (mid-thigh) – 90% x 3 x 4
- Back Squat – 70% x 6, 75% x 6 x 4
- SLDL – 3 x 5
- Back Squat Jump – 20% (of Back Squat) x 5 x 4

Tuesday
- Jerk Technique Primer
- Jerk – 70% x 2, 75% x 2, 80% x 2 x 4
- Power Clean – 70% x 2, 75% x 2, 80% x 2 x 4
- Push Press – 70% x 3, 75% x 3 x 4
- Upper Body Push Bodybuilding

Wednesday
- Clean Technique Primer
- Clean – 70% x 2, 75% x 2, 80% x 2 x 4
- Clean Pull on Riser – 100% x 3 x 4
- Halting Clean Deadlift (mid-thigh) – 90% x 3 x 4
- Front Squat – 70% x 4, 75% x 4 x 3
- Good Morning – 3 x 5
- Depth Jump – 4 x 6

Thursday
- Snatch or Jerk Technique Primer
- Power Snatch – 70% x 2, 75% x 2, 80% x 2 x 4
- Power Jerk – 70% x 2, 75% x 2, 80% x 2 x 4
- Overhead Squat – 70% x 2, 75% x 2 x 4
- Snatch Push Press – 70% (of Snatch) x 5, 75% x 4 x 4
- Upper Body Pull Bodybuilding

Saturday
- Snatch, Clean or Jerk Technique Primer
- Snatch + Snatch Balance – 1+1RM
- Clean & Jerk – 2+1 or 1+2RM
- Block Snatch Pull (knee) – 110% x 3, 115% x 3 x 3
- Back Squat – 70% x 3, 80% x 3, 85% x 3 x 3
- Depth Jump – 4 x 5
- Upper Body Push & Pull Bodybuilding

Week 6

Monday
- Snatch Technique Primer
- Snatch – 70% x 2, 75% x 2, 80% x 2, 85% x 2 x 2
- Snatch Pull on Riser – 105% x 3 x 3
- Halting Snatch Deadlift (mid-thigh) – 95% x 3 x 3
- Back Squat – 70% x 6, 75% x 6, 80% x 6 x 3
- SLDL – 3 x 5
- Back Squat Jump – 20% (of Back Squat) x 5 x 4

Tuesday
- Jerk Technique Primer
- Jerk – 70% x 2, 75% x 2, 80% x 2, 85% x 2 x 2
- Power Clean – 70% x 2, 75% x 2, 80% x 2, 85% x 2 x 2
- Push Press – 70% x 3, 75% x 3, 80% x 3 x 3
- Upper Body Push Bodybuilding

Wednesday
- Clean Technique Primer
- Clean – 70% x 2, 75% x 2, 80% x 2, 85% x 2 x 2
- Clean Pull on Riser – 105% x 3 x 3
- Halting Clean Deadlift (mid-thigh) – 95% x 3 x 3
- Front Squat – 70% x 4, 75% x 4, 80% x 4 x 2
- Good Morning – 3 x 5
- Depth Jump – 4 x 6

Thursday
- Snatch or Jerk Technique Primer
- Power Snatch – 70% x 2, 75% x 2, 80% x 2, 85% x 2 x 2
- Power Jerk – 70% x 2, 75% x 2, 80% x 2, 85% x 2 x 2
- Overhead Squat – 70% x 2, 75% x 2, 80% x 2 x 2
- Snatch Push Press – 70% (of Snatch) x 5, 75% x 4, 80% x 4 x 3
- Upper Body Pull Bodybuilding

Saturday
- Snatch, Clean or Jerk Technique Primer
- Snatch + Snatch Balance – 1+1RM
- Clean & Jerk – 2+1 or 1+2RM
- Block Clean Pull (knee) – 115% x 3 x 3
- Back Squat – 70% x 3, 80% x 3, 85% x 3, 90% x 3
- Depth Jump – 3 x 5
- Upper Body Push & Pull Bodybuilding

Week 7

Monday
- Snatch Technique Primer
- Snatch – 70% x 2, 75% x 2, 80% x 2, 85% x 2, 2RM
- Snatch Pull on Riser – 105% x 3, 110% x 3 x 2
- Halting Snatch Deadlift (mid-thigh) – 95% x 3, 100% x 3 x 2
- Back Squat – 70% x 6, 75% x 6, 80% x 6, 6RM
- SLDL – 2 x 5
- Back Squat Jump – 20% (of Back Squat) x 3 x 3

Tuesday
- Jerk Technique Primer
- Jerk – 70% x 2, 75% x 2, 80% x 2, 85% x 2, 2RM
- Power Clean – 70% x 2, 75% x 2, 80% x 2, 85% x 2, 2RM
- Push Press – 70% x 3, 75% x 3, 80% x 3, 3RM
- Upper Body Push Bodybuilding

Wednesday
- Clean Technique Primer
- Clean – 70% x 2, 75% x 2, 80% x 2, 85% x 2, 2RM
- Clean Pull on Riser – 105% x 3, 110% x 3 x 2
- Halting Clean Deadlift (mid-thigh) – 95% x 3, 100% x 3 x 2
- Front Squat – 70% x 4, 75% x 4, 80% x 4, 85% x 4
- Good Morning – 2 x 5
- Depth Jump – 3 x 5

Thursday
- Snatch or Jerk Technique Primer
- Power Snatch – 70% x 2, 75% x 2, 80% x 2, 85% x 2, 2RM
- Power Jerk – 70% x 2, 75% x 2, 80% x 2, 85% x 2, 2RM
- Overhead Squat – 70% x 2, 75% x 2, 80% x 2, 85% x 2
- Snatch Push Press – 70% (of Snatch) x 5, 75% x 4, 80% x 4, 85% x 4 x 2
- Upper Body Pull Bodybuilding

Saturday
- Snatch, Clean or Jerk Technique Primer
- Snatch + Snatch Balance – 1+1RM
- Clean & Jerk – 2+1 or 1+2RM
- Block Snatch Pull (knee) – 120% x 3 x 3
- Back Squat – 75% x 3, 85% x 3, 90% x 3, 3RM
- Depth Jump – 3 x 5
- Upper Body Push & Pull Bodybuilding

Week 8

Monday
- Snatch Technique Primer
- Snatch – 70% x 2, 75% x 2 x 4
- Snatch Pull on Riser – 95% x 3 x 3
- Halting Snatch Deadlift (mid-thigh) – 80% x 3 x 3
- Back Squat – 70% x 5, 75% x 5 x 3
- Back Squat Jump – 20% (of Back Squat) x 3 x 3

Tuesday
- Jerk Technique Primer
- Jerk – 70% x 2, 75% x 2 x 3
- Power Clean – 70% x 2, 75% x 2 x 3
- Push Press – 70% x 3, 75% x 3 x 3
- Upper Body Push Bodybuilding

Wednesday
- Clean Technique Primer
- Clean – 70% x 2, 75% x 2 x 3
- Clean Pull on Riser – 95% x 3 x 3
- Halting Clean Deadlift (mid-thigh) – 80% x 3 x 3
- Front Squat – 70% x 4 x 3
- Depth Jump – 3 x 4

Thursday
- Snatch or Jerk Technique Primer
- Power Snatch – 70% x 2, 75% x 2 x 3
- Power Jerk – 70% x 2, 75% x 2 x 3
- Overhead Squat – 70% x 2 x 3
- Snatch Push Press – 70% (of Snatch) x 5, 75% x 4 x 3
- Upper Body Pull Bodybuilding

Saturday
- Snatch, Clean or Jerk Technique Primer
- Snatch + Snatch Balance – 1+1RM
- Clean & Jerk – 2+1 or 1+2RM
- Block Clean Pull (knee) – 105% x 3 x 3
- Back Squat – 70% x 3, 75% x 3, 80% x 3
- Back Squat Jump – 20% (of Back Squat) x 5 x 3
- Upper Body Push & Pull Bodybuilding

Mesocycle 3: Competition

Week 9

Monday
- Snatch Technique Primer
- Snatch – HS; (85% (of HS) x 1, 90% x 1, 95% x 1) x 2
- Clean & Jerk – 70% x 1+1, 75% x 1+1, 80% x 1+1, 85% x 1+1 x 3
- Front Squat – 70% x 3, 80% x 3, 85% x 3 x 3
- Good Morning – 3 x 5
- Back Squat Jump – 20% (of Back Squat) x 3 x 3

Tuesday
- Power Snatch – 70% x 1, 75% x 1, 80% x 1, 85% x 1 x 3
- Jerk Technique Primer
- Power Clean + Power Jerk – HS; 85% (of HS) x 1+1, 90% x 1+1, 95% x 1+1
- Clean Pull – 100% x 2, 105% x 2, 110% x 2 x 2, 90% x 2

Wednesday
- Snatch – 70% x 1, 75% x 1, 80% x 1, 85% x 1 x 3
- Clean Technique Primer
- Clean & Jerk – HS; (85% (of HS) x 1+1, 90% x 1+1, 95% x 1+1) x 2
- Back Squat – 75% x 3 x 4
- Box Jump – 4 x 3

Thursday
- Snatch Technique Primer
- Power Snatch – HS; 85% (of HS) x 1, 90% x 1, 95% x 1
- Power Clean + Power Jerk – 70% x 1+1, 75% x 1+1, 80% x 1+1, 85% x 1+1 x 3
- Snatch Pull – 100% x 2, 105% x 2, 110% x 2 x 2, 90% x 2
- Good Morning – 3 x 5

Saturday
- Technique Primer
- Snatch – HS; (90% (of HS) x 1, 95% x 1, HS) x 2
- Clean & Jerk – HS; (90% (of HS) x 1+1, 95% x 1+1, HS) x 2
- Clean Pull – 90% x 2, 100% x 2, 105% x 2, 80% x 2
- Front Squat – 80% x 3, 85% x 3, 90% x 3 x 2
- Squat Box Jump – 4 x 3

Week 10

Monday
- Snatch Technique Primer
- Snatch – HS: (85% (of HS) x 1, 90% x 1, 95% x 1) x 2
- Clean & Jerk – 70% x 1+1, 75% x 1+1, 80% x 1+1, 85% x 1+1, 90% x 1+1
- Front Squat – 70% x 3, 80% x 3, 85% x 3, 90% x 2 x 3
- Back Squat Jump – 20% (of Back Squat) x 3 x 3

Tuesday
- Power Snatch – 70% x 1, 75% x 1, 80% x 1, 85% x 1, 90% x 1
- Jerk Technique Primer
- Power Clean + Power Jerk – HS: 85% (of HS) x 1+1, 90% x 1+1, 95% x 1+1
- Clean Pull – 100% x 2, 110% x 2, 115% x 2, 90% x 2

Wednesday
- Snatch – 70% x 1, 75% x 1, 80% x 1, 85% x 1, 90% x 1
- Clean Technique Primer
- Clean & Jerk – HS: (85% (of HS) x 1+1, 90% x 1+1, 95% x 1+1) x 2
- Back Squat – 75% x 3, 80% x 3 x 3
- Box Jump – 3 x 3

Thursday
- Snatch Technique Primer
- Power Snatch – HS: 85% (of HS) x 1, 90% x 1, 95% x 1
- Power Clean + Power Jerk – 70% x 1+1, 75% x 1+1, 80% x 1+1, 85% x 1+1, 90% x 1+1
- Snatch Pull – 100% x 2, 110% x 2, 115% x 2, 90% x 2

Saturday
- Technique Primer
- Snatch – HS: (90% (of HS) x 1, 95% x 1, HS) x 2
- Clean & Jerk – HS: (90% (of HS) x 1+1, 95% x 1+1, HS) x 2
- Snatch Pull – 90% x 2, 100% x 2, 105% x 2
- Front Squat – HS: 85% (of HS) x 1, 90% x 1, 95% x 1
- Squat Box Jump – 3 x 3

Week 11

Monday
- Snatch Technique Primer
- Snatch – HS: 85% (of HS) x 1, 90% x 1, 95% x 1
- Clean & Jerk – 70% x 1+1, 75% x 1+1, 80% x 1+1, 85% x 1+1, 90% x 1+1
- Front Squat – 70% x 2, 80% x 2, 85% x 2 x 3
- Back Squat Jump – 20% (of Back Squat) x 3 x 3

Tuesday
- Power Snatch – 70% x 1, 75% x 1, 80% x 1, 85% x 1, 90% x 1 x 2
- Jerk Technique Primer
- Power Clean + Power Jerk – 70% x 1+1, 75% x 1+1, 80% x 1+1, 85% x 1+1, 90% x 1+1 x 2
- Clean Pull – 90% x 2, 95% x 2, 100% x 2, 90% x 2

Wednesday
- Snatch – 70% x 1, 75% x 1, 80% x 1, 85% x 1 x 3
- Clean Technique Primer
- Clean & Jerk – 70% x 1+1, 75% x 1+1, 80% x 1+1, 85% x 1+1 x 3
- Back Squat – 75% x 3 x 3
- Box Jump – 3 x 3

Thursday
- Snatch Technique Primer
- Power Snatch – 70% x 1, 75% x 1, 80% x 1, 85% x 1 x 3
- Power Clean + Power Jerk – 70% x 1+1, 75% x 1+1, 80% x 1+1, 85% x 1+1 x 3
- Snatch Pull – 90% x 2, 95% x 2, 100% x 2, 90% x 2

Saturday
- Technique Primer
- Snatch – HS: 90% (of HS) x 1, 95% x 1
- Clean & Jerk – To Opener
- Clean Pull – 85% x 2, 90% x 2, 95% x 2, 100% x 2
- Front Squat – 70% x2, 80% x 2, 85% x 2 x 2
- Squat Box Jump – 3 x 3

Week 12

Monday
- Snatch Technique Primer
- Snatch – 70% x 1, 75% x 1, 80% x 1, 85% x 1, 90% x 1 x 3
- Clean & Jerk – 70% x 1+1, 75% x 1+1, 80% x 1+1, 85% x 1+1 x 3
- Clean Pull – 90% x 2 x 3
- Back Squat – 70% x 3, 75% x 3 x 3

Wednesday
- Snatch – 70% x 1, 75% x 1, 80% x 1, 85% x 1 x 3
- Clean Technique Primer
- Clean & Jerk – 70% x 1+1, 75% x 1+1, 80% x 1+1 x 3
- Snatch Pull – 85% x 2 x 3
- Front Squat – 75% x 2 x 3

Thursday
- Snatch – 70% x 1 x 5
- Power Clean & Jerk – 70% x 1+1 x 5

Saturday
- Competition

Program **Skill Level 5**

The Level 5 classification represents the highest level of US national competition. These lifters have significant weightlifting training experience, have a fairly high level of technical proficiency and consistency, and optimal mobility overall. They will also be able to tolerate high levels of volume, average intensity and training frequency, and will have a relatively large amount of competition experience, and may be competing at least at the lower international level, or at least be in range of making an international team.

These lifters will typically be training 6 days per week, possibly with twice-daily training, with minimal GPP work, mostly consisting of jump training and bodybuilding work. Macrocycles will typically be approximately 12-16 weeks in duration, varying as needed based on the competition schedule. They will be able to rely on objective relative intensity prescriptions based on accurate maxima. Bear in mind that the percentages in the sample program may need to be adjusted for certain athletes.

These training programs will have distinct preparation and competition mesocycles, the latter of which may emphasize frequent, heavy single competition lifts, as these lifters should be at a level of technical proficiency that allows such training to be effective.

Mesocycle 1: Preparation

Week 1

Monday

AM
- Snatch Technique Primer
- Snatch Pull + Hang Snatch Pull (knee) + Hang Snatch (knee) – 70% x 1+1+2 x 6
- Snatch Pull on Riser – 90% x 4, 95% x 4 x 3
- Depth Jump – 3 x 8

PM
- Clean Pull + Hang Clean Pull (knee) + Hang Clean (knee) – 70% x 1+1+2 x 6
- Clean Segment Deadlift (1", knee) – 80% x 3 x 3
- Back Squat – 70% x 8 x 4
- SLDL – 3 x 5

Tuesday
- Power Clean – 70% x 3, 75% x 3 x 5
- Jerk – 70% x 3, 75% x 3 x 5
- Push Press – 70% x 5 x 5
- Upper Body Push Bodybuilding

Wednesday

AM
- Clean Technique Primer
- Clean Pull + Hang Clean Pull (below knee) + Hang Clean (below knee) – 70% x 1+1+2, 75% x 1+1+2 x 5
- Clean Pull on Riser – 90% x 4, 95% x 4 x 3
- Box Jump – 4 x 3

PM
- Snatch Pull + Hang Snatch Pull (below knee) + Hang Snatch (below knee) – 70% x 1+1+2, 75% x 1+1+2 x 5
- Snatch Segment Deadlift (1", knee) – 80% x 3 x 3
- Front Squat – 70% x 5 x 4
- Good Morning – 3 x 5

Thursday
- Power Snatch – 70% x 3, 75% x 3 x 5
- Power Jerk – 70% x 3, 75% x 3 x 5
- Overhead Squat – 70% x 3, 80% x 3 x 5
- Upper Body Pull Bodybuilding

Friday

AM
- Technique Primer
- Snatch – 70% x 1 x 5
- Clean & Jerk – 70% x 1+1 x 5

PM
- Technique Primer
- Snatch – HS
- Clean & Jerk – HS
- Depth Jump – 4 x 6

Saturday
- Drop to Split – 4 x 5
- Snatch Push Press – 75% (of snatch) x 5 x 5
- Back Squat – 70% x 5, 75% x 5, 80% x 5 x 3
- Upper Body Push & Pull Bodybuilding

Week 2

Monday

AM
- Snatch Technique Primer
- Snatch Pull + Hang Snatch Pull (knee) + Hang Snatch (knee) – 70% x 1+1+2, 75% x 1+1+2 x 4
- Snatch Pull on Riser – 90% x 4, 100% x 4 x 2
- Depth Jump – 3 x 6

PM
- Clean Pull + Hang Clean Pull (knee) + Hang Clean (knee) – 70% x 1+1+2, 75% x 1+1+2 x 4
- Clean Segment Deadlift (1", knee) – 80% x 3, 85% x 3 x 2
- Back Squat – 70% x 8 x 2, 75% x 8 x 2
- SLDL – 2 x 5

Tuesday
- Power Clean – 70% x 3, 75% x 3, 80% x 3 x 3
- Jerk – 70% x 3, 75% x 3, 80% x 3 x 3
- Push Press – 70% x 5, 75% x 5 x 4
- Upper Body Push Bodybuilding

Wednesday

AM
- Clean Technique Primer
- Clean Pull + Hang Clean Pull (below knee) + Hang Clean (below knee) – 70% x 1+1+2, 75% x 1+1+2, 80% x 1+1+2 x 3
- Clean Pull on Riser – 90% x 4, 100% x 4 x 2
- Box Jump – 4 x 3

PM
- Snatch Pull + Hang Snatch Pull (below knee) + Hang Snatch (below knee) – 70% x 1+1+2, 75% x 1+1+2, 80% x 1+1+2 x 3
- Snatch Segment Deadlift (1", knee) – 80% x 3, 85% x 3 x 2
- Front Squat – 70% x 5 x 2, 75% x 5 x 2
- Good Morning – 2 x 5

Thursday
- Power Snatch – 70% x 3, 75% x 3, 80% x 3 x 3
- Power Jerk – 70% x 3, 75% x 3, 80% x 3 x 3
- Upper Body Pull Bodybuilding

Friday

AM
- Technique Primer
- Snatch – 70% x 1 x 3
- Clean & Jerk – 70% x 1+1 x 3

PM
- Technique Primer
- Snatch – HS
- Clean & Jerk – HS
- Box Jump – 4 x 3

Saturday
- Drop to Split – 4 x 5
- Snatch Push Press + Overhead Squat – 75% (of snatch) x 5+1 x 2, 80% x 5+1 x 3
- Back Squat – 70% x 5, 75% x 5, 80% x 5, 85% x 5 x 2
- Upper Body Push & Pull Bodybuilding

Week 3

Monday

AM
- Snatch Technique Primer
- Snatch Pull + Hang Snatch Pull (knee) + Hang Snatch (knee) – 70% x 1+1+2, 75% x 1+1+2, 1+1+2RM
- Snatch Pull on Riser – 90% x 4, 100% x 4, 105% x 4 x 2
- Depth Jump – 4 x 6

PM
- Clean Pull + Hang Clean Pull (knee) + Hang Clean (knee) – 70% x 2(1+1), 75% x 2(1+1), 2(1+1)RM
- Clean Segment Deadlift (1", knee) – 85% x 3 x 3
- Back Squat – 70% x 8, 75% x 8 x 3
- SLDL – 3 x 5

Tuesday
- Power Clean – 70% x 3, 75% x 3, 80% x 3, 3RM
- Jerk – 70% x 3, 75% x 3, 80% x 3, 3RM
- Push Press – 70% x 5, 75% x 5, 80% x 5, 5RM
- Upper Body Push Bodybuilding

Wednesday

AM
- Clean Technique Primer
- Clean Pull + Hang Clean Pull (below knee) + Hang Clean (below knee) – 70% x 1+1+2, 75% x 1+1+2, 80% x 1+1+2, 1+1+2RM
- Clean Pull on Riser – 90% x 4, 100% x 4, 105% x 4 x 2
- Box Jump – 4 x 3

PM

- Snatch Pull + Hang Snatch Pull (below knee) + Hang Snatch (below knee) – 70% x 1+1+2, 75% x 1+1+2, 80% x 1+1+2, 1+1+2RM
- Snatch Segment Deadlift (1", knee) – 85% x 3 x 3
- Front Squat – 70% x 5, 75% x 5 x 3
- Good Morning – 3 x 5

Thursday

- Power Snatch – 70% x 3, 75% x 3, 80% x 3, 3RM
- Power Jerk – 70% x 3, 75% x 3, 80% x 3, 3RM
- Overhead Squat – 70% x 3, 75% x 3, 80% x 3, 3RM
- Upper Body Pull Bodybuilding

Friday

AM

- Technique Primer
- Snatch – 70% x 1 x 5
- Clean & Jerk – 70% x 1+1 x 5

PM

- Technique Primer
- Snatch – HS: 85% x 1, 90% x 1
- Clean & Jerk – HS: 85% x 1+1, 90% x 1+1
- Depth Jump – 4 x 6

Saturday

- Drop to Split – 4 x 5
- Snatch Push Press – 75% (of snatch) x 5, 80% x 5, 85% x 5 x 3
- Back Squat – 70% x 5, 80% x 5, 85% x 5, 5RM
- Upper Body Push & Pull Bodybuilding

Week 4

Monday

AM

- Snatch Technique Primer
- Snatch Pull + Hang Snatch Pull (knee) + Hang Snatch (knee) – 70% x 1+1+2 x 5
- Snatch Pull on Riser – 85% x 3 x 3

PM

- Clean Pull + Hang Clean Pull (knee) + Hang Clean (knee) – 70% x 1+1+2 x 5
- Clean Pull – 85% x 3 x 3
- Back Squat – 70% x 5 x 4
- SLDL – 3 x 5

Tuesday

- Power Clean – 70% x 2 x 5
- Jerk – 70% x 2 x 5
- Push Press – 70% x 3 x 4
- Upper Body Push Bodybuilding

Wednesday

AM

- Clean Technique Primer
- Clean Pull + Hang Clean Pull (below knee) + Hang Clean (below knee) – 70% x 1+1+2 x 5
- Clean Pull on Riser – 80% x 3 x 3
- Box Jump – 4 x 3

PM

- Snatch Pull + Hang Snatch Pull (below knee) + Hang Snatch (below knee) – 70% x 1+1+2 x 5
- Snatch Pull – 85% x 3 x 3
- Front Squat – 70% x 5 x 4
- Good Morning – 3 x 5

Thursday

- Power Snatch – 70% x 2 x 5
- Power Jerk – 70% x 2 x 5
- Overhead Squat – 70% x 2 x 5
- Upper Body Pull Bodybuilding

Friday

AM

- Technique Primer
- Snatch – 70% x 1 x 5
- Clean & Jerk – 70% x 1+1 x 5

PM

- Technique Primer
- Snatch – 70% x 1, (75% x 1, 80% x 1, 85% x 1) x 3
- Clean & Jerk – 70% x 1+1, (75% x 1+1, 80% x 1+1, 85% x 1+1) x 3
- Box Jump – 4 x 3

Saturday

- Drop to Split – 4 x 5
- Snatch Push Press – 75% (of snatch) x 3 x 4
- Back Squat – 70% x 5, 75% x 5 x 4
- Upper Body Push & Pull Bodybuilding

Mesocycle 2: Preparation

Week 5

Monday

AM
- Snatch Technique Primer
- Snatch Pull + Hang Snatch (knee) – 70% x 1+2, 75% x 1+2 x 6
- Snatch Pull on Riser – 90% x 3, 100% x 3 x 4
- Depth Jump – 3 x 8

PM
- Clean Pull + Hang Clean (knee) – 70% x 1+2, 75% x 1+2 x 6
- Halting Clean Deadlift (mid-thigh) – 85% x 3 x 4
- Back Squat – 70% x 6, 75% x 6 x 4
- SLDL – 3 x 5

Tuesday
- Power Clean – 70% x 3, 75% x 3, 80% x 2 x 5
- Jerk – 70% x 3, 75% x 3, 80% x 2 x 5
- Push Press – 70% x 5, 75% x 3 x 5
- Upper Body Push Bodybuilding

Wednesday

AM
- Clean Technique Primer
- Clean Pull + Hang Clean (below knee) – 70% x 1+2, 75% x 1+2, 80% x 1+2 x 5
- Clean Pull on Riser – 90% x 3, 100% x 3 x 4
- Box Jump – 4 x 3

PM
- Snatch Pull + Hang Snatch (below knee) – 70% x 1+2, 75% x 1+2, 80% x 1+2 x 5
- Halting Snatch Deadlift (mid-thigh) – 85% x 3 x 4
- Front Squat – 73% x 4 x 4
- Good Morning – 3 x 5

Thursday
- Power Snatch – 70% x 2, 75% x 2, 80% x 2 x 5
- Power Jerk – 70% x 2, 75% x 2, 80% x 2 x 5
- Overhead Squat – 70% x 3, 80% x 3, 85% x 2 x 5
- Upper Body Pull Bodybuilding

Friday

AM
- Technique Primer
- Snatch – 70% x 1 x 5
- Clean & Jerk – 70% x 1+1 x 5

PM
- Technique Primer
- Snatch – HS
- Clean & Jerk – HS
- Depth Jump – 4 x 6

Saturday
- Push Jerk Behind the Neck in Split – 4 x 5
- Drop to Split – 4 x 5
- Snatch Push Press – 75% (of snatch) x 5, 80% x 4 x 5
- Back Squat – 70% x 3, 80% x 3, 85% x 3 x 3
- Upper Body Push & Pull Bodybuilding

Week 6

Monday

AM
- Snatch Technique Primer
- Snatch Pull + Hang Snatch (knee) – 70% x 1+2, 75% x 1+2, 80% x 1+2 x 4
- Snatch Pull on Riser – 90% x 3, 100% x 3, 105% x 3 x 2
- Depth Jump – 3 x 8

PM
- Clean Pull + Hang Clean (knee) – 70% x 1+2, 75% x 1+2, 80% x 1+2 x 4
- Halting Clean Deadlift (mid-thigh) – 85% x 3, 90% x 3 x 2
- Back Squat – 70% x 6, 75% x 6, 78% x 6 x 3
- SLDL – 3 x 5

Tuesday
- Power Clean – 70% x 3, 75% x 3, 80% x 2, 85% x 2 x 3
- Jerk – 70% x 3, 75% x 3, 80% x 2, 85% x 2 x 3
- Push Press – 70% x 5, 75% x 3 x 2, 80% x 3 x 3
- Upper Body Push Bodybuilding

Wednesday

AM
- Clean Technique Primer
- Clean Pull + Hang Clean (below knee) – 70% x 1+2, 75% x 1+2, 80% x 1+2, 85% x 1+2 x 3
- Clean Pull on Riser – 90% x 3, 100% x 3, 105% x 3 x 2
- Box Jump – 4 x 3

PM
- Snatch Pull + Hang Snatch (below knee) – 70% x 1+2, 75% x 1+2, 80% x 1+2, 85% x 1+2 x 3
- Halting Snatch Deadlift (mid-thigh) – 85% x 3, 90% x 3 x 2
- Front Squat – 73% x 4, 75% x 4 x 3
- Good Morning – 3 x 5

Thursday
- Power Snatch – 70% x 2, 75% x 2, 80% x 2, 85% x 2 x 3
- Power Jerk – 70% x 2, 75% x 2, 80% x 2, 85% x 2 x 3
- Overhead Squat – 70% x 3, 80% x 3, 85% x 2, 90% x 2 x 3
- Upper Body Pull Bodybuilding

Friday

AM
- Technique Primer
- Snatch – 70% x 1 x 5
- Clean & Jerk – 70% x 1+1 x 5

PM
- Technique Primer
- Snatch – HS
- Clean & Jerk – HS
- Depth Jump – 3 x 6

Saturday
- Push Jerk Behind the Neck in Split – 4 x 5
- Drop to Split – 4 x 5
- Snatch Push Press – 70% (of snatch) x 5, 75% x 5, 80% x 4, 85% x 4 x 3
- Back Squat – 70% x 3, 80% x 3, 85% x 3, 88% x 3 x 2
- Upper Body Push & Pull Bodybuilding

Week 7

Monday

AM
- Snatch Technique Primer
- Snatch Pull + Hang Snatch (knee) – 70% x 1+2, 75% x 2+1, 80% x 1+2, 1+2RM
- Snatch Pull on Riser – 90% x 3, 100% x 3, 110% x 3
- Depth Jump – 3 x 6

PM
- Clean Pull + Hang Clean (knee) – 70% x 1+2, 75% x 2+1, 80% x 1+2, 1+2RM
- Halting Clean Deadlift (mid-thigh) – 90% x 3 x 3
- Back Squat – 70% x 6, 75% x 6, 78% x 6, 80% x 6 x 2
- SLDL – 2 x 5

Tuesday
- Power Clean – 70% x 3, 75% x 3, 80% x 2, 85% x 2, 2RM
- Jerk – 70% x 3, 75% x 3, 80% x 2, 85% x 2, 2RM
- Push Press – 70% x 5, 75% x 3 x 2, 80% x 3, 3RM
- Upper Body Push Bodybuilding

Wednesday

AM
- Clean Technique Primer
- Clean Pull + Hang Clean (below knee) – 70% x 1+2, 75% x 1+2, 80% x 1+2, 85% x 1+2, 1+2RM
- Clean Pull on Riser – 90% x 3, 100% x 3, 110% x 3
- Box Jump – 3 x 3

PM
- Snatch Pull + Hang Snatch (below knee) – 70% x 1+2, 75% x 1+2, 80% x 1+2, 85% x 1+2, 1+2RM
- Halting Snatch Deadlift (mid-thigh) – 90% x 3 x 3
- Front Squat – 73% x 4, 75% x 4, 77% x 4 x 2
- Good Morning – 2 x 5

Thursday
- Power Snatch – 70% x 2, 75% x 2, 80% x 2, 85% x 2, 2RM
- Power Jerk – 70% x 2, 75% x 2, 80% x 2, 85% x 2, 2RM
- Overhead Squat – 70% x 3, 80% x 3, 85% x 2, 90% x 2, 2RM
- Upper Body Pull Bodybuilding

Friday

AM
- Technique Primer
- Snatch – 70% x 1 x 5
- Clean & Jerk – 70% x 1+1 x 5

PM
- Technique Primer
- Snatch – HS
- Clean & Jerk – HS
- Depth Jump – 3 x 5

Saturday
- Push Jerk Behind the Neck in Split – 3 x 5
- Drop to Split – 3 x 5
- Snatch Push Press – 70% (of snatch) x 5, 75% x 5, 80% x 4, 85% x 4, 90% x 4 x 2
- Back Squat – 70% x 3, 80% x 3, 85% x 3, 88% x 3, 3RM
- Upper Body Push & Pull Bodybuilding

Week 8

Monday

AM
- Snatch Technique Primer
- Snatch Pull + Hang Snatch (knee) – 70% x 1+2, 75% x 1+2 x 4
- Snatch Pull on Riser – 85% x 3
- Box Jump – 4 x 3

PM

- Clean Pull + Hang Clean (knee) – 70% x 1+2, 75% x 1+2 x 4
- Clean Pull – 85% x 3 x 3
- Back Squat – 70% x 4 x 2, 75% x 4 x 2
- SLDL – 2 x 5

Tuesday

- Power Clean – 70% x 2, 75% x 2 x 4
- Jerk – 70% x 2, 75% x 2 x 4
- Push Press – 70% x 5, 75% x 3 x 3
- Upper Body Push Bodybuilding

Wednesday

AM

- Clean Technique Primer
- Clean Pull + Hang Clean (below knee) – 70% x 1+2, 75% x 1+2 x 4
- Clean Pull on Riser – 85% x 3 x 3
- Box Jump – 3 x 3

PM

- Snatch Pull + Hang Snatch (below knee) – 70% x 1+2, 75% x 1+2 x 4
- Snatch Pull – 85% x 3 x 3
- Front Squat – 70% x 3 x 4
- Good Morning – 2 x 5

Thursday

- Power Snatch – 70% x 2, 75% x 2 x 4
- Power Jerk – 70% x 2, 75% x 2 x 4
- Overhead Squat – 70% x 2, 75% x 2 x 4
- Upper Body Pull Bodybuilding

Friday

AM

- Technique Primer
- Snatch – 70% x 1 x 5
- Clean & Jerk – 70% x 1+1 x 5

PM

- Technique Primer
- Snatch – 70% x 1, (75% x 1, 80% x 1, 85% x 1) x 3
- Clean & Jerk – 70% x 1+1, (75% x 1+1, 80% x 1+1, 85% x 1+1) x 3
- Depth Jump – 3 x 5

Saturday

- Push Jerk Behind the Neck in Split – 3 x 5
- Drop to Split – 3 x 5
- Snatch Push Press – 70% (of snatch) x 3, 75% x 3 x 4
- Back Squat – 70% x 3, 75% x 3, 80% x 3 x 2
- Upper Body Push & Pull Bodybuilding

Mesocycle 3: Preparation/Transition

Week 9

Monday

AM

- Clean Technique Primer
- Power Clean + Hang Clean (knee) – 70% (of Power Clean) x 1+2, 75% x 1+2 x 4
- Clean High-Pull – 75% x 3 x 3
- Box Jump – 4 x 3

PM

- Snatch – 70% x 1 x 5 OTM, 75% x 1 x 5 OTM, 80% x 1 x 5 OTM, HS
- Snatch Pull – 100% x 3, 105% x 3 x 3
- Back Squat – 70% x 4, 80% x 4 x 4
- SLDL – 3 x 5

Tuesday

- Jerk Technique Primer
- Jerk – 70% x 1 x 5 OTM, 75% x 1 x 5 OTM, 80% x 1 x 5 OTM, HS
- Segment Power Clean (knee) + Power Clean – 70% x 1+1, 75% x 1+1 x 5
- Push Press – 70% x 3, 80% x 3 x 4
- Upper Body Push Bodybuilding

Wednesday

AM

- Snatch Technique Primer
- Power Snatch + Hang Snatch (knee) – 70% x 1+2, 75% x 1+2 x 4
- Snatch High-Pull – 75% x 3 x 3
- Box Jump – 4 x 3

PM

- Clean – 70% x 1 x 5 OTM, 75% x 1 x 5 OTM, 80% x 1 x 5 OTM, HS
- Clean Pull – 100% x 3, 105% x 3 x 3
- Front Squat – 70% x 3, 75% x 3 x 4
- Good Morning – 3 x 5

Thursday

- Jerk Technique Primer
- Power Jerk – 70% x 1 x 5 OTM, 75% x 1 x 5 OTM, 80% x 1 x 5 OTM, HS
- Segment Power Snatch (knee) + Power Snatch – 70% (of Power Snatch) x 1+1, 75% x 1+1 x 5
- Snatch Balance – 70% x 2, 80% x 2 x 4
- Upper Body Pull Bodybuilding

Friday

AM
- Technique Primer
- Snatch – 70% x 1 x 5
- Clean & Jerk – 70% x 1+1 x 5

PM
- Technique Primer
- Snatch – HS
- Clean & Jerk – HS
- Depth Jump – 3 x 5

Saturday
- Power Jerk + Jerk – 70% x 2+1, 75% x 2+1 x 5
- Jump to Split – 4 x 4
- Snatch Push Press – 70% (of snatch) x 3, 80% x 3 x 4
- Front Squat – 70% x 3, 80% x 3, 85% x 3 x 3
- Upper Body Push & Pull Bodybuilding

Week 10

Monday

AM
- Clean Technique Primer
- Power Clean + Hang Clean (knee) – 70% (of Power Clean) x 1+1, 75% x 1+1, 80% x 1+1 x 3
- Clean High-Pull – 75% x 2, 80% x 2 x 2
- Box Jump – 4 x 3

PM
- Snatch – 73% x 1 x 5 OTM, 78% x 1 x 5 OTM, 83% x 1 x 5 OTM, HS
- Snatch Pull – 100% x 3, 105% x 3, 110% x 3 x 2
- Back Squat – 70% x 4, 80% x 4, 83% x 4 x 3
- SLDL – 3 x 4

Tuesday
- Jerk Technique Primer
- Jerk – 73% x 1 x 5 OTM, 78% x 1 x 5 OTM, 83% x 1 x 5 OTM, HS
- Segment Power Clean (knee) + Power Clean – 70% x 1+1, 75% x 1+1, 80% x 1+1 x 3
- Push Press – 70% x 3, 80% x 3, 85% x 3 x 3
- Upper Body Push Bodybuilding

Wednesday

AM
- Snatch Technique Primer
- Power Snatch + Hang Snatch (knee) – 70% x 1+1, 75% x 1+1, 80% x 1+1 x 3
- Snatch High-Pull – 75% x 2, 80% x 2 x 2
- Box Jump – 4 x 3

PM
- Clean – 73% x 1 x 5 OTM, 78% x 1 x 5 OTM, 83% x 1 x 5 OTM, HS
- Clean Pull – 100% x 3, 105% x 3, 110% x 3 x 2
- Front Squat – 70% x 3, 75% x 3, 78% x 3 x 3
- Good Morning – 3 x 4

Thursday
- Jerk Technique Primer
- Power Jerk – 73% x 1 x 5 OTM, 78% x 1 x 5 OTM, 83% x 1 x 5 OTM, HS
- Segment Power Snatch (knee) + Power Snatch – 70% (of Power Snatch) x 1+1, 75% x 1+1, 80% x 1+1 x 3
- Snatch Balance – 70% x 2, 80% x 2, 85% x 2 x 3
- Upper Body Pull Bodybuilding

Friday

AM
- Technique Primer
- Snatch – 70% x 1 x 5
- Clean & Jerk – 70% x 1+1 x 5

PM
- Technique Primer
- Snatch – HS
- Clean & Jerk – HS
- Depth Jump – 3 x 5

Saturday
- Power Jerk + Jerk – 70% x 1+1, 75% x 1+1, 80% x 1+1 x 3
- Jump to Split – 4 x 3
- Snatch Push Press – 70% (of snatch) x 3, 80% x 3, 85% x 3 x 3
- Front Squat – 70% x 3, 80% x 3, 85% x 3, 88% x 3 x 2
- Upper Body Push & Pull Bodybuilding

Week 11

Monday

AM
- Clean Technique Primer
- Power Clean + Hang Clean (knee) – 70% (of Power Clean) x 1+1, 75% x 1+1, 80% x 1+1, 85% x 1+1
- Clean High-Pull – 80% x 2 x 3
- Box Jump – 3 x 3

PM
- Snatch – 75% x 1 x 5 OTM, 80% x 1 x 5 OTM, 85% x 1 x 5 OTM, HS
- Snatch Pull – 105% x 3, 110% x 3, 115% x 3
- Back Squat – 70% x 4, 80% x 4, 4RM
- SLDL – 2 x 4

Tuesday
- Jerk Technique Primer
- Jerk – 75% x 1 x 5 OTM, 80% x 1 x 5 OTM, 85% x 1 x 5 OTM, HS
- Segment Power Clean (knee) + Power Clean – 70% x 1+1, 75% x 1+1, 80% x 1+1, 85% x 1+1
- Push Press – 70% x 3, 80% x 3, 85% x 3, 3RM
- Upper Body Push Bodybuilding

Wednesday

AM
- Snatch Technique Primer
- Power Snatch + Hang Snatch (knee) – 70% x 1+1, 75% x 1+1, 80% x 1+1, 85% x 1+1
- Snatch High-Pull – 80% x 2 x 3
- Box Jump – 3 x 3

PM
- Clean – 75% x 1 x 5 OTM, 80% x 1 x 5 OTM, 85% x 1 x 5 OTM, HS
- Clean Pull – 105% x 3, 110% x 3, 115% x 3
- Front Squat – 70% x 3, 75% x 3, 78% x 3, 80% x 3
- Good Morning – 2 x 4

Thursday
- Jerk Technique Primer
- Power Jerk – 75% x 1 x 5 OTM, 80% x 1 x 5 OTM, 85% x 1 x 5 OTM, HS
- Segment Power Snatch (knee) + Power Snatch – 70% (of Power Snatch) x 1+1, 75% x 1+1, 80% x 1+1, 85% x 1+1
- Snatch Balance – 70% x 2, 80% x 2, 85% x 2, 2RM
- Upper Body Pull Bodybuilding

Friday

AM
- Technique Primer
- Snatch – 70% x 1 x 4
- Clean & Jerk – 70% x 1+1 x 4

PM
- Technique Primer
- Snatch – HS
- Clean & Jerk – HS
- Depth Jump – 3 x 4

Saturday
- Power Jerk + Jerk – 70% x 1+1, 75% x 1+1, 80% x 1+1, 85% x 1+1
- Jump to Split – 4 x 3
- Snatch Push Press – 70% (of snatch) x 3, 80% x 3, 85% x 3, 90% x 3
- Front Squat – 70% x 3, 80% x 3, 85% x 3, 88% x 3, 3RM
- Upper Body Push & Pull Bodybuilding

Week 12

Monday

AM
- Clean Technique Primer
- Power Clean + Hang Clean (knee) – 70% (of Power Clean) x 1+1 x 4
- Clean High-Pull – 70% x 3 x 3
- Box Jump – 4 x 3

PM
- Snatch – (70% x 2, 75% x 1, 80% x 1) x 3
- Snatch Pull – 90% x 3, 95% x 3, 100% x 3
- Back Squat – 70% x 3, 75% x 3 x 3

Tuesday
- Jerk Technique Primer
- Jerk – (70% x 2, 75% x 1, 80% x 1) x 3
- Segment Power Clean (knee) + Power Clean – 70% x 1+1 x 4
- Push Press – 70% x 3 x 4
- Upper Body Push Bodybuilding

Wednesday

AM
- Snatch Technique Primer
- Power Snatch + Hang Snatch (knee) – 70% x 1+1 x 4
- Snatch High-Pull – 70% x 3 x 3
- Box Jump – 4 x 3

PM
- Clean – (70% x 2, 75% x 1, 80% x 1) x 3
- Clean Pull – 90% x 3, 95% x 3, 100% x 3
- Front Squat – 70% x 3 x 4

Thursday
- Jerk Technique Primer
- Power Jerk – (70% x 2, 75% x 1, 80% x 1) x 3
- Segment Power Snatch (knee) + Power Snatch – 70% (of Power Snatch) x 1+1 x 4
- Snatch Balance – 70% x 2 x 4
- Upper Body Pull Bodybuilding

Friday

AM
- Technique Primer
- Snatch – 70% x 1 x 5
- Clean & Jerk – 70% x 1+1 x 5

PM
- Technique Primer
- Snatch – 70% x 1, 75% x 1, 80% x 1, 85% x 1 x 5
- Clean & Jerk – 70% x 1+1, 75% x 1+1, 80% x 1+1, 85% x 1+1 x 5
- Back Squat Jump – 20% (of Back Squat) x 3 x 4

Saturday
- Power Jerk + Jerk – 70% x 1+1 x 4
- Drop to Split – 4 x 3
- Snatch Push Press – 70% (of snatch) x 3, 75% x 3 x 3
- Front Squat – 70% x 3, 75% x 3 x 3
- Upper Body Push & Pull Bodybuilding

Mesocycle 4: Competition

Week 13

Monday
- Snatch Technique Primer
- Snatch – HS; (85% (of HS) x 1, 90% x 1, 95% x 1) x 3
- Clean & Jerk - HS; (85% (of HS) x 1+1, 90% x 1+1, 95% x 1+1) x 3
- Clean Pull – 100% x 2, 110% x 2, 115% x 2 x 2, 90% x 2
- Front Squat – 70% x 3, 80% x 3, 85% x 3 x 4
- Good Morning – 3 x 5
- Depth Jump – 4 x 8

Tuesday
- Power Snatch – HS; (85% (of HS) x 1, 90% x 1, 95% x 1) x 2
- Jerk Technique Primer
- Power Clean & Jerk – HS; (85% (of HS) x 1+1, 90% x 1+1, 95% x 1+1) x 2
- Snatch High-Pull – 70% x 3 x 5

Wednesday
- Snatch – HS; (85% (of HS) x 1, 90% x 1, 95% x 1) x 2
- Clean Technique Primer
- Clean & Jerk - HS; (85% (of HS) x 1+1, 90% x 1+1, 95% x 1+1) x 2
- Snatch Pull – 100% x 2, 110% x 2, 115% x 2 x 2, 90% x 2
- Back Squat – 75% x 3 x 5
- Box Jump – 5 x 3

Thursday
- Snatch Technique Primer
- Power Snatch – HS; (85% (of HS) x 1, 90% x 1, 95% x 1) x 2
- Power Clean & Jerk – HS; (85% (of HS) x 1+1, 90% x 1+1, 95% x 1+1) x 2
- Clean High-Pull – 70% x 3 x 5
- Good Morning – 3 x 5

Saturday
- Technique Primer
- Snatch – HS; (90% (of HS) x 1, 95% x 1, HS) x 3
- Clean & Jerk – HS; (90% (of HS) x 1+1, 95% x 1+1, HS) x 3
- Snatch Pull – 95% x 2, 105% x 2, 110% x 2 x 2, 90% x 2
- Front Squat – 70% x 3, 80% x 3, 85% x 3, 90% x 2 x 3
- Back Squat Jump – 20% (of Back Squat) x 5 x 4

Week 14

Monday
- Snatch Technique Primer
- Snatch – HS; (85% (of HS) x 1, 90% x 1, 95% x 1) x 2
- Clean & Jerk - HS; (85% (of HS) x 1+1, 90% x 1+1, 95% x 1+1) x 2
- Clean Pull – 105% x 2, 115% x 2, 120% x 2 x 2, 90% x 2
- Front Squat – 70% x 3, 80% x 3, 85% x 3, 90% x 2 x 3
- Good Morning – 3 x 4
- Depth Jump – 4 x 6

Tuesday
- Power Snatch – HS; 85% (of HS) x 1, 90% x 1, 95% x 1
- Jerk Technique Primer
- Power Clean & Jerk – HS; 85% (of HS) x 1+1, 90% x 1+1, 95% x 1+1
- Snatch High-Pull – 70% x 3, 75% x 2 x 2, 70% x 3

Wednesday
- Snatch – HS; 85% (of HS) x 1, 90% x 1, 95% x 1
- Clean Technique Primer
- Clean & Jerk - HS; 85% (of HS) x 1+1, 90% x 1+1, 95% x 1+1
- Snatch Pull – 105% x 2, 115% x 2, 120% x 2 x 2, 90% x 2
- Back Squat – 75% x 3 x 2, 80% x 2 x 3
- Box Jump – 5 x 3

Thursday
- Snatch Technique Primer
- Power Snatch – HS; 85% (of HS) x 1, 90% x 1, 95% x 1
- Power Clean & Jerk – HS; 85% (of HS) x 1+1, 90% x 1+1, 95% x 1+1
- Clean High-Pull – 70% x 3, 75% x 2 x 2, 70% x 3
- Good Morning – 3 x 4

Saturday
- Technique Primer
- Snatch – HS; (90% (of HS) x 1, 95% x 1, HS) x 2
- Clean & Jerk – HS; (90% (of HS) x 1+1, 95% x 1+1, HS) x 2
- Clean Pull – 95% x 2, 105% x 2, 110% x 2 x 2, 90% x 2
- Front Squat – 70% x 3, 80% x 3, 85% x 3, 90% x 2, HS
- Back Squat Jump – 20% (of Back Squat) x 5 x 4

Week 15

Monday
- Snatch Technique Primer
- Snatch – HS; (85% (of HS) x 1, 90% x 1, 95% x 1) x 2
- Clean & Jerk - HS; (85% (of HS) x 1+1, 90% x 1+1, 95% x 1+1) x 2
- Clean Pull – 90% x 2, 95% x 2, 100% x 2 x 2, 80% x 2
- Front Squat – 70% x 3, 80% x 3, 85% x 2 x 3
- Depth Jump – 4 x 6

Tuesday
- Power Snatch – 70% x 1, 75% x 1, 80% x 1, 85% x 1 x 3
- Jerk Technique Primer
- Power Clean & Jerk – HS; 85% (of HS) x 1+1, 90% x 1+1, 95% x 1+1

Wednesday
- Snatch – HS; 85% (of HS) x 1, 90% x 1, 95% x 1
- Clean Technique Primer
- Clean & Jerk - HS; 85% (of HS) x 1+1, 90% x 1+1, 95% x 1+1
- Snatch Pull – 90% x 2, 95% x 2, 100% x 2 x 2, 80% x 2
- Back Squat – 75% x 3 x 5
- Box Jump – 5 x 3

Thursday
- Snatch Technique Primer
- Power Snatch – HS; 85% (of HS) x 1, 90% x 1, 95% x 1
- Power Clean & Jerk – 70% x 1+1, 75% x 1+1, 80% x 1+1, 85% x 1+1

Saturday
- Technique Primer
- Snatch – HS
- Clean & Jerk – To Opener
- Snatch Pull – 90% x 2, 100% x 2, 105% x 2, 110% x 2, 80% x 2
- Front Squat – 70% x 3, 80% x 3, 85% x 2 x 3
- Back Squat Jump – 20% (of Back Squat) x 3 x 4

Week 16

Monday
- Snatch Technique Primer
- Snatch – 70% x 2, 75% x 1, 80% x 1, 85% x 1, 90% x 1 x 3
- Clean & Jerk – 70% x 1+1, 75% x 1+1, 80% x 1+1, 85% x 1+1 x 3
- Clean Pull – 90% x 2 x 4
- Back Squat – 75% x 3 x 4

Wednesday
- Snatch – 70% x 2, 75% x 1, 80% x 1, 85% x 1 x 3
- Clean & Jerk - 70% x 1+1, 75% x 1+1, 80% x 1+1 x 3
- Snatch Pull – 85% x 2 x 4
- Front Squat – 75% x 2 x 4

Thursday
- Snatch – 70% x 1 x 5
- Power Clean & Jerk – 70% x 1+1 x 5

Saturday
- Competition

Program **Beginner Template**

The following template is intended for beginning lifters with a reasonable foundation of general athleticism—that is, not in need of serious fundamental work on mobility, stability and work capacity.

Each stage is somewhat more technically demanding than the previous. For example, the first stage uses snatches and cleans from the hang and jerks from behind the neck and progresses to the regular classic lifts. Positions and mechanics are emphasized early on to build a foundation for the lifter to progress with the classic lifts and assistance exercises.

Each training day has a technique primer for the classic lift (snatch, clean or jerk) that will be the focus of that day; Saturday's will be a primer of the athlete or coach's choice. This exercise should be chosen for each athlete to address individual need and encourage better execution of the classic lift to follow. These exercises can be changed each time if desired, or can be kept the same for as long as is needed or effective. These are lightweight, technique exercises and should not cause significant fatigue. Examples of these technique primers are light snatch balances for an athlete who is not aggressive overhead in the snatch; muscle cleans for an athlete who needs to improve the mechanics of the clean turnover; or jerk dip squats for an athlete who fails to maintain the proper balance and position during the dip and drive of the jerk.

Proper positions and posture should be emphasized and reinforced at all times. Snatches and jerks should be held in the receiving position for 3 seconds before standing to strengthen the positions and improve stability and positioning.

Weights must be determined by feel. In the first week of each stage, weights should be challenging, but comfortably within the athlete's limits. Each week, the goal will be to add weight. After 3-4 weeks of each stage, the athlete will proceed to the next stage, again starting with conservative weights for the prescribed sets and reps and building up the weight over the course of 3-4 weeks. This will provide a pro-gression of reduced volume and increased weight on average over the 9-12 weeks of the cycle.

On Saturdays, the snatch and clean & jerk will be taken up gradually to the heaviest weight with which the athlete is comfortable that day for a single rep. Small weight increases and relatively short rest periods (1-2 minutes) are recommended to improve consistency among sets. Athletes should aim to accumulate about 15 total reps above approximately 60% of max (this must of course be estimated based on effort for most beginners, who will not have established or accurate 1RMs). If this number of reps has not been achieved while working up to the heavy single, back-off singles at a somewhat reduced weight should be done after the heavy single to make up the difference. Making successful lifts is the priority over weight.

This basic template can be repeated with minor modifications to exercise variations each time to best address the changing needs of the athlete.

Stage 1

Monday
- Snatch Technique Primer
- Mid-Hang Snatch - 5 x 3
- Halting Snatch Deadlift (mid-thigh) - 5 x 3
- Back Squat - 3 x 8
- Back Extensions – 3 x 10
- Abs

Tuesday
- Jerk Technique Primer
- Jerk Behind the Neck - 5 x 3
- Front Squat - 3 x 5
- Press - 3 x 10
- DB row - 3 x 10
- Back Extensions – 3 x 10
- Abs

Thursday
- Clean Technique Primer
- Mid-Hang Clean - 5 x 3
- Halting Clean Deadlift (mid-thigh) - 5 x 3
- Back Squat - 3 x 6 (lighter than Monday)
- Back Extensions – 3 x 10
- Abs

Saturday
- Choice Technique Primer
- Snatch - heavy single (15 total reps)
- Clean & Jerk - heavy single (15 total reps)
- Front Squat - 3 x 3
- Back Extensions – 3 x 10
- Abs

Stage 2

Monday
- Snatch Technique Primer
- Snatch - 5 x 2
- Halting Snatch Deadlift (mid-thigh) + Snatch Pull - 5 x (1+2)
- Back Squat - 3 x 6
- Back Extensions – 3 x 10
- Abs

Tuesday
- Jerk Technique Primer
- Jerk - 5 x 2
- Front Squat - 3 x 3
- Push Press - 3 x 6
- DB row or Pull-up - 3 x 10
- Back Extensions – 3 x 10
- Abs

Thursday
- Clean Technique Primer
- Clean - 5 x 2
- Halting Clean Deadlift (mid-thigh) + Clean Pull - 5 x (1+2)
- Back Squat - 3 x 5 (lighter than Monday)
- Back Extensions – 3 x 10
- Abs

Saturday
- Choice Technique Primer
- Snatch - heavy single (15 total reps)
- Clean & Jerk - heavy single (15 total reps)
- Front Squat - 3 x 2
- Back Extensions – 3 x 10
- Abs

Stage 3

Monday
- Snatch Technique Primer
- Snatch – 8 x 1
- Snatch Pull - 5 x 3
- Back Squat - 3 x 5
- Back Extensions – 3 x 10
- Abs

Tuesday
- Jerk Technique Primer
- Jerk – 8 x 1
- Front Squat - 3 x 2
- Push Press - 3 x 4
- DB row or Pull-up - 3 x 10
- Back Extensions – 3 x 10
- Abs

Thursday
- Clean Technique Primer
- Clean – 8 x 1
- Clean Pull - 5 x 3
- Back Squat - 3 x 3 (lighter than Monday)
- Back Extensions – 3 x 10
- Abs

Saturday
- Choice Technique Primer
- Snatch - heavy single (15 total reps)
- Clean & Jerk - heavy single (15 total reps)
- Front Squat - 3 x 1
- Back Extensions – 3 x 10
- Abs

Program **Simple 3-Day Template**

The following is a 3-day per week training template that keeps programming very simple and flexible. This can be used by master lifters or other individuals who have limited recovery capacity, limited time or are trying to balance other training with weightlifting. It can also be used simply as a starting point for building more extensive programming.

The snatch, clean and jerk can be the classic lifts as written, or any variation based on the needs of the athlete with regard to position strength and technical problems. This includes variations like powers, hangs, complexes, etc.

Snatch and clean pulls can be done as pulls as written, or any pulling-related exercise such as halting deadlifts, partial pulls, segment pulls and pull complexes can be substituted as appropriate. Again, exercises should be chosen to address specific needs with regard to technique and strength rather than at random simply for the sake of variation.

The push press on day 2 can be any kind of upper body pressing exercise that is determined to be most effective: push press behind the neck, press, incline bench press, snatch push press, etc. Similarly, the overhead squat on day 2 can be replaced with a snatch balance variation, complex of snatch balance and overhead squat, snatch push press and overhead squat, etc.

Front squats and back squats on days 1 and 3 can be done with the rep and set numbers deemed appropriate for the athlete and stage of the program. A good average would be 3 reps for the front squat and 5 reps for the back squat, 3-5 sets for each. Early on, sets of 8-10 in the back squat and 4-6 in the front squat might be used if appropriate.

The first week should employ fairly conservative weights, and then those weights increased gradually over the course of 3-4 weeks with uniform rep and set numbers. On the last week of a given block, max lifts can be tested as desired. In a subsequent block, rep numbers can be reduced and the starting weights for the first week increased according to this reduction and the improved ability of the lifter.

Day 1
- Snatch
- Snatch Pull
- Front Squat

Day 2
- Jerk
- Push Press
- Overhead Squat

Day 3
- Clean & Jerk
- Clean Pull
- Back Squat

Program **Masters Program**

This program is a very general idea of what master lifters may find productive, created with a forty-something athlete with average recovery ability and training experience in mind. Athletes with extensive weightlifting backgrounds will likely be capable of and even require more work; those with minimal or no weightlifting backgrounds may need to reduce the volume somewhat.

There is a simple rotation in terms of intensity and volume among staple exercises to attempt to achieve balance, with two days of heavier training and two days of lighter training each week. This basic template can be used with gradually increasing intensity for 2-4 weeks, followed by a recovery week with weights kept to 60-70%. After this, some change to the exercises or reps can be made to focus on an athlete's present needs.

Masters lifters may also find variations of the Simple Template effective.

Week 1

Monday
- Clean Pull - 4 x 3
- Back Squat - 5 x 3
- Snatch Push Press - 4 x 5
- Abs

Tuesday
- Snatch - 80% x 1 x 3
- Power Clean & Power Jerk - 75% x 2(1+1) x 4
- Back Extensions
- Abs

Thursday
- Snatch Pull - 3 x 3
- Front Squat - 3 x 2
- Overhead Squat - 4 x 3
- Push Press - 3 x 5
- Abs

Friday
- Clean & Jerk - 80% x 1+1 x 3
- Power Snatch - 75% x 2 x 4
- Back Extensions
- Abs

Week 2

Monday
- Snatch Pull - 4 x 3
- Front Squat - 5 x 3
- Overhead Squat - 3 x 2
- Push Press - 5 x 5
- Abs

Tuesday
- Clean & Jerk - 80% x 1+1 x 3
- Power Snatch - 75% x 2 x 4
- Back Extensions
- Abs

Thursday
- Clean Pull - 3 x 3
- Back Squat - 3 x 2
- Snatch Push Press - 3 x 5
- Abs

Friday
- Snatch - 80% x 1 x 3
- Power Clean & Power Jerk - 75% x 2(1+1) x 4
- Back Extensions
- Abs

Recovery Week

Monday
- Snatch – 5 x 1
- Snatch Pull – 3 x 2
- Back Squat – 3 x 3

Wednesday
- Power Snatch – 5 x 1
- Power Clean & Power Jerk – 5 x 1+1
- Press – 3 x 5

Friday
- Clean & Jerk – 5 x 1+1
- Clean Pull – 3 x 2
- Front Squat – 3 x 3

Program Weight Gain Program

The following program intends to help the athlete gain functional bodyweight. It involves generally higher repetition numbers, and relatively high volume, along with a significant volume of bodybuilding exercises.

Loading should be controlled by feel with the goal being to start with fairly conservative weights and increase weekly for 3-4 weeks before inserting a recovery week of lower volume and intensity. The exercises in each new block following a recovery week should be changed in some way, whether to different variations of the same exercise, or simply to the repetition numbers.

For squats, the first sets should be fairly heavy, with the last higher-rep sets lighter but each set heavier than the previous, aiming to finish the last set with close to a maximal effort for the repetition count. Back squat 5s on Monday should start around 70-75% depending on how accustomed the lifter is to this rep count in the squat. Front squat triples on Friday should start around 75-80%, again depending on the athlete's conditioning.

Power snatch, power clean and jerk triples should begin around 70% in the first week. Deadlifts on risers may range from about 85-105% of the lifter's best snatch or clean depending on technical proficiency and general pulling strength. If the lifter needs to emphasize squatting strength over pulling strength, these should be kept somewhat lighter to allow more work in the squats.

In all cases, it's advisable to err on the side of lower intensity when beginning this program and build longer rather than attempting to begin heavier and grind to a halt more quickly.

On Friday, the snatch and clean & jerk can be taken to heavy singles, which will on most weeks not be particularly high percentages of the lifter's maxes. Following the heavy single, the weight should be reduced 10-20% so 5 more singles can be performed, either at a uniform weight or ascending weights each set.

The bodybuilding exercises used should change every week. The total repetition count for each day is approximate and should be split between 2-3 exercises with sets of 10-15 reps (e.g., 4 sets of 10 on Exercise 1 and 4 sets of 10 on Exercise 2 to reach 80 total reps). At least one of these exercises per day per body part should be taken to failure on each set.

Lower body bodybuilding may be squatting, lunging, or split squatting variations, as well as exercises like leg curls and extensions, or calf raises. Monday can be any of these, while Friday should involve at least 1 unilateral exercise.

More information on bodybuilding training can be found in the Accessory Work chapter. Ab work can be done according to the Ab Matrix provided in the same chapter.

It should be kept in mind that in order for weight to be gained on any program, the athlete's nutrition must be in order to support it. Details on gaining weight are covered in the Nutrition section of the book. Sleep is also critical to allow maximal recovery during this program.

Weekly Template

Monday
- Back Squat – 4 x 5; 3 x 10
- SLDL – 4 x 8
- Leg Bodybuilding – 80 total reps (2-3 exercises, sets of 10-15)
- Abs

Tuesday
- Jerk – 5 x 3
- Push Press – 5 x 6
- Upper Body Push Bodybuilding – 80 total reps (2-3 exercises, sets of 10-15)
- Abs

Wednesday
- Power Clean – 5 x 3
- Clean Deadlift on Riser – 4 x 5
- Upper Body Pull Bodybuilding – 80 total reps (2-3 exercises, sets of 10-15)
- Abs

Friday
- Snatch – HS; 5 x 1
- Clean & Jerk – HS; 5 x 1+1
- Front Squat – 4 x 3; 3 x 8
- Unilateral Leg Bodybuilding – 80 total reps (2-3 exercises, sets of 10-15)
- Abs

Saturday
- Power Snatch – 5 x 3
- Snatch Deadlift on Riser – 4 x 5
- Upper Body Push & Pull Bodybuilding – 100 total reps (2 exercises for each, sets of 10-15)
- Abs

Recovery Week

Monday
- Back Squat – 3 x 3
- SLDL – 3 x 5
- Leg Bodybuilding – 40 total reps (2 exercises, sets of 10-15)
- Abs

Tuesday
- Jerk – 4 x 2
- Push Press – 4 x 3
- Upper Body Push Bodybuilding – 40 total reps (2 exercises, sets of 10-15)
- Abs

Wednesday
- Power Clean – 4 x 2
- Clean Deadlift on Riser – 3 x 3
- Upper Body Pull Bodybuilding – 40 total reps (2-3 exercises, sets of 10-15)
- Abs

Friday
- Snatch – 75-85% x 1 x 5
- Clean & Jerk – 75-85% x 1+1 x 5
- Front Squat – 3 x 2
- Unilateral Leg Bodybuilding – 40 total reps (2-3 exercises, sets of 10-15)
- Abs

Saturday
- Power Snatch – 4 x 2
- Snatch Deadlift on Riser – 3 x 3
- Upper Body Push & Pull Bodybuilding – 50 total reps (1-2 exercises for each, sets of 10-15)
- Abs

Program **Bulgarian Program**

This is a very simple Bulgarian-style program with minimal volume, but maximal intensity. Each day, each lift is taken up to the heaviest single rep the athlete can manage that day. The second squat workout of the day includes back-off sets—the lifter will select weights for these doubles by feel, always aiming to beat the previous best double, but understanding this will not be possible every day or week. On Monday, Wednesday and Friday, there are also back-off singles for the snatch and clean & jerk. Weights for these will also need to be selected by feel day to day. The ideal approach is to drop the weight around 10% from the heavy single and then try to work back up to beat that heavy single within 5 sets. On days when the lifter is confident this isn't possible, these 5 singles can be done at a uniform weight at a lower percentage, or can be ascending weights simply starting at a lower percentage rather than attempting to exceed the preceding heavy single.

Ab and back work should be done daily. Days can be split into two workouts if the athlete wishes, splitting between the snatch and clean & jerk.

This structure can be repeated essentially indefinitely, and as a competition approaches, 1-2 weeks of reduced squatting and volume can be used to taper slightly. In these weeks, the first squat workout of each day and the squat back-off sets can be removed, and in the final week, the back-off sets for all exercises removed.

Monday
- Front Squat – HS
- Snatch – HS; 5x1
- Clean & Jerk – HS; 5x1
- Back Squat – HS; 2x2
- Abs

Tuesday
- Back Squat – HS
- Snatch – HS
- Clean & Jerk – HS
- Front Squat – HS; 2x2
- Abs

Wednesday
- Front Squat – HS
- Snatch – HS; 5x1
- Clean & Jerk – HS; 5x1
- Back Squat – HS; 2x2
- Abs

Thursday
- Back Squat – HS
- Snatch – HS
- Clean & Jerk – HS
- Front Squat – HS; 2x2
- Abs

Friday
- Front Squat – HS
- Snatch – HS; 5x1
- Clean & Jerk – HS; 5x1
- Back Squat – HS; 2x2
- Abs

Saturday
- Back Squat – HS
- Snatch – HS
- Clean & Jerk – HS
- Front Squat – HS; 2x2
- Abs

Program **5-Week Front Squat Cycle**

This program has produced some amazing increases in lifters' front squats in only five weeks (as much as 20-30kg for some athletes), and although not specifically intended to do so, in many cases has also increased lifters' snatch and clean & jerk numbers considerably as well. It's a moderate amount of volume that most intermediate to advanced lifters will be able to handle productively. It is necessary, however, for lifter's to have accurate 1RMs for their lifts in order for the program to be effective.

Week 1

Monday
- Snatch – 75% x 3 x 5
- Jerk – 75% x 3 x 5
- Front Squat – 75% x 3 x 5
- Snatch Deadlift – 100% x 5 x 3
- Abs

Tuesday
- Power Snatch + Snatch Push Press + Overhead Squat – 70% x 3+3+3 x 3, 75% x 3+3+3 x 2
- Power Clean + Power Jerk – 70% x 2(1+1) x 3, 75% x 2(1+1) x 2
- Snatch Pull – 90% x 3 x 2, 95% x 3 x 3
- Abs

Wednesday
- Clean – 75% x 3 x 5
- Jerk Behind the Neck – 75% x 3 x 5
- Back Squat – 70% x 2 x 5
- Clean Pull – 90% x 3 x 2, 95% x 3 x 2
- Abs

Thursday
- Power Clean + Push Press (% of Push Press) – 75% x 2(2+1) x 5
- Snatch Push Press + Snatch Balance (% of Snatch) – 70% x 3+1 x 5
- Snatch Pull – 90% x 3 x 5
- Abs

Saturday
- Front Squat – 80% x 3 x 5
- Snatch – Heavy Single
- Clean & Jerk – Heavy Single
- Clean Deadlift – 100% x 5 x 3
- Abs

Week 2

Monday
- Clean – 75% x 3 x 3, 80% x 2 x 2
- Jerk Behind the Neck – 75% x 3 x 3, 80% x 3 x 2
- Back Squat – 70% x 2 x 5
- Snatch Deadlift – 100% x 5, 105% x 5 x 2
- Abs

Tuesday
- Power Snatch + Snatch Push Press + Overhead Squat – 70% x 3+3+3, 75% x 3+3+3 x 4
- Power Clean + Power Jerk – 70% x 2(1+1), 75% x 2(1+1) x 4
- Snatch Pull – 95% x 3 x 2, 100% x 3 x 3
- Abs

Wednesday
- Front Squat – 85% x 2 x 5
- Snatch – 75% x 3 x 3, 80% x 2 x 2
- Jerk – 75% x 3 x 3, 80% x 2 x 2
- Clean Pull – 95% x 3 x 2, 100% x 3 x 3
- Abs

Thursday
- Power Clean + Push Press (% of Push Press) – 75% x 2(2+1) x 3, 80% x 2(2+1) x 2
- Snatch Push Press + Snatch Balance (% of Snatch) – 70% x 3+1 x 2, 75% x 3+1 x 3
- Snatch Pull – 95% x 3 x 5
- Abs

Saturday
- Snatch – Heavy Single
- Clean & Jerk – Heavy Single
- Clean Deadlift – 100% x 5 x 3
- Back Squat – 70% x 2 x 5
- Abs

Week 3

Monday
- Front Squat – 85% x 3 x 4
- Snatch – 75% x 3 x 1, 80% x 2 x 4
- Jerk – 75% x 3 x 1, 80% x 2 x 4
- Clean Pull – 100% x 3 x 4
- Abs

Tuesday
- Power Snatch + Snatch Push Press + Overhead Squat – 70% x 3+3+3, 75% x 3+3+3 x 2, 80% x 3+3+3 x 2
- Power Clean + Power Jerk – 70% x 2+1, 75% x 2+1 x 2, 80% x 2+1 x 2
- Snatch Pull – 95% x 3 x 4
- Abs

Wednesday
- Clean – 75% x 3 x 1, 80% x 2 x 4
- Jerk Behind the Neck – 75% x 3, 80% x 2 x 4
- Snatch Pull – 100% x 3 x 4
- Back Squat – 70% x 2 x 5
- Abs

Thursday
- Power Clean + Push Press (% of Push Press) – 75% x 2(2+1), 80% x 2(2+1) x 4
- Snatch Push Press + Snatch Balance (% of Snatch) – 70% x 3+1, 75% x 3+1 x 2, 80% x 3+1 x 2
- Clean Pull – 95% x 3 x 4
- Abs

Saturday
- Front Squat – 90% x 1 x 5
- Snatch – Heavy Single
- Clean & Jerk – Heavy Single
- Snatch Pull – 100% x 3 x 3
- Abs

Week 4

Monday
- Clean & Jerk – 75% x 2+1, 80% x 1+1 x 2, 85% x 1+1 x 2
- Clean Pull – 95% x 3, 100% x 3, 105% x 2 x 3
- Back Squat – 70% x 2 x 5
- Abs

Tuesday
- Power Snatch + Overhead Squat – 70% x 2+1, 75% x 2+1, 80% x 2+1, 85% x 1+1 x 3
- Power Clean + Power Jerk – 70% x 2+1, 75% x 2+1, 80% x 1+1, 85% x 1+1 x 3
- Snatch Pull – 95% x 2 x 2, 100% x 2 x 2
- Abs

Wednesday
- Front Squat – 90% x 2 x 3
- Snatch – 75% x 2, 80% x 2, 85% x 1 x 3
- Jerk – 75% x 2, 80% x 2, 85% x 1 x 3
- Snatch Pull – 100% x 3 x 2, 105% x 2 x 2
- Abs

Thursday
- Power Snatch – 75% x 2 x 2, 80% x 1 x 4
- Power Clean + Power Jerk – 75% x 2+1 x 2, 80% x 1+1 x 4
- Clean Pull – 95% x 2 x 2, 100% x 2 x 2
- Abs

Saturday
- Snatch – Heavy Single
- Clean & Jerk – Heavy Single
- Clean Pull – 105% x 3 x 3
- Back Squat – 70% x 2 x 5
- Abs

Week 5

Monday
- Front Squat – 95% x 1 x 3
- Snatch – 70% x 2, 75% x 2, 80% x 1, 85% x 1 x 3
- Clean & Jerk – 70% x 1+1, 75% x 1+1, 80% x 1+1 x 2
- Clean Pull – 85% x 2, 90% x 2, 95% x 2
- Abs

Tuesday
- Power Snatch – 70% x 1 x 3, 75% x 1 x 3
- Power Clean + Power Jerk – 70% x 1+1 x 3, 75% x 1+1 x 3
- Abs

Wednesday
- Snatch – 70% x 2, 75% x 2, 80% x 1 x 3
- Clean & Jerk – 70% x 1+1, 75% x 1+1, 80% x 1+1
- Snatch Pull – 85% x 2, 90% x 2, 95% x 2
- Abs

Thursday
- Power Snatch – 70% x 1 x 3, 75% x 1 x 3
- Power Clean + Power Jerk – 70% x 1+1 x 3, 75% x 1+1 x 3
- Abs

Saturday
- Front Squat – Text Max
- Snatch – Heavy Single
- Clean & Jerk – Heavy Single

Program **10-Week Volume Squat Cycle**

This is a 10-week squatting program for increasing both leg strength and size, as well as work capacity. Included is "Week 0" which can be used as an introductory week. If the individual is accustomed to fairly high-volume squatting already, this week may not be necessary.

Accompanying training should be conservative in terms of intensity and volume to accommodate the need for recovery from the squatting work. How much can be managed in addition to this program varies significantly among individuals. The volume of additional work can be kept relative to that of the squatting, i.e. increasing gradually to week 4 and then tapering off. Week 9 volume should be very low, and week 10 should involve very little work to allow the athlete to recover as much as possible for the front squat max attempt on Saturday—dropping all work other than squatting and possibly including some unweighted squat jumps is one option.

This front squat max will not be 100% accurate because of the timing. The cycle can also be used with back and front squats switched if the athlete needs to prioritize the front squat.

Week 0

Monday
- Back Squat – 50% x 4 x 3

Tuesday
- Front Squat – 50% x 2 x 3

Wednesday
- Back Squat – 50% x 2 x 3

Thursday
- Front Squat – 50% x 5 x 3

Friday
- Back Squat – 50% x 2 x 3

Saturday
- Back Squat – 50% x 2 x 3

Week 1

Monday
- Back Squat – 65% x 6 x 4

Tuesday
- Front Squat – 60% x 2 x 3

Wednesday
- Back Squat – 60% x 2 x 3

Thursday
- Front Squat – 65% x 5 x 4

Friday
- Back Squat – 60% x 2 x 3

Saturday
- Back Squat – 65% x 2 x 3

Week 2

Monday
- Back Squat – 70% x 6 x 6

Tuesday
- Front Squat – 60% x 2 x 3

Wednesday
- Back Squat – 60% x 2 x 3

Thursday
- Front Squat – 70% x 5 x 6

Friday
- Back Squat – 60% x 2 x 3

Saturday
- Back Squat – 70% x 2 x 3

Week 3

Monday
- Back Squat – 70% x 6 x 8

Tuesday
- Front Squat – 60% x 2 x 3

Wednesday
- Back Squat – 60% x 2 x 3

Thursday
- Front Squat – 70% x 5 x 8

Friday
- Back Squat – 60% x 2 x 3

Saturday
- Back Squat – 70% x 2 x 3

Week 4

Monday
- Back Squat – 70% x 6 x 10

Tuesday
- Front Squat – 60% x 2 x 3

Wednesday
- Back Squat – 60% x 2 x 3

Thursday
- Front Squat – 70% x 5 x 10

Friday
- Back Squat – 60% x 2 x 3

Saturday
- Back Squat – 70% x 2 x 3

Week 5

Monday
- Back Squat – 75% x 6 x 8

Tuesday
- Front Squat – 60% x 2 x 3

Wednesday
- Back Squat – 60% x 2 x 3

Thursday
- Front Squat – 75% x 4 x 8

Friday
- Back Squat – 60% x 2 x 3

Saturday
- Back Squat – 70% x 2 x 3

Week 6

Monday
- Back Squat – 80% x 5 x 6

Tuesday
- Front Squat – 60% x 2 x 3

Wednesday
- Back Squat – 60% x 2 x 3

Thursday
- Front Squat – 78% x 4 x 6

Friday
- Back Squat – 60% x 2 x 3

Saturday
- Back Squat – 70% x 2 x 3

Week 7

Monday
- Back Squat – 85% x 4 x 4

Tuesday
- Front Squat – 60% x 2 x 3

Wednesday
- Back Squat – 60% x 2 x 3

Thursday
- Front Squat – 81% x 4 x 4

Friday
- Back Squat – 60% x 2 x 3

Saturday
- Back Squat – 70% x 2 x 3

Week 8

Monday
- Back Squat – 90% x 3 x 3

Tuesday
- Front Squat – 60% x 2 x 3

Wednesday
- Back Squat – 60% x 2 x 3

Thursday
- Front Squat – 84% x 3 x 3

Friday
- Back Squat – 60% x 2 x 3

Saturday
- Back Squat – 70% x 2 x 3

Week 9

Monday
- Back Squat – 95% x 2 x 2

Tuesday
- Front Squat – 60% x 2 x 3

Wednesday
- Front Squat – 87% x 2 x 2

Thursday
- Back Squat – 60% x 2 x 3

Friday
- Back Squat – 60% x 2 x 3

Saturday
- Back Squat – 70% x 2 x 3

Week 10

Monday
- Back Squat – Text Max

Tuesday
- Front Squat – 50% x 2 x 2

Wednesday
- Front Squat – 60% x 2 x 2

Thursday
- Front Squat – 60% x 1 x 2

Friday
- Front Squat – 50% x 1 x 3

Saturday
- Front Squat – Test Max

Program **On-The-Minute Cycle**

This program provides one example of how to incorporate on-the-minute singles in the snatch, clean and jerk for an intermediate to advanced weightlifter. For exercises on the minute, each set will begin exactly 1 minute after the previous set was begun—that is, there will be less than 1 minute of rest between sets. This kind of training is typically effective for improving technical consistency in the competition lifts, as well as conditioning lifters for potentially fast-paced warm-up situations in competition.

Series of OTM weights are performed with a continuously running clock. For example, if lifting 5 singles at 70%, 5 singles at 75%, and 5 singles at 80%, the fifteenth set will begin on minute 14 (the first set begins at minute 0). Weight changes must be done within the 1 minute time limit. If a series of OTM scts is followed by "HS", the lifter, after completing the first 15 sets, can then proceed off the clock to a heavy single. Generally this should only be done if there were no misses during the first 15 singles, but exceptions can be made if sensible in the coach's judgment. These off-the-clock sets should still be done with relatively short rest periods—typically around 2 minutes.

Weights in bold can be increased if the lifter is feeling strong that day, but not to maximal effort.

Week 1

Monday
- Snatch - 70% x 1 x 5 OTM, 75% x 1 x 5 OTM, 80% x 1 x 5 OTM
- Snatch Pull - 85% x 3 x 3
- Segment Snatch Deadlift (knee) + Floating Snatch Deadlift - 80% x 3+1 x 3
- Back Squat (5 sec eccentric on rep 1) - 70% x 5 x 3
- Abs

Tuesday
- Jerk - 70% x 1 x 5 OTM, 75% x 1 x 5 OTM, 80% x 1 x 5 OTM
- Push Press - 70% x 5 x 5
- Back Squat Jump (% of Back Squat) - 25% x 3 x 3
- Abs

Wednesday
- Clean - 70% x 1 x 5 OTM, 75% x 1 x 5 OTM, 80% x 1 x 5 OTM
- Clean Pull - 85% x 3 x 3
- Segment Clean Deadlift (knee) + Floating Clean Deadlift - 80% x 3+1 x 3
- Pause Back Squat - 60% x 3 x 3
- Abs

Thursday
- Power Clean - 70% x 3 x 5
- Power Jerk - 70% x 3 x 5
- SLDL – 3 x 5
- Abs

Saturday
- Snatch - 70% x 1, 75% x 1, 80% x 1, 80% x 1 x 2
- Clean & Jerk - 70% x 1+1, 75% x 1+1, 80% x 1+1, 80% x 1+1 x 2
- Front Squat - 75% x 3 x 3
- Good Morning – 3 x 5
- Abs

Week 2

Monday
- Snatch – 73% x 1 x 5 OTM, 78% x 1 x 5 OTM, 83% x 1 x 5 OTM , HS
- Snatch Pull - 85% x 3, 90% x 3 x 2
- Segment Snatch Deadlift (knee) + Floating Snatch Deadlift - 80% x 3+1, 85% x 3+1 x 2
- Back Squat (5 sec eccentric on rep 1) - 70% x 5, 75% x 5 x 2
- Abs

Tuesday
- Jerk 73% x 1 x 5 OTM, 78% x 1 x 5 OTM, 83% x 1 x 5 OTM, HS
- Push Press - 70% x 5 x 2, 75% x 5 x 3
- Back Squat Jump - 25% x 3 x 3
- Abs

Wednesday
- Clean - 73% x 1 x 5 OTM, 78% x 1 x 5 OTM, 83% x 1 x 5 OTM, HS
- Clean Pull - 85% x 3, 90% x 3 x 2
- Segment Clean Deadlift (knee) + Floating Clean Deadlift - 80% x 3+1, 85% x 3+1 x 2
- Pause Back Squat - 65% x 3 x 3
- Abs

Thursday
- Power Clean - 70% x 3 x 2, 75% x 3 x 3
- Power Jerk - 70% x 3 x 2, 75% x 3 x 3
- SLDL – 3 x 5
- Abs

Saturday
- Snatch - 70% x 1, 75% x 1, 80% x 1, 85% x 1, 85% x 1 x 2
- Clean & Jerk - 70% x 1+1, 75% x 1+1, 80% x 1+1, 85% x 1+1, 85% x 1+1 x 2
- Front Squat - 75% x 3, 80% x 3 x 2
- Good Morning – 3 x 5
- Abs

Week 3

Monday
- Snatch - 75% x 1 x 5 OTM, 80% x 1 x 5 OTM, 85% x 1 x 5 OTM, HS
- Snatch Pull - 90% x 3 x 3
- Segment Snatch Deadlift (knee) + Floating Snatch Deadlift - 85% x 3+1 x 3
- Back Squat (5 sec eccentric on rep 1) - 75% x 5 x 2, 75% x 5
- Abs

Tuesday
- Jerk 75% x 1 x 5 OTM, 80% x 1 x 5 OTM, 85% x 1 x 5 OTM, HS
- Push Press - 75% x 5, 75% x 5 x 4
- Back Squat Jump - 25% x 3 x 3
- Abs

Wednesday
- Clean - 75% x 1 x 5 OTM, 80% x 1 x 5 OTM, 85% x 1 x 5 OTM, HS
- Clean Pull - 90% x 3 x 3
- Segment Clean Deadlift (knee) + Floating Clean Deadlift - 85% x 3+1 x 3
- Pause Back Squat - 68% x 3 x 3
- Abs

Thursday
- Power Clean - 75% x 3, 75% x 3 x 4
- Power Jerk - 75% x 3, 75% x 3 x 4
- SLDL - 3 x 5
- Abs

Saturday
- Snatch - 70%x1, 75%x1, 80%x1, 85%x1, 90%x1 x 2
- Clean & Jerk - 70%x1+1, 75%x1+1, 80%x1+1, 85%x1+1, 90%x1+1 x 2
- Front Squat - 80% x 3 x 3
- Good Morning – 3 x 5
- Abs

Week 4

Monday
- Snatch - 75% x 1 x 5 OTM
- Snatch Pull - 85% x 3 x 3
- Back Squat - 75% x 3 x 3
- Abs

Tuesday
- Jerk - 75% x 1 x 5 OTM
- Push Press - 70% x 3 x 3
- Abs

Wednesday
- Clean - 75% x 1 x 5 OTM
- Clean Pull - 85% x 3 x 3
- Pause Back Squat - 65% x 2 x 3
- Abs

Thursday
- Power Clean - 75% x 1 x 5
- Power Jerk - 75% x 1 x 5
- Abs

Saturday
- Snatch - 70% x 1, 75% x 1, 80% x 1 x 4
- Clean & Jerk - 70% x 1+1, 75% x 1+1, 80% x 1+1 x 4
- Front Squat - 75% x 2, 80% x 2 x 2
- Abs

Week 5

Monday
- Snatch - 78% x 1 x 5 OTM, 83% x 1 x 5 OTM, 88% x 1 x 5 OTM, HS
- Snatch Pull - 90% x 3, 95% x 3 x 2
- Segment Snatch Deadlift (knee) + Floating Snatch Deadlift - 85% x 3+1, 90% x 3+1 x 2
- Back Squat (5 sec eccentric on rep 1) - 80% x 3 x 3
- Abs

Tuesday
- Jerk 78% x 1 x 5 OTM, 83% x 1 x 5 OTM, 88% x 1 x 5 OTM, HS
- Push Press - 80% x 3 x 5
- Back Squat Jump - 25% x 3 x 3
- Abs

Wednesday
- Clean - 78% x 1 x 5 OTM, 83% x 1 x 5 OTM, 88% x 1 x 5 OTM, HS
- Clean Pull - 90% x 3, 95% x 3 x 2
- Segment Clean Deadlift (knee) + Floating Clean Deadlift - 85% x 3+1, 90% x 3+1 x 2
- Pause Back Squat - 70% x 2 x 3
- Abs

Thursday
- Power Clean - 80% x 2 x 5
- Power Jerk - 80% x 2 x 5
- SLDL – 3 x 5
- Abs

Saturday
- Snatch - HS
- Clean & Jerk - HS
- Front Squat - 85% x 2 x 3
- Good Morning – 3 x 5
- Abs

Week 6

Monday
- Snatch - 80% x 1 x 5 OTM, 85% x 1 x 5 OTM, 90% x 1 x 5 OTM, HS
- Snatch Pull - 95% x 3 x 3
- Segment Snatch Deadlift (knee) + Floating Snatch Deadlift - 90% x 2+1 x 3
- Back Squat - 80% x 3, 85% x 3 x 2
- Abs

Tuesday
- Jerk - 80% x 1 x 5 OTM, 85% x 1 x 5 OTM, 90% x 1 x 5 OTM, HS
- Push Press - 80% x 3 x 2, 83% x 3 x 3
- Back Squat Jump - 25% x 3 x 3
- Abs

Wednesday
- Clean - 80% x 1 x 5 OTM, 85% x 1 x 5 OTM, 90% x 1 x 5 OTM, HS
- Clean Pull - 95% x 3 x 3
- Segment Clean Deadlift (knee) + Floating Clean Deadlift - 90% x 2+1 x 3
- Pause Back Squat - 70% x 2 x 3
- Abs

Thursday
- Power Clean - 80% x 2 x 2, 85% x 2 x 3
- Power Jerk - 80% x 2 x 2, 85% x 2 x 3
- SLDL – 3 x 5
- Abs

Saturday
- Snatch - HS
- Clean & Jerk - HS
- Front Squat - 85% x 2 x 2, 90% x 2
- Good Morning – 3 x 5
- Abs

Week 7

Monday
- Snatch - 82% x 1 x 5 OTM, 87% x 1 x 5 OTM, 92% x 1 x 5 OTM, HS
- Snatch Pull - 95% x 3, 100% x 3, 95% x 3
- Segment Snatch Deadlift (knee) + Floating Snatch Deadlift - 90% x 2+1, 95% x 2+1, 90% x 2+1
- Back Squat - 85% x 3 x 3
- Abs

Tuesday
- Jerk - 85% x 1 x 5 OTM, 87% x 1 x 5 OTM, 92% x 1 x 5 OTM, HS
- Push Press - 83% x 3 x 5
- Back Squat Jump - 25% x 3 x 3
- Abs

Wednesday
- Clean - 82% x 1 x 5 OTM, 87% x 1 x 5 OTM, 92% x 1 x 5 OTM, HS
- Clean Pull - 95% x 3, 100% x 3, 95% x 3
- Segment Clean Deadlift (knee) + Floating Clean Deadlift - 90% x 2+1, 95% x 2+1, 90% x 2+1
- Pause Back Squat - 70% x 2, 75% x 2, 70% x 2
- Abs

Thursday
- Power Clean - 85% x 2 x 5
- Power Jerk - 85% x 2 x 5
- SLDL – 3 x 5
- Abs

Saturday
- Snatch - HS
- Clean & Jerk - HS
- Front Squat - 85% x 2, 90% x 2 x 2
- Good Morning – 3 x 5
- Abs

Week 8

Monday
- Snatch - 75% x 1 x 2, 80% x 1 x 3
- Snatch Pull - 85% x 3, 90% x 3 x 2
- Back Squat - 75% x 3, 80% x 3 x 2
- Abs

Tuesday
- Jerk - 75% x 1 x 2, 80% x 1 x 3
- Push Press - 70% x 3, 75% x 3 x 2
- Abs

Wednesday
- Clean - 75% x 1 x 2, 80% x 1 x 3
- Clean Pull - 85% x 3, 90% x 3 x 2
- Pause Back Squat - 65% x 2, 70% x 2 x 2
- Abs

Thursday
- Power Clean - 75% x 1 x 2, 80% x 1 x 3
- Power Jerk - 75% x 1 x 2, 80% x 1 x 3
- Abs

Saturday
- Snatch - 70% x 1, 75% x 1, 80% x 1, 85% x 1 x 2
- Clean & Jerk - 70% x 1, 75% x 1, 80% x 1, 85% x 1 x 2
- Front Squat - 80% x 2 x 3
- Abs

Week 9

Monday
- Snatch - HS; 75% x 2 x 3 OTM (% of HS)
- Clean & Jerk - HS; 75% x 2+1 x 3 OTM (% of HS)
- Back Squat - HS; 75% x 3 x 3 (% of HS)
- Abs

Tuesday
- Power Snatch - 75% x 1 x 10 OTM
- Power Clean + Power Jerk - 75% x 1+1 x 10 OTM
- Abs

Wednesday
- Clean & Jerk - HS; 75% x 2+1 x 3 OTM (% of HS)
- Snatch - HS; 75% x 2 x 3 OTM (% of HS)
- Pause Back Squat - HS; 75% x 3 x 3 (% of HS)
- Abs

Thursday
- Power Clean + Power Jerk - 75% x 1+1 x 10 OTM
- Power Snatch - 75% x 1 x 10 OTM
- Abs

Saturday
- Snatch - HS; 80% x 1 x 3 OTM (% of HS)
- Clean & Jerk - HS; 80% x 1 x 3 OTM (% of HS)
- Front Squat - HS; 80% x 2 x 2 (% of HS)
- Abs

Week 10

Monday
- Snatch - HS; 80% x 1 x 3 OTM (% of HS)
- Clean & Jerk - HS; 80% x 1+1 x 3 OTM (% of HS)
- Back Squat - HS; 80% x 2 x 3 (% of HS)
- Abs

Tuesday
- Power Snatch - 75% x 1 x 10 OTM
- Power Clean + Power Jerk - 75% x 1+1 x 10 OTM
- Abs

Wednesday
- Clean & Jerk - HS; 80% x 2+1 x 3 OTM (% of HS)
- Snatch - HS; 80% x 2 x 3 OTM (% of HS)
- Pause Back Squat - HS; 80% x 2 x 3 (% of HS)
- Abs

Thursday
- Power Clean + Power Jerk - 75% x 1+1 x 10 OTM
- Power Snatch - 75% x 1 x 10 OTM
- Abs

Saturday
- Snatch - HS; 85% x 1 x 3 OTM (% of HS)
- Clean & Jerk - HS; 85% x 1+1 x 3 OTM (% of HS)
- Front Squat - HS; 85% x 2 x 3 (% of HS)
- Abs

Week 11

Monday
- Snatch - HS; 85% x 2 x 3 OTM (% of HS)
- Clean & Jerk - HS; 85% x 2+1 x 3 OTM (% of HS)
- Back Squat - HS; 85% x 2 x 3 (% of HS)
- Abs

Tuesday
- Power Snatch - 75% x 1 x 10 OTM
- Power Clean + Power Jerk - 75% x 1+1 x 10 OTM
- Abs

Wednesday
- Clean & Jerk - HS; 85% x 2+1 x 3 OTM (% of HS)
- Snatch - HS; 85% x 1 x 3 OTM (% of HS)
- Pause Back Squat - HS; 85% x 2 x 3 (% of HS)
- Abs

Thursday
- Power Clean + Power Jerk - 75% x 1+1 x 10 OTM
- Power Snatch - 75% x 1 x 10 OTM
- Abs

Saturday
- Snatch - HS; 85% x 2 x 3 OTM (% of HS)
- Clean & Jerk - HS; 85% x 2+1 x 3 OTM (% of HS)
- Front Squat - HS; 90% x 2 x 3 (% of HS)
- Abs

Week 12

Monday
- Snatch - 70% x 1, 75% x 1, 80% x 1, 85% x 1 x 3
- Clean & Jerk - 70% x 1, 75% x 1, 80% x 1, 85% x 1
- Back Squat - 70% x 2, 75% x 2, 80% x 2, 85% x 2
- Abs

Tuesday
- Power Snatch - 70% x 1 x 5
- Power Clean + Power Jerk - 70% x 1+1 x 5
- Abs

Wednesday
- Snatch - 70% x 1, 75% x 1, 80% x 1 x 3
- Power Clean + Jerk - 70% x 1, 75% x 1, 80% x 1
- Front Squat - 70% x 2, 75% x 2, 80% x 1, 85% x 1
- Abs

Thursday
- Power Snatch - 60% x 1 x 5
- Power Clean + Power Jerk - 60% x 1+1 x 5
- Abs

Saturday
- Snatch - Max
- Clean & Jerk - Max
- Front Squat - Max

Program Risers, Waves & Positions

This program is appropriate for higher intermediate and advanced lifters, and is an example of the use of daily maximums with back-off sets, wave loading with varying reps and ascending intensities, and on-the-minute lifts.

Percentages that follow HS or RM sets are of the preceding HS or RM, not the lifter's absolute maximum unless otherwise noted. The basic goal is for the lifter to try to beat the previous week's intensities in these exercises, but this will not necessarily occur, and lifters and coaches will need to make sure that decisions on intensities are based on accurate evaluations on the lifter's present state, not only on desired numbers.

Series of OTM weights are performed with a continuously running clock. For example, if lifting 5 singles at 70%, 5 singles at 75%, and 5 singles at 80%, the fifteenth set will begin on minute 14 (the first set begins at minute 0). Weight changes must be done within the 1 minute time limit. If a series of OTM sets is followed by "HS", the lifter, after completing the first 15 sets, can then proceed off the clock to a heavy single. Generally this should only be done if there were no misses during the first 15 singles, but exceptions can be made if sensible in the coach's judgment. These off the clock sets should still be done with relatively short rest periods—typically around 2 minutes.

Technique primers are included each day. These should be performed with light weights and the focus kept entirely on proper execution and position.

Week 1

Monday
- Technique Primer: Muscle Snatch + Tall Snatch - 3 x 3+3
- 3-Position Snatch (floor, knee, mid-thigh) - RM; 95%, 90% (% of RM)
- Snatch Pull on Riser - 105% x 5, 110% x 5, 115% x 5
- Back Squat - 70% x 5, 80% x 1, 72% x 5, 82% x 1, 74% x 5, 84% x 1
- Back Squat Jump - 20% x 3 x 5 (% of Back Squat)
- Abs

Tuesday
- Technique Primer: Tall Jerk + Push Jerk Behind the Neck in Split - 3 x 3+3
- Pause Jerk + Jerk - 2+1RM; 95%, 90% (% of RM)
- Power Clean - 70% x 3 x 5
- Push Press Behind the Neck - 70% x 5 x 4 (% of Push Press)
- Abs

Wednesday
- Technique Primer: Muscle Clean + Tall Clean - 3 x 3+3
- 3-Position Clean (floor, knee, mid-thigh) - RM; 95%, 90% (% of RM)
- Clean Pull on Riser - 105% x 5, 110% x 5, 115% x 5
- Front Squat - 70% x 3 x 4
- SLDL - 50% x 5 x 3 (% of Back Squat)
- Abs

Thursday
- Technique Primer: Muscle Snatch + Push Jerk in Snatch - 3 x 3+3
- Power Snatch - 70% x 3 x 5
- Power Jerk - 70% x 3 x 5
- Snatch Push Press + OHS - 70% x 5+1 x 4 (% of OHS or Snatch)
- Back Squat Jump - 20% x 3 x 5
- Abs

Saturday
- Technique Primer of Choice: 3-4 sets of 2-3 reps
- Snatch + Snatch Balance + OHS - 1+1+1RM; 95% x 1+1+1, 90% x 1+1+1
- Clean + Power Jerk + Jerk - 1+1+1RM; 95% x 1+1+1, 90% x 1+1+1
- Back Squat - 5RM; 50% x 10 (% of max Back Squat)
- Good Morning - 20% x 5 x 3 (% of Back Squat)
- Abs

Week 2

Monday
- Technique Primer: Muscle Snatch + Tall Snatch - 3 x 3+3
- 3-Position Snatch (floor, knee, mid-thigh) - RM
- Snatch Pull on Riser - 108% x 5, 113% x 5, 118% x 5
- Back Squat - 73% x 5, 83% x 1, 75% x 5, 85% x 1, 77% x 5, 87% x 1
- Back Squat Jump - 20% x 3 x 5
- Abs

Tuesday
- Technique Primer: Tall Jerk + Push Jerk Behind the Neck in Split - 3 x 3+3
- Pause Jerk + Jerk - 2+1RM
- Power Clean - 70% x 3, 75% x 3 x 3
- Push Press Behind the Neck - 70%x5, 75%x5x3
- Abs

Wednesday
- Technique Primer: Muscle Clean + Tall Clean - 3 x 3+3
- 3-Position Clean (floor, knee, mid-thigh) RM
- Clean Pull on Riser - 108% x 5, 113% x 5, 118% x 5
- Front Squat - 70% x 3, 73% x 3 x 2
- SLDL - 50% x 5, 53% x 5 x 2
- Abs

Thursday
- Technique Primer: Muscle Snatch + Push Jerk in Snatch - 3 x 3+3
- Power Snatch - 70% x 3, 75% x 3 x 3
- Power Jerk - 70% x 3, 75% x 3 x 3
- Snatch Push Press + OHS - 70% x 5+1, 75% x 5+1 x 3 (% of OHS or Snatch)
- Back Squat Jump - 20% x 3 x 5
- Abs

Saturday
- Technique Primer of Choice: 3-4 sets of 2-3 reps
- Snatch + Snatch Balance + OHS - 1+1+1RM
- Clean + Power Jerk + Jerk - 1+1+1RM
- Back Squat - 5RM; 53% x 10 (% of max Back Squat)
- Good Morning - 20% x 5, 23% x 5 x 2
- Abs

Week 3

Monday
- Technique Primer: Muscle Snatch + Tall Snatch - 3 x 3+3
- 3-Position Snatch (floor, knee, mid-thigh) - RM; 95%, 90% (% of RM)
- Snatch Pull on Riser - 110% x 5, 115% x 5, 120% x 5
- Back Squat - 75% x 5, 85% x 1, 77% x 5, 87% x 1, 79% x 5, 89% x 1
- Back Squat Jump - 20% x 3 x 5
- Abs

Tuesday
- Technique Primer: Tall Jerk + Push Jerk Behind the Neck in Split - 3 x 3+3
- Pause Jerk + Jerk - 2+1RM; 95%, 90% (% of RM)
- Power Clean - 3RM
- Push Press Behind the Neck - 5RM
- Abs

Wednesday
- Technique Primer: Muscle Clean + Tall Clean - 3 x 3+3
- 3-Position Clean (floor, knee, mid-thigh) - RM; 95%, 90% (% of RM)
- Clean Pull on Riser - 110% x 5, 115% x 5, 120% x 5
- Front Squat - 73% x 3 x 3
- SLDL - 53% x 5 x 3
- Abs

Thursday
- Technique Primer: Muscle Snatch + Push Jerk in Snatch - 3 x 3+3
- Power Snatch - 3RM
- Power Jerk - 3RM
- Snatch Push Press + OHS - 5+1RM
- Back Squat Jump - 20% x 3 x 5
- Abs

Saturday
- Technique Primer of Choice: 3-4 sets of 2-3 reps
- Snatch + Snatch Balance + OHS - 1+1+1RM; 95%, 90% (% of RM)
- Clean + Power Jerk + Jerk - 1+1+1RM; 95%, 90% (% of RM)
- Back Squat - 5RM; 55% x 10 (% of max Back Squat)
- Good Morning - 23% x 5 x 3
- Abs

Week 4

Monday
- Technique Primer: Muscle Snatch + Tall Snatch - 3 x 3+3
- 2-Position Snatch (floor, knee) - 70% x 4 sets
- Snatch Pull - 100% x 3 x 3
- Back Squat - 70% x 3, 80% x 1, 70% x 3, 80% x 1, 70%x3, 80%x1
- Back Squat Jump - 20% x 3 x 3
- Abs

Tuesday
- Technique Primer: Tall Jerk + Push Jerk Behind the Neck in Split - 3 x 3+3
- Pause Jerk + Jerk - 70% x 1+1 x 4
- Power Clean - 70% x 2 x 4
- Push Press - 70% x 3 x 4
- Abs

Wednesday
- Technique Primer: Muscle Clean + Tall Clean - 3 x 3+3
- 2-Position Clean (floor, knee) - 70% x 4 sets
- Clean Pull - 100% x 3 x 3
- Front Squat - 70% x 2 x 3
- SLDL - 50% x 4 x 2
- Abs

Thursday
- Technique Primer: Muscle Snatch + Push Jerk in Snatch - 3 x 3+3
- Power Snatch - 70% x 2 x 4
- Power Jerk - 70% x 2 x 4
- Snatch Push Press + OHS - 70% x 3+1 x 4 (% of OHS or snatch)
- Back Squat Jump - 20% x 3 x 3
- Abs

Saturday
- Technique Primer of Choice: 3-4 sets of 2-3 reps
- Snatch + OHS - 1+1RM; 95%, 90% (% of RM)
- Clean + Front Squat + Jerk - 1+1+1RM; 95%, 90% (% of RM)
- Back Squat - 75% x 3 x 3
- Good Morning - 23% x 4 x 2
- Abs

Week 5

Monday
- Technique Primer: Muscle Snatch + Tall Snatch - 3 x 3+3
- 2-Position Snatch (floor, knee) - RM; 95%, 90% (% of RM)
- Snatch Pull on Riser - 110% x 3, 115% x 3, 120% x 3
- Back Squat - 75% x 3, 85% x 1, 77% x 3, 87% x 1, 79% x 3, 89% x 1
- Back Squat Jump - 20% x 3 x 3
- Abs

Tuesday
- Technique Primer: Tall Jerk + Push Jerk Behind the Neck in Split - 3 x 3+3
- Pause Jerk + Jerk - 1+1)RM; 95%, 90% (% of RM)
- Power Clean - 75% x 2 x 5
- Push Press - 75% x 3 x 4
- Abs

Wednesday
- Technique Primer: Muscle Clean + Tall Clean - 3 x 3+3
- 2-Position Clean (floor, knee) - RM; 95%, 90% (% of RM)
- Clean Pull - 110% x 3, 115% x 3, 120% x 3
- Front Squat - 75% x 3 x 3
- SLDL - 55% x 4 x 3
- Abs

Thursday
- Technique Primer: Muscle Snatch + Push Jerk in Snatch - 3 x 3+3
- Power Snatch - 75% x 2 x 5
- Power Jerk - 75% x 2 x 5
- Snatch Push Press + OHS - 75% x 3+1 x 4 (% of OHS or snatch)
- Back Squat Jump - 20% x 3 x 5
- Abs

Saturday
- Technique Primer of Choice: 3-4 sets of 2-3 reps
- Snatch + OHS - 1+1RM; 95%, 90% (% of RM)
- Clean + Jerk - 1+2RM; 95%, 90% (% of RM)
- Back Squat - 3RM; 57% x 10 (% of max Back Squat)
- Good Morning - 25% x 4 x 3
- Abs

Week 6

Monday
- Technique Primer: Muscle Snatch + Tall Snatch - 3 x 3+3
- 2-Position Snatch (floor, knee) - RM
- Snatch Pull - 113% x 3, 118% x 3, 123% x 3
- Back Squat - 77% x 3, 87% x 1, 79% x 3, 89% x 1, 81% x 3, 91% x 1
- Back Squat Jump - 20% x 3 x 5
- Abs

Tuesday
- Technique Primer: Tall Jerk + Push Jerk Behind the Neck in Split - 3 x 3+3
- Pause Jerk + Jerk - 1+1RM
- Power Clean - 75% x 2, 80% x 2 x 3
- Push Press - 75% x 3, 80% x 3 x 2
- Abs

Wednesday
- Technique Primer: Muscle Clean + Tall Clean - 3 x 3+3
- 2-Position Clean (floor, knee) - RM
- Clean Pull - 113% x 3, 118% x 3, 123% x 3
- Front Squat - 75% x 3, 77% x 3 x 2
- SLDL - 55% x 4, 57% x 4 x 2
- Abs

Thursday
- Technique Primer: Muscle Snatch + Push Jerk in Snatch - 3 x 3+3
- Power Snatch - 75% x 2, 80% x 2 x 3
- Power Jerk - 75% x 2, 80% x 2 x 3
- Snatch Push Press + OHS - 75% x 3+1, 80% x 3+1 x 3 (% of OHS or snatch)
- Back Squat Jump - 20% x 3 x 5
- Abs

Saturday
- Technique Primer of Choice: 3-4 sets of 2-3 reps
- Snatch + OHS - 1+1RM
- Clean + Jerk - 1+2RM
- Back Squat - 3RM; 59% x 10 (% of max Back Squat)
- Good Morning - 25% x 4, 27% x 4 x 2
- Abs

Week 7

Monday
- Technique Primer: Muscle Snatch + Tall Snatch - 3 x 3+3
- 2-Position Snatch (floor, knee) - RM
- Snatch Pull - 115% x 3, 120% x 3, 125% x 3
- Back Squat - 79% x 3, 89% x 1, 81% x 3, 91% x 1, 83% x 3, 93% x 1
- Back Squat Jump - 20% x 3 x 5
- Abs

Tuesday
- Technique Primer: Tall Jerk + Push Jerk Behind the Neck in Split - 3 x 3+3
- Pause Jerk + Jerk - 1+1RM
- Power Clean - 2RM
- Push Press - 3RM
- Abs

Wednesday
- Technique Primer: Muscle Clean + Tall Clean - 3 x 3+3
- 2-Position Clean (floor, knee) - RM
- Clean Pull - 115% x 3, 120% x 3, 125% x 3
- Front Squat - 77% x 3 x 3
- SLDL - 57% x 4 x 3
- Abs

Thursday
- Technique Primer: Muscle Snatch + Push Jerk in Snatch - 3 x 3+3
- Power Snatch - 2RM
- Power Jerk - 2RM
- Snatch Push Press + OHS - 3+1RM
- Back Squat Jump - 20% x 3 x 5
- Abs

Saturday
- Technique Primer of Choice: 3-4 sets of 2-3 reps
- Snatch + OHS - 1+1RM
- Clean + Jerk - 1+2RM
- Back Squat - 3RM; 61% x 10 (% of max Back Squat)
- Good Morning - 27% x 4 x 3
- Abs

Week 8

Monday
- Technique Primer: Muscle Snatch + Tall Snatch - 3 x 3+3
- Snatch - 70% x 1 x 5 OTM, 72% x 1 x 5 OTM, 74% x 1 x 5 OTM
- Snatch Pull - 110% x 2 x 4, 90% x 2
- Front Squat - 80% x 2, 85% x 2, 90% x 2 x 2
- Abs

Tuesday
- Technique Primer: Tall Jerk + Push Jerk Behind the Neck in Split - 3 x 3+3
- Jerk - 70% x 1 x 5 OTM, 72% x 1 x 5 OTM, 74% x 1 x 5 OTM
- Power Clean - 70% x 1 x 3 OTM, 72% x 1 x 3 OTM, 74% x 1 x 3 OTM
- Good Morning - 25% x 4 x 3
- Abs

Wednesday
- Technique Primer: Muscle Clean + Tall Clean - 3 x 3+3
- Clean - 70% x 1 x 5 OTM, 72% x 1 x 5 OTM, 74% x 1 x 5 OTM
- Clean Pull - 110% x 2 x 5
- Back Squat - 80% x 2 x 4
- Abs

Thursday
- Technique Primer: Muscle Snatch + Push Jerk in Snatch - 3 x 3+3
- Power Snatch -70% x 1 x 3 OTM, 72% x 1 x 3 OTM, 74% x 1 x 3 OTM
- Power Jerk - 70% x 1 x 3 OTM, 72% x 1 x 3 OTM, 74% x 1 x 3 OTM
- Good Morning - 20% x 5 x 3
- Abs

Saturday
- Technique Primer of Choice: 3-4 sets of 2-3 reps
- Snatch - HS; 95% x 1, 90% x 1 (% of HS)
- Clean + Jerk - HS; 95% x 1+1, 90% x 1+1 (% of HS)
- Front Squat - 75% x 2, 80% x 2 x 3
- Abs

Week 9

Monday
- Technique Primer: Muscle Snatch + Tall Snatch - 3 x 3+3
- Snatch - 70% x 1 x 5 OTM, 73% x 1 x 5 OTM, 76% x 1 x 5 OTM, HS
- Snatch Pull - 120% x 2 x 4, 90% x 2
- Front Squat - HS; 90% x 1, 95% x 1
- Abs

Tuesday
- Technique Primer: Tall Jerk + Push Jerk Behind the Neck in Split - 3 x 3+3
- Jerk - 70% x 1 x 5 OTM, 73% x 1 x 5 OTM, 76% x 1 x 5 OTM, HS
- Power Clean - 70% x 1 x 3 OTM, 73% x 1 x 3 OTM, 76% x 1 x 3 OTM, HS
- Good Morning - 25% x 4, 27% x 4 x 2
- Abs

Wednesday
- Technique Primer: Muscle Clean + Tall Clean - 3 x 3+3
- Clean - 70% x 1 x 5 OTM, 73% x 1 x 5 OTM, 76% x 1 x 5 OTM, HS
- Clean Pull - 120% x 2 x 4, 90% x 2
- Back Squat - HS; 90% x 1, 95% x 1
- Abs

Thursday
- Technique Primer: Muscle Snatch + Push Jerk in Snatch - 3 x 3+3
- Power Snatch -70% x 1 x 3 OTM, 73% x 1 x 3 OTM, 76% x 1 x 3 OTM, HS
- Power Jerk - 70% x 1 x 3 OTM, 73% x 1 x 3 OTM, 76% x 1 x 3 OTM, HS
- Good Morning - 20% x 5 x 3
- Abs

Saturday
- Technique Primer of Choice: 3-4 sets of 2-3 reps
- Snatch - HS; 95% x 1, 90% x 1 (% of HS)
- Clean + Jerk - HS; 95% x 1+1, 90% x 1+1 (% of HS)
- Front Squat - 75% x 2, 80% x 2, 85% x 2 x 2
- Abs

Week 10

Monday
- Technique Primer: Muscle Snatch + Tall Snatch - 3 x 3+3
- Snatch - 73%x1x5 OTM, 76%x1x5 OTM, 79%x1x5 OTM, HS
- Snatch Pull - 120%x2, 125%x2x3, 90%x2
- Front Squat - HS; 90%x1, 95%x1 (% of HS)
- Abs

Tuesday
- Technique Primer: Tall Jerk + Push Jerk Behind the Neck in Split - 3 x 3+3
- Jerk - 73% x 1 x 5 OTM, 76% x 1 x 5 OTM, 79% x 1 x 5 OTM, HS
- Power Clean - 73% x 1 x 3 OTM, 76% x 1 x 3 OTM, 79% x 1 x 3 OTM, HS
- Good Morning - 27% x 4 x 3
- Abs

Wednesday
- Technique Primer: Muscle Clean + Tall Clean - 3 x 3+3
- Clean - 73% x 1 x 5 OTM, 76% x 1 x 5 OTM, 79% x 1 x 5 OTM, HS
- Clean Pull - 120% x 2, 125% x 2 x 3, 90% x 2
- Back Squat - HS; 90% x 1, 95% x 1 (% of HS)
- Abs

Thursday
- Technique Primer: Muscle Snatch + Push Jerk in Snatch - 3 x 3+3
- Power Snatch -73% x 1 x 3 OTM, 76% x 1 x 3 OTM, 79% x 1 x 3 OTM, HS
- Power Jerk - 73% x 1 x 3 OTM, 76% x 1 x 3 OTM, 79% x 1 x 3 OTM, HS
- Good Morning - 22% x 5 x 3
- Abs

Saturday
- Technique Primer of Choice: 3-4 sets of 2-3 reps
- Snatch - HS; 90% x 1 (% of HS)
- Clean + Jerk - HS; 90% x 1+1 (% of HS)
- Front Squat - 75% x 2, 80% x 2, 85% x 2, 90% x 2
- Abs

Week 11

Monday
- Technique Primer: Muscle Snatch + Tall Snatch - 3 x 3+3
- Snatch - 65% x 1 x 4 OTM, 70% x 1 x 4 OTM, 75% x 1 x 4 OTM, HS
- Snatch Pull - 110% x 2, 115% x 2 x 2, 90% x 2
- Front Squat - HS; 90% x 1 (% of HS)
- Abs

Tuesday
- Technique Primer: Tall Jerk + Push Jerk Behind the Neck in Split - 3 x 3+3
- Jerk - 65% x 1 x 4 OTM, 70% x 1 x 4 OTM, 75% x 1 x 4 OTM, HS
- Power Clean - HS
- Good Morning - 27% x 4 x 2, 29% x 4
- Abs

Wednesday
- Technique Primer: Muscle Clean + Tall Clean - 3 x 3+3
- Clean - 65% x 1 x 4 OTM, 70% x 1 x 4 OTM, 75% x 1 x 4 OTM, HS
- Clean Pull - 110% x 2, 115% x 2 x 2, 90% x 2
- Back Squat - HS; 90% x 1 (% of HS)
- Abs

Thursday
- Technique Primer: Muscle Snatch + Push Jerk in Snatch - 3 x 3+3
- Power Snatch -HS
- Power Jerk - HS
- Good Morning - 22% x 5 x 2, 24% x 5
- Abs

Saturday
- Technique Primer of Choice: 3-4 sets of 2-3 reps
- Snatch - HS
- Clean + Jerk - HS
- Front Squat - 75% x 2, 80% x 2, 85% x 2 x 2
- Abs

Week 12

Monday
- Snatch - 70% x 1, 75% x 1, 80% x 1, 85% x 1 x 3
- Clean & Jerk - 70% x 1+1, 75% x 1+1, 80% x 1+1, 85% x 1+1 x 3
- Back Squat - 70% x 2, 75% x 2, 80% x 2, 85% x 2
- Abs

Tuesday
- Snatch - 70% x 1, 75% x 1, 80% x 1 x 3
- Clean & Jerk - 70% x 1+1, 75% x 1+1, 80% x 1+1 x 3

Wednesday
- Snatch - 70% x 1, 75% x 1 x 5
- Clean & Jerk - 70% x 1+1, 75% x 1+1 x 5
- Front Squat - 70% x 2, 75% x 1, 80% x 1
- Abs

Thursday
- Snatch - 70% x 1 x 5
- Clean & Jerk - 70% x 1+1 x 5

Saturday
- Snatch - MAX
- Clean & Jerk - MAX
- Front Squat - MAX

Program **Double Day Squats & Heavy Weights**

This is an extremely demanding training program for more advanced lifters. It has produced remarkable increases in many lifters' squat numbers, as well as in the snatch and clean & jerk. Intensity is determined nearly entirely by feel day to day rather than by prescription, and will primarily be maximal efforts. A transition week is included and is recommended before starting the cycle proper to help prepare the lifter for the frequent high intensity.

While the goal is to lift as heavy as possible each day, actual failed lifts, in the squat in particular, should be avoided as much as possible. This will improve the effect by reducing the recovery demand. However, it's imperative the lifter get as close to maximum each day, which will fluctuate, sometimes dramatically.

Back-off sets after heavy singles or rep maxes should be ascending weights when possible, working up to a rep max for the day, again trying to avoid actual failure. Percentages that follow heavy singles or rep maxes are of those weights, not of the lifter's absolute maximum.

The goal each day is to try to beat, by at least 1kg, what has been done to date in the cycle. This means that warm-up set weights need to be carefully selected to set the lifter up to reach these target weights; if identical jumps are taken every day, there is an excellent chance of the lifter simply repeating the same top weight every workout or week and effectively making no progress.

This program does not need to be done in two workouts per day—"double day squats" refers to the two squat sessions per workout. However, the days can be split into two workouts if desired.

Finally, this program should be done without the athlete sitting down during workouts. This will help keep the lifter engaged and focused, and will keep the pace relatively high.

Transition Week

Monday
- Front Squat - 80% x 1
- Snatch - HS; 80% (of HS) x 1 x 3
- Segment Snatch Pull (knee) + Snatch Pull - 90% (of sn) x 1+2 x 4
- Back Squat - 90% x 1, 75% x 3 x 3
- Good Morning - 3 x 5 (very light)

Tuesday
- Muscle Snatch - 3x3
- Mid-Hang Snatch - 70% x 2 x 5
- Power Clean + Power Jerk - 75% x 1+1 x 5
- Front Squat - 90% x 1, 75% x 2 x 3

Wednesday
- Front Squat - 80% x 1
- Clean & Jerk - HS; 80% (of HS) x 2+1 x 3
- Segment Clean Pull (knee) + Clean Pull - 90% (of clean) x 1+2 x 4
- Back Squat - 90% x 1
- Pause Back Squat - 70% (of squat) x 3 x 3
- Good Morning - 3 x 5 (heavier than Monday)

Thursday
- Back Squat - 80% x 1
- Power Snatch - 75% x 2 x 5
- Mid-Hang Clean - 70% x 2 x 5
- Push Press - 3 x 5
- Front Squat - HS; 75% (of HS) x 3 x 3

Saturday
- Front Squat - HS
- Snatch - HS
- Clean & Jerk - HS
- Back Squat - HS
- Pause Back Squat - 70% (of back squat HS) x 3 x 3
- Good Morning - 3x5

Week 1

Monday
- Front Squat - HS
- Snatch - HS; 3 x 2
- Segment Snatch Pull (knee) + Snatch pull - 5 x 1+2
- Back Squat - HS; 4 x 3
- Good Morning - 3 x 5

Tuesday
- Back Squat - HS
- High-Hang Snatch - 5 x 2
- Power Clean + Power Jerk - 5 x 2+1
- Front Squat - HS; 3 x 3

Wednesday
- Front Squat - HS
- Clean & Jerk - HS; 3 x 2+1
- Segment Clean Pull (knee) + Clean Pull - 5 x 1+2
- Back Squat - HS
- Pause Back Squat - 4 x 3
- Good Morning - 3 x 5

Thursday
- Back Squat - HS
- Jerk Behind the Neck - 5 x 2
- High-Hang Clean - 5 x 2
- Push Press - 4 x 5
- Front Squat - HS; 3 x 3

Saturday
- Front Squat - HS
- Snatch - HS
- Clean & Jerk - HS
- Back Squat - HS
- Pause Back Squat - 4 x 3
- Good Morning - 3 x 5

Week 2

Monday
- Front Squat - HS
- Snatch - HS; 3 x 2
- Segment Snatch Pull (knee) + Snatch Pull - 5 x 2+1
- Back Squat - HS; 4 x 3
- Good Morning - 3 x 5

Tuesday
- Back Squat - HS
- High-Hang Snatch - 5 x 2
- Power Clean + Power Jerk - 5 x 2+1
- Front Squat - HS; 3 x 2

Wednesday
- Front Squat - HS
- Clean & Jerk - HS; 3 x 2+1
- Segment Clean Pull (knee) + Clean Pull - 5 x 1+2
- Back Squat - HS
- Pause Back Squat - 4 x 3
- Good Morning - 3 x 5

Thursday
- Back Squat - HS
- Jerk Behind the Neck - 5 x 2
- High-Hang Clean - 5 x 2
- Push Press - 4 x 5
- Front Squat - HS; 3 x 3

Saturday
- Front Squat - HS
- Snatch - HS
- Clean & Jerk - HS
- Back Squat - HS
- Pause Back Squat - 4 x 3
- Good Morning - 3 x 5

Week 3

Monday
- Front Squat - HS
- Snatch – HS; 5 x 1
- Snatch Pull - 5 x 3
- Back Squat - HS; 4 x 3
- Good Morning - 3 x 5

Tuesday
- Back Squat - HS
- Hang Snatch (knee) - 5 x 2
- Power Clean + Power Jerk - 5 x 1+1
- Front Squat - HS; 3 x 3

Wednesday
- Front Squat - HS
- Clean & Jerk - HS; 5 x 1+1
- Clean Pull - 5 x 3
- Back Squat - HS
- Pause Back Squat - 4 x 3
- Good Morning - 3 x 5

Thursday
- Back Squat - HS
- Jerk Behind the Neck - 5 x 2
- Hang Clean (knee) - 5 x 2
- Push Press - 4 x 5
- Front Squat - HS; 3 x 3

Saturday
- Front Squat - HS
- Snatch - HS
- Clean & Jerk - HS
- Back Squat - HS
- Pause Back Squat - 4 x 3
- Good Morning - 3 x 5

Week 4

Monday
- Snatch - HS
- Snatch Pull - 4 x 3
- Back Squat - HS; 3 x 2
- Good Morning - 3 x 5

Tuesday
- Power Snatch + Snatch Push Press - 5 x 1+3
- Power Clean + Power Jerk - 5 x 1+1
- Front Squat - HS; 3 x 2

Wednesday
- Clean & Jerk - HS
- Clean Pull - 4 x 3
- Back Squat - HS; 3 x 2
- Good Morning - 3 x 5

Thursday
- Power Snatch - 5 x 2
- Power Clean + Push Press - 5 x 1+3
- Front Squat - HS; 3 x 2

Saturday
- Snatch - HS
- Clean & Jerk - HS
- Back Squat - HS; 3 x 2
- Good Morning - 3 x 5

Week 5

Monday
- Front Squat - HS
- Snatch - HS; 3 x 2
- Snatch Deadlift to knee + Deadlift knee to hip + Snatch Pull - 5 x 2+2+1
- Back Squat - HS; 4 x 3
- Good Morning - 3 x 5

Tuesday
- Back Squat - HS
- Snatch High-Pull + Hang Power Snatch (below knee) + Overhead Squat - 5 x 1+1+1
- Power Clean + Front Squat + Jerk - 5 x 1+1+1
- Snatch Push Press - 4 x 5
- Front Squat - HS; 3 x 3

Wednesday
- Front Squat - HS
- Clean & Jerk - HS; 3 x 2+1
- Clean Deadlift to knee + Deadlift knee to hip + Clean Pull - 5 x 2+2+1
- Back Squat - HS
- Pause Back Squat - 4 x 3
- Good Morning - 3 x 5

Thursday
- Back Squat - HS
- Jerk - 3 x (3, 2, 1)
- Power Clean - 5 x 2
- Push Press - 4 x 5
- Front Squat - HS; 3 x 3

Saturday
- Front Squat - HS
- Snatch - HS
- Clean & Jerk - HS
- Back Squat - HS
- Pause Back Squat - 4 x 3
- Good Morning - 3 x 5

Week 6

Monday
- Front Squat - HS
- Snatch - HS; 3 x 2
- Snatch Deadlift to knee + Deadlift knee to hip + Snatch Pull - 5 x 2+2+1
- Back Squat - HS; 4 x 3
- Good Morning - 3 x 5

Tuesday
- Back Squat - HS
- Snatch High-Pull + Hang Power Snatch (below knee) + Overhead Squat - 5 x 1+1+1
- Power Clean + Front Squat + Jerk - 5 x 1+1+1
- Snatch Push Press - 4 x 5
- Front Squat - HS; 3 x 3

Wednesday
- Front Squat - HS
- Clean & Jerk - HS; 3 x 2+1
- Clean Deadlift to knee + Deadlift knee to hip + Clean Pull - 5 x 2+2+1
- Back Squat - HS
- Pause Back Squat - 4 x 3
- Good Morning - 3 x 5

Thursday
- Back Squat - HS
- Jerk - 3 x (3, 2, 1)3
- Power Clean - 5 x 2
- Push Press - 4 x 5
- Front Squat - HS; 3 x 3

Saturday
- Front Squat - HS
- Snatch - HS
- Clean & Jerk - HS
- Back Squat - HS
- Pause Back Squat - 4 x 3
- Good Morning - 3 x 5

Week 7

Monday
- Front Squat - HS
- Snatch - HS; 3 x 1
- Snatch Deadlift to knee + Deadlift knee to hip + Snatch Pull - 4 x 2+2+1
- Back Squat - HS; 3 x 3
- Good Morning - 3 x 5

Tuesday
- Back Squat - HS
- Snatch High-Pull + Hang Power Snatch (below knee) + OHS - 5 x 1+1+1
- Power Clean + Jerk - 5 x 1+1
- Snatch Push Press - 4 x 5
- Front Squat - HS; 3 x 3

Wednesday
- Front Squat - HS
- Clean & Jerk - HS; 3 x 1+1
- Clean Deadlift to knee + Deadlift knee to hip + Clean Pull - 4 x 2+2+1
- Back Squat - HS
- Pause Back Squat - 3 x 3
- Good Morning - 3 x 5

Thursday
- Back Squat - HS
- Jerk - 3 x (2, 2, 1)
- Power Clean - 5 x 2
- Push Press - 4 x 5
- Front Squat - HS; 3 x 3

Saturday
- Front Squat - HS
- Snatch - HS
- Clean & Jerk - HS
- Back Squat - HS
- Pause Back Squat - 3 x 3
- Good Morning - 3 x 5

Week 8

Monday
- Snatch - (75% x 2, 80% x 1, 85% x 1) x 3
- Snatch Pull - 90% x 3, 95% x 3, 100% x 3
- Back Squat - 75% x 2, 80% x 2, 85% x 2 x 2
- Good Morning - 3 x 5

Tuesday
- Power Snatch - 70% x 2 x 2, 75% x 2 x 2, 80% x 2 x 2
- Power Clean + Jerk - 70% x 2, 75% x 2, 80% x 2 x 3
- Front Squat - 85% x 1, 75% x 2 x 3

Wednesday
- Clean & Jerk - (75% x 2+1, 80% x 1+1, 85% x 1+1) x 3
- Clean Pull - 90% x 3, 95% x 3, 100% x 3
- Back Squat - 90% x 1
- Pause Back Squat - 70% x 2 x 3
- Good Morning - 3 x 5

Thursday
- Jerk - 70% x 2, 75% x 2, 80% x 2 x 3
- Power clean - 70% x 2 x 2, 75% x 2 x 3
- Front Squat - 85% x 1, 75% x 2 x 3

Saturday
- Snatch - HS
- Clean & Jerk - HS
- Back Squat - 90% x 1
- Pause Back Squat - 75% x 2 x 3
- Good Morning - 3 x 5

Week 9

Monday
- Snatch - HS; (90% x 1, 95% x 1) x 3
- Clean & Jerk - HS; (90% x 1+1, 95% x 1+1) x 3
- Snatch Pull - 105% x 2 x 4
- Front Squat - 70% x 2, 80% x 2, 85% x 2, 90% x 2 x 3

Tuesday
- Hang Power Snatch - 60% x 2, 65% x 2, 70% x 2 x 3
- Hang Power Clean - 60% x 2, 65% x 2, 70% x 2 x 3

Wednesday
- Snatch - 70% x 1, 80% x 1, 85% x 1, 90% x 1, 95% x 1, 80% x 2 x 2
- Clean & Jerk - 70% x 1+1, 80% x 1+1, 85% x 1+1, 90% x 1+1, 95% x 1+1, 80% x 2+1 x 2
- Snatch Pull - 100% x 3 x 2, 105% x 2 x 2
- Back Squat - 70% x 1, 80% x 1, 85% x 1, 90% x 1, 95% x 1, 80% x 3 x 3

Thursday
- Power Snatch - HS; (90% x 1, 95% x 1, 100% x 1) x 3
- Power Clean + Jerk - HS; (90% x 1+1, 95% x 1+1, 100% x 1+1) x 3
- Clean Pull - 100% x 3 x 3, 105% x 3 x 2

Saturday
- Snatch - 70% x 2, 80% x 2, 85% x 2 x 4
- Clean & Jerk - 70% x 2(1+1), 80% x 2(1+1), 85% x 2(1+1) x 3
- Clean Pull - 95% x 2 x 2, 105% x 2 x 3
- Front Squat - 70% x 2, 80% x 2, (85% x 2, 90% x 1, 95% x 1) x 3

Week 10

Monday
- Snatch - HS; (90% x 1, 95% x 1) x 3
- Clean & Jerk - HS; (90% x 1, 95% x 1) x 3
- Snatch Pull - 110% x 2 x 5
- Front Squat - HS; (90% x 1, 95% x 1) x 3

Tuesday
- Technique Work of Choice
- Hang Power Snatch - 60% x 2, 65% x 2, 70% x 2 x 3
- Hang Power Clean - 60% x 2, 65% x 2, 70% x 2 x 3

Wednesday
- Snatch - HS
- Clean & Jerk - HS
- Clean Pull - 105% x 2 x 5
- Back Squat - HS; (90% x 1, 95% x 1) x 3

Thursday
- Power Snatch - HS; (90% x 1, 95% x 1) x 3
- Power Clean + Jerk - HS; (90% x 1, 95% x 1) x 3
- Snatch High-Pull - 100% x 2 x 4

Saturday
- Snatch - 60% x 2, 70% x 2, 80% x 2, 85% x 2 x 2, 90% x 2 x 2
- Clean & Jerk - 60% x 2(1+1), 70% x 2(1+1), 80% x 2(1+1), 85% x 2+1 x 2, 90% x 2+1 x 2
- Snatch Pull - 110% x 2 x 5
- Front Squat - 60% x 2, 70% x 2, 80% x 2, 85% x 2 x 2, 90% x 2 x 2

Week 11

Monday
- Snatch - HS; (90% x 1, 95% x 1) x 3 (% of HS)
- Clean & Jerk - HS; (90% x 1+1, 95% x 1+1) x 3 (% of HS)
- Snatch Pull - 100% x 2 x 5
- Front Squat - HS; 90% x 1 x 5 (% of HS)

Tuesday
- Technique Work of Choice
- Power Snatch - 60% x 2, 65% x 2, 70% x 1 x 8
- Power Clean + Power Jerk - 60% x 1+1, 65% x 1+1, 70% x 1+1 x 8

Wednesday
- Snatch - HS; 90% x 2 x 3 (% of PR)
- Clean & Jerk - HS; 90% x 1+1 x 3 (% of PR)
- Clean Pull - 95% x 2 x 5
- Back Squat - HS; 90% x 2 x 3 (% of PR)

Thursday
- Power Snatch - HS; (90% x 1, 95% x 1) x 3 (% of HS)
- Power Clean + Jerk - HS; (90% x 1, 95% x 1) x 3 (% of HS)
- Clean Pull - 100% x 2 x 5

Saturday
- Snatch - 70% x 2, 75% x 2, 80% x 2, 85% x 2 x 3
- Clean & Jerk - 70% x 2(1+1), 75% x 2(1+1), 80% x 2(1+1), 85% x (2+1) x 2, 90% x (2+1) x 2
- Snatch Pull - 110% x 2 x 5
- Front Squat - 70% x 2, 80% x 2, 85% x 2 x 2, 90% x 2 x 2

Week 12

Monday
- Snatch - 70% x 1, 80% x 1, 85% x 1, 90% x 1, 85% x 1 x 2
- Clean & Jerk - 70% x 1+1, 80% x 1+1, 85% x 1+1, 90% x 1+1, 85% x 1+1 x 2
- Clean Pull - 90% x 2, 95% x 2 x 2
- Back Squat - 75% x 3, 80% x 2, 85% x 2 x 2

Tuesday
- Power Snatch - 60% x 2, 65% x 2, 70% x 2, 75% x 1 x 3
- Power Clean + Jerk - 60% x 2(1+1), 65% x 2(1+1), 70% x 2(1+1), 75% x 1+1 x 3

Wednesday
- Snatch - 75% x 2, 80% x 1 x 3
- Power Clean + Jerk - 75% x 1+1 x 3
- Snatch Pull - 90% x 2 x 3
- Front Squat - 75% x 2, 80% x 1 x 2

Thursday
- Power Snatch - 60% x 1 x 5
- Power Clean + Jerk - 60% x 1+1 x 5

Saturday
- Snatch - HS
- Clean & Jerk - HS

Introduction to Supplemental Exercises

This section of the book contains information on a wide array of weightlifting training exercises, ranging from technique-oriented lifts to strength lifts, and many that can serve both purposes. Because of the lack of a centralized system of weightlifting, there are often multiple names in use around the world for a single exercise. The names in this section are the most commonly used, unless the common usage is deemed erroneous or confusing, and in many cases, additional "also known as" names are listed to help cover differences among sources.

In some cases, the precise execution of the exercise is contended by different sources. While the most significant of these have explanations regarding such contention, the descriptions of the exercises that follow are the preference of the author. Exercises exist to achieve certain training goals—their names are material only insofar as allowing effective communication. As long as the athlete understands what the coach's intention is (it is the combined responsibility of both to ensure this), the names themselves are incidental.

Photographs have not been included for these exercises, as very few can be accurately represented in the medium. However, video demonstrations of all of the included exercises can be found on the Catalyst Athletics website.

Modified & Hybrid Exercises

In many situations, new exercises are created by a coach to serve a very specific need, and a name may not exist, although there is always a reasonable chance that exercise has been performed by another athlete somewhere at some point, so caution should be used by coaches and athletes with regard to naming them or taking credit for their creation.

Often such exercises are hybridizations of two or more existing lifts, or slight modifications of an existing lift. For example, we may want an athlete to perform a halting snatch deadlift without allowing the bar to touch the floor between reps, but ensure complete range of motion—the athlete will then be performing what can be called a *floating halting snatch deadlift on riser*. If the athlete is familiar with all of the terms used, it will be obvious what the coach wants. There is no need to create a new name for the exercise; there are far too many potential hybridizations and modifications to allow such naming to make sense. Coaches and athletes simply need to be familiar with common terminology, and terminology specific to each coach/program, to allow clear communication.

Complexes

Commonly multiple exercises will be combined into a series in a single set. These are known as *complexes*. The number of reps and the sequence can be modified for different purposes depending on the intent and use. For example, the complex *Snatch Pull + Snatch + Overhead Squat* can be performed with quite a few variations in repetition numbers.

Snatch Pull + Snatch + Overhead Squat – 80% (of snatch) x 1+1+1 x 5

would mean that in each set the lifter performs 1 snatch pull, then 1 snatch, then 1 overhead squat, and does this series for 5 sets at 80% of his or her best snatch (the intensity prescriptions in complexes need to be assigned to a specific lift; in this case, we are using the 1RM snatch to calculate the intensity. If the complex is commonly used by that coach or athlete, a percentage of the best performance in that complex can also be used to prescribe intensity if desired.).

Snatch Pull + Snatch + Overhead Squat – 75% (of snatch) x 2(1+1+1) x 5

would mean that in each set the lifter performs 1 snatch pull, then 1 snatch, then 1 overhead squat, then 1 snatch pull, then 1 snatch, then 1 overhead squat, and does this series for 5 sets at 75% of his or her best snatch.

The volume of a complex is the total number of reps performed. In the first example above, this would be 3 repetitions per set (1+1+1); in the second example, it would be 6 reps per set. It's important to measure the volume properly, as it is very misleading and inaccurate to consider, as some lifters and coaches do, a complex as one rep.

Snatch Exercises

2-Position / 3-Position Power Snatch

The 2-position or 3-position power snatch is simply 2-3 power snatches performed from 2-3 progressive (increasing or decreasing height) starting positions consecutively. Typically the set will start from the floor and move to progressively higher hang positions; for example, from the floor, then from the knee, then from mid-thigh). This forces the lifter to produce more power/force on subsequent reps after having been fatigued by the preceding rep(s) and having less time and space to lift the subsequent reps. The starting positions should be chosen with reason—that is, the exercise should serve a purpose that the chosen positions address.

The order of the positions may be reversed in cases in which technique is more of a priority than power and aggression. That is, for a less technically-proficient lifter, beginning in a higher hang position in which the lifter is more comfortable and progressively working down to the floor can help improve technique at the lower starting positions.

Purpose: If performed bottom to top, the 2-position or 3-position power snatch helps primarily with rate of force development, more aggressive and complete extension at the top of the pull, and more aggressive turnover of the bar. If performed from the top down, it can serve as more of a technique exercise that reinforces proper position in the pull at the hang positions chosen, or to gradually prepare a learning lifter to lift from the floor.

Programming: When using the 2-position or 3-position power snatch in a training program, it's important to note the starting positions. Intensities will typically range from 70-85%, but the exercise can also be taken to maximal effort.

Variations: Variations of the 2-position and 3-position power snatch include different hang positions, pauses in the hang position, or pauses in the receiving position.

2-Position / 3-Position Snatch

The 2-position or 3-position snatch is simply 2-3 snatches performed from 2-3 progressive (increasing or decreasing height) starting positions consecutively. Typically the set will start from the floor and move to progressively higher hang positions; for example, from the floor, then from the knee, then from mid-thigh). This forces the lifter to produce more power/force on subsequent reps after having been fatigued by the preceding rep(s) and having less time and space to lift the subsequent reps. The starting positions should be chosen with reason—that is, the exercise should serve a purpose that the chosen positions address.

The order of the positions may be reversed in cases in which technique is the purpose. That is, for a less technically-proficient lifter, beginning in a higher hang position in which the lifter is more comfortable and progressively working down to the floor can help improve technique at the lower starting positions.

Purpose: If performed bottom to top, the 2-position or 3-position snatch helps primarily with rate of force development, more aggressive and complete extension at the top of the pull, and more aggressive turnover of the bar. If performed from the top down, it can serve as more of a technique exercise that reinforces proper position in the pull at the hang positions chosen, or to gradually prepare a learning lifter to lift from the floor.

Programming: When using the 2-position or 3-position snatch in a training program, it's important to note the starting positions. Intensities will typically range from 70-85%, but the exercise can also be taken to maximal effort.

Variations: Variations of the 2-position and 3-position snatch include different hang positions, pauses in the hang position, or pauses in the receiving position.

Barksi Snatch

The Barksi snatch, named for Bob Bednarksi, is simply a high-hang snatch triple performed without using straps. The lifter will perform 3 consecutive high-hang snatches without using straps and without setting the bar down between reps.

Notes: Not all coaches and athletes agree what constitutes "high hang". Typically this is a bar starting height above mid-thigh, but it may or may not involve a forward lean of the torso (i.e. it may be a bend at the knees only or nearly so). Clarify when prescribing or performing.

Purpose: This exercise is a great snatch grip strength developer, and will also help in improving the aggressiveness and completeness of the final extension and turnover.

Programming: The Barksi snatch would be used as a snatch variation on lighter training days or as a lighter exercise in addition to heavier snatch training.

Variations: The Barksi snatch can be performed as power snatches, and without the hook grip for even greater grip work.

Block Power Snatch

The block power snatch is an exercise that can serve a number of purposes depending on the lifter's or coach's goals. The block power snatch should be performed identically to the power snatch except that the bar begins resting on blocks instead of the floor. The most common starting heights are at the knee and below the knee.

AKA: Power snatch from blocks, power snatch off blocks.

Notes: When lifting from the blocks, the pressure on the feet prior to the bar being separated from the blocks will need to be farther back toward the heels than it would be during a lift from the floor when the

barbell is at the same height, or in the starting position of a hang power snatch from the same starting height.

Purpose: The block power snatch will force the lifter to accelerate the bar more rapidly because of the limited distance available to accelerate, and because it's beginning from a dead stop with no prior stretch or tensioning of the lifting muscles as would occur from a hang position. This means it can be a good choice for training speed and rate of force development. The generally limited weight also means it can serve as a good exercise for lighter training days, especially during periods when squatting is very heavy and the demand on the legs needs to be kept minimal (except for athletes who are capable of power snatching more from a certain block height than from the floor).

Programming: The block power snatch is appropriate for lighter training days or in addition to heavier snatch training. The power receiving position and higher starting position reduce the possible intensity, meaning that even if performed maximally, the exercise will have less of an effect on the athlete's systemic fatigue and recovery. Use 1-3 reps per set. Intensities will typically range between 70-90%.

Variations: The block power snatch can be performed from blocks of any height to emphasize specific positions or limit pulling distance.

Block Snatch

The block snatch should be performed identically to the snatch except that the bar begins resting on blocks instead of the floor. The most common block heights are at the knee and below the knee.

AKA: Snatch from blocks, snatch off blocks.

Notes: When lifting from the blocks, the pressure on the feet prior to the bar being separated from the blocks will need to be farther back toward the heels than it would be during a lift from the floor when the barbell is at the same height, or in the starting position of a hang power snatch from the same starting height.

Purpose: The block snatch will force the lifter to accelerate the bar more rapidly because of the limited distance available to accelerate, and because it's beginning from a dead stop with no prior stretch or tensioning of the lifting muscles as would occur from a hang position. This means it can be a good choice for training speed and rate of force development. It can also be used during periods of time when the loading on the back and legs needs to be reduced somewhat. Additionally, lifting from the blocks rather than from the floor reduces the loading on the back and legs, meaning that it's less taxing on the lifter and may allow more frequent lifting at a given intensity.

Programming: The block snatch is appropriate for lighter training days, or it can be a primary snatch exercise if performed heavy. Some lifters will be able to snatch more from certain block heights than they can from the floor—this is not necessarily a problem, although it can be an indicator of technical or strength issues in the pull from the floor.

The block snatch may be used as a way for a lifter who has a problem lifting from the floor to train the snatch heavy while this problem is being addressed; it can also be a way to train the snatch heavy but with somewhat reduced loading on the back and legs to reduce the overall fatigue of the training. Use 1-3 reps per set. Intensities will range from 70-100%.

Variations: The block snatch can be performed from blocks of any height. It can also be combined in a complex with snatch pulls. Straps may or may not be used depending on what's appropriate for the athlete at the time.

Block Snatch High-Pull

The block snatch high-pull should be performed identically to the snatch high-pull except that the bar begins resting on blocks instead of the floor. The most common block heights are at the knee and below the knee.

AKA: Snatch high-pull from blocks, snatch high-pull off blocks.

Notes: When lifting from the blocks, the pressure on the feet prior to the bar being separated from the blocks will need to be farther back toward the heels than it would be during a lift from the floor when the barbell is at the same height, or in the starting position of a hang snatch high-pull from the same starting height.

Purpose: The block snatch high-pull is a way to

train the final extension and upper body movement of the snatch high-pull with reduced fatigue and overall training load on the athlete, or to give the legs and back a break during periods of very heavy training or when needing to reduce loading for recovery purposes. It can also be used as a way to emphasize upper body strength development for the initial pull down in the third pull by reducing the contribution of the legs to the barbell's acceleration and elevation.

Programming: The block snatch high-pull is used for essentially the same reasons as the snatch high-pull, but can be substituted if there is a need for reducing the load on the legs and back, reducing the overall training load during a recovery period, or creating variety. It may also be used as more of an upper body strengthening exercise by reducing the contribution of the lower body. Use 3-5 reps per set, typically around 70-85% of the lifter's best snatch.

Variations: The block snatch high-pull can be performed from blocks of any height. To add grip strengthening to the exercise, it can be performed without straps.

Block Snatch Pull

The block snatch pull should be performed identically to the snatch pull except that the bar begins resting on blocks instead of the floor. The most common block heights are at the knee and below the knee.

AKA: Snatch pull from blocks, snatch pull off blocks.

Notes: When lifting from the blocks, the pressure on the feet prior to the bar being separated from the blocks will need to be farther back toward the heels than it would be during a lift from the floor when the barbell is at the same height, or in the starting position of a hang snatch pull from the same starting height.

Purpose: The block snatch pull is a way to train the final extension with reduced fatigue and overall training load on the athlete, to give the legs and back a break during periods of very heavy training or when needing to reduce loading for recovery purposes. It can also be used simply for variety if an athlete is doing frequent pulling in a training cycle, in which case it would be used in addition to snatch pulls, probably on different days. Finally, it can be used to significantly overload the snatch pull by removing the portion of the pull where the lifter struggles the most (from the floor to the knee, typically).

Programming: Use 3-5 reps per set, typically around 90-120% of the lifter's best snatch. For the heaviest overloading, weights may be as heavy as 130% or more of the lifter's snatch.

Clean-Grip Snatch

The clean-grip snatch is a fairly obscure exercise, but it can be useful and even fun when implemented appropriately. Exactly as the name implies, the clean-grip snatch is simply a snatch performed with a narrow grip (about the width of the athlete's clean grip in most cases). The narrower grip means that the bar will contact the body below the hips, meaning that the athlete will need to work even harder to keep the bar close to the body. Additionally, the narrower grip will mean the bar needs to travel higher and the body needs to travel lower to fix it overhead. The athlete will need to focus on pulling the elbows high and out to the sides during the turnover.

AKA: Close-grip snatch, narrow-grip snatch.

Notes: The narrower grip significantly increases the demand on mobility; this exercise should only be performed by athletes who are capable of a clean-grip overhead squat.

Purpose: The clean-grip snatch can be used for different reasons, such as improving turnover strength, mobility, and maintaining proximity of the bar to the body. It can also be used simply for variety, as a way to break the monotony common in weightlifting training. Finally, it can be used in cases of wrist injuries that prevent the lifter from snatching with the normal wide grip.

Programming: The clean-grip snatch is typically used as an exercise on lighter training days between heavy snatch sessions, or as a temporary substitute for snatches during a period of recovery or injury. It may even be used as a technique primer to encourage a more aggressive third pull.

Variations: The clean-grip snatch is sometimes performed without allowing the bar to touch the body on its way up in order to increase the strength development of the turnover motion.

Dip Snatch

The terminology gets somewhat confusing, as this exercise is called a high-hang snatch or hip snatch by some coaches. The athlete will begin standing in the tall position—standing fully erect with the bar held at arms' length. He or she will bend smoothly at the knees only as for a jerk dip, then quickly and aggressively transition in the bottom of the dip and extend the hips and knees together to finish the pull of the snatch. The feet should remain flat throughout the dip. This lift is meant to be done with an elastic dip and drive just like a jerk—there should be no pause in the bottom of the dip. The bar must be kept as close to the body as possible throughout the lift.

AKA: High-hang snatch, hip snatch.

Notes: Straps can be used for this lift and may even be helpful to encourage lifters to relax the arms during the upward extension.

Purpose: The primary purpose of this exercise is to train the leg drive of the snatch extension for lifters who are overly reliant on hip extension to the detriment of adequate leg extension. These lifters will typically reach the hips too far forward through the bar and not get enough upward force into it. It's also helpful to get lifters to remain flat-footed longer through the second pull, to help lifters keep the bar closer to their bodies both in the second and third pulls, and to focus on proper arm mechanics in the pull under (i.e. elbows high and to the sides).

Programming: The dip snatch can serve as a lighter snatch exercise on light training days, replacing power snatches or other hang snatch variations to force a reduction in intensity and allow recovery between heavier training days. It's also an excellent technique primer to be used to reinforce technique before a snatch training session. Use 1-3 reps per set. Intensities can range from 60-85% or more.

Variations: The dip snatch can be performed with a pause in the dip position if needed to ensure balance and position (making it a snatch from power position), but this should generally be only as an introductory stage to the exercise, and would then be called a snatch from power position. It can also be performed as a power snatch.

Drop Snatch

The drop snatch is a dynamic snatch receiving position exercise that adds more demand on technique, precision and speed to the overhead squat. It is one of three snatch balance exercises whose names are often confused with each other or used interchangeably. It's execution is described in the Learning the Snatch chapter.

AKA: Snatch balance (incorrectly).

Notes: Because there is no upward drive on the bar preceding the downward punch of the body, drop snatch weights will be limited relative to the snatch balance and heaving snatch balance, but with quick and aggressive lifters, can still be significant. If a lifter maintains the hook grip overhead in the snatch, it should also be used in the drop snatch.

Purpose: The drop snatch is a good choice of exercises to develop speed and aggression in the final part of the snatch turnover, to develop precision in bar and foot placement and posture in the snatch turnover, and to develop strength and confidence in the receiving position of the snatch.

Programming: The drop snatch can be used as a technique primer before snatch training sessions or as a light technique exercise any time, but most often will be used as a fairly heavily loaded training exercise after snatches or on days between primary snatch training sessions. Use sets of 1-5 reps, usually from 70-100% of the lifter's best snatch. Because there is no upward leg drive before the push under the bar, weights will be limited relative to the snatch balance and heaving snatch balance. Intensities should not be allowed to exceed what the lifter can handle with a properly executed lift—in this case, receipt in a relatively deep squat.

Variations: Drop snatches with the feet planted on the floor in the receiving position rather than being lifted and relocated can be used for athletes who have trouble consistently moving their feet correctly or who need a simpler introduction to the exercise.

Everett Snatch Pull

The Everett snatch pull is a remedial exercise to strengthen and teach the ability to keep the bar in immediate proximity to the body during the pull of the snatch. The athlete will stand with a barbell in a snatch-width grip and move down into the mid-hang position. Without changing the position of the body, the lifter will slowly allow the arms to move until they're hanging vertically from the shoulders (allowing the bar to move forward away from the legs); from this vertical arm position, the athlete will engage the lats and shoulders to move the bar back against the thighs without changing the position of the rest of the body. As the bar moves into light contact with the thighs, he or she will push with the legs against the floor and extend the hips to perform the final extension of a snatch pull.

AKA: Snatch push back + hang snatch pull.

Notes: Using straps will allow a looser grip on the bar, which will typically allow the athlete to relax the arms and focus more on engaging the lats and shoulders.

Purpose: This is a remedial exercise to help individuals who have problems controlling the path of the bar above the knees due to either strength or a misunderstanding of technique or timing. The movement will strengthen the back, lats and shoulders to improve the lifter's ability to stay over the bar and keep it close to the body, and also teach the lifter how to engage the lats to maintain that proximity of the bar.

Programming: The Everett snatch pull can be performed immediately prior to snatches in a workout as a technique primer to help the performance of the subsequent snatches. It can also be performed toward the end of a training session if being used as more of a strength exercise. Sets of 3-5 reps are appropriate.

Variations: The lift can be done with or without the snatch pull; if the focus is strength in staying over the bar and keeping it close to the body, the exercise can be limited to the movement of the bar out and back to the body in the hang position. If performing the complete movement with the snatch pull, it can be done with or without a pause after moving the bar back to the legs.

Floating Snatch Deadlift

The first rep of the floating snatch deadlift will be the same as a snatch deadlift. After standing, the lifter will return to the starting position under control and bring the plates as close to the floor as possible without allowing them to touch, then begin the next rep from this position without setting the bar down on the floor. The lifter should pause momentarily in the bottom position between reps.

AKA: No-touch snatch deadlift, hang snatch deadlift.

Notes: The tempo should be controlled in this movement, particularly during the eccentric portion. Because the primary purpose is to build postural strength and balance, using a more controlled tempo is more effective by allowing the lifter to make adjustments as necessary to maintain the proper position and balance and to maintain constant tension.

Purpose: The floating snatch deadlift is a good exercise to develop pulling strength in the snatch, strengthen the proper posture, and emphasize strength in the bottom range of the pull (from the floor to the knee), particularly to train the correct position and posture during that pull.

Programming: Generally the floating snatch deadlift should be done for 2-6 reps per set with anywhere from 80%-110% of the lifter's best snatch depending on the lifter and how it fits into the program. In any case, the weight should not exceed what the lifter can do with proper positioning or it is failing to achieve the intended purpose. As a heavy strength exercise, it should normally be placed toward the end of a workout.

Variations: The floating snatch deadlift can be performed standing on a riser to allow the same range of motion that would be possible from the floor, but without the bar ever resting on the floor. The lift can also be done as a halting snatch deadlift or snatch segment deadlift, and a longer pause can be added in the bottom position.

Floating Snatch Deadlift on Riser

The floating snatch deadlift on riser is identical to the floating snatch deadlift, but the athlete is standing on a riser. The athlete needs to set the starting position properly with the same arm orientation and back angle—the only difference should be that the hips and knees are bent more to accommodate the deficit. The correct posture must be maintained on the way up, and the lifter should attempt to maintain the same posture on the way down. Each rep will stop with the bottom of the plates level with the top of the riser so that the range of motion is identical to that of a deadlift from the floor but without the weight being supported.

AKA: Riser floating snatch deadlift, no-touch snatch deadlift on riser, hang snatch deadlift on riser.

Notes: The tempo should be controlled in this movement, particularly during the eccentric portion. Because the primary purpose is to build postural strength and balance, using a more controlled tempo is more effective by allowing the lifter to make adjustments as necessary to maintain the proper position and balance and to maintain constant tension. Riser height can be anywhere from 1"-4". If the riser is being used only to allow full depth starting position, the height is unimportant; if the riser is being used to further strengthen the pull from the floor during the first rep, a higher riser may be appropriate.

Purpose: The floating snatch deadlift on riser is a good exercise to develop pulling strength in the snatch, and emphasize strength in the bottom range of the pull (from the floor to the knee), particularly to train the correct position and posture during that pull. The advantage over the floating snatch deadlift is that standing on the riser allows the bar to move down to the same position it would be during a normal pull from the floor but without resting on the floor.

Programming: Generally the floating snatch deadlift on riser should be done for 2-6 reps per set with anywhere from 80%-110% of the lifter's best snatch depending on the lifter and how it fits into the program. In any case, the weight should not exceed what the lifter can do with proper positioning or it is failing to achieve the intended purpose. As a heavy strength exercise, it should normally be placed toward the end of a workout.

Variations: The floating snatch deadlift on riser can be performed as a halting snatch deadlift or snatch segment deadlift, and a longer pause can be added in the bottom position.

Floating Snatch Pull

The floating snatch pull is a variation of the snatch pull in which the bar doesn't return all the way to the floor between reps. The first rep of each set will be the same as a snatch pull. After reaching full extension, the athlete will return to the starting position under control and bring the plates as close to the floor as possible without allowing them to touch. The next rep will begin from this position, without setting the bar down on the floor, after a momentary pause.

AKA: No-touch snatch pull, hang snatch pull.

Purpose: The floating snatch pull is a good exercise to develop pulling strength in the snatch, and emphasize strength in the bottom range of the pull (from the floor to the knee), particularly to train the correct position and posture during that pull.

Programming: Generally the floating snatch pull should be done for 2-5 reps per set anywhere from 80%-110% of the lifter's best snatch depending on the lifter and how it fits into the program. In any case, the weight should not exceed what the lifter can do with reasonably proper positioning and speed in the final extension and maintenance of the proper position at the bottom in between reps. As a strength exercise, it should be placed toward the end of a workout, but because it also involves some speed and technique, it's generally best placed before more basic strength work like squats.

Variations: The floating snatch pull can be performed standing on a riser to allow the same range of motion that would be possible from the floor, but without the bar ever resting on the floor. The lift can also be done as a snatch high-pull, and a longer pause can be added in the bottom position.

Floating Snatch Pull on Riser

The floating snatch pull on riser is identical the snatch pull on riser, with the exception that the bar does not return all the way to the floor after the first rep. After reaching full extension, the athlete will return to a position at which the bottom of the plates are even with the top of the riser—in other words, this position is identical to the starting position from the

floor, but in this case the weights are not in contact with the platform. Subsequent reps start from this position after a momentary pause.

AKA: No-touch snatch pull on riser, hang snatch pull on riser, riser hang snatch pull, riser floating snatch pull.

Notes: Riser heights can be anywhere from 1"-4" depending on the athlete's ability (based on height and mobility) or the degree of challenge desired. The athlete can also stand on bumper plates or any other hard, flat, stable surface. Riser heights should not exceed what allows the lifter to set a proper starting position.

Purpose: The floating snatch pull on riser is a good exercise to develop pulling strength in the snatch, and emphasize strength in the bottom range of the pull (from the floor to the knee), particularly to train the correct position and posture during that pull. The advantage over the floating snatch pull is that the lifter can achieve the same starting position as in the snatch while still preventing the weights from resting on the floor.

Programming: Generally the floating snatch pull should be done for 2-5 reps per set anywhere from 80%-110% of the lifter's best snatch depending on the lifter and how it fits into the program. In any case, the weight should not exceed what the lifter can do with reasonably proper positioning and speed in the final extension and maintenance of the proper position at the bottom in between reps. As a strength exercise, it should be placed toward the end of a workout, but because it also involves some speed and technique, it's generally best placed before more basic strength work like squats.

Variations: The floating snatch pull on riser can be performed as a snatch high-pull, with a longer pause in the bottom position, with or without straps, and with a slow eccentric movement. Slower eccentric speeds in particular will increase the strengthening of pulling posture and back arch strength.

Halting Snatch Deadlift

The halting snatch deadlift is a pull variation that stops short of full extension at the top to strengthen and reinforce the position of the lifter over the bar during the pull of the snatch. The athlete will perform a snatch deadlift up to the designated height (usually mid-thigh), keeping the shoulders over the bar, and hold this position for 3 seconds before returning the bar to the floor.

Notes: Halting snatch deadlifts can be performed without a pause in the top position (i.e. just stopping at a point prior to full extension but not holding the position at that point), but this limits the potential effectiveness of the exercise.

Purpose: The halting snatch deadlift is primarily a tool to strengthen an athlete to allow him or her to be able to stay over the bar long enough during the pull of the snatch. It also helps reinforce position and balance earlier in the pull because it's typically performed at a more controlled speed. Finally, it can help improve the lifter's timing of the initiation of the second pull in the snatch.

Programming: Generally the halting snatch deadlift should be done for 2-6 reps per set with a 2-3 second pause and anywhere from 80%-110% of the lifter's best snatch depending on the lifter and how it fits into the program. In any case, the weight should not exceed what the lifter can do with proper positioning or it is failing to achieve the intended purpose. As a heavy strength exercise, it should normally be placed toward the end of a workout.

Variations: The halting snatch deadlift can be performed standing on a riser, with the pause at different points, or with different pause times. The lift can also be done with either a static start or dynamic start. Multiple pause positions may be used, turning the exercise into a halting snatch segment deadlift.

Halting Snatch Deadlift on Riser

The halting snatch deadlift on riser is identical to the halting snatch deadlift with the exception that the lifter is standing on a riser or platform. The key is ensuring that the starting position is set properly with the same back angle and arm orientation that would be used from the floor—the only difference should be more bending of the knees and hips to account for the deficit.

Notes: Riser heights can be anywhere from 1"-4" depending on the athlete's ability (based on height and mobility) or the degree of challenge desired. The

athlete can also stand on bumper plates or any other hard, flat, stable surface. Riser heights should not exceed what allows the lifter to set a proper starting position.

Purpose: The halting snatch deadlift is primarily a tool to strengthen an athlete to allow him or her to be able to stay over the bar long enough during the pull of the snatch. It also helps reinforce position and balance earlier in the pull because it's typically performed at a more controlled speed. Finally, it can help improve the lifter's timing of the initiation of the second pull in the snatch.

Lifts from risers are used primarily to strengthen the legs for the pull from the floor, and to help train the proper balance, posture and initial movement from the floor. They can also be used simply for variety, and as a way to introduce more demand from the lift earlier in a training cycle that can then be reduced over time by reducing the riser height and/or eliminating the riser.

Programming: Generally the halting snatch deadlift on riser should be done for 2-6 reps per set with a 3 second pause and anywhere from 80%-110% of the lifter's best snatch depending on the lifter and how it fits into the program. In any case, the weight should not exceed what the lifter can do with proper positioning or it is failing to achieve the intended purpose. As a heavy strength exercise, it should normally be placed toward the end of a workout.

Variations: The halting snatch deadlift can be performed on the floor, with the pause at different points, and with different pause times. The lift can also be done with either a static start or dynamic start. Multiple pause positions may be done, turning the exercise into a halting snatch segment deadlift on riser.

Hang Power Snatch

The hang power snatch is performed identically to the power snatch, but with a starting position at some point above the floor. Hang positions include High-Hang: Upper thigh; Mid-hang: Mid-thigh; Hang: Top of knee caps; Knee: Bar at knee caps; Below knee: Bar below patellar tendon.

Notes: Straps are commonly used for the hang

power snatch, particularly for multiple-rep sets, but newer lifters and those with grip weakness are discouraged from using straps to force grip strengthening. The hang position needs to be specified when prescribing the hang snatch. Generally if no qualifier is present, a hang snatch is done from a starting position with the bar just above the knee.

Purpose: The purpose of the hang power snatch can vary depending on its application. It can be an exercise to help teach beginners to snatch that is often easier than lifting from the floor because of the abbreviated movement and the ability to ensure proper positioning and balance at the start of the second pull, and the power receiving position reduces the demand on mobility. As a training exercise, the common purpose is to develop better force production in the extension and more aggressiveness in the pull under due to the limited time and distance to accelerate and elevate the bar, and the limited movement down under the bar. Another purpose is use as a lighter snatch variation for lighter training days (weights naturally limited relative to the power snatch, and somewhat less work for the legs and back due to both the hang start and power receiving position to allow more recovery for subsequent training sessions).

Programming: Hang power snatch reps should be kept to 1-3 per set. If being used for technique work, weights should remain light (around 75% or lighter); for work on aggressiveness in the extension and/or pull under the bar, heavier weights should be used (75% and above); for use as a lighter snatch variation on a lighter training day, weights can be as heavy or light as needed for the athlete at that time, but a loose guideline would be about 70-80%; for more speed work, weights should generally be in the 65-75% range.

Variations: The hang power snatch can be done from any hang position—any starting point above the floor itself qualifies as a hang power snatch. The lift can be done with or without a pause in the hang position (i.e. with a countermovement or from a dead stop). The lift can be done with or without straps, and can be done without the hook grip to emphasize grip strength.

Hang Snatch

The hang snatch is performed identically to the snatch, but with a starting position at some point above the floor. Hang positions include High-Hang: Upper thigh; Mid-hang: Mid-thigh; Hang: Top of knee caps; Knee: Bar at knee caps; Below knee: Bar below patellar tendon.

Notes: Straps are commonly used for hang snatch variations, particularly for multiple-rep sets, but newer lifters and those with grip weakness are discouraged from using straps to force grip strengthening. The hang position needs to be specified when prescribing the hang snatch. Generally if no qualifier is present, a hang snatch is done from a starting position with the bar just above the knee.

Purpose: The purpose of the hang snatch can vary depending on its application. It can be an exercise to help teach beginners to snatch that is often easier than lifting from the floor because of the abbreviated movement and the ability to ensure proper positioning and balance at the start of the second pull. As a training exercise, the common purpose is to develop better force production in the extension and more aggressiveness in the pull under due to the limited time and distance to accelerate and elevate the bar. Another purpose is use as a lighter snatch variation (often an alternative to the power snatch) for lighter training days (weights naturally limited for most lifters relative to the snatch, and somewhat less work for the legs and back to allow more recovery for subsequent training sessions).

Programming: Hang snatch reps should be kept to 1-3 per set. If being used for technique work, weights should remain light (around 75% or lighter); for work on aggressiveness in the extension and/or pull under the bar, heavier weights should be used (75% and above); for use as a lighter snatch variation on a lighter training day, weights can be as heavy or light as needed for the athlete at that time, but a loose guideline would be about 70-80%.

Variations: The hang snatch can be done from any hang position—any starting point above the floor itself qualifies as a hang snatch. The lift can be done with or without a pause in the hang position (i.e. with a countermovement or from a dead stop). The lift can be done with or without straps, and can be done without the hook grip to emphasize grip strength.

Heaving Snatch Balance

The execution of the heaving snatch balance was described in detail in the Learning the Snatch chapter of the book.

Notes: If the athlete maintains the hook grip when overhead in the snatch, the hook grip should be used in the heaving snatch balance.

Purpose: The heaving snatch balance develops strength in the receiving position for the snatch with the elements of speed, timing and precision like the snatch balance, but the static foot position helps reinforce the proper receiving position and balance, helps the lifter practice maintaining tension against the bar at all times, and can help improve mobility. It will also help with confidence getting under heavy snatch weights.

Programming: The heaving snatch balance should be performed with sets of 1-5 reps, typically anywhere from 70-100% or more of the lifter's best snatch (less technically proficient lifters will be able to use greater weights relative to their snatches due to low snatch weights). The exercise is usually performed best in the middle of a training session, after any snatch, clean or jerk exercises that demand more speed and technique, but before more strength-oriented exercises like pulls and squats. It can be performed before snatches with light weights as a technique primer.

Variations: Two other variations of the snatch balance exist, but are really considered different exercises—the drop snatch and the snatch balance. The most common variation of the heaving snatch balance itself is adding a 3 second pause in the bottom position before standing.

Hang Snatch Pull

The hang snatch pull is a variation of the snatch pull that begins in the hang position instead of with the bar on the floor. The lifter will stand with the bar in a snatch grip at arms' length, then hinge at the hips and bend the knees until the bar is at the prescribed hang position. He or she will accelerate the bar upward aggressively with violent leg and hip extension, keeping the bar close to the body and allowing it to contact at the hip. The movement should be directed vertically with a focus on extending the body upward, although to maintain balance, it will be leaned back slightly. The arms are not engaged in the movement, but remain relaxed in extension. The shoulders should be shrugged up after the completion of leg and hip extension to continue the bar's upward path and allow it to stay against the body. The aggressiveness of the push against the ground should result in the lifter's heels rising off the floor as the extension is completed. The lifter will return the bar to the hang position for the next rep with the same posture used to lift it.

Hang Positions: High-Hang: Upper thigh; Mid-hang: Mid-thigh; Hang: Top of knee caps; Knee: Bar at knee caps; Below knee: Bar just below knees

Purpose: The hang snatch pull can be used to focus on the final extension of the pull, to reduce the loading on the legs and back for recovery purposes, or for practice and strengthening of posture and balance in a specific position.

Programming: Generally the hang snatch pull should be done for 2-5 reps per set anywhere from 80%-110% of the lifter's best snatch depending on the lifter and how it fits into the program. It's generally used as a lighter snatch pull variation during periods of lighter training, as way to train the final extension of the pull, or as part of a complex with other clean pull variations. As a strength exercise, it should be placed toward the end of a workout, but because it also involves some speed and technique, it's generally best placed before more basic strength work like squats. With lighter weights, it can be used before snatches as a technique primer.

Variations: The hang snatch pull can be performed from different hang positions (commonly below the knee or at the knee), with or without straps, with a pause in the hang position, and with a prescribed eccentric speed.

High-Pull Snatch

The high-pull snatch is simply a snatch in which the athlete delays the squat under the bar until after he or she has started pulling the elbows up to over-emphasize upward extension.

Purpose: The high-pull snatch can be used as a remedial or technique exercise to emphasize a longer or more complete extension for lifters who have a tendency to cut the pull short, and especially quit pushing with the legs against the floor too early. It can also be used to reinforce the proper arm mechanics of the pull under the bar. This exercise should not be used for lifters who have bad habits of engaging the arms too early or hesitating at the top of the extension.

Programming: The high-pull snatch should be done for 1-3 reps per set with relatively light weights. It can be done after primary technique and speed-oriented lifts (e.g. snatch, clean or jerk), or it can be done before snatches as a technique primer.

Variations: The high-pull snatch can be done with or without straps, without moving the feet from the floor, or from the hang or blocks.

Hip Snatch

The athlete will stand tall with the bar in a snatch grip. He or she will hinge at the hips and bend the knees slightly, keeping the bar against the crease of the hips, and initiate the hang snatch from this position.

AKA: Snatch from hip.

Notes: Typically hip snatches are done with a countermovement; that is, the lifter moves into the hang position and then immediately snatches with no pause in the hang position. Straps are commonly used for hang snatch variations, particularly for multiple-rep sets, but newer lifters and those with grip weakness are discouraged from using straps to force grip strengthening.

Purpose: The purpose of the hip snatch is to force an extremely aggressive final extension in the pull and to practice the proper position and balance at this stage of the lift, in particular the placement of the bar in the crease of the hips. It will also help improve the pull under the bar due to the limited ability of the athlete to accelerate and elevate the bar first.

Programming: Hip snatch reps should be kept to 1-3 per set. If being used for technique work, weights should remain light (around 70% of the snatch or lighter); for work on aggressiveness in the

extension and/or pull under the bar, heavier weights should be used (70% and above); for use as a lighter snatch variation on a lighter training day, weights can be as heavy or light as needed for the athlete at that time, but a loose guideline would be about 70-80%.

Variations: The hip snatch can be done with or without a countermovement, and with or without straps or the hook grip.

Muscle Snatch

The muscle snatch is possibly one of the most underused and commonly incorrectly-performed exercises in weightlifting. Its commonly poor execution may contribute to its underuse, as if it's done improperly, it doesn't serve the purpose it should. The athlete will initiate the lift in the same way as the snatch. Once complete upward extension is reached, rather than repositioning the feet and pulling down into a squat under the barbell, the lifter will keep the knees straight and the body extended and pull the elbows up as high as possible and out to the sides, keeping the bar in immediate proximity to the body. Once the elbows reach maximal height, the lifter will turn the arms over to bring the bar the rest of the way up and back into the proper overhead position, punching straight up against the bar and finishing in a tight, aggressive overhead position. The legs must remain straight once extended in the pull. Constant tension against the bar should be maintained throughout the movement to make sure the bar is moving continuously—there should be no pausing or hesitation during the lift.

Notes: A muscle snatch is only legitimate if the elbows never drop from their elevated position during the turnover (approximately shoulder height). If the elbows drop, the movement is not a muscle snatch; it's an awkward snatch-grip clean and press, and it will not serve the intended purpose. It's helpful to think of the movement as a snatch high-pull with an added turnover of the bar afterward. This will help reinforce the idea of lifting the elbows high and to the sides before the turnover, and reinforce a single continuous motion.

Purpose: The muscle snatch is helpful at lighter weights to learn and reinforce the proper upper body mechanics of the turnover (third pull) of the snatch.

At more challenging weights, the muscle snatch will help strengthen the turnover of the snatch.

Programming: The muscle snatch can be performed early in a training session as a technique primer, or as a training exercise. It can also be performed at the end of a training session as accessory work. Use 3-5 reps per set generally, although the muscle snatch can also be done for heavy singles and doubles.

Variations: The muscle snatch can be performed from the hang or from blocks. Straps can be used if desired, but doing the lift without straps will help with grip strength and help the lifter practice the transition from the hook grip to a hookless grip if that lifter releases the hook grip in the snatch. They can also be done without a hook grip to help grip strength.

Overhead Squat

The overhead squat is the most basic snatch receiving position strength exercise. Its execution is described in detail in the Receiving Position chapter of the Snatch section of the book.

Purpose: The overhead squat can serve as part of a learning progression for the snatch (learning the proper receiving position), a simple strength builder for the upper body and trunk in particular to help in the snatch, and a mobility exercise to improve a lifter's bottom position for the snatch.

Programming: Overhead squats should typically be done for sets of 1-3 reps. If being used as a strength exercise, they should be performed toward the end of a workout after more speed and technique dependent exercises, but before more basic strength work such as squats. They can be performed before snatches with light weights as a technique primer, or to help warm up and stretch for the snatch.

Variations: The most common variation of the overhead squat includes a pause in the bottom position to further train stability, strength and balance, or can be performed as a 1¼ squat. The overhead squat is also very commonly combined into a complex with snatch push presses preceding it.

Power Snatch

The power snatch is the most basic variation of the snatch; the only difference is the height at which the bar is received. The lift is performed identically to the snatch until the third pull. The athlete will need to elevate the bar adequately and pull under quickly enough to fix the bar overhead before squatting below parallel. The bar must be locked out overhead and all downward movement stopped with the lifter's thighs above horizontal. More information on the power snatch can be found in the Learning the Snatch chapter of the book.

Notes: Coaches and athletes sometimes have different definitions of what constitutes a "power" receiving position. Most commonly, anything received with the thighs horizontal or higher is considered a power lift. Others will require the knee to be bent to no more than 90 degrees, and others will count only lifts with the thighs above horizontal (i.e. a lift with thighs exactly horizontal is too low). Some lifters will also intentionally receive power snatches with a much wider foot stance than in the snatch. This makes arresting the downward movement easier, but also means that the lift cannot continue into a full squat if the bar isn't elevated adequately.

Purpose: The power snatch can be used to train speed, force production and aggression in both the second pull and the third pull by limiting the amount of time and distance the lifter has available to get under the bar, or as a lighter snatch variation for lighter training days. The power snatch can also be useful as part of a learning progression for beginners, or as a variation for individuals who are not mobile enough to sit into a deep overhead squat.

Programming: Power snatches should generally be programmed with 1-3 reps. They can be performed at maximal effort for training or testing at this rep range. Even at maximal weight, the power snatch can serve as a lighter exercise for lighter training days between full heavy snatch days. For speed training, weights of 60-75% are more appropriate, and for general use in lighter training days, 70-80% weights are typical.

Variations: The primary variations of the power snatch include hang power snatches and block power snatches. Straps can be used if appropriate.

Power Snatch into Overhead Squat

The power snatch into overhead squat is a hybrid exercise that combines a power snatch and overhead squat into a single exercise, but is different from a power snatch + overhead squat complex. The lifter will perform a power snatch as usual, but hold in the power receiving position for 2-3 seconds, and then sit directly into an overhead squat and recover to standing.

Notes: This exercise is not the same as a power snatch + overhead squat complex because the athlete never stands completely between the power snatch and squat.

Purpose: The primary purpose of the exercise is to allow the athlete to practice a better receiving position for the snatch by meeting the bar in a relatively high position with the proper stance, posture and resistance against the bar. It can be thought of as a snatch with a pause partway under the bar. It can also help force athletes to use the same receiving stance in the power snatch as in the snatch.

Programming: The power snatch into overhead squat should generally be programmed with 1-3 reps. It can be performed for maximal effort singles like a power snatch would be, but generally 2-3 reps at sub-maximal weights is more appropriate as it's more of a technical exercise. Typically intensity will be about 70-85% of the lifter's best power snatch.

Variations: The power snatch into overhead squat can be combined in a complex with a snatch following it to first practice meeting the bar properly, and then put that technique to use in a subsequent snatch.

Press in Snatch

The press in snatch is a mobility and strength exercise for the receiving position of the snatch. With a snatch-width grip and the bar resting behind the neck, the lifter will sit into the bottom of a squat. From this bottom position, he or she will press the bar straight up into the proper overhead position, making sure to lock the elbows securely and squeeze the shoulder blades together aggressively. Ideally this overhead position is held momentarily before returning the bar to the back of the neck at a controlled speed (the athlete should not allow the to bar crash back down). Subsequent reps can be touch-and-go without completely resetting the bar on the back, but making sure it touches the traps. The squat stance should be exactly what is used in the snatch with the feet flat and the balance correct. The trunk should be held rigidly throughout the set in exactly the same posture used when receiving the snatch.

AKA: Sots press (incorrectly).

Notes: This exercise is only appropriate for lifters whose mobility allows the movement to be done without pain and in a reasonably close to correct position. While it will help improve mobility and posture to some extent, the athlete needs to be in range for it to be effective and not harmful to the shoulders. If the lifter maintains the hook grip overhead in the snatch, he or she should use it in the press in snatch.

Purpose: The press in snatch helps improve snatch receiving position mobility in the ankles, hips, thoracic spine and shoulders. It also helps improve trunk stability strength, back extension strength (particularly mid and upper back), upper body overhead strength, balance in the receiving position, and accuracy in the overhead position.

Programming: The press in snatch is most commonly used at the beginning of a training session before snatches to reinforce and prepare the receiving position. Sets of 3-5 reps are appropriate; weights need to be determined based on the abilities of the lifter, and may be limited to the empty barbell. If they will be done with heavy loading, they can be performed toward the end of a training session as more of a strength exercise to prevent overly fatiguing the upper body prior to performing heavy snatches. In any case, weights should not exceed what can be done while maintaining the proper position and balance.

Variations: The press in snatch can be started from the top down (i.e. the athlete sits into the squat with the bar already overhead and then lowers and presses); it can be done with prescribed pauses in the overhead position (usually 2-3 seconds); and it can be done with completely resetting the bar on the back and beginning each rep from a dead stop.

Pressing Snatch Balance

The pressing snatch balance is a snatch receiving position exercise that can be used as a teaching drill or mobility exercise. Its execution is described in detail in the Receiving Position chapter of the Snatch section.

Notes: If the athlete maintains the hook grip overhead in the snatch, the hook grip should be used in the pressing snatch balance.

Purpose: The pressing snatch balance is primarily a teaching drill to introduce the snatch balance and to help athletes develop a sense of position for the snatch. It can also be used as an active stretch.

Programming: The pressing snatch balance can be performed with sets of 3-5 reps. The exercise can be performed at the beginning of a training session as part of a warm-up, or immediately before snatches or related exercises like overhead squats or snatch balances as a technique primer or specific warm-up.

Variations: There are three other variations of the snatch balance that are considered distinct exercises: the drop snatch, the heaving snatch balance and the snatch balance. The most common variation is adding a 2-3 second pause in the bottom position before standing.

Push Jerk in Snatch

The push jerk in snatch is a variation of the press in snatch that allows more weight to be used. With a snatch-width grip and the bar resting behind the neck, the athlete will sit into the bottom of a squat. From this bottom position, he or she will push with the legs up into a low partial squat to drive the bar up before pushing up against it with the arms. As the arms are punching against the bar, the athlete will sit back into the full squat position to allow a quick elbow extension that is completed at approximately the same time the bottom of the squat is reached again. The squat stance should be exactly what is used in the snatch with the feet flat and the balance correct. The trunk should be held rigidly throughout the set in exactly the same posture wanted when receiving the snatch.

AKA: Push in snatch, push press in snatch.

Notes: This exercise is only appropriate for lifters whose mobility allows the movement to be done smoothly and without pain. While it will help improve mobility and posture to some extent, the athlete needs to be in range for it to be effective and not harmful to the shoulders. The exercise could be considered a variation of the heaving snatch balance in which the lifter never stands above a low partial squat.

Purpose: Just like the press in snatch, the push jerk in snatch helps improve snatch receiving position mobility in the ankles, hips, thoracic spine and shoulders. It also helps improve trunk stability and strength, back extension strength (particularly mid and upper back), upper body overhead strength and stability, balance in the receiving position, and accuracy in the overhead position. However, it allows the use of more weight than the press in snatch.

Programming: With light weights, the push jerk in snatch can be used in the same way as the press in snatch—as a warm-up drill or technique primer to prepare the lifter for the upcoming snatch training session. If using heavy weights for more strength development, it should be used after primary lifts like snatch, clean and jerk variations, and can be done before or after strength exercises like pulls and squats. Sets of 2-5 reps are appropriate.

Variations: The push jerk in snatch can be done as a continuous series of reps, immediately changing directions and driving back up from the squat each time, or can be done as a series of distinct reps in which the lifter pauses in the bottom of the squat momentarily before beginning the next rep.

Segment Snatch

The segment snatch is performed identically to the snatch with the exception that there are one or more pauses included during the pull. The athlete will begin the lift as usual and pause and hold in the first prescribed position for 3 seconds. If more than one pause position is being used, the lifter will move to it and hold again. After the final pause position, the lifter will complete the snatch as usual directly from the final pause position (no countermovement).

AKA: Pause snatch.

Purpose: The primary purpose of the segment snatch is to reinforce certain positions during the pull and strengthen the athlete to improve his or her ability to achieve those positions during the snatch, or to reinforce the movement into or between certain positions. It can also be used as a hang snatch variation to limit the distance and time the lifter has to accelerate and elevate the bar, improving rate of force development and aggressiveness. It can be used as a lighter variation on easier training days, or to also work on speed. Finally, if done without straps, it will improve grip strength for the snatch due to the additional time the lifter must hold the bar and the added acceleration.

Programming: Sets of 1-3 reps at weights anywhere from 70-100% of the lifter's best snatch can be used (the less technically proficient the lifter is, the higher percentage of the snatch he or she will be able to do as a segment snatch). Weights should not exceed what can be done with proper positions and movement, as it then defeats the purpose of the exercise. Pauses of 3 seconds are typical, but can be shorter or longer.

Variations: The primary variations of the segment snatch involve different pause positions. Most common is at the knee, but others include 1" off the floor, below the knee, and mid-thigh. Multiple pauses can be used as well—for example, 1" off the floor to ensure proper balance and posture, then mid-thigh to train staying over the bar long enough in the pull. Straps can be used if appropriate, or for maximal grip work, it can be done with no hook grip.

Segment Power Snatch

The segment power snatch is performed identically to the power snatch with the exception that there are one or more pauses included during the pull. The athlete will begin the lift as usual and pause and hold in the first prescribed position for 3 seconds. If more than one pause position is being used, the lifter will move to it and hold again. After the final pause position, the lifter will complete the power snatch as usual directly from the final pause position (no countermovement).

AKA: Pause power snatch.

Purpose: The primary purpose of the segment power snatch is to reinforce certain positions during the pull and strengthen the athlete to improve his

or her ability to achieve those positions during the snatch, or to reinforce the movement into or between certain positions. It can also be used as a hang power snatch variation to limit the distance and time the lifter has to accelerate and elevate the bar, improving rate of force development and aggressiveness. As a power snatch instead of a snatch, it can be used as a lighter variation on easier training days, or to also work on speed. Finally, if done without straps, it will improve grip strength for the snatch due to the additional time the lifter must hold the bar and the added acceleration.

Programming: Sets of 1-3 reps at weights anywhere from 70-100% of the lifter's best power snatch can be used (the less technically proficient the lifter is, the higher percentage of the power snatch he or she will be able to do as a segment power snatch). Weights should not exceed what can be done with proper positions and movement, as it then defeats the purpose of the exercise. Pauses of 3 seconds are typical, but can be shorter or longer.

Variations: The primary variations of the segment power snatch involve different pause positions. Most common is at the knee, but others include 1" off the floor, below the knee, and mid-thigh. Multiple pauses can be used as well—for example, 1" off the floor to ensure proper balance and posture, then mid-thigh to train staying over the bar long enough in the pull. Straps can be used if appropriate, or for maximal grip work, it can be done with no hook grip.

Slow Pull Snatch

The slow pull snatch is simply a snatch in which the athlete performs the first pull at a lower than natural speed. The athlete will take 3 or more seconds to move from the floor to mid-thigh, ensuring perfect position and balance. As the bar reaches mid-thigh, without slowing down or hesitating, the lifter will accelerate the bar aggressively with violent leg and hip extension to complete the snatch.

Purpose: The slow pull snatch can be used as a remedial or technique exercise to train the athlete to properly time the initiation of the second pull and to maintain the proper position over the bar until that point. As a training exercise, the slower speed will produce greater strengthening of the pulling posture, and because the second pull is being initiated with less existing upward momentum of the bar, it will force great power production and aggressiveness in both the final extension and the pull under the bar.

Programming: The slow pull snatch should be done for 1-3 reps per set with weights that allow the proper timing and position. It can be done with light weights before snatches as a technique primer, or it can be used as its own training exercise with more difficult weights (70-80% generally, but can be taken as heavy as a maximum single).

Variations: The slow pull snatch can be done without moving the feet from the floor, standing on a riser, as a power snatch, or in a complex followed by a snatch at regular speed. Snatch pulls can also be done with this reduced initial pull speed.

Snatch Balance

The snatch balance is a dynamic snatch receiving position exercise that adds more demand on technique, precision and speed to the overhead squat. Its execution is described in detail in the Receiving Position chapter of the Snatch section of the book.

AKA: Drop snatch (incorrectly).

Notes: If the athlete maintains the hook grip overhead in the snatch, the hook grip should also be used in the snatch balance.

Purpose: The snatch balance develops strength in the receiving position for the snatch like the overhead squat, but also adds the elements of speed, timing, precision and aggression. It will help train proper footwork for the snatch (transitioning from the pulling to receiving stance and reconnecting the feet flat on the floor), and help with confidence and aggression getting under heavy snatch weights.

Programming: The snatch balance should be performed with sets of 1-3 reps, typically anywhere from 70-100% or more of the lifter's best snatch (less technically proficient lifters will be able to use greater weights relative to their snatches due to low snatch weights). The exercise is usually performed best in the middle of a training session, after any snatch, clean or jerk exercises that demand more speed and technique, but before more strength-oriented exercises like pulls and squats. They can be performed before snatches with light weights as a

technique primer.

Variations: There are three other variations of the snatch balance that are considered distinct exercises: the drop snatch, the heaving snatch balance and the pressing snatch balance. The most common variation is adding a 2-3 second pause in the bottom position before standing.

Snatch Bench Pull

The snatch bench pull is a fairly rare partial pull variation that uses spring of the bar to increase speed. Use either a sturdy bench or a set of staircase blocks to support the center of the bar at the desired height (below the knee to mid-thigh). After setting the grip with straps and establishing the starting position tightly while straddling the bench or stair blocks, the lifter will perform a snatch pull. After completing the extension, the lifter will return the bar under control to the bench or block, but with enough downward speed (it doesn't take much) that the bar bends somewhat and whips back up. The next rep should be timed to move with this upward rebound of the bar so that it moves more easily from the bottom position and with more speed.

AKA: Snatch bounce pull, snatch staircase block pull, snatch pull on stairs.

Purpose: The snatch bench pull allows speed at the top of the pull that wouldn't normally be achievable with the weights in question due to the rebound of the bar. This allows the lifter to get the feel for pulling heavier weights at a speed that they would be unable to achieve from a dead stop from the floor or blocks. It can also be used with more moderate weights to work on speed at the top of the pull.

Programming: Generally the snatch bench pull should be done for 2-5 reps per set anywhere from 90%-120% of the lifter's best snatch depending on the lifter and how it fits into the program. It should be performed after the primary snatch work in the training session and before more basic strength work. Depending on the goal, it can be performed before or after standard snatch pulls or snatch deadlifts.

Variations: Because the initial rep begins from a dead stop, making it far more difficult with heavy weights, a recommended variation is to start the bar on a set of blocks immediately behind the bench or stair blocks—the athlete will lift the bar from the blocks, walk into position straddling the bench or stairs, and then begin the set from the top, allowing the use of the rebound for all reps in the set. The exercise can also be done as a snatch high-pull.

Snatch Deadlift

The snatch deadlift is a pull variation with a controlled speed into a standing position rather than a complete upward acceleration with extension onto the balls of the feet like the snatch pull. The athlete will set the snatch starting position tightly and initiate the lift by pushing with the legs against the floor. He or she will shift the weight back slightly more toward the heels as the bar separates from the floor, and maintain approximately the same back angle until the bar is at mid-thigh. At mid-thigh, the shoulders should be at least slightly in front of the bar. The lifter will finish extending the knees and hips to achieve a standing position with the bar at arms' length, making sure to keep the quads, glutes and abs tight. The legs should be extended vertically with the shoulders slightly behind the hips in the final position. The bar should be returned to the floor under control and with the same posture used to lift it.

Notes: The speed of the snatch deadlift will not be maximal. It should not be performed intentionally slowly unless for specific reasons, but its speed should be secondary to perfect posture and balance. Straps are used for the lift unless a lifter is intentionally using the lift to also train grip strength. Often after reaching the top, lifters will return the bar to the floor by dropping it. Lowering the bar with some control in the same posture used to lift the bar, even if not a particularly slow speed, will increase the effectiveness of the exercise.

Purpose: The snatch deadlift is the most basic strength development lift for the pull of the snatch. Lifters will be able to manage somewhat heavier weights with better positions than in the snatch pull, and the slower speed will allow more focus on posture, position and balance, so that these things can also be strengthened and practiced. In addition to a basic strength builder, the snatch deadlift can be used as a remedial exercise to practice balance and position in the pull, or as part of a learning progression

for the snatch.

Programming: Generally the snatch deadlift should be done for 2-6 reps per set anywhere from 80%-120% or more of the lifter's best snatch depending on the lifter and how it fits into the program. In any case, the weight should not exceed what the lifter can do with reasonably proper positioning—if being used for posture, position and balance training, weights need to be controlled to allow perfect positioning and movement. As a heavy strength exercise, it should be placed toward the end of a workout. With lighter weights, it can be used before snatches as a technique primer.

Variations: The snatch deadlift can be performed standing on a riser, with either a static start or dynamic start, with or without straps, as a partial deadlift from blocks, and with prescribed concentric and/or eccentric speeds. Slower eccentric speeds in particular will increase the strengthening of pulling posture and back arch strength.

Snatch Deadlift on Riser

The snatch deadlift on riser is identical to the snatch deadlift with the exception that the lifter is standing on a riser. The athlete will set the starting position the same way he or she would on the floor, but with more flexion of the knees and hips—that is, the angle of the back and arms and the balance over the feet will be the same, but the shoulders and hips will be lower relative to the feet because of the riser. It's also important to initiate the lift in the same way— by pushing with the legs against the floor, which because of the riser, will feel more similar to a squat.

AKA: Deficit snatch deadlift, snatch deadlift from deficit.

Notes: Riser heights can be anywhere from 1"-4" depending on the athlete's ability (based on height and mobility) or the degree of challenge desired. The athlete can also stand on bumper plates or any other hard, flat, stable surface. Riser heights should not exceed what allows the lifter to set a proper starting position.

Purpose: Lifts from risers are used primarily to strengthen the legs for the pull from the floor, and to help train the proper balance, posture and initial movement from the floor. They can also be used simply for variety, and as a way to introduce more demand from the lift earlier in a training cycle that can then be reduced over time by reducing the riser height and/or eliminating the riser.

Programming: Generally the snatch deadlift on riser should be done for 2-6 reps per set anywhere from 80%-120% or more of the lifter's best snatch depending on the lifter and how it fits into the program. In any case, the weight should not exceed what the lifter can do with reasonably proper positioning—if being used for posture, position and balance training, weights need to be controlled to allow perfect positioning and movement. As a heavy strength exercise, it should be placed toward the end of a workout. With lighter weights, it can be used before snatches as a technique primer.

Variations: The snatch deadlift on riser can be performed with either a static start or dynamic start, with or without straps, and with prescribed concentric and/or eccentric speeds. Slower eccentric speeds in particular will increase the strengthening of pulling posture and back arch strength. The lift can also be done without allowing the bar to touch the floor after the first rep, turning it into a floating snatch deadlift on riser.

Snatch Deadlift to Power Position

The snatch deadlift to power position is a snatch deadlift variation that stops in the snatch power position rather than a completely standing position. The athlete will set the snatch starting position tightly and initiate the lift by pushing with the legs against the floor, shift the weight back slightly more toward the heels as the bar separates from the floor, and maintain approximately the same back angle until the bar is at mid-thigh. As the bar moves up the thigh, the lifter will bring the slightly-bent knees forward under the bar and lift the chest until the trunk is vertical and the knees still bent to the same degree—this is the finish position of the lift (the power position) with slightly more weight on the heels than the balls of the feet. The bar should be returned to the floor under control with the same posture used to lift it.

Notes: The lift should be performed at a controlled speed to improve strengthening of proper posture and balance. Straps should be used un-

less a lifter is intentionally using the lift to also train grip strength.

Purpose: The snatch deadlift to power position is useful as a remedial exercise for lifters who have difficulty reaching this position during the snatch. It can be performed with relatively light weights as a strictly technique-oriented exercise or technique primer, or can be used as an alternative to snatch deadlifts for a primary pulling strength exercise for athletes who need to work on the position.

Programming: Generally the snatch deadlift to power position should be done for 2-6 reps per set anywhere from 80%-120% of the lifter's best snatch depending on the lifter and how it fits into the program. In any case, the weight should not exceed what the lifter can do with proper positioning—if being used for posture, position and balance training, weights need to be controlled to allow perfect positioning and movement. As a heavy strength exercise, it should be placed toward the end of a workout. With lighter weights, it can be used before snatches as a technique primer.

Variations: The snatch deadlift to power position can be performed standing on a riser, with either a static start or dynamic start, with or without straps, as a partial deadlift from blocks, and with prescribed concentric and/or eccentric speeds. Slower eccentric speeds in particular will increase the strengthening of pulling posture and back arch strength.

Snatch from Power Position

The snatch from power position can be useful as both a technique drill and a training exercise for lifters with specific technical remediation needs or weaknesses. The lifter will begin standing in the tall position—standing fully erect with the bar held at arms' length—then bend smoothly at the knees only as if for a jerk so that the trunk is vertical, feet flat on the floor, and the bar against the hip. This is the starting position for the exercise—it begins from a static start, rather than having a countermovement like a dip snatch. From the dip position, the athlete will drive hard against the floor with the legs and extend the hips to perform a snatch, completing the rest of the lift as usual.

Purpose: The primary purposes of this exercise

are to train the leg drive of the snatch extension for lifters who are overly reliant on hip extension to the detriment of adequate leg extension, and/or to train the power position for lifters who tend to fail to reach this position in the snatch. It's also helpful to get lifters to remain flat-footed longer through the pull, to help lifters keep the bar close to their bodies both in the second and third pulls, and to focus on proper arm mechanics in the pull under (i.e. elbows high and to the sides).

Programming: The snatch from power position can serve as a lighter snatch exercise on light training days, replacing power snatches or other hang snatch variations to force a reduction in intensity and allow recovery between heavier training days. It's also an excellent technique primer to be used to reinforce technique before a snatch training session. Use 1-3 reps per set.

Variations: The snatch from power position can be performed with a countermovement, which makes it a dip snatch, or can be performed as a power snatch.

Snatch High-Pull

The snatch high-pull is identical to the snatch pull with the exception of a continued upward pull of the bar with the arms following the extension of the body. After executing the knee and hip extension of a snatch pull with maximal acceleration, the lifter will keep the legs straight and driving against the floor and pull the elbows as high as possible and out to the sides. The fully extended position should be maintained by continuing the pressure against the floor until the bar stops moving upward. The goal is to elevate the elbows as much as possible—the lifter should focus on lifting the elbows rather than the bar in order to ensure proper movement and final position. Depending on the weight, the elbows may not actually reach maximal height, but that is always the goal. Technically, if the arms are engaged and pulling following the extension of the body in the pull, the exercise is considered a high-pull.

Notes: Straps should be used on all pulls unless intentionally training the grip. The grip security provided by straps will allow maximal acceleration.

Purpose: The snatch high-pull is an exercise for training strength, speed, power, posture and balance in the extension of the snatch in the same way the snatch pull does, but with the added training of the mechanics and strength of the arms that will be used in the third pull. Because of the continued upward pull to maximal height, the snatch high-pull also helps reinforce more aggressive, complete and vertically-oriented extension. In addition to a training exercise for the pull of the snatch, the snatch high-pull can be used to teach and train the proper initial movement of the arms for the third pull.

Programming: Generally the snatch high-pull should be done for 2-5 reps per set anywhere from 70%-85% of the lifter's best snatch. This weight range will allow most athletes to get the elbows to maximal height. High-pulls can still be prescribed with heavier weights as long as maximal elbow height is not desired. As a strength exercise, it should be placed toward the end of a workout, but because it also involves some speed and technique, it's generally best placed before more basic strength work like squats. With lighter weights, it can be used before snatches as a technique primer.

Variations: The snatch high-pull can be performed standing on a riser, from blocks, with either a static start or dynamic start, with or without straps, with pauses on the way up, maintaining flat feet, and with prescribed concentric and/or eccentric speeds. Slower eccentric speeds in particular will increase the strengthening of pulling posture and back arch strength.

Snatch High-Pull on Riser

The snatch high-pull on riser is identical to the snatch high-pull with the exception that the lifter is standing on a riser or platform. The athlete will set the starting position the same way he or she would on the floor, but with more flexion of the knees and hips—that is, the angle of the back and arms and the balance over the feet will be the same, but the shoulders and hips will be lower relative to the feet because of the riser. It's also important to initiate the lift in the same way—by pushing with the legs against the floor, which because of the riser, will feel more similar to a squat.

AKA: Riser snatch high-pull, deficit snatch high-pull, snatch high-pull from deficit.

Notes: Riser heights can be anywhere from 1"-4" depending on the athlete's ability (based on height and mobility) or the degree of challenge desired. The athlete can also stand on bumper plates or any other hard, flat, stable surface. Riser heights should not exceed what allows the lifter to set a proper starting position.

Purpose: The snatch high-pull on riser serves the same purposes as the snatch high-pull— training strength, speed, power, posture and balance in the extension of the snatch in the same way the snatch pull does, but with the added training of the mechanics and strength of the arms that will be used in the third pull. The addition of the riser will further strengthen the legs for the pull from the floor. Snatch high-pulls on riser can also be used simply for variety, and as a way to introduce more demand from the lift earlier in a training cycle that can then be reduced over time by reducing the riser height and/or eliminating the riser.

Programming: Generally the snatch high-pull on riser should be done for 2-5 reps per set anywhere from 70%-85% of the lifter's best snatch. This weight range will allow most athletes to get the elbows to maximal height. High-pulls can still be prescribed with heavier weights as long as maximal elbow height is not desired. In any case, the weight should not exceed what the lifter can do with reasonably proper positioning and speed in the final extension, and in particular what he or she can set and maintain proper pulling posture with. As a strength exercise, it should be placed toward the end of a workout, but because it also involves some speed and technique, it's generally best placed before more basic strength work like squats.

Variations: The snatch high-pull on riser can be performed with different riser heights, with either a static start or dynamic start, with or without straps, with pauses on the way up, maintaining flat feet, and with prescribed concentric and/or eccentric speeds. Slower eccentric speeds in particular will increase the strengthening of pulling posture and back arch strength. The lift can also be done without allowing the bar to touch the floor after the first rep, turning it into a floating snatch high-pull on riser.

Snatch Lift-off

The snatch lift-off is simply a snatch pull that stops at the knee. Generally this lift is performed as quickly as possible but ensuring proper position and balance, and the barbell is returned immediately to the floor after reaching the knee rather than being held in this position.

AKA: Snatch deadlift to knee, snatch pull to knee, halting snatch deadlift.

Notes: Straps should be used for this exercise.

Purpose: The snatch lift-off strengthens the pull of the snatch from the floor and can help the lifter practice the proper position and shifting of weight as the bar leaves the floor, as well as train acceleration in the initial lift.

Programming: Generally the snatch lift-off should be done for 2-5 reps per set with anywhere from 80%-120% (or more) of the lifter's best snatch depending on the lifter and how it fits into the program. In any case, the weight should not exceed what the lifter can do with proper positioning or it is failing to achieve the intended purpose. As a heavy strength exercise, it should normally be placed toward the end of a workout, and should be placed after conventional pulls unless being used primarily to reinforce proper posture and movement for subsequent pulls.

Variations: The snatch lift-off can be performed with a static or dynamic start. If a lifter uses a dynamic start in the snatch, this would be the typical way to start the snatch lift-off. However, if additional strength work and in particular familiarity with the starting position is desired, a static start is a good idea. A pause can also be performed at knee height to strengthen the posture in this position (making it more of a halting snatch deadlift), and a slow eccentric can be performed after each rep or only the last rep of each set. The lift-off can also be performed standing on a riser.

Snatch Long Pull

The snatch long pull is simply a muscle snatch in which the bar is not allowed to make contact with the body on the way up, and generally is done without straps or the hook grip. This limits the contribution of the legs and hips to the elevation of the bar and forces the upper body to do more of the work. The athlete will perform a muscle snatch but prevent the barbell from touching the body at the hips without allowing excessive distance. The elbows should be lifted as high as possible and out to the sides; once they reach maximal height, the arms can be turned over to bring the bar the rest of the way up and back into the proper overhead position, and punched straight up against the bar and to finish in a tight, aggressive overhead position. The legs must remain straight once extended in the pull. Constant tension against the bar should be maintained throughout the movement, making sure the bar is moving continuously—there should be no pausing or hesitation during the lift.

AKA: Muscle snatch.

Notes: The elbows should never drop from their elevated position during the turnover. It's helpful to think of the movement as a snatch high-pull (but without letting the bar touch the body) with an added turnover of the bar afterward. This will help reinforce the idea of lifting the elbows high and to the sides before the turnover.

Purpose: The snatch long pull is helpful at lighter weights to learn and reinforce the proper upper body mechanics of the turnover (third pull) of the snatch. At more challenging weights, the snatch long pull will help strengthen the turnover of the snatch. Relative to the muscle snatch, it will demand more work by the upper body.

Programming: The snatch long pull can be performed early in a training session as a technique primer, or as a training exercise. It can also be performed at the end of a training session as accessory work. Use 3-5 reps per set generally, although the snatch long pull can also be done for heavy singles and doubles.

Variations: The snatch long pull can be performed as a muscle snatch by allowing the bar to contact the body at the hips as it does in the snatch. The snatch long pull can also be performed from the hang or from blocks. Straps can be used if desired, but generally the lift should be done without straps or the hook grip. If practice of the mechanics and timing of the release of the hook grip in the snatch is needed, the lifter can include it in the snatch long pull.

Snatch on Riser

The snatch on riser is performed identically to the snatch, but with the lifter standing on a riser or platform. The athlete will set the starting position the same way he or she would on the floor, but with more flexion of the knees and hips—that is, the angle of the back and arms and the balance over the feet will be the same, but the shoulders and hips will be lower relative to the feet because of the riser. It's also important to initiate the lift in the same way—by pushing with the legs against the floor, which because of the riser, will feel more similar to a squat.

AKA: Riser snatch, snatch from deficit, deficit snatch.

Notes: Riser heights can be anywhere from 1"-4" depending on the athlete's ability (based on height and mobility) or the degree of challenge desired. The athlete can also stand on bumper plates or any other hard, flat, stable surface. Be sure there is enough surface area for the athlete to receive the lift with his or her normal foot position so there is no risk of slipping off, and that the riser is stable on the platform.

Purpose: Lifts from risers are used primarily to strengthen the legs for the pull from the floor, and to help train the proper balance, posture and initial movement from the floor. They can also be used simply for variety, and as a way to introduce more demand from the snatch earlier in a training cycle that can then be reduced over time by reducing the riser height and/or eliminating the riser.

Programming: Snatches on riser should generally be programmed with 1-3 reps. Heavy weights and even maximal lifts can be done if the athlete is technically proficient and adequately mobile to set a proper starting position. Riser lifts are appropriate for preparation mesocycles, and generally should not be included close to competition.

Variations: Variations of the riser snatch include different riser heights, not allowing the bar to touch the floor after the first rep, and power snatches.

Snatch Power Jerk

The lifter will secure the bar behind the neck as for a back squat but with a snatch grip, the feet at approximately hip-width and the toes turned out slightly. If the lifter holds the hook grip overhead in the snatch, he or she should also use the hook grip here. The lifter will bend slightly at the knees only, keeping the trunk vertical and the weight toward the heels, then transition immediately at the bottom of this dip and drive aggressively with the legs against the floor to accelerate the barbell upward. As the legs finish extending, the lifter will begin pushing against the bar with the arms, quickly lifting the feet and transitioning them into the squat stance, punching the arms into a locked-out overhead position as he or she sits into a partial squat. The athlete will secure and stabilize the bar overhead before recovering into a standing position with the bar still overhead. The thighs must remain above horizontal in the squat for the lift to qualify as a power jerk.

AKA: Snatch power jerk behind the neck, snatch-grip power jerk.

Notes: Any snatch pressing or jerking exercise is normally started behind the neck, so it's usually unnecessary to specify *behind the neck* when prescribing such lifts. Because the bar and the trunk begin in the same place and orientation respectively that they should be in when the bar is overhead, the bar path should be perfectly vertical and the trunk should remain in the same orientation (inclined forward very slightly).

Purpose: The snatch power jerk is primarily used as a way to get the bar into place overhead in preparation for overhead squats, but it can also be used to train and strengthen the proper overhead position for the snatch, and as an alternative to snatch balances for an athlete who because of injury cannot squat.

Programming: If being used to secure a bar overhead for a subsequent overhead squat, the snatch power jerk will just be a single. If using it to strengthen the snatch overhead position, sets of 3-5 reps are suggested with weights starting around 70% of the lifter's best snatch or overhead squat, and typically the receiving position should be held for 2-3 seconds. Generally this exercise should be performed following any snatch variants and possibly before clean variants depending on what the intended emphasis of the workout is.

Variations: The snatch power jerk can be performed without the feet leaving the floor, in which case it becomes a snatch push jerk.

Snatch Press

The lifter will stand with the barbell behind the neck as it would be in a back squat, but with a snatch grip. Keeping the shoulder blades squeezed back together and the trunk stabilized tightly, the athlete will press the bar straight up into the proper snatch overhead position, locking it in tightly before lowering the bar for the next rep.

AKA: Snatch grip press behind the neck.

Notes: Athletes who cannot press smoothly from behind the neck should avoid this exercise until they've achieved better mobility.

Purpose: The snatch press is a simple upper body strength exercise for the snatch, and can be used as a teaching or remedial drill to reinforce the proper snatch overhead position.

Programming: The snatch press can be done with anywhere from 3-10 reps per set. Weights should generally be such that the exercise can be performed fairly smoothly—that is, the athlete shouldn't need to grind through it with changes from ideal positions. Heavy weights can be used by lifters with excellent mobility and shoulder stability and strength. Those with less than optimal mobility should keep weights low. As a strength exercise, it should be placed toward the end of a workout. With lighter weights (or an empty bar), it can be used before snatches as a warm-up for the shoulders, elbows and wrists, or as a technique primer to reinforce the proper snatch overhead position.

Variations: The snatch press can be done with touch-and-go reps, or by completely resetting the bar on the back and starting each rep from a dead stop. It can also be done seated.

Snatch Pull

The snatch pull is the most common snatch-related strength exercise. The lifter will set the snatch starting position tightly and initiate the lift by pushing with the legs against the floor, shifting the weight back slightly more toward the heels as the bar separates from the floor, and maintaining approximately the same back angle until the bar is at mid-thigh. At mid-thigh, the shoulders should be at least slightly in front of the bar. The lifter will accelerate the bar aggressively with violent leg and hip extension, keeping the bar close to the body and allowing it to contact at the hips. The movement should be directed vertically with a focus on extending the body upward, although to maintain balance, it will be leaned back slightly. The arms are not engaged in the movement, but remain relaxed in extension. The shoulders should be shrugged up after the completion of leg and hip extension to continue the bar's upward path and allow it to stay against the body. The aggressiveness of the push against the ground should result in the lifter's heels rising off the floor as the extension is completed.

AKA: Snatch extension.

Notes: Straps should be used on all pulls unless intentionally training the grip. The grip security provided by straps will allow maximal acceleration.

Purpose: The snatch pull is a basic and important exercise for training the extension of the snatch in terms of strength, speed, power, posture and balance. Lifters will be able to manage heavier weights than in the snatch, which allows the development of strength to push weights in the snatch, and it can be used at somewhat lighter weights to train speed and acceleration. The snatch pull can also be used as a remedial exercise to practice balance and position in the pull, or as part of a learning progression for the snatch.

Programming: Generally the snatch pull should be done for 2-5 reps per set anywhere from 80%-110% of the lifter's best snatch depending on the lifter and how it fits into the program. In any case, the weight should not exceed what the lifter can do with reasonably proper positioning and speed in the final extension. As a strength exercise, it should be placed toward the end of a workout, but because it also involves some speed and technique, it's generally best placed before more basic strength work like squats. With lighter weights, it can be used before snatches as a technique primer.

Variations: The snatch pull can be performed standing on a riser, from blocks or the hang, with either a static start or dynamic start, with or without straps, with pauses on the way up, maintaining flat feet, and with prescribed concentric and/or eccentric speeds. Slower eccentric speeds in particular will in-

crease the strengthening of pulling posture and back arch strength.

Snatch Pull-Down

The snatch pull-down is identical to the snatch high-pull with the exception that rather than pulling with the arms to continue lifting the bar upward after the extension of the body, the athlete pulls with the arms to move his or her body down toward the bar. As the legs and hips reach full extension, the lifter will pull the elbows up and to the sides aggressively, keeping the bar in immediate proximity to the body, but stop pushing against the floor with the legs, so this action of the arms moves the body down toward the bar. The trunk should be kept upright as it moves down rather than allowing the chest to lean down toward the bar. The feet can remain in contact with the floor, or they can be picked up and transitioned into the squat position as the pull down is initiated. It's important that full extension of the legs and hips is achieved before the athlete moves down.

AKA: Chinese snatch pull.

Notes: This is not a recommended exercise for beginning lifters or lifters who have the habit of cutting their extension short in the snatch, as it's difficult to perform correctly with full extension, and if done incorrectly, will further reinforce the bad habit of not finishing the pull. It's also important that the athlete maintains proper balance and an upright posture when pulling down to prevent the creation of bad habits in the actual snatch.

Purpose: The snatch pull-down is an exercise for training strength, speed, power, posture and balance in the extension of the snatch in the same way the snatch pull does, but with the added training of the mechanics and strength of the arms that will be used in the third pull like the snatch high-pull does, and additionally trains the timing and mechanics of the movement of the body down under the bar. The work of the arms can also be performed with heavier loading in the pull than can be used in a traditional snatch high-pull because the bar is not elevated past the height of a standard snatch pull.

Programming: Generally the snatch pull-down should be done for 2-5 reps per set anywhere from

80%-110% of the lifter's best snatch. As a strength exercise, it should be placed toward the end of a workout, but because it also involves some speed and technique, it's generally best placed before more basic strength work like squats.

Variations: The snatch pull-down can be performed with or without movement of the feet from the pulling to receiving position, standing on a riser, from blocks, with either a static start or dynamic start, with or without straps, with pauses on the way up, maintaining flat feet, and with prescribed concentric and/or eccentric speeds. Slower eccentric speeds in particular will increase the strengthening of pulling posture and back arch strength.

Snatch Pull on Riser

The snatch pull on riser is identical to the snatch pull with the exception that the lifter is standing on a riser or platform. The athlete will set the starting position the same way he or she would on the floor, but with more flexion of the knees and hips—that is, the angle of the back and arms and the balance over the feet will be the same, but the shoulders and hips will be lower relative to the feet because of the riser. It's also important to initiate the lift in the same way—by pushing with the legs against the floor, which because of the riser, will feel more similar to a squat. The bar should be returned to the floor under control and with the same posture used to lift it.

AKA: Riser snatch pull, deficit snatch pull, snatch pull from deficit.

Notes: Riser heights can be anywhere from 1"-4" depending on the athlete's ability (based on height and mobility) or the degree of challenge desired. The athlete can also stand on bumper plates or any other hard, flat, stable surface. Riser heights should not exceed what allows the lifter to set a proper starting position.

Purpose: The snatch pull on riser serves the same purposes as the snatch pull, but the addition of the riser will further strengthen the legs for the pull from the floor. They can also be used simply for variety, and as a way to introduce more demand from the lift earlier in a training cycle that can then be reduced over time by reducing the riser height and/or eliminating the riser.

Programming: Generally the snatch pull on riser should be done for 2-5 reps per set anywhere from 80%-110% of the lifter's best snatch depending on the lifter and how it fits into the program. In any case, the weight should not exceed what the lifter can do with reasonably proper positioning and speed in the final extension, and in particular what he or she can set and maintain proper pulling posture with. As a strength exercise, it should be placed toward the end of a workout, but because it also involves some speed and technique, it's generally best placed before more basic strength work like squats.

Variations: The snatch pull on riser can be performed with different riser heights, with either a static start or dynamic start, with or without straps, with pauses on the way up, maintaining flat feet, and with prescribed concentric and/or eccentric speeds. Slower eccentric speeds in particular will increase the strengthening of pulling posture and back arch strength. The lift can also be done without allowing the bar to touch the floor after the first rep, turning it into a floating snatch pull on riser.

Snatch Push Press

The lifter will stand with the barbell behind the neck as it would be in a back squat, but with a snatch grip. Keeping the shoulder blades squeezed back together and the trunk stabilized tightly, the lifter will dip smoothly at the knees and drive hard against the floor with the legs to accelerate and elevate the bar. As the bar leaves the shoulders, he or she will continue pressing it with the arms straight up into the proper snatch overhead position while keeping the legs straight, locking it in tightly before lowering it for the next rep. Unless doing otherwise for a specific reason, the bar should be driven as hard as possible with the legs to achieve maximal acceleration and elevation. The lifter should reset in a standing position before starting each rep.

AKA: Snatch-grip push press, snatch-grip push press behind the neck.

Notes: Snatch pressing variations are normally done from behind the neck, so it's unnecessary to specify *behind the neck* when prescribing them. Remaining flat-footed during a snatch push press indicates that the leg drive was not powerful enough or was ceased prematurely. If the lifter maintains the hook grip overhead in the snatch, it should be used in the snatch push press.

Purpose: The snatch push press uses leg drive to move more weight into the overhead position and increase the strength development of the arms for the snatch receiving position. The greater weights relative to the snatch press also mean more work for the upper back and trunk. The snatch push press is also commonly used to move the bar into the overhead position for overhead squats, or in a complex with overhead squats.

Programming: The snatch push press should generally be done in sets of 3-5 reps. Typical weights will be 70-80% of the lifter's best snatch. As a strength exercise, it should be placed toward the end of a workout. With lighter weights (or an empty bar), it can be used before snatches as a warm-up for the shoulders, elbows and wrists.

Variations: Rather than starting each rep from a still standing position, sets can be done continuously, using a bend of the legs to absorb the return of a rep to the shoulders as the dip before the leg drive of the next rep. Pauses in the overhead position, typically of 2-3 seconds, can also be used.

Snatch Segment Deadlift

The snatch segment deadlift is a pull variation that includes one or more pauses on the way up to strengthen and reinforce the position of the lifter during the pull of the snatch. The lifter will perform a snatch deadlift up to the first designated pause position and hold for 3 seconds, then move to the next pause position(s) and hold (if they exist), finishing the lift in a fully standing position, then return the bar to the floor under control.

AKA: Pause snatch deadlift.

Notes: The movement and the positions in the pauses must be correct for the exercise to be effective. If weights exceed what the lifter can do properly, the exercise can even be counterproductive by strengthening and reinforcing incorrect positions.

Purpose: The snatch segment deadlift is primarily a tool to strengthen an athlete to allow him or her to maintain proper positioning during the pull of the snatch. The pauses further increase the pos-

tural strengthening effect and practice of balance by allowing the athlete to focus specifically on problem areas, and increasing the time the positions are under tension.

Programming: Generally the snatch segment deadlift should be done for 2-5 reps per set with 2-3 second pauses and anywhere from 70%-110% or more of the lifter's best snatch depending on the lifter and how it fits into the program. In any case, the weight should not exceed what the lifter can do with proper positioning or it is failing to achieve the intended purpose. As a heavy strength exercise, it should normally be placed toward the end of a workout. Common pause positions are 1 inch off the floor, the knee, and mid-thigh.

Variations: The snatch segment deadlift can be performed standing on a riser, with different pause positions, and different pause durations. The lift can also be done with either a static start or dynamic start, and with a slow eccentric movement.

Snatch Segment Pull

The snatch segment pull is a pull variation that includes one or more pauses on the way up to strengthen and reinforce the position of the lifter during the pull of the snatch. The lifter will perform a snatch deadlift up to the first designated pause position and hold for 3 seconds, then move to the next pause position(s) and hold (if they exist). Following the final pause position, the athlete will complete a snatch pull directly from that pause position with no countermovement, then return the bar to the floor under control.

AKA: Pause snatch pull.

Notes: The movement and the positions in the pauses must be correct for the exercise to be effective. If weights exceed what the lifter can do properly, the exercise can even be counterproductive by strengthening and reinforcing incorrect positions.

Purpose: The snatch segment pull is primarily a tool to strengthen an athlete to allow him or her to maintain proper positioning during the pull of the snatch. The pauses further increase the strengthening effect and practice of position by allowing the athlete to focus specifically on problem areas, and increasing the time the positions are under tension.

The segment pull adds the element of speed in the finish unlike the segment deadlift.

Programming: Generally the snatch segment pull should be done for 2-5 reps per set with 2-3 second pauses and anywhere from 70%-110% of the lifter's best snatch depending on the lifter and how it fits into the program. In any case, the weight should not exceed what the lifter can do with proper positioning and reasonable speed in the finish or it is failing to achieve the intended purpose. As a speed-strength exercise, it should normally be placed after technical and speed work like the classic lifts, but before pure strength work like squats. Common pause positions are 1 inch off the floor, the knee, and mid-thigh.

Variations: The snatch segment pull can be performed standing on a riser, with different pause positions, and different pause durations. The lift can also be done with either a static start or dynamic start, and with a slow eccentric movement.

Snatch Shrug

The snatch shrug is a snatch pull variation that involves only the final vertical extension of the movement. With a snatch grip, the lifter will take the bar from high blocks or pulling stands and start in a fully standing position. He or she will dip at the knees and drive against the ground with the legs, extending the body vertically and shrugging the bar up as the legs finish extending. The goal is to extend the body maximally and vertically. The lifter must actively keep the bar against the body throughout the movement.

AKA: High-hang snatch pull, dip snatch pull.

Notes: Generally the snatch shrug is performed primarily with movement at the knees, with the trunk remaining essentially vertical throughout. However, some minimal inclination of the trunk is acceptable, although in the hang position, the bar should remain very high on the thighs.

Purpose: The snatch shrug is useful for training the final aggressive extension of the legs in the pull of the snatch. It can also serve as a pull variation that taxes the lifter less than a full pull to be used to reduce the loading on an athlete during periods of recovery, or can be loaded beyond what the lifter is capable of handling properly with a full snatch pull

to overload the movement to a greater extent.

Programming: Generally the snatch shrug should be done for 3-6 reps with anywhere from 100-120% or more of the lifter's best snatch, although this range can be exceeded where appropriate. It should usually be performed after primary and speed-oriented lifts like the competition lifts or variants, and before pure strength work like squats. However, it can also be performed at the end of workouts because of its relatively limited requirement of speed and precision.

Variations: The snatch shrug can be performed directly from blocks or stands if they're high enough. It can also be performed without a countermovement from a dead stop in the bent-knee position.

Snatch Transition Deadlift

The snatch transition deadlift is a remedial exercise to train and reinforce the shifting of the knees under the bar and the maintenance of proximity of the bar to the body during the scoop. Starting in a standing position with a snatch grip, the lifter will bend the knees slightly while keeping the trunk vertical to simulate the power position during the second pull—this will be the finish position of each rep. The lifter will slowly hinge at the hips and push the knees back to bring the bar down along the thighs until the bar is just below the knee caps, the shins are vertical, and the shoulders are directly above or very slightly in front of the bar—this is the bottom of each rep. At a slow tempo, the lifter will shift between these two end positions, maintaining balance over the feet and keeping the bar in light contact with the thighs.

AKA: Snatch transition.

Notes: This exercise should only be used in rare cases in which a lifter has developed a habit of completely extending the knees prior to the second pull or is somehow preventing the scoop from occurring naturally.

Purpose: The snatch transition deadlift is intended for remediation in cases of lifters who have found a way to avoid allowing the scoop or double knee bend from occurring naturally. This is very unusual and consequently this exercise won't be a common one.

Programming: The snatch transition deadlift

should be done with moderate weights for 3-6 reps to ensure the body is being strengthened in the correct positions.

Snatch with No Brush

The snatch with no brush is a tricky snatch variation that can help strengthen the turnover and encourage better leg drive in the pull. The lifter will simply perform a snatch without allowing the bar to touch the body during the extension. This will require a more vertically-oriented extension of the body. Despite not contacting the body, the barbell should still be kept close to the body throughout the lift.

AKA: Snatch with no touch, snatch with no contact.

Purpose: The snatch with no brush will force a more aggressive and vertical extension with the legs, and a more aggressive pull under the bar.

Programming: Sets of 1-3 reps are appropriate, with weights ranging broadly from very light in the case of technique work (such as a technique primer before a snatch training session) to maximal. It can also be used as a naturally lighter snatch variation on lighter training days.

Variations: The most common variation is to also use no hook grip during the lift, which reinforces the need to be aggressive with the grip on the pull under the bar and turnover and maintain tension longer. Another variation includes keeping the feet planted on the floor.

Snatch with No Jump

The lifter will simply perform a snatch while keeping the feet planted on the floor throughout the movement. The feet should begin in the receiving position since they will not move. A very slight and brief lift of the heels is acceptable, but it should be avoided as much as possible. It's important that the athlete still make the effort to completely extend the knees and hips in the pull.

AKA: Flat-footed snatch, snatch with no feet, no feet snatch, no jump snatch.

Notes: Sometimes snatches with no jump are done without the hook grip to force a somewhat more controlled extension.

Purpose: The first reason to use a snatch with no jump is to correct a lifter who tends to roll to the balls of the feet and lift the heels too soon in the extension of the snatch. The second is to correct excessive lifting of the feet during the transition under the bar. Additionally, it can be helpful to correct any type of imbalances during the pull or turnover of the lift because the athlete's base can't move to compensate for unintended displacement of the center of mass.

Programming: This exercise can be used as a technique primer or as a standalone technique exercise. Typically in the latter case, it would be used on lighter training days between heavier snatch training sessions. In any case, sets of 1-3 reps are appropriate.

Variations: Any snatch variation can be performed with the feet planted flat on the floor.

Split Snatch

The split snatch was the traditional form of the snatch until the 1950s and 1960s when the squat style now used today began to take over. Its primary use now is by masters lifters with limited mobility or injuries. Execution of the split snatch is described in detail in the Learning the Snatch chapter.

Purpose: The primary modern use of the split snatch is to make snatching possible for masters lifters or those otherwise limited in the receiving position by immobility or injuries. However, the lift can also be used as a way to include more split footwork training for the jerk without adding additional exercises—for example, a lifter who needs split practice may perform split snatches where another athlete would perform power snatches, thereby addressing both purposes with a single exercise. In this case, the split position needs to match the jerk split position rather than being the more aggressive split used in deep split snatches.

Programming: If the split snatch is the main snatch variation used by the athlete, the programming for the lift is the same as for the squat snatch. It can also be used in a similar manner as the power snatch as a less taxing snatch variation for lighter training days, or as a split footwork technique exercise. In any case, sets of 1-3 reps are recommended.

Stage Snatch

The stage snatch is an exercise that progressively builds from 2 or more partial pulling movements into a complete snatch. The exact partial movements can be prescribed differently and specifically for each athlete at a given time to achieve certain goals. A basic example would be a snatch pull to the knee, then a snatch pull, and then a snatch.

Notes: Stage snatch is simply another way to write a complex of certain progressively more extensive pull or deadlift movements and a complete snatch.

Purpose: The stage snatch is useful for reinforcing proper balance, position and timing in the pull of the snatch. It might be thought of as having technique primers built into the sets of snatches themselves rather than being performed in isolation before a snatch workout. It can be used in this way as a technique exercise, or with heavier loading it can serve to improve speed, explosiveness and aggression in the snatch by fatiguing the lifter prior to the snatch itself.

Programming: The stage snatch can be used as a warm-up for snatches, as a lighter snatch variation between heavier snatch workouts, or as a primary heavy snatch variation during preparation mesocycles. Because each set is really 3 reps already, the stage snatch should only be performed with 1-2 reps per set (which is really 3-6 reps). Intensities will range from 70% and up.

Tall Snatch

The lifter will stand tall with a snatch grip, the bar hanging at arms' length and the feet in the pulling position. He or she will then pull the elbows up and out aggressively, pick up the feet, and pull down as quickly as possible while replacing the feet flat on the floor in the receiving position and locking the bar overhead in a squat. The athlete should attempt to lock the bar out overhead as quickly as possible, although it will be near the bottom of the squat. The feet should reconnect flat with the floor.

AKA: Snatch pull-unders, dead-hang snatch.

Notes: This exercise is very intimidating at first and often seems impossible to lifters who have never performed it previously. The longer the athlete stands and thinks about it, the harder it will seem—lifters should get set and go immediately.

Purpose: The tall snatch can help train and reinforce the proper mechanics of the pull under the bar, and train speed, aggressiveness, confidence and precision in the turnover.

Programming: The tall snatch is a great technique primer prior to a snatch training session for athletes who have a weak, slow pull under the bar, or who need to focus on proper footwork in the third pull. It can also be used at essentially any time in a program to strengthen the pull under or improve its speed and aggression. Sets of 1-3 reps are appropriate, and weights will be extremely light. Lifters should be careful of increasing the weight too much and unintentionally changing the exercise into a dip snatch or high-hang snatch. Like any technical exercise, improper execution defeats the purpose.

Variations: The tall snatch can be started on flat feet or standing up on the balls of the feet.

Clean Exercises

2-Position / 3-Position Clean

The 2-position or 3-position clean is simply 2-3 cleans performed from 2-3 progressive (increasing or decreasing height) starting positions consecutively. Typically the set will start from the floor and move to progressively higher hang positions; for example, from the floor, then from the knee, then from mid-thigh). This forces the lifter to produce more power/force on subsequent reps after having been fatigued by the preceding rep(s), as well as having less time and space to accelerate subsequent reps. The starting positions should be chosen with reason—that is, the exercise should serve a purpose that the chosen positions address.

The order of the positions may be reversed in cases in which technique is the purpose. That is, for a less technically-proficient lifter, beginning in a higher hang position in which the lifter is more comfortable and progressively working down to the floor will help the lifter improve the lift from lower starting positions.

Purpose: If performed bottom to top, the 2-position or 3-position clean helps primarily with rate of force development, more aggressive and complete extension at the top of the pull, and more aggressive turnover of the bar. If performed from the top down, it can serve as more of a technique exercise that reinforces proper position in the pull at the hang position chosen, or to gradually prepare a learning lifter to lift from the floor.

Programming: When using the 2-position or 3-position clean in a training program, it's important to note the starting positions. Intensities will typically range from 70-85%, but the exercise can also be taken to maximal effort.

Variations: Variations of the 2-position and 3-position clean include different hang positions, pauses in the hang position, or pauses in the receiving position.

2-Position / 3-Position Power Clean

The 2-position or 3-position power clean is simply 2-3 power cleans performed from 2-3 progressive (increasing or decreasing height) starting positions consecutively. Typically the set will start from the floor and move to progressively higher hang positions; for example, from the floor, then from the knee, then from mid-thigh). This forces the lifter to produce more power/force on subsequent reps after having been fatigued by the preceding rep(s), as well as having less time and space to accelerate subsequent reps. The starting positions should be chosen with reason—that is, the exercise should serve a purpose that the chosen positions address.

The order of the positions may be reversed in cases in which technique is the purpose. That is, for a less technically-proficient lifter, beginning in a higher hang position in which the lifter is more comfortable and progressively working down to the floor will help the lifter improve the lift from lower starting positions.

Purpose: If performed bottom to top, the 2-position or 3-position power clean helps primarily with rate of force development, more aggressive and complete extension at the top of the pull, and more aggressive turnover of the bar. If performed from the top down, it can serve as more of a technique exercise that reinforces proper position in the pull at the hang position chosen, or to gradually prepare a learning lifter to lift from the floor.

Programming: When using the 2-position or 3-position power clean in a training program, it's important to note the starting positions. Intensities will typically range from 70-85%, but the exercise can also be taken to maximal effort.

Variations: Variations of the 2-position and 3-position power clean include different hang positions, pauses in the hang position, or pauses in the receiving position.

Barksi Clean

The Barksi clean, named for Bob Bednarksi, is simply a high-hang clean triple performed without using straps. The lifter will perform 3 consecutive high-hang cleans without using straps and without setting the bar down between reps.

Notes: Not all coaches and athletes agree what constitutes "high hang". Typically this is a bar starting height above mid-thigh, but it may or may not involve a forward lean of the torso (i.e. it may be a bend at the knees only or nearly so). Clarify when prescribing or performing.

Purpose: This exercise is a great clean grip strength developer, and will also help in improving the aggressiveness and completeness of the final extension and turnover.

Programming: The Barksi clean can be used as a clean variation on lighter training days or as a lighter exercise in addition to heavier clean training.

Variations: The Barksi clean can be performed as power cleans or without the hook grip for even greater grip work.

Block Clean

The block clean should be performed identically to the clean except that the bar begins resting on blocks instead of the floor. The most common block heights are at the knee and below the knee.

AKA: Clean from blocks, clean off blocks.

Notes: When lifting from the blocks, the pressure on the feet prior to the bar being separated from the blocks will need to be farther back toward the heels than it would be during a lift from the floor when the barbell is at the same height, or in the starting position of a hang clean from the same starting height.

Purpose: The block clean will force the lifter to

accelerate the bar more rapidly because of the limited distance available to accelerate, and because it's beginning from a dead stop with no prior stretch or tensioning of the lifting muscles as would occur from a hang position. This means it can be a good choice for training speed and rate of force development. It can also be used during periods of time when the loading on the back and legs needs to be reduced somewhat. Additionally, lifting from the blocks rather than from the floor reduces the loading on the back and legs, meaning that it's less taxing on the lifter.

Programming: The block clean is an appropriate clean variation for lighter training days, or it can be a primary clean exercise if performed heavy. Some lifters will be able to clean more from certain block heights than they can from the floor—this is not necessarily a problem, although it can be an indicator of technical or strength issues in the pull from the floor.

The block clean may be used as a way for a lifter who has a problem lifting from the floor to train the clean heavy while this problem is being addressed; it can also be a way to train the clean heavy but with somewhat reduced loading on the back and legs to reduce the overall fatigue of the training. Use 1-3 reps per set.

Variations: The block clean can be performed from blocks of any height. It can also be combined in a complex with clean pulls.

Block Clean High-Pull

The block clean high-pull should be performed identically to the clean high-pull except that the bar begins resting on blocks instead of the floor. The most common block heights are knee and below the knee.

AKA: Clean high-pull from blocks, clean high-pull off blocks.

Notes: When lifting from the blocks, the pressure on the feet prior to the bar being separated from the blocks will need to be farther back toward the heels than it would be during a lift from the floor when the barbell is at the same height, or in the starting position of a hang clean high-pull from the same starting height.

Purpose: The block clean high-pull is a way to train the final extension and upper body movement of the clean high-pull with reduced fatigue and overall training load on the athlete, or to give the legs and back a break during periods of very heavy training or when needing to reduce loading for recovery purposes. It can also be used as a way to emphasize upper body strength development for the initial pull down in the third pull by reducing the contribution of the legs to the barbell's acceleration and elevation.

Programming: The block clean high-pull would be used for essentially the same reasons as the clean high-pull, but would be substituted if there is a need for reducing the load on the legs and back, or reducing the overall training load during a recovery period. It may also be used as more of an upper body strengthening exercise by reducing the contribution of the lower body. Use 3-5 reps per set, typically around 70-85% of the lifter's best clean.

Variations: The block clean high-pull can be performed from blocks of any height. To add grip strengthening to the exercise, it can be performed without straps.

Block Clean Pull

The block clean pull should be performed identically to the clean pull except that the bar begins resting on blocks instead of the floor. The most common block heights are knee and below the knee.

AKA: Clean pull from blocks, clean pull off blocks.

Notes: When lifting from the blocks, the pressure on the feet prior to the bar being separated from the blocks will need to be farther back toward the heels than it would be during a lift from the floor when the barbell is at the same height, or in the starting position of a hang clean pull from the same starting height.

Purpose: The block clean pull is a way to train the final extension with reduced fatigue and overall training load on the athlete, to give the legs and back a break during periods of very heavy training or when needing to reduce loading for recovery purposes. It can also be used simply for variety if an athlete is doing frequent pulling in a training cycle, in which case it would be used in addition to clean pulls, probably on different days. Finally, it can be used to significantly overload the clean pull by removing the portion of the pull where the lifter struggles the most

(from the floor to the knee, typically).

Programming: Use 3-5 reps per set, typically around 90-120% of the lifter's best clean. For the heaviest overloading, weights may be as heavy as 130% or more of the lifter's clean.

Block Power Clean

The block power clean should be performed identically to the power clean except that the bar begins resting on blocks instead of the floor. The most common block heights are at the knee and below the knee.

AKA: Power clean from blocks, power clean off blocks.

Notes: When lifting from the blocks, the pressure on the feet prior to the bar being separated from the blocks will need to be farther back toward the heels than it would be during a lift from the floor when the barbell is at the same height, or in the starting position of a hang power clean from the same starting height.

Purpose: The block power clean will force the lifter to accelerate the bar more rapidly because of the limited distance available to accelerate, and because it's beginning from a dead stop with no prior stretch or tensioning of the lifting muscles as would occur from a hang position. This means it can be a good choice for training speed and rate of force development. The naturally limited weight also means it can serve as a good exercise for lighter training days, especially during periods when squatting is very heavy and the demand on the legs needs to be kept minimal.

Programming: The block power clean is an appropriate clean variation for lighter training days, or as a variation of the power clean to force more aggression and speed in the extension and turnover. The power receiving position and higher starting position reduce the possible intensity, meaning that even if performed maximally, the exercise will have less of an effect on the athlete's systemic fatigue and recovery. Use 1-3 reps per set.

Variations: The block power clean can be performed from blocks of any height.

Clean Bench Pull

Use either a sturdy bench or a set of staircase blocks to support the center of the bar at the desired height (below the knee to mid-thigh). After setting the grip with straps and establishing the starting position tightly while straddling the bench or stair blocks, the lifter will perform a clean pull. After completing the extension, the lifter will return the bar under control to the bench or block, but with enough downward speed (it doesn't take much) that the bar bends somewhat and whips back up. The next rep should be timed to move with this upward rebound of the bar so that it moves more easily from the bottom position and with more speed.

AKA: Clean bounce pull, clean staircase block pull, clean pull on stairs.

Purpose: The clean bench pull allows speed at the top of the pull that wouldn't normally be achievable with the weights in question due to the rebound of the bar. This allows the lifter to get the feel for pulling heavier weights at a speed that they would be unable to achieve from a dead stop from the floor or blocks. It can also be used with more moderate weights to work on speed at the top of the pull.

Programming: The clean bench pull should be done for 2-5 reps per set anywhere from 90%-120% of the lifter's best clean depending on the lifter and how it fits into the program. It should be performed after the primary clean work in the training session and before more basic strength work. Depending on the goal, it can be performed before or after standard clean pulls or clean deadlifts.

Variations: Because the initial rep begins from a dead stop, making it far more difficult with heavy weights, a recommended variation is to start the bar on a set of blocks immediately behind the bench or stair blocks—the athlete will lift the bar from the blocks, walk into position straddling the bench or stairs, and then begin the set from the top, allowing the use of the rebound for all reps in the set. The exercise can also be done as a clean high-pull.

Clean Deadlift

The clean deadlift is a pull variation with a controlled speed into a standing position rather than a complete upward acceleration with extension onto the balls of the feet like the clean pull. The athlete will set the clean starting position tightly and initiate the lift by pushing with the legs against the floor. He or she will shift the weight back slightly more toward the heels as the bar separates from the floor, and maintain approximately the same back angle until the bar is at mid-thigh. At mid-thigh, the shoulders should be at least slightly in front of the bar. The lifter will finish extending the knees and hips to achieve a standing position with the bar at arms' length, making sure to keep the quads, glutes and abs tight. The legs should be extended vertically with the shoulders slightly behind the hips in the final position. The bar should be returned to the floor under control and with the same posture used to lift it.

Notes: The speed of the clean deadlift will not be maximal. It should not be performed intentionally slowly unless for specific reasons, but its speed should be secondary to perfect posture and balance. Straps are used for the lift unless a lifter is intentionally using the lift to also train grip strength. Often after reaching the top, lifters will return the bar to the floor by dropping it. Lowering the bar with some control in the same posture used to lift the bar, even if not a particularly slow speed, will increase the effectiveness of the exercise.

Purpose: The clean deadlift is the most basic strength development lift for the pull of the clean. Lifters will be able to manage somewhat heavier weights with better positions than in the clean pull, and the slower speed will allow more focus on posture, position and balance, so that these things can also be strengthened and practiced. In addition to a basic strength builder, the clean deadlift can be used as a remedial exercise to practice balance and position in the pull, or as part of a learning progression for the clean.

Programming: Generally the clean deadlift should be done for 2-6 reps per set anywhere from 80%-120% or more of the lifter's best clean depending on the lifter and how it fits into the program. In any case, the weight should not exceed what the lifter can do with reasonably proper positioning—if being used for posture, position and balance training, weights need to be controlled to allow perfect positioning and movement. As a heavy strength exercise, it should be placed toward the end of a workout. With lighter weights, it can be used before snatches as a technique primer.

Variations: The clean deadlift can be performed standing on a riser, with either a static start or dynamic start, with or without straps, as a partial deadlift from blocks, and with prescribed concentric and/or eccentric speeds. Slower eccentric speeds in particular will increase the strengthening of pulling posture and back arch strength.

Clean Deadlift on Riser

The clean deadlift on riser is identical to the clean deadlift with the exception that the lifter is standing on a riser. The athlete will set the starting position the same way he or she would on the floor, but with more flexion of the knees and hips—that is, the angle of the back and arms and the balance over the feet will be the same, but the shoulders and hips will be lower relative to the feet because of the riser. It's also important to initiate the lift in the same way—by pushing with the legs against the floor, which because of the riser, will feel more similar to a squat.

AKA: Deficit clean deadlift, clean deadlift from deficit.

Notes: Riser heights can be anywhere from 1"-4" depending on the athlete's ability (based on height and mobility) or the degree of challenge desired. The athlete can also stand on bumper plates or any other hard, flat, stable surface. Riser heights should not exceed what allows the lifter to set a proper starting position.

Purpose: Lifts from risers are used primarily to strengthen the legs for the pull from the floor, and to help train the proper balance, posture and initial movement from the floor. They can also be used simply for variety, and as a way to introduce more demand from the lift earlier in a training cycle that can then be reduced over time by reducing the riser height and/or eliminating the riser.

Programming: Generally the clean deadlift on riser should be done for 2-6 reps per set anywhere

from 80%-120% or more of the lifter's best clean depending on the lifter and how it fits into the program. In any case, the weight should not exceed what the lifter can do with reasonably proper positioning—if being used for posture, position and balance training, weights need to be controlled to allow perfect positioning and movement. As a heavy strength exercise, it should be placed toward the end of a workout. With lighter weights, it can be used before cleans as a technique primer.

Variations: The clean deadlift on riser can be performed with either a static start or dynamic start, with or without straps, and with prescribed concentric and/or eccentric speeds. Slower eccentric speeds in particular will increase the strengthening of pulling posture and back arch strength. The lift can also be done without allowing the bar to touch the floor after the first rep, turning it into a floating clean deadlift on riser.

Clean Deadlift to Power Position

The clean deadlift to power position is a clean deadlift variation that stops in the clean power position rather than a completely standing position. The athlete will set the clean starting position tightly and initiate the lift by pushing with the legs against the floor, shift the weight back slightly more toward the heels as the bar separates from the floor, and maintain approximately the same back angle until the bar is at mid-thigh. As the bar moves up the thigh, the lifter will bring the slightly-bent knees forward under the bar and lift the chest until the trunk is vertical and the knees still bent to the same degree—this is the finish position of the lift (the power position) with slightly more weight on the heels than the balls of the feet. The bar should be returned to the floor under control with the same posture used to lift it.

Notes: The lift should be performed at a controlled speed to improve strengthening of proper posture and balance. Straps should be used unless a lifter is intentionally using the lift to also train grip strength.

Purpose: The clean deadlift to power position is useful as a remedial exercise for lifters who have difficulty reaching this position during the clean. It can be performed with relatively light weights as a strictly technique-oriented exercise or technique primer, or can be used as an alternative to clean deadlifts for a primary pulling strength exercise for athletes who need to work on the position.

Programming: Generally the clean deadlift to power position should be done for 2-6 reps per set anywhere from 80%-120% of the lifter's best clean depending on the lifter and how it fits into the program. In any case, the weight should not exceed what the lifter can do with proper positioning—if being used for posture, position and balance training, weights need to be controlled to allow perfect positioning and movement. As a heavy strength exercise, it should be placed toward the end of a workout. With lighter weights, it can be used before cleans as a technique primer.

Variations: The clean deadlift to power position can be performed standing on a riser, with either a static start or dynamic start, with or without straps, as a partial deadlift from blocks, and with prescribed concentric and/or eccentric speeds. Slower eccentric speeds in particular will increase the strengthening of pulling posture and back arch strength.

Clean from Power Position

The clean from power position can be useful as both a technique drill and a training exercise for lifters with specific technical remediation needs or weaknesses. The lifter will begin standing in the tall position—standing fully erect with the bar held at arms' length—then bend smoothly at the knees only as if for a jerk so that the trunk is vertical, feet flat on the floor, and the bar against the upper thighs. This is the starting position for the exercise—it begins from a static start, rather than having a countermovement like a dip clean. From the dip position, the athlete will drive hard against the floor with the legs and extend the hips to perform a clean, completing the rest of the lift as usual.

Purpose: The primary purposes of this exercise are to train the leg drive of the clean extension for lifters who are overly reliant on hip extension to the detriment of adequate leg extension, and/or to train the power position for lifters who tend to fail to reach this position in the clean. It's also helpful to get lifters to remain flat-footed longer through the pull,

to help lifters keep the bar close to their bodies both in the second and third pulls, and to focus on proper arm mechanics in the pull under (i.e. elbows high and to the sides).

Programming: The clean from power position can serve as a clean exercise on light training days, replacing power clean or other hang clean variations to force a reduction in intensity and allow recovery between heavier training days. It's also an excellent technique primer to be used to reinforce technique before a clean training session. Use 1-3 reps per set.

Variations: The clean from power position can be performed with a countermovement, which makes it a dip clean, or can be performed as a power clean.

Clean High-Pull

The clean high-pull is identical to the clean pull with the exception of a continued upward pull of the bar with the arms following the extension of the body. After executing the knee and hip extension of a clean pull with maximal acceleration, the lifter will keep the legs straight and driving against the floor and pull the elbows as high as possible and out to the sides. The fully extended position should be maintained by continuing the pressure against the floor until the bar stops moving upward. The goal is to elevate the elbows as much as possible—the lifter should focus on lifting the elbows rather than the bar in order to ensure proper movement and final position. Depending on the weight, the elbows may not actually reach maximal height, but that is always the goal. Technically, if the arms are engaged and pulling following the extension of the body in the pull, the exercise is considered a high-pull.

Notes: Straps should be used on all pulls unless intentionally training the grip. The grip security provided by straps will allow maximal acceleration.

Purpose: The clean high-pull is an exercise for training strength, speed, power, posture and balance in the extension of the clean in the same way the clean pull does, but with the added training of the mechanics and strength of the arms that will be used in the third pull. Because of the continued upward pull to maximal height, the clean high-pull also helps reinforce more aggressive, complete and vertically-oriented extension. In addition to a training exercise for the pull of the clean, the clean high-pull can be used to teach and train the proper initial movement of the arms for the third pull.

Programming: Generally the clean high-pull should be done for 2-5 reps per set anywhere from 70%-85% of the lifter's best clean. This weight range will allow most athletes to get the elbows to maximal height. High-pulls can still be prescribed with heavier weights as long as maximal elbow height is not desired. As a strength exercise, it should be placed toward the end of a workout, but because it also involves some speed and technique, it's generally best place before more basic strength work like squats. With lighter weights, it can be used before cleans as a technique primer.

Variations: The clean high-pull can be performed standing on a riser, from blocks, with either a static start or dynamic start, with or without straps, with pauses on the way up, maintaining flat feet, and with prescribed concentric and/or eccentric speeds. Slower eccentric speeds in particular will increase the strengthening of pulling posture and back arch strength.

Clean High-Pull on Riser

The clean high-pull on riser is identical to the clean high-pull with the exception that the lifter is standing on a riser or platform. The athlete will set the starting position the same way he or she would on the floor, but with more flexion of the knees and hips—that is, the angle of the back and arms and the balance over the feet will be the same, but the shoulders and hips will be lower relative to the feet because of the riser. It's also important to initiate the lift in the same way—by pushing with the legs against the floor, which because of the riser, will feel more similar to a squat.

AKA: Riser clean high-pull, deficit clean high-pull, clean high-pull from deficit.

Notes: Riser heights can be anywhere from 1"-4" depending on the athlete's ability (based on height and mobility) or the degree of challenge desired. The athlete can also stand on bumper plates or any other hard, flat, stable surface. Riser heights should not exceed what allows the lifter to set a proper starting position.

Purpose: The clean high-pull on riser serves the same purposes as the clean high-pull— training strength, speed, power, posture and balance in the extension of the clean in the same way the clean pull does, but with the added training of the mechanics and strength of the arms that will be used in the third pull. The addition of the riser will further strengthen the legs for the pull from the floor. Clean high-pulls on riser can also be used simply for variety, and as a way to introduce more demand from the lift earlier in a training cycle that can then be reduced over time by reducing the riser height and/or eliminating the riser.

Programming: Generally the clean high-pull on riser should be done for 2-5 reps per set anywhere from 70%-85% of the lifter's best clean. This weight range will allow most athletes to get the elbows to maximal height. High-pulls can still be prescribed with heavier weights as long as maximal elbow height is not desired. In any case, the weight should not exceed what the lifter can do with reasonably proper positioning and speed in the final extension, and in particular what he or she can set and maintain proper pulling posture with. As a strength exercise, it should be placed toward the end of a workout, but because it also involves some speed and technique, it's generally best placed before more basic strength work like squats.

Variations: The clean high-pull on riser can be performed with different riser heights, with either a static start or dynamic start, with or without straps, with pauses on the way up, maintaining flat feet, and with prescribed concentric and/or eccentric speeds. Slower eccentric speeds in particular will increase the strengthening of pulling posture and back arch strength. The lift can also be done without allowing the bar to touch the floor after the first rep, turning it into a floating clean high-pull on riser.

Clean-Jerk

The clean-jerk is a hybrid exercise that combines the clean and jerk into a single movement. Note that this is not the same thing as a clean & jerk, which is two distinct movements. The lifter will perform a clean, making sure to rack it with as close to a full grip as possible (to be as close to a jerk rack position as allowable), and accelerating up through the squat recovery as much as possible. As the lifter reaches the standing position, he or she will continue driving hard against the floor with the legs to push the bar up off the shoulders, moving directly into a split jerk.

Notes: If the lifter is unable to rack a clean with a jerk rack position, he or she will need to get as close as possible and shift the position as he or she reaches the top of the squat to allow a transition into the jerk.

Purpose: This exercise can be used to train a more aggressive recovery in the clean, a more accurate turnover in the clean, and strengthen the drive of the jerk by tiring the legs more prior to the final extension.

Programming: Sets of 1-3 reps are suggested with weights anywhere from 70% to the lifter's maximum jerk. Generally this exercise should be performed following any snatch variants and before heavier clean variants depending on what the intended emphasis of the workout is.

Variations: This movement can be followed by a second normal jerk or clean & jerk, and the clean can be taken from the hang or blocks.

Clean Lift-off

The clean lift-off is simply a clean pull that stops at the knee. Generally this lift is performed as quickly as possible but ensuring proper position and balance, and the barbell is returned immediately to the floor after reaching the knee rather than being held in this position.

AKA: Clean deadlift to knee, clean pull to knee, halting clean deadlift.

Notes: Straps should be used for this exercise.

Purpose: The clean lift-off strengthens the pull of the clean from the floor and can help the lifter practice the proper position and shifting of weight as the bar leaves the floor, as well as train acceleration in the initial lift.

Programming: Generally the clean lift-off should be done for 2-5 reps per set with anywhere from 80%-120% (or more) of the lifter's best clean depending on the lifter and how it fits into the program. In any case, the weight should not exceed what the lifter can do with proper positioning or it is failing to achieve the intended purpose. As a heavy strength exercise, it should normally be placed toward the end

of a workout, and should be placed after conventional pulls unless being used primarily to reinforce proper posture and movement for subsequent pulls.

Variations: The clean lift-off can be performed with a static or dynamic start. If a lifter uses a dynamic start in the clean, this would be the typical way to start the clean lift-off. However, if additional strength work and in particular familiarity with the starting position is desired, a static start is a good idea. A pause can also be performed at knee height to strengthen the posture in this position (making it more of a halting clean deadlift), and a slow eccentric can be performed after each rep or only the last rep of each set. The lift-off can also be performed standing on a riser.

Clean Long Pull

The clean long pull is simply a muscle clean in which the bar is not allowed to make contact with the body on the way up, and is generally done without the hook grip. This limits the contribution of the legs and hips to the elevation of the bar and forces the upper body to do more of the work. The athlete will perform a muscle clean but prevent the barbell from touching the body at the upper thigh without allowing excessive distance. The elbows should be lifted as high as possible and out to the sides; once they reach maximal height, the arms can be turned over to bring the bar the rest of the way up and back into the proper clean rack position. The legs must remain straight once extended in the pull. Constant tension against the bar should be maintained throughout the movement, making sure the bar is moving continuously—there should be no pausing or hesitation during the lift.

AKA: Muscle clean.

Notes: It's helpful to think of the movement as a clean high-pull (but without letting the bar touch the body) with an added turnover of the bar afterward. This will help reinforce the idea of lifting the elbows high and to the sides before the turnover.

Purpose: The clean long pull is helpful at lighter weights to learn and reinforce the proper upper body mechanics of the turnover (third pull) of the clean. At more challenging weights, the clean long pull will help strengthen the turnover of the clean. Relative to the muscle clean, it will demand more work by the upper body.

Programming: The clean long pull can be performed early in a training session as a technique primer, or as a training exercise. It can also be performed at the end of a training session as accessory work. Use 3-5 reps per set generally, although the clean long pull can also be done for heavy singles and doubles.

Variations: The clean long pull can be performed as a muscle clean by allowing the bar to contact the body at the hips as it does in the clean. The clean long pull can also be performed from the hang or from blocks.

Clean on Riser

The clean on riser is performed identically to the clean, but with the lifter standing on a riser or platform. The athlete will set the starting position the same way he or she would on the floor, but with more flexion of the knees and hips—that is, the angle of the back and arms and the balance over the feet will be the same, but the shoulders and hips will be lower relative to the feet because of the riser. It's also important to initiate the lift in the same way—by pushing with the legs against the floor, which because of the riser, will feel more similar to a squat.

AKA: Riser clean, clean from deficit, deficit clean.

Notes: Riser heights can be anywhere from 1"-4" depending on the athlete's ability (based on height and mobility) or the degree of challenge desired. The athlete can also stand on bumper plates or any other hard, flat, stable surface. Be sure there is enough surface area for the athlete to receive the lift with his or her normal foot position so there is no risk of slipping off, and that the riser is stable on the platform.

Purpose: Lifts from risers are used primarily to strengthen the legs for the pull from the floor, and to help train the proper balance, posture and initial movement from the floor. They can also be used simply for variety, and as a way to introduce more demand from the clean earlier in a training cycle that can then be reduced over time by reducing the riser height and/or eliminating the riser.

Programming: Cleans on riser should generally be programmed with 1-3 reps. Heavy weights

and even maximal lifts can be done if the athlete is technically proficient and adequately mobile to set a proper starting position. Riser lifts are appropriate for preparation mesocycles, and generally should not be included close to competition.

Variations: Variations of the riser clean include different riser heights, not allowing the bar to touch the floor after the first rep, and power cleans.

Clean Pull

The clean pull is the most common clean-related strength exercise. The lifter will set the clean starting position tightly and initiate the lift by pushing with the legs against the floor, shifting the weight back slightly more toward the heels as the bar separates from the floor, and maintaining approximately the same back angle until the bar is at mid-thigh. At mid-thigh, the shoulders should be at least slightly in front of the bar. The lifter will accelerate the bar aggressively with violent leg and hip extension, keeping the bar close to the body and allowing it to contact at the hips. The movement should be directed vertically with a focus on extending the body upward, although to maintain balance, it will be leaned back slightly. The arms are not engaged in the movement, but remain relaxed in extension. The shoulders should be shrugged up after the completion of leg and hip extension to continue the bar's upward path and allow it to stay against the body. The aggressiveness of the push against the ground should result in the lifter's heels rising off the floor as the extension is completed.

AKA: Clean extension.

Notes: Straps should be used on all pulls unless intentionally training the grip. The grip security provided by straps will allow maximal acceleration.

Purpose: The clean pull is a basic and important exercise for training the extension of the clean in terms of strength, speed, power, posture and balance. Lifters will be able to manage heavier weights than in the clean, which allows the development of strength to push weights in the clean, and it can be used at somewhat lighter weights to train speed and acceleration. The clean pull can also be used as a remedial exercise to practice balance and position in the pull, or as part of a learning progression for the clean.

Programming: Generally the clean pull should be done for 2-5 reps per set anywhere from 80%-110% of the lifter's best clean depending on the lifter and how it fits into the program. In any case, the weight should not exceed what the lifter can do with reasonably proper positioning and speed in the final extension. As a strength exercise, it should be placed toward the end of a workout, but because it also involves some speed and technique, it's generally best placed before more basic strength work like squats. With lighter weights, it can be used before cleans as a technique primer.

Variations: The clean pull can be performed standing on a riser, from blocks or the hang, with either a static start or dynamic start, with or without straps, with pauses on the way up, maintaining flat feet, and with prescribed concentric and/or eccentric speeds. Slower eccentric speeds in particular will increase the strengthening of pulling posture and back arch strength.

Clean Pull-Down

The clean pull-down is identical to the clean high-pull with the exception that rather than pulling with the arms to continue lifting the bar upward after the extension of the body, the athlete pulls with the arms to move his or her body down toward the bar. As the legs and hips reach full extension, the lifter will pull the elbows up and to the sides aggressively, keeping the bar in immediate proximity to the body, but stop pushing against the floor with the legs, so this action of the arms moves the body down toward the bar. The trunk should be kept upright as it moves down rather than allowing the chest to lean down toward the bar. The feet can remain in contact with the floor, or they can be picked up and transitioned into the squat position as the pull down is initiated. It's important that full extension of the legs and hips is achieved before the athlete moves down.

AKA: Chinese clean pull.

Notes: This is not a recommended exercise for beginning lifters or lifters who have the habit of cutting their extension short in the clean, as it's difficult to perform correctly with full extension, and if done incorrectly, will further reinforce the bad habit of not

finishing the pull. It's also important that the athlete maintains proper balance and an upright posture when pulling down to prevent the creation of bad habits in the actual clean.

Purpose: The clean pull-down is an exercise for training strength, speed, power, posture and balance in the extension of the clean in the same way the clean pull does, but with the added training of the mechanics and strength of the arms that will be used in the third pull like the clean high-pull does, and additionally trains the timing and mechanics of the movement of the body down under the bar. The work of the arms can also be performed with heavier loading in the pull than can be used in a traditional clean high-pull because the bar is not elevated past the height of a standard clean pull.

Programming: Generally the clean pull-down should be done for 2-5 reps per set anywhere from 80%-110% of the lifter's best clean. As a strength exercise, it should be placed toward the end of a workout, but because it also involves some speed and technique, it's generally best placed before more basic strength work like squats.

Variations: The clean pull-down can be performed with or without movement of the feet from the pulling to receiving position, standing on a riser, from blocks, with either a static start or dynamic start, with or without straps, with pauses on the way up, maintaining flat feet, and with prescribed concentric and/or eccentric speeds. Slower eccentric speeds in particular will increase the strengthening of pulling posture and back arch strength.

Clean Pull on Riser

The clean pull on riser is identical to the clean pull with the exception that the lifter is standing on a riser or platform. The athlete will set the starting position the same way he or she would on the floor, but with more flexion of the knees and hips—that is, the angle of the back and arms and the balance over the feet will be the same, but the shoulders and hips will be lower relative to the feet because of the riser. It's also important to initiate the lift in the same way—by pushing with the legs against the floor, which because of the riser, will feel more similar to a squat. The bar should be returned to the floor under control and with the same posture used to lift it.

AKA: Riser clean pull, deficit clean pull, clean pull from deficit.

Notes: Riser heights can be anywhere from 1"-4" depending on the athlete's ability (based on height and mobility) or the degree of challenge desired. The athlete can also stand on bumper plates or any other hard, flat, stable surface. Riser heights should not exceed what allows the lifter to set a proper starting position.

Purpose: The clean pull on riser serves the same purposes as the clean pull, but the addition of the riser will further strengthen the legs for the pull from the floor. They can also be used simply for variety, and as a way to introduce more demand from the lift earlier in a training cycle that can then be reduced over time by reducing the riser height and/or eliminating the riser.

Programming: Generally the clean pull on riser should be done for 2-5 reps per set anywhere from 80%-110% of the lifter's best clean depending on the lifter and how it fits into the program. In any case, the weight should not exceed what the lifter can do with reasonably proper positioning and speed in the final extension, and in particular what he or she can set and maintain proper pulling posture with. As a strength exercise, it should be placed toward the end of a workout, but because it also involves some speed and technique, it's generally best placed before more basic strength work like squats.

Variations: The clean pull on riser can be performed with different riser heights, with either a static start or dynamic start, with or without straps, with pauses on the way up, maintaining flat feet, and with prescribed concentric and/or eccentric speeds. Slower eccentric speeds in particular will increase the strengthening of pulling posture and back arch strength. The lift can also be done without allowing the bar to touch the floor after the first rep, turning it into a floating clean pull on riser.

Clean Rack Support

The clean rack support is a simple static exercise to strengthen the clean rack position and trunk for the clean. The lifter will set up a bar in a power rack 2-3 inches below the height at which it would be when on the shoulders in a standing position. The lifter will move under the bar into the clean rack position and stand to lift the bar off the pins. The lifter will hold the positions for 3-10 seconds, actively maintaining a strong rack position, before returning the bar to the pins.

Notes: It's important to keep the shoulders lifted slightly in a proper rack position to prevent compression of the carotid arteries and dizziness. For longer holds, lifters will need to release some of their air as well.

Purpose: The clean rack support strengthens the clean rack position, upper back and trunk, and can help with confidence by getting the lifter accustomed to the feel of heavy weights in the rack position.

Programming: This exercise should be placed at or near the end of a workout. Use weights of 100% and above of the lifter's best clean for holds of 3-10 seconds.

Clean Segment Deadlift

The clean segment deadlift is a pull variation that includes one or more pauses on the way up to strengthen and reinforce the position of the lifter during the pull of the clean. The lifter will perform a clean deadlift up to the first designated pause position and hold for 3 seconds, then move to the next pause position(s) and hold (if they exist), finishing the lift in a fully standing position, then return the bar to the floor under control.

AKA: Pause clean deadlift.

Notes: The movement and the positions in the pauses must be correct for the exercise to be effective. If weights exceed what the lifter can do properly, the exercise can even be counterproductive by strengthening and reinforcing incorrect positions.

Purpose: The clean segment deadlift is primarily a tool to strengthen an athlete to allow him or her to maintain proper positioning during the pull of the clean. The pauses further increase the postural strengthening effect and practice of balance by allowing the athlete to focus specifically on problem areas, and increasing the time the positions are under tension.

Programming: Generally the clean segment deadlift should be done for 2-5 reps per set with

2-3 second pauses and anywhere from 70%-110% or more of the lifter's best clean depending on the lifter and how it fits into the program. In any case, the weight should not exceed what the lifter can do with proper positioning or it is failing to achieve the intended purpose. As a heavy strength exercise, it should normally be placed toward the end of a workout. Common pause positions are 1 inch off the floor, the knee, and mid-thigh.

Variations: The clean segment deadlift can be performed standing on a riser, with different pause positions, and different pause durations. The lift can also be done with either a static start or dynamic start, and with a slow eccentric movement.

Clean Segment Pull

The clean segment pull is a pull variation that includes one or more pauses on the way up to strengthen and reinforce the position of the lifter during the pull of the clean. The lifter will perform a clean deadlift up to the first designated pause position and hold for 3 seconds, then move to the next pause position(s) and hold (if they exist). Following the final pause position, the athlete will complete a clean pull directly from that pause position with no countermovement, then return the bar to the floor under control.

AKA: Pause clean pull.

Notes: The movement and the positions in the pauses must be correct for the exercise to be effective. If weights exceed what the lifter can do properly, the exercise can even be counterproductive by strengthening and reinforcing incorrect positions.

Purpose: The clean segment pull is primarily a tool to strengthen an athlete to allow him or her to maintain proper positioning during the pull of the clean. The pauses further increase the strengthening effect and practice of position by allowing the athlete to focus specifically on problem areas, and increasing the time the positions are under tension. The segment pull adds the element of speed in the finish unlike the segment deadlift.

Programming: Generally the clean segment pull should be done for 2-5 reps per set with 2-3 second pauses and anywhere from 70%-110% of the lifter's best clean depending on the lifter and how it fits into the program. In any case, the weight should not ex-

ceed what the lifter can do with proper positioning and reasonable speed in the finish or it is failing to achieve the intended purpose. As a speed-strength exercise, it should normally be placed after technical and speed work like the classic lifts, but before pure strength work like squats. Common pause positions are 1 inch off the floor, the knee, and mid-thigh.

Variations: The clean segment pull can be performed standing on a riser, with different pause positions, and different pause durations. The lift can also be done with either a static start or dynamic start, and with a slow eccentric movement.

Clean Shrug

The clean shrug is a clean pull variation that involves only the final vertical extension of the movement. With a clean grip, the lifter will take the bar from high blocks or pulling stands and start in a fully standing position. He or she will dip at the knees and drive against the ground with the legs, extending the body vertically and shrugging the bar up as the legs finish extending. The goal is to extend the body maximally and vertically. The lifter must actively keep the bar against the body throughout the movement.

AKA: High-hang clean pull, dip clean pull.

Notes: Generally the clean shrug is performed primarily with movement at the knees, with the trunk remaining essentially vertical throughout. However, some minimal inclination of the trunk is acceptable, although in the hang position, the bar should remain very high on the thighs.

Purpose: The clean shrug is useful for training the final aggressive extension of the legs in the pull of the clean. It can also serve as a pull variation that taxes the lifter less than a full pull to be used to reduce the loading on an athlete during periods of recovery, or can be loaded beyond what the lifter is capable of handling properly with a full clean pull to overload the movement to a greater extent.

Programming: Generally the clean shrug should be done for 3-6 reps with anywhere from 100-120% or more of the lifter's best clean, although this range can be exceeded where appropriate. It should usually be performed after primary and speed-oriented lifts like the competition lifts or variants, and before pure strength work like squats. However, it can also be performed at the end of workouts because of its relatively limited requirement of speed and precision.

Variations: The clean shrug can be performed directly from blocks or stands if they're high enough. It can also be performed without a countermovement from a dead stop in the bent-knee position.

Clean Transition Deadlift

The clean transition deadlift is a remedial exercise to train and reinforce the shifting of the knees under the bar and the maintenance of proximity of the bar to the body during the scoop. Starting in a standing position with a clean grip, the lifter will bend the knees slightly while keeping the trunk vertical to simulate the power position during the second pull—this will be the finish position of each rep. The lifter will slowly hinge at the hips and push the knees back to bring the bar down along the thighs until the bar is just below the knee caps, the shins are vertical, and the shoulders are directly above or very slightly in front of the bar—this is the bottom of each rep. At a slow tempo, the lifter will shift between these two end positions, maintaining balance over the feet and keeping the bar in light contact with the thighs.

AKA: Clean transition.

Notes: This exercise should only be used in rare cases in which a lifter has developed a habit of completely extending the knees prior to the second pull or is somehow preventing the scoop from occurring naturally.

Purpose: The clean transition deadlift is intended for remediation in cases of lifters who have found a way to avoid allowing the scoop or double knee bend from occurring naturally. This is very unusual and consequently this exercise won't be a common one.

Programming: The clean transition deadlift should be done with moderate weights for 3-6 reps to ensure the body is being strengthened in the correct positions.

Clean with No Brush

The clean with no brush is a tricky clean variation that can help strengthen the turnover and encourage better leg drive in the pull. The lifter will simply perform a clean without allowing the bar to touch the body during the extension. This will require a more vertically-oriented extension of the body. Despite not contacting the body, the barbell should still be kept close to the body throughout the lift.

AKA: Clean with no touch, clean with no contact.

Purpose: The clean with no brush will force a more aggressive and vertical extension with the legs, and a more aggressive pull under the bar.

Programming: Sets of 1-3 reps are appropriate, with weights ranging broadly from very light in the case of technique work (such as a technique primer before a clean training session) to maximal. It can also be used as a naturally lighter clean variation on lighter training days.

Variations: The most common variation is to also use no hook grip during the lift, which reinforces the need to be aggressive with the grip on the pull under the bar and turnover and maintain tension longer. Another variation includes keeping the feet planted on the floor.

Clean with No Jump

The lifter will simply perform a clean while keeping the feet planted on the floor throughout the movement. The feet should begin in the receiving position since they will not move. A very slight and brief lift of the heels is acceptable, but it should be avoided as much as possible. It's important that the athlete still make the effort to completely extend the knees and hips in the pull.

AKA: Flat-footed clean, clean with no feet, no feet clean, no jump clean.

Notes: Sometimes cleans with no jump are done without the hook grip to force a somewhat more controlled extension.

Purpose: The first reason to use a clean with no jump is to correct a lifter who tends to roll to the balls of the feet and lift the heels too soon in the extension of the clean. The second is to correct excessive lifting of the feet during the transition under the bar. Additionally, it can be helpful to correct any type of imbalances during the pull or turnover of the lift because the athlete's base can't move to compensate for unintended displacement of the center of mass.

Programming: This exercise can be used as a

technique primer or as a standalone technique exercise. Typically in the latter case, it would be used on lighter training days between heavier clean training sessions. In any case, sets of 1-3 reps are appropriate.

Variations: Any clean variation can be performed with the feet planted flat on the floor

Dip Clean

The terminology gets somewhat confusing, as this exercise is sometimes called a high-hang clean or hip clean by some coaches. The athlete will begin standing in the tall position—standing fully erect with the bar held at arms' length. He or she will bend smoothly at the knees only as for a jerk dip, then quickly and aggressively transition in the bottom of the dip and extend the hips and knees together to finish the pull of the clean. The feet should remain flat throughout the dip. This lift is meant to be done with an elastic dip and drive just like a jerk—there should be no pause in the bottom of the dip. The bar must be kept as close to the body as possible throughout the lift.

AKA: High-hang clean, hip clean.

Purpose: The primary purpose of this exercise is to train the leg drive of the clean extension for lifters who are overly reliant on hip extension to the detriment of adequate leg extension. These lifters will typically reach the hips too far forward through the bar and not get enough upward force into the bar. It's also helpful to get lifters to remain flat-footed longer through the second pull, to help lifters keep the bar closer to their bodies both in the second and third pulls, and to focus on proper arm mechanics in the pull under (i.e. elbows high and to the sides).

Programming: The dip clean can serve as a lighter clean exercise, replacing power cleans or other hang clean variations to force a reduction in intensity and allow recovery between heavier training days. It's also an excellent technique primer to be used to reinforce technique before a clean training session. Use 1-3 reps per set. Intensities can range from 60-85%.

Variations: The dip clean can be performed with a pause in the dip position if needed to ensure balance and position (making it a clean from power position), but this should generally be only as an introductory stage to the exercise. It can also be performed as a power snatch.

Everett Clean Pull

The Everett clean pull is a remedial exercise to strengthen and teach the ability to keep the bar in immediate proximity to the body during the pull of the clean. The athlete will stand with a barbell in a clean grip and move down into the mid-hang position. Without changing the position of the body, the lifter will slowly allow the arms to move until they're hanging vertically from the shoulders (allowing the bar to move forward away from the legs); from this vertical arm position, the athlete will engage the lats and shoulders to move the bar back against the thighs without changing the position of the rest of the body. As the bar moves into light contact with the thighs, he or she will push with the legs against the floor and extend the hips to perform the final extension of a clean pull.

AKA: Clean push back + hang clean pull.

Notes: Using straps will allow a looser grip on the bar, which will typically allow the athlete to relax the arms and focus more on engaging the lats and shoulders.

Purpose: This is a remedial exercise to help individuals who have problems controlling the path of the bar above the knees due to either strength or a misunderstanding of technique or timing. The movement will strengthen the back, lats and shoulders to improve the lifter's ability to stay over the bar and keep it close to the body, and also teach the lifter how to engage the lats to maintain that proximity of the bar.

Programming: The Everett clean pull can be performed immediately prior to cleans in a workout as a technique primer to help the performance of the subsequent cleans. It can also be performed toward the end of a training session if being used as more of a strength exercise. Sets of 3-5 reps are appropriate.

Variations: The lift can be done with or without the clean pull; if the focus is strength in staying over the bar and keeping it close to the body, the exercise can be limited to the movement of the bar out and back to the body in the hang position. If performing the complete movement with the clean pull, it can be done with or without a pause after moving the bar back to the legs.

Floating Clean Deadlift

The first rep of the floating clean deadlift will be the same as a clean deadlift. After standing, the lifter will return to the starting position under control and bring the plates as close to the floor as possible without allowing them to touch, then begin the next rep from this position without setting the bar down on the floor. The lifter should pause momentarily in the bottom position between reps.

AKA: No-touch clean deadlift, hang clean deadlift.

Notes: The tempo should be controlled in this movement, particularly during the eccentric portion. Because the primary purpose is to build postural strength and balance, using a more controlled tempo is more effective by allowing the lifter to make adjustments as necessary to maintain the proper position and balance and train it as intended.

Purpose: The floating clean deadlift is a good exercise to develop pulling strength in the snatch, strengthen the proper posture, and emphasize strength in the bottom range of the pull (from the floor to the knee), particularly to train the correct position and posture during that pull.

Programming: Generally the floating clean deadlift should be done for 2-6 reps per set with anywhere from 80%-110% of the lifter's best clean depending on the lifter and how it fits into the program. In any case, the weight should not exceed what the lifter can do with proper positioning or it is failing to achieve the intended purpose. As a heavy strength exercise, it should normally be placed toward the end of a workout.

Variations: The floating clean deadlift can be performed standing on a riser to allow the same range of motion that would be possible from the floor, but without the bar ever resting on the floor. The lift can also be done as a halting clean deadlift or clean segment deadlift, and a longer pause can be added in the bottom position.

Floating Clean Deadlift on Riser

The floating clean deadlift on riser is identical to the floating clean deadlift, but the athlete is standing on a riser. The athlete needs to set the starting position properly with the same arm orientation and back angle—the only difference should be that the hips and knees are bent more to accommodate the deficit. The correct posture must be maintained on the way up, and the lifter should maintain the same posture on the way down. Each rep will stop with the bottom of the plates level with the top of the riser so that the range of motion is identical to that of a deadlift from the floor but without the weight being supported.

AKA: Riser floating clean deadlift, no-touch clean deadlift on riser, hang clean deadlift on riser.

Notes: The tempo should be controlled in this movement, particularly during the eccentric portion. Because the primary purpose is to build postural strength and balance, using a more controlled tempo is more effective by allowing the lifter to make adjustments as necessary to maintain the proper position and balance and train it as intended. Riser height can be anywhere from 1"-4". If the riser is being used only to allow a full depth starting position, the height is unimportant; if the riser is being used to further strengthen the pull from the floor during the first rep, a higher riser may be appropriate.

Purpose: The floating clean deadlift on riser is a good exercise to develop pulling strength in the clean, and emphasize strength in the bottom range of the pull (from the floor to the knee), particularly to train the correct position and posture during that pull. The advantage over the floating clean deadlift is that standing on the riser allows the bar to move down to the same position it would be during a normal pull from the floor but without resting on the floor.

Programming: Generally the floating clean deadlift on riser should be done for 2-6 reps per set with anywhere from 80%-110% of the lifter's best clean depending on the lifter and how it fits into the program. In any case, the weight should not exceed what the lifter can do with proper positioning or it is failing to achieve the intended purpose. As a heavy strength exercise, it should normally be placed toward the end of a workout.

Variations: The floating clean deadlift on riser can be performed as a halting clean deadlift or clean segment deadlift, and a longer pause can be added in the bottom position.

Floating Clean Pull

The floating clean pull is a variation of the clean pull in which the bar doesn't return all the way to the floor between reps. The first rep of each set will be the same as a clean pull. After reaching full extension, the athlete will return to the starting position under control and bring the plates as close to the floor as possible without allowing them to touch. The next rep will begin from this position, without setting the bar down on the floor, after a momentary pause.

AKA: No-touch clean pull, hang clean pull.

Purpose: The floating clean pull is a good exercise to develop pulling strength in the clean, and emphasize strength in the bottom range of the pull (from the floor to the knee), particularly to train the correct position and posture during that pull.

Programming: Generally the floating clean pull should be done for 2-5 reps per set anywhere from 80%-110% of the lifter's best clean depending on the lifter and how it fits into the program. In any case, the weight should not exceed what the lifter can do with reasonably proper positioning and speed in the final extension and maintenance of the proper position at the bottom in between reps. As a strength exercise, it should be placed toward the end of a workout, but because it also involves some speed and technique, it's generally best placed before more basic strength work like squats.

Variations: The floating clean pull can be performed standing on a riser to allow the same range of motion that would be possible from the floor, but without the bar ever resting on the floor. The lift can also be done as a clean high-pull, and a longer pause can be added in the bottom position.

Floating Clean Pull on Riser

The floating clean pull on riser is identical the clean pull on riser, with the exception that the bar does not return all the way to the floor after the first rep. After reaching full extension, the athlete will return to a position in which the bottom of the plates are even with the top of the riser—in other words, this position is identical to the starting position from the floor, but in this case the weights are not in contact with the platform. Subsequent reps start from this position after a momentary pause.

AKA: No-touch clean pull on riser, hang clean pull on riser, riser hang clean pull, riser floating clean pull.

Notes: Riser heights can be anywhere from 1"-4" depending on the athlete's ability (based on height and mobility) or the degree of challenge desired. The athlete can also stand on bumper plates or any other hard, flat, stable surface. Riser heights should not exceed what allows the lifter to set a proper starting position.

Purpose: The floating clean pull on riser is a good exercise to develop pulling strength in the clean, and emphasize strength in the bottom range of the pull (from the floor to the knee), particularly to train the correct position and posture during that pull. The advantage over the floating clean pull is that the lifter can achieve the same starting position as in the clean while still preventing the weights from resting on the floor.

Programming: Generally the floating clean pull should be done for 2-5 reps per set anywhere from 80%-110% of the lifter's best clean depending on the lifter and how it fits into the program. In any case, the weight should not exceed what the lifter can do with reasonably proper positioning and speed in the final extension and maintenance of the proper position at the bottom in between reps. As a strength exercise, it should be placed toward the end of a workout, but because it also involves some speed and technique, it's generally best placed before more basic strength work like squats.

Variations: The floating clean pull can be performed as a clean high-pull, with a longer pause in the bottom position, with or without straps, and with a slow eccentric movement. Slower eccentric speeds in particular will increase the strengthening of pulling posture and back arch strength.

Halting Clean Deadlift

The halting clean deadlift is a pull variation that stops short of full extension at the top to strengthen and reinforce the position of the lifter over the bar during the pull of the clean. The athlete will perform a clean deadlift up to the designated height (usually mid-thigh), keeping the shoulders over the bar, and hold this position for 3 seconds before returning the bar to the floor.

Notes: Halting clean deadlifts can be performed without a pause in the top position (i.e. just stopping at a point prior to full extension but not holding the position at that point), but this limits the potential effectiveness of the exercise.

Purpose: The halting clean deadlift is primarily a tool to strengthen an athlete to allow him or her to be able to stay over the bar long enough during the pull of the clean. It also helps reinforce position and balance earlier in the pull because it's typically performed at a more controlled speed. Finally, it can help improve the lifter's timing of the initiation of the second pull in the clean.

Programming: Generally the halting clean deadlift should be done for 2-6 reps per set with a 2-3 second pause and anywhere from 80%-110% of the lifter's best clean depending on the lifter and how it fits into the program. In any case, the weight should not exceed what the lifter can do with proper positioning or it is failing to achieve the intended purpose. As a heavy strength exercise, it should normally be placed toward the end of a workout.

Variations: The halting clean deadlift can be performed standing on a riser, with the pause at different points, or with different pause times. The lift can also be done with either a static start or dynamic start. Multiple pause positions may be used, turning the exercise into a halting clean segment deadlift.

Halting Clean Deadlift on Riser

The halting clean deadlift on riser is identical to the halting clean deadlift with the exception that the lifter is standing on a riser or platform. The key is ensuring that the starting position is set properly with the same back angle and arm orientation that would be used from the floor—the only difference should be more bending of the knees and hips to account for the deficit.

Notes: Riser heights can be anywhere from 1"-4" depending on the athlete's ability (based on height and mobility) or the degree of challenge desired. The athlete can also stand on bumper plates or any other hard, flat, stable surface. Riser heights should not exceed what allows the lifter to set a proper start-ing position.

Purpose: The halting clean deadlift is primarily a tool to strengthen an athlete to allow him or her to be able to stay over the bar long enough during the pull of the clean. It also helps reinforce position and balance earlier in the pull because it's typically performed at a more controlled speed. Finally, it can help improve the lifter's timing of the initiation of the second pull in the clean.

Lifts from risers are used primarily to strengthen the legs for the pull from the floor, and to help train the proper balance, posture and initial movement from the floor. They can also be used simply for variety, and as a way to introduce more demand from the lift earlier in a training cycle that can then be reduced over time by reducing the riser height and/or eliminating the riser.

Programming: Generally the halting clean deadlift on riser should be done for 2-6 reps per set with a 3 second pause and anywhere from 80%-110% of the lifter's best clean depending on the lifter and how it fits into the program. In any case, the weight should not exceed what the lifter can do with proper positioning or it is failing to achieve the intended purpose. As a heavy strength exercise, it should normally be placed toward the end of a workout.

Variations: The halting clean deadlift can be performed on the floor, with the pause at different points, and with different pause times. The lift can also be done with either a static start or dynamic start. Multiple pause positions may be done, turning the exercise into a halting clean segment deadlift on riser.

Hang Clean

The hang clean is performed identically to the clean, but with a starting position at some point above the floor. Hang positions include High-Hang: Upper thigh; Mid-hang: Mid-thigh; Hang: Top of knee caps; Knee: Bar at knee caps; Below knee: Bar below patellar tendon.

Notes: Straps are not recommended for hang clean or any clean variations because of the risk of wrist injury. The hang position needs to be specified when prescribing the hang clean. Generally if no qualifier is present, a hang snatch is done from a starting position with the bar just above the knee.

Purpose: The purpose of the hang clean can vary depending on its application. It can be an exercise to help teach beginners to clean that is often easier than lifting from the floor because of the abbreviated movement and the ability to ensure proper positioning and balance at the start of the second pull. As a training exercise, the common purpose is to develop better force production in the extension and more aggressiveness in the pull under due to the limited time and distance to accelerate and elevate the bar. Another purpose is use as a lighter clean variation (often an alternative to the power clean) for lighter training days (weights naturally limited for most lifters relative to the clean, and somewhat less work for the legs and back to allow more recovery for subsequent training sessions).

Programming: Hang clean reps should be kept to 1-3 per set. If being used for technique work, weights should remain light (around 75% or lighter); for work on aggressiveness in the extension and/or pull under the bar, heavier weights should be used (75% and above); for use as a lighter clean variation on a lighter training day, weights can be as heavy or light as needed for the athlete at that time, but a loose guideline would be about 70-80%.

Variations: The hang clean can be done from any hang position—any starting point above the floor itself qualifies as a hang clean. It can be done with or without a pause in the hang position (i.e. with a countermovement or from a dead stop), and without the hook grip to emphasize grip strength.

Hang Clean Pull

The hang clean pull is a variation of the clean pull that begins in the hang position instead of with the bar on the floor. The lifter will stand with the bar in a clean grip at arms' length, then hinge at the hips and bend the knees until the bar is at the prescribed hang position. He or she will accelerate the bar upward aggressively with violent leg and hip extension, keeping the bar close to the body and allowing it to contact at the upper thighs. The movement should be directed vertically with a focus on extending the body upward, although to maintain balance, it will be leaned back slightly. The arms are not engaged in the movement, but remain relaxed in extension. The

shoulders should be shrugged up after the completion of leg and hip extension to continue the bar's upward path and allow it to stay against the body. The aggressiveness of the push against the ground should result in the lifter's heels rising off the floor as the extension is completed. The lifter will return the bar to the hang position for the next rep with the same posture used to lift it.

Hang Positions: High-Hang: Upper thigh; Mid-hang: Mid-thigh; Hang: Top of knee caps; Knee: Bar at knee caps; Below knee: Bar below patellar tendons.

Purpose: The hang clean pull can be used to focus on the final extension of the pull, to reduce the loading on the legs and back for recovery purposes, or for practice and strengthening of posture and balance in a specific position.

Programming: Generally the hang clean pull should be done for 2-5 reps per set anywhere from 80%-110% of the lifter's best clean depending on the lifter and how it fits into the program. It's generally used as a lighter clean pull variation during periods of lighter training, as way to train the final extension of the pull, or as part of a complex with other clean pull variations. As a strength exercise, it should be placed toward the end of a workout, but because it also involves some speed and technique, it's generally best placed before more basic strength work like squats. With lighter weights, it can be used before cleans as a technique primer.

Variations: The hang clean pull can be performed from different hang positions (commonly below the knee or at the knee), with or without straps, with a pause in the hang position, and with a prescribed eccentric speed.

Hang Power Clean

The hang power clean is performed identically to the power clean, but with a starting position at some point above the floor. Hang positions include High-Hang: Upper thigh; Mid-hang: Mid-thigh; Hang: Top of knee caps; Knee: Bar at knee caps; Below knee: Bar below patellar tendons.

Notes: The use of straps is discouraged with this and any clean variation because of the risk of wrist injury.

Purpose: The purpose of the hang power clean

should remain light (around 70% of the clean or lighter); for work on aggressiveness in the extension and/or pull under the bar, heavier weights should be used (70% and above); for use as a lighter clean variation on a lighter training day, weights can be as heavy or light as needed for the athlete at that time, but a loose guideline would be about 70-80%.

Variations: The hip clean can be done with or without a countermovement, and with or without the hook grip.

Muscle Clean

The muscle clean is a much less commonly used exercise than its snatch counterpart, the muscle snatch, but can be very useful in many cases. The lifter will start with the bar on the floor in the clean starting position, making sure the elbows are oriented to the sides (arms internally rotated), then lift the bar as he or she would for a clean until reaching the top of the upward extension of the body. At this point, rather than repositioning the feet and pulling down into a squat under the barbell as would be done in a clean, the athlete will keep the knees straight and the body extended and pull the elbows up as high as possible and out to the sides, keeping the bar in immediate proximity to the body. Once the elbows reach maximal height, the lifter will bring them around the bar and into the clean rack position quickly but smoothly. The legs must remain straight once extended in the pull, and the bar must move continuously with constant tension—there should be no pausing or hesitation during the lift.

Notes: It's helpful to think of the movement as a clean high-pull with an added turnover of the bar afterward. This will help reinforce the idea of lifting the elbows high and to the sides before the turnover. If the elbows don't move properly, the purpose of the exercise is defeated.

Purpose: The muscle clean is helpful at lighter weights to learn and reinforce the proper upper body mechanics of the third pull of the clean—in particular, it's useful for learning how to deliver the bar precisely and smoothly into the rack position for lifters who have a tendency to allow the bar to crash on them. At more challenging weights, the muscle clean will help strengthen the third pull of the clean.

Programming: The muscle clean can be performed early in a training session as a technique primer, or as a training exercise. It can also be performed at the end of a training session as accessory work. Use 3-5 reps per set generally, although the muscle clean can also be done for heavy singles and doubles.

Variations: The muscle clean can be performed from the hang or from blocks, and can also be done without a hook grip to strengthen the grip.

Power Clean

The power clean is the most basic variation of the clean; the only difference is the height at which the bar is received. The lift is performed identically to the clean until the third pull. The athlete will need to elevate the bar adequately and pull under quickly enough to fix the bar in the rack position before squatting below parallel. The bar must be racked and all downward movement stopped with the lifter's thighs above horizontal. More information on the power clean can be found in the Learning the Clean chapter of the book.

Notes: Coaches and athletes sometimes have different definitions of what constitutes a "power" receiving position. Most commonly, anything received with the thighs horizontal or higher is considered a power lift. Others will require the knee to be bent to no more than 90 degrees, and others will count only lifts with the thighs above horizontal (i.e. a lift with thighs exactly horizontal is too low). Some lifters will also intentionally receive power cleans with a much wider foot stance than in the clean. This makes arresting the downward movement easier, but also means that the lift cannot continue into a full squat if the bar isn't elevated adequately.

Purpose: The power clean can be used to train speed and force production in both the second pull and the third pull by limiting the amount of time and distance the lifter has available to get under the bar, or as a lighter clean variation for lighter training days. The power clean can also be useful as part of a learning progression for beginners, or as a variation for individuals who are not mobile enough to sit into a deep front squat.

Programming: Power cleans should generally be programmed with 1-3 reps. They can be performed

can vary depending on its application. It can be an exercise to help teach beginners to clean that is often easier than lifting from the floor because of the abbreviated movement and the ability to ensure proper positioning and balance at the start of the second pull, and the power receiving position reduces the demand on mobility. As a training exercise, the common purpose is to develop better force production in the extension and more aggressiveness in the pull under due to the limited time and distance to accelerate and elevate the bar, and the limited movement down under the bar. Another purpose is use as a lighter clean variation for lighter training days (weights naturally limited relative to the power clean, and somewhat less work for the legs and back due to both the hang start and power receiving position to allow more recovery for subsequent training sessions).

Programming: Hang power clean reps should be kept to 1-3 per set. If being used for technique work, weights should remain light (around 75% or lighter); for work on aggressiveness in the extension and/or pull under the bar, heavier weights should be used (75% and above); for use as a lighter clean variation on a lighter training day, weights can be as heavy or light as needed for the athlete at that time, but a loose guideline would be about 70-80%; for more speed work, weights should generally be in the 65-75% range.

Variations: The hang power clean can be done from any hang position—any starting point above the floor itself qualifies as a hang power clean. The lift can be done with or without a pause in the hang position (i.e. with a countermovement or from a dead stop). It can also be done without the hook grip to emphasize grip strength.

High-Pull Clean

The high-pull clean is simply a clean in which the athlete delays the squat under the bar until after he or she has started pulling the elbows up to over-emphasize upward extension.

Purpose: The high-pull clean can be used as a remedial or technique exercise to emphasize a longer or more complete extension for lifters who have a tendency to cut the pull short, and especially quit pushing with the legs against the floor too ear-

ly. It can also be used to reinforce the proper arm mechanics of the pull under the bar. This exercise should not be used for lifters who have bad habits of engaging the arms too early or hesitating at the top of the extension.

Programming: The high-pull clean should be done for 1-3 reps per set with relatively light weights. It can be done after primary technique and speed-oriented lifts (e.g. snatch, clean or jerk), or it can be done before cleans as a technique primer.

Variations: The high-pull clean can be done without moving the feet from the floor, or from the hang or blocks.

Hip Clean

The athlete will stand tall with the bar in a clean grip. He or she will hinge at the hips and bend the knees slightly, keeping the bar near the crease of the hips (as close to it as possible), and initiate the hang clean from this position. Typically hip cleans are done with a countermovement; that is, the lifter moves into the hang position and then immediately cleans with no pause in the hang position.

AKA: Clean from hip.

Notes: The hip clean is a less useful exercise than the hip snatch due to the fact that the narrower grip of the clean typically means that the bar naturally contacts the lifter's body on the upper thigh rather than the crease of the hips as it would in the snatch. This means that in reality, the bar isn't actually tucked into the hips in this exercise, making it more of a high-hang clean, or that the athlete will bend the elbows to tuck the bar into the hip, which will both encourage bad habits in the clean and reduce the exercise's utility due to the difference in position relative to the clean. Straps should not be used because of the injury risk.

Purpose: The purpose of the hip clean is to force an extremely aggressive final extension in the and to practice the proper position and balance this stage of the lift, in particular the placement the bar in the crease of the hips. It will also help prove the pull under the bar due to the limited of the athlete to accelerate and elevate the bar

Programming: Hip clean reps should be 1-3 per set. If being used for technique work,

can vary depending on its application. It can be an exercise to help teach beginners to clean that is often easier than lifting from the floor because of the abbreviated movement and the ability to ensure proper positioning and balance at the start of the second pull, and the power receiving position reduces the demand on mobility. As a training exercise, the common purpose is to develop better force production in the extension and more aggressiveness in the pull under due to the limited time and distance to accelerate and elevate the bar, and the limited movement down under the bar. Another purpose is use as a lighter clean variation for lighter training days (weights naturally limited relative to the power clean, and somewhat less work for the legs and back due to both the hang start and power receiving position to allow more recovery for subsequent training sessions).

Programming: Hang power clean reps should be kept to 1-3 per set. If being used for technique work, weights should remain light (around 75% or lighter); for work on aggressiveness in the extension and/or pull under the bar, heavier weights should be used (75% and above); for use as a lighter clean variation on a lighter training day, weights can be as heavy or light as needed for the athlete at that time, but a loose guideline would be about 70-80%; for more speed work, weights should generally be in the 65-75% range.

Variations: The hang power clean can be done from any hang position—any starting point above the floor itself qualifies as a hang power clean. The lift can be done with or without a pause in the hang position (i.e. with a countermovement or from a dead stop). It can also be done without the hook grip to emphasize grip strength.

High-Pull Clean

The high-pull clean is simply a clean in which the athlete delays the squat under the bar until after he or she has started pulling the elbows up to over-emphasize upward extension.

Purpose: The high-pull clean can be used as a remedial or technique exercise to emphasize a longer or more complete extension for lifters who have a tendency to cut the pull short, and especially quit pushing with the legs against the floor too ear-

ly. It can also be used to reinforce the proper arm mechanics of the pull under the bar. This exercise should not be used for lifters who have bad habits of engaging the arms too early or hesitating at the top of the extension.

Programming: The high-pull clean should be done for 1-3 reps per set with relatively light weights. It can be done after primary technique and speed-oriented lifts (e.g. snatch, clean or jerk), or it can be done before cleans as a technique primer.

Variations: The high-pull clean can be done without moving the feet from the floor, or from the hang or blocks.

Hip Clean

The athlete will stand tall with the bar in a clean grip. He or she will hinge at the hips and bend the knees slightly, keeping the bar near the crease of the hips (as close to it as possible), and initiate the hang clean from this position. Typically hip cleans are done with a countermovement; that is, the lifter moves into the hang position and then immediately cleans with no pause in the hang position.

AKA: Clean from hip.

Notes: The hip clean is a less useful exercise than the hip snatch due to the fact that the narrower grip of the clean typically means that the bar naturally contacts the lifter's body on the upper thigh rather than the crease of the hips as it would in the snatch. This means that in reality, the bar isn't actually tucked into the hips in this exercise, making it more of a high-hang clean, or that the athlete will bend the elbows to tuck the bar into the hip, which will both encourage bad habits in the clean and reduce the exercise's utility due to the difference in position relative to the clean. Straps should not be used because of the injury risk.

Purpose: The purpose of the hip clean is to force an extremely aggressive final extension in the pull and to practice the proper position and balance at this stage of the lift, in particular the placement of the bar in the crease of the hips. It will also help improve the pull under the bar due to the limited ability of the athlete to accelerate and elevate the bar first.

Programming: Hip clean reps should be kept to 1-3 per set. If being used for technique work, weights should remain light (around 70% of the clean or lighter); for work on aggressiveness in the extension and/or pull under the bar, heavier weights should be used (70% and above); for use as a lighter clean variation on a lighter training day, weights can be as heavy or light as needed for the athlete at that time, but a loose guideline would be about 70-80%.

Variations: The hip clean can be done with or without a countermovement, and with or without the hook grip.

Muscle Clean

The muscle clean is a much less commonly used exercise than its snatch counterpart, the muscle snatch, but can be very useful in many cases. The lifter will start with the bar on the floor in the clean starting position, making sure the elbows are oriented to the sides (arms internally rotated), then lift the bar as he or she would for a clean until reaching the top of the upward extension of the body. At this point, rather than repositioning the feet and pulling down into a squat under the barbell as would be done in a clean, the athlete will keep the knees straight and the body extended and pull the elbows up as high as possible and out to the sides, keeping the bar in immediate proximity to the body. Once the elbows reach maximal height, the lifter will bring them around the bar and into the clean rack position quickly but smoothly. The legs must remain straight once extended in the pull, and the bar must move continuously with constant tension—there should be no pausing or hesitation during the lift.

Notes: It's helpful to think of the movement as a clean high-pull with an added turnover of the bar afterward. This will help reinforce the idea of lifting the elbows high and to the sides before the turnover. If the elbows don't move properly, the purpose of the exercise is defeated.

Purpose: The muscle clean is helpful at lighter weights to learn and reinforce the proper upper body mechanics of the third pull of the clean—in particular, it's useful for learning how to deliver the bar precisely and smoothly into the rack position for lifters who have a tendency to allow the bar to crash on them. At more challenging weights, the muscle clean will help strengthen the third pull of the clean.

Programming: The muscle clean can be performed early in a training session as a technique primer, or as a training exercise. It can also be performed at the end of a training session as accessory work. Use 3-5 reps per set generally, although the muscle clean can also be done for heavy singles and doubles.

Variations: The muscle clean can be performed from the hang or from blocks, and can also be done without a hook grip to strengthen the grip.

Power Clean

The power clean is the most basic variation of the clean; the only difference is the height at which the bar is received. The lift is performed identically to the clean until the third pull. The athlete will need to elevate the bar adequately and pull under quickly enough to fix the bar in the rack position before squatting below parallel. The bar must be racked and all downward movement stopped with the lifter's thighs above horizontal. More information on the power clean can be found in the Learning the Clean chapter of the book.

Notes: Coaches and athletes sometimes have different definitions of what constitutes a "power" receiving position. Most commonly, anything received with the thighs horizontal or higher is considered a power lift. Others will require the knee to be bent to no more than 90 degrees, and others will count only lifts with the thighs above horizontal (i.e. a lift with thighs exactly horizontal is too low). Some lifters will also intentionally receive power cleans with a much wider foot stance than in the clean. This makes arresting the downward movement easier, but also means that the lift cannot continue into a full squat if the bar isn't elevated adequately.

Purpose: The power clean can be used to train speed and force production in both the second pull and the third pull by limiting the amount of time and distance the lifter has available to get under the bar, or as a lighter clean variation for lighter training days. The power clean can also be useful as part of a learning progression for beginners, or as a variation for individuals who are not mobile enough to sit into a deep front squat.

Programming: Power cleans should generally be programmed with 1-3 reps. They can be performed at maximal effort for training or testing at this rep range. Even at maximal weight, the power clean can serve as a lighter exercise for lighter training days between full heavy clean days. For speed training, weights of 60-75% are more appropriate, and for general use in lighter training days, 70-80% weights are typical.

Variations: The primary variations of the power clean include hang power cleans and block power cleans. It can also be done without the hook grip for a grip strength emphasis.

Power Clean into Front Squat

The power clean into front squat is a hybrid exercise that combines a power clean and front squat into a single exercise, but is different from a power clean + front squat complex. The lifter will perform a power clean as usual, but hold in the power receiving position for 2-3 seconds, and then sit directly into a front squat and recover to standing.

Notes: This exercise is not the same as a power clean + front squat complex because the athlete never stands completely between the power clean and squat.

Purpose: The primary purpose of the exercise is to allow the athlete to practice a better receiving position for the clean by meeting the bar in a relatively high position with the proper stance, posture and resistance against the bar. It can be thought of as a clean with a pause partway under the bar. It can also help force athletes to use the same receiving stance in the power clean as in the clean.

Programming: The power clean into front squat should generally be programmed with 1-3 reps. It can be performed for maximal effort singles like a power clean would be, but generally 2-3 reps at submaximal weights is more appropriate as it's more of a technical exercise. Typically intensity will be about 70-85% of the lifter's best power clean.

Variations: The power clean into front squat can be combined in a complex with a clean following it to first practice meeting the bar properly, and then put that technique to use in a subsequent clean.

Press in Clean

The press in clean is a mobility and strength exercise for the receiving position of the clean. With a clean grip and the bar in the jerk rack position, the lifter will sit into the bottom of a squat. From this bottom position, he or she will press the bar up into the proper jerk overhead position, making sure to press in a direct line by getting the head back out of the way, locking the elbows securely and squeezing the shoulder blades together aggressively. The overhead position should be held momentarily before returning the bar to the rack position at a controlled speed. The bar does not need to be completely reset in the rack position before subsequent reps as long as the bar is brought all the way down to touch the shoulders between reps. The squat stance should be exactly what is used in the clean with the feet flat and balance correct. The trunk should be held rigidly throughout the set in exactly the same posture used when receiving the clean.

AKA: Sots press (for Viktor Sots).

Notes: This exercise can be done even by lifters who are not mobile enough to bring the bar all the way into the overhead position—the attempt to do so will be an active stretch for the upper and lower body. However, if there is pain associated with the effort, it should be avoided.

Purpose: The press in clean helps improve clean receiving position mobility in the ankles, hips, thoracic spine and shoulders. It also helps improve trunk stability and strength, back extension strength (particularly mid and upper back), upper body overhead strength, and balance in the receiving position.

Programming: The press in clean is most commonly used at the beginning of a training session before cleans to reinforce and prepare the receiving position. Sets of 3-5 reps are appropriate; weights need to be determined based on the abilities of the lifter, and may be limited to the empty barbell.

Variations: The press in clean can be started from the top down (i.e. the athlete will sit into the squat with the bar already overhead and then lower and press); it can be done with prescribed pauses in the overhead position (usually 2-3 seconds); and it can be done with completely resetting the bar in the rack position and beginning each rep from a dead stop.

Segment Clean

The segment clean is performed identically to the clean with the exception that there are one or more pauses included during the pull. The athlete will begin the lift as usual and pause and hold in the first prescribed position for 3 seconds. If more than one pause position is being used, the lifter will move to it and hold again. After the final pause position, the lifter will complete the clean as usual directly from the final pause position (no countermovement).

AKA: Pause clean.

Purpose: The primary purpose of the segment clean is to reinforce certain positions during the pull and strengthen the athlete to improve his or her ability to achieve those positions during the clean, or to reinforce the movement into or between certain positions. It can also be used as a hang clean variation to limit the distance and time the lifter has to accelerate and elevate the bar, improving rate of force development and aggressiveness. It can be used as a lighter clean variation on easier training days. Finally, the additional time the lifter must hold the bar and the additional acceleration will increase the grip strengthening effect.

Programming: Sets of 1-3 reps at weights anywhere from 70-100% of the lifter's best clean can be used (the less technically proficient the lifter is, the higher percentage of the clean he or she will be able to do as a segment clean). Weights should not exceed what can be done with proper positions and movement, as it then defeats the purpose of the exercise. Pauses of 3 seconds are typical, but can be shorter or longer.

Variations: The primary variations of the segment clean involve different pause positions. Most common is at the knee, but others include 1" off the floor, below the knee, and mid-thigh. Multiple pauses can be used as well—for example, 1" off the floor to ensure proper balance and posture, then mid-thigh to train staying over the bar long enough in the pull. It can be done without the hook grip or for even more grip work.

Segment Power Clean

The segment power clean is performed identically to the power clean with the exception that there are one or more pauses included during the pull. The athlete will begin the lift as usual and pause and hold in the first prescribed position for 3 seconds. If more than one pause position is being used, the lifter will move to it and hold again. After the final pause position, the lifter will complete the power clean as usual directly from the final pause position (no countermovement).

AKA: Pause power clean.

Purpose: The primary purpose of the segment power clean is to reinforce certain positions during the pull and strengthen the athlete to improve his or her ability to achieve those positions during the clean, or to reinforce the movement into or between certain positions. It can also be used as a hang power clean variation to limit the distance and time the lifter has to accelerate and elevate the bar, improving rate of force development and aggressiveness. As a power clean instead of a clean, it can be used as a lighter variation on easier training days, or to also work on speed. Finally, the additional time the lifter must hold the bar and the additional acceleration will increase the grip strengthening effect.

Programming: Sets of 1-3 reps at weights anywhere from 70-100% of the lifter's best power clean can be used (the less technically proficient the lifter is, the higher percentage of the power clean he or she will be able to do as a segment power clean). Weights should not exceed what can be done with proper positions and movement, as it then defeats the purpose of the exercise. Pauses of 3 seconds are typical, but can be shorter or longer.

Variations: The primary variations of the segment power clean involve different pause positions. Most common is at the knee, but others include 1" off the floor, below the knee, and mid-thigh. Multiple pauses can be used as well—for example, 1" off the floor to ensure proper balance and posture, then mid-thigh to train staying over the bar long enough in the pull. It can be done without the hook grip or for even more grip work.

Slow Pull Clean

The slow pull clean is simply a clean in which the athlete performs the first pull at a lower than natural speed. The athlete will take 3 or more seconds to move from the floor to mid-thigh, ensuring perfect position and balance. As the bar reaches mid-thigh, without slowing down or hesitating, the lifter will accelerate the bar aggressively with violent leg and hip extension to complete the clean.

Purpose: The slow pull clean can be used as a remedial or technique exercise to train the athlete to properly time the initiation of the second pull and to maintain the proper position over the bar until that point. As a training exercise, the slower speed will produce greater strengthening of the pulling posture, and because the second pull is being initiated with less existing upward momentum of the bar, it will force great power production and aggressiveness in both the final extension and the pull under the bar.

Programming: The slow pull clean should be done for 1-3 reps per set with weights that allow the proper timing and position. It can be done with light weights before cleans as a technique primer, or it can be used as its own training exercise with more difficult weights (70-80% generally, but can be taken as heavy as a maximum single).

Variations: The slow pull clean can be done without moving the feet from the floor, standing on a riser, as a power clean, or in a complex followed by a clean at regular speed. Clean pulls can also be done with this reduced initial pull speed.

Split Clean

The split clean was the traditional form of the clean until the 1950s and 1960s when the squat style now used today began to take over. Its primary use now is by masters lifters with limited mobility or injuries. Execution of the split clean is described in detail in the Learning the Clean chapter.

Purpose: The primary modern use of the split clean is to make cleaning possible for masters lifters or those otherwise limited in the receiving position by immobility or injuries. However, the lift can

also be used as a way to include more split footwork training for the jerk without adding additional exercises—for example, a lifter who needs split practice may perform split cleans where another athlete would perform power cleans, thereby addressing both purposes with a single exercise. In this case, the split position needs to match the jerk split position rather than being the more aggressive split used in deep split cleans.

Programming: If the split clean is the main clean variation used by the athlete, the programming for the lift is the same as for the squat clean. It can also be used in a similar manner as the power clean as a less taxing clean variation for lighter training days, or as a split footwork technique exercise. In any case, sets of 1-3 reps are recommended.

Stage Clean

The stage clean is an exercise that progressively builds from 2 or more partial pulling movements into a complete clean. The exact partial movements can be prescribed differently and specifically for each athlete at a given time to achieve certain goals. A basic example would be a clean pull to the knee, then a clean pull, and then a clean.

Notes: Stage clean is simply another way to write a complex of certain progressively more extensive pull or deadlift movements and a complete clean.

Purpose: The stage clean is useful for reinforcing proper balance, position and timing in the pull of the clean. It might be thought of as having technique primers built into the sets of cleans themselves rather than being performed in isolation before a clean workout. It can be used in this way as a technique exercise, or with heavier loading it can serve to improve speed, explosiveness and aggression in the clean by fatiguing the lifter prior to the clean itself.

Programming: The stage clean can be used as a warm-up for cleans, as a lighter clean variation between heavier clean workouts, or as a primary heavy clean variation during preparation mesocycles. Because each set is really 3 reps already, the stage clean should only be performed with 1-2 reps per set (which is really 3-6 reps). Intensities will range from 70% and up.

Tall Clean

The lifter will stand tall with a clean grip, the bar hanging at arms' length and the feet in the pulling position. He or she will then pull the elbows up and out aggressively, pick up the feet, and pull down as quickly as possible while replacing the feet flat on the floor in the receiving position and receiving the bar in the clean rack position. The athlete should attempt to rack the bar as quickly as possible, although it will be near the bottom of the squat. The feet should reconnect flat with the floor.

AKA: Clean pull-under, dead-hang clean.

Notes: This exercise is very intimidating at first and often seems impossible to lifters who have never performed it previously. The longer the athlete stands and thinks about it, the harder it will seem—lifters should get set and go immediately.

Purpose: The tall clean can help train and reinforce the proper mechanics of the pull under the bar, and train speed, aggressiveness, confidence and precision in the turnover.

Programming: The tall clean is a great technique primer prior to a clean training session for athletes who have a weak, slow pull under the bar, who need to focus on proper footwork in the third pull, or who need to improve the precision of the turnover. It can also be used at essentially any time in a program to strengthen the pull under or improve its speed and aggression. Sets of 1-3 reps are appropriate, and weights will be extremely light. Lifters should be careful of increasing the weight too much and unintentionally changing the exercise into a dip clean or high-hang clean. Like any technical exercise, improper execution defeats the purpose.

Variations: The tall clean can be started on flat feet or standing up on the balls of the feet.

Jerk Exercises

Drop to Split

The lifter will place the barbell behind the neck as for a back squat, being sure to use a fairly narrow grip and actively pulling the bar tightly against the body to ensure it doesn't shift during the exercise. The athlete will jump the feet out quickly into the jerk split position and absorb the weight tightly, making sure to land in the proper position with the weight balanced approximately evenly between the front and back foot, and keeping the trunk tight and upright. He or she will then recover by stepping back about a third of the way with the front foot, then stepping the back foot up to meet it.

AKA: Split drop.

Notes: This exercise can be very intimidating and may need to be introduced to a lifter with very light weights, although eventually heavy weights will be possible. If heavier weights are desired, the jump to split is more appropriate.

Purpose: The drop to split trains quick and accurate foot transition into the split position. It also strengthens the split receiving position for the jerk, which can often be a weakness that limits an athlete's jerk.

Programming: The drop to split should be done after the jerk and variants, but can be done before more strength-oriented work like squatting and pulling. Weights of up to 100% and more of the athlete's best jerk may be used for 1-5 reps, although 2-3 reps will be most common. Weights will be lighter than used in the jump to split. It can also be done with light weights before a jerk workout as a technique primer to practice footwork for 3-5 reps.

Variations: The drop to split can be done with a dip and drive of the legs first to create more time and space to split the feet. This will increase the weight

that can be used somewhat, and the lift can then more accurately be called a jump to split. It can be started from flat feet or on the toes.

Front Squat-Jerk

The front squat-jerk is a hybrid exercise that combines the front squat and jerk into a single movement. Note that this is not the same thing as a front squat + jerk, which is a complex of two distinct movements. The lifter will perform a front squat with the bar in the jerk rack position, accelerating up through the squat recovery as much as possible. As the lifter reaches the standing position, he or she will continue driving hard against the floor with the legs to push the bar up off the shoulders, then move the feet into the split position as he or she punches down under the bar into a locked-out overhead position. The lift can be thought of simply as a jerk that begins with a full squat rather than the normal dip and drive.

Notes: If the lifter is unable to front squat with a jerk rack position, he or she should get as close as possible and shift the position as he or she reaches the top of the squat to transition smoothly into the jerk.

Purpose: This exercise can be used to train more aggressive leg drive in the jerk and strengthen the drive by tiring the legs more prior to the final extension.

Programming: Sets of 1-3 reps are suggested with weights anywhere from 70% to the lifter's maximum jerk. Generally this exercise should be performed following any snatch variants and possibly before clean variants depending on what the intended emphasis of the workout is.

Variations: This movement can also be performed as a back squat with a jerk behind the neck.

Front Squat-Push Press

The front squat-push press is a hybrid exercise that combines the front squat and push press into a single movement. Note that this is not the same thing as a front squat + push press, which is a complex of two distinct movements. The lifter will perform a front squat with the bar in the jerk rack position, accelerating up through the squat recovery as much as possible. As he or she reaches the standing position, the lifter will continue driving hard against the floor with the legs to push the bar up off the shoulders and push it into the overhead position with the arms in the same way as a push press. This is simply a push press that begins with a full squat rather than the normal dip and drive.

Notes: If the lifter is unable to front squat with a jerk rack position, he or she should get as close as possible and shift the position as he or she reaches the top of the squat to transition smoothly into the push press.

Purpose: This exercise can be used as a warm-up, as a way to train more aggressive acceleration in the recovery of the squat, and as a way to train leg drive speed and aggressiveness for the clean or jerk.

Programming: As a warm-up or training exercise, sets of 3-5 reps are usually suggested, although singles and doubles may have a place if taking the weight up as heavy as possible. Used as a warm-up at the beginning of a training session, weights should remain light. If used as a training exercise, it should be placed after snatch, clean and jerk variants but before basic strength work with less of a speed component such as squats.

Variations: This movement can also be performed as a back squat with a push press behind the neck, or with a snatch grip push press behind the neck.

Jerk Balance

The jerk balance is a teaching drill, a remediation exercise, and a training exercise for the split jerk. Its execution is described in detail in the Learning the Jerk chapter.

Notes: The most common errors in this exercise are diving the chest forward and leaning too much weight on the front foot rather than stepping into the split with the front foot and hips and remaining equally balanced between the feet. The trunk should remain approximately vertical (only inclining forward slightly as required by a proper overhead position) and the weight evenly balanced between the front and back feet.

Purpose: The jerk balance is useful for teaching and practicing the proper movement of the body under the bar during the split jerk for athletes who have a habit of diving the head and chest through and leaving the hips behind the bar. It's also helpful for teaching better balance between the feet in the split position rather than overloading the front leg.

Programming: The jerk balance can be used as a technique primer before jerk training sessions, or as technique work at any other time. If used as a primer, light weights (as little as an empty bar) should be used. Sets of 2-5 reps are suggested with weights anywhere from 40%-70% of the lifter's maximum, but heavier weights should only be allowed if the lift is being done correctly—not only will it not be helpful if not done properly, it will reinforce the very problems it's supposed to correct.

Jerk Behind the Neck

The athlete will place the bar on the top of the traps with a jerk grip (as for a back squat) and the feet in the drive position with the weight balanced slightly more toward the heels and the full foot in contact with the floor. The lifter will bend slightly at the knees only, keeping the trunk vertical and the weight near the heels, and transition immediately at the bottom of this dip to drive aggressively with the legs against the floor to accelerate the barbell upward. As he or she finishes the extension of the legs, the athlete will begin pushing against the bar with the arms, quickly lifting the feet and transitioning them into the split position, punching the arms into a locked-out overhead position. The lifter will secure and stabilize the bar overhead before recovering from the split into a standing position with the bar still overhead.

AKA: Jerk bnk, BTN jerk, behind the neck jerk.

Notes: With the bar starting behind the neck, it

is already in the plane it should be in when overhead, and the trunk is already very slightly inclined as it should be in the overhead position, so the bar and trunk have directly vertical paths. The most common errors in this exercise are leaning the trunk forward and pushing the hips back during the dip. While the trunk will begin and remain inclined forward slightly because of the placement of the bar behind the neck, it's important that it not lean farther forward in the dip.

Purpose: The jerk behind the neck can serve a few purposes. Because the bar and trunk begin in the same positions they will need to end up in the receiving position, the direct paths simplify the movement and the exercise can serve as a good teaching or remediation exercise for lifters who have trouble getting the bar behind the neck overhead when jerking from the front. It can also be a substitute for the jerk during periods of injury or pain in the wrists, shoulders or elbows that prevent jerking from the front. Some lifters will be stronger and more confident from behind the neck, making the jerk behind the neck a way for them to get more weight overhead to develop both overhead strength and confidence in the jerk. Finally, often lifters will be able to better feel the proper timing of the push with the arms from behind the neck.

Programming: The jerk behind the neck can be programmed in the same way as the jerk—usually 1-3 reps from 70% up to the lifter's maximum jerk, and sometimes beyond. It can also be used as a technique primer with light weights, or as light technique work at any time.

Variations: Jerks from behind the neck can be done with any of the jerk receiving positions: split, power, push and squat.

Jerk Dip

The lifter will place the bar in the jerk rack position with the feet in the jerk drive stance. He or she will perform the dip of a jerk with maximal downward speed and brake as abruptly as possible at the bottom. It's critical that the position and balance be correct. Typically this exercise is done only for a single rep following cleans or front squats, but if done for multiple reps, the lifter should recover from the bottom of each dip at a natural pace—there is no explosive upward drive component. The braking at the bottom is the most important element of the exercise—if braking is not adequately quick, the weight and downward speed should reduced until it is appropriately abrupt.

Notes: The speed at which a lifter dips in this exercise may exceed the speed at which he or she dips during an actual jerk depending on the jerk style (i.e. strength or elastic). This is intentional in order to create more downward force for the legs to absorb and arrest.

Purpose: The jerk dip is intended to strengthen the bottom of the dip and train the legs to stop the downward force abruptly in order to improve the ability of the lifter to take advantage of the elastic rebound.

Programming: The jerk dip can be performed in isolation from a rack for 1-5 reps, but most commonly it's performed for a single rep at the end of a set of cleans or front squats as a some bonus work for the jerk. Weights can be very heavy and exceed the lifter's maximum jerk as long as the position, balance and timing are correct.

Variations: There are a few variations of the jerk dip that are considered distinct exercises (described in this chapter).

Jerk Dip Squat

The lifter will place the bar in the jerk rack position and the feet in the jerk drive position. Maintaining the same upright posture and balance used in the dip of the jerk, the lifter will bend at the knees only with a smooth and controlled tempo and stand again with the same controlled tempo, trying to maintain constant tension throughout the movement. This is not a quick, springy movement like the actual dip and drive of a jerk, but a controlled strength movement.

Notes: Avoid the temptation to load this exercise so heavily that the athlete changes the depth and position of the dip—it's only effective if the movement is correct.

Purpose: The jerk dip squat is a basic dip and drive strength exercise that helps develop strength and balance in the upright posture and knees-only movement needed for a solid jerk, and helps teach and reinforce the proper balance in the movement. It also strengthens the trunk and rack position.

Programming: The jerk dip squat can be used at very light weights to teach and practice the proper dip position and movement, or it can be done with very heavy weights, usually 80-110% and more of the lifter's best jerk, to strengthen the movement and position and build confidence. Dip squats can also be combined with jerks, clean & jerks, or cleans to create complexes that emphasize that part of the movement (e.g. clean + 3 jerk dip squats + jerk or clean + jerk dip squat).

Variations: There are a few variations of the jerk dip squat that are considered distinct exercises (described in this chapter). A pause can be added in the bottom of the dip or tempos can be assigned.

Jerk Drive

The lifter will place the bar in the jerk rack position with the feet in the jerk drive position. The athlete will dip and drive just as he or she does for the jerk, and push the bar up off the shoulders with the arms as high as possible after completing the leg drive (this will only be a few inches at most with heavy weights). It's important the lifter pull his or her head back out of the way just as would be done in the jerk to ensure the bar can move up rather than forward. The lifter will absorb the weight back onto the shoulders with a bend of the legs and reset in the standing position for the next rep.

AKA: Half jerk.

Notes: This exercise is often very difficult to perform correctly—many athletes will push the bar forward off of the shoulders, which makes it ineffective and even counterproductive. If the athlete can't perform it correctly, a different exercise such as a jerk dip squat should be used.

Purpose: The jerk drive strengthens the dip position and trains the explosiveness of the transition and upward drive with heavier weights than can be handled for the same number of reps or with the same frequency as the jerk itself. If done correctly, it can also train and reinforce the proper balance and dip position for the jerk and strengthen the posture.

Programming: The jerk drive can be performed from a rack for 3-5 reps with weights anywhere from 70%-100% or more of the lifter's best jerk. Weights can be very heavy as long as the position and balance are correct and the bar is pushed up rather than forward.

Variations: There are a few variations of the jerk drive that are considered distinct exercises (described in this chapter).

Jerk Rack Support

The jerk rack support is a simple static exercise to strengthen the jerk rack position, trunk and upper back for the jerk. The lifter will set up a bar in a power rack 2-3 inches below the height at which it would be when on the shoulders in a standing position. The lifter will step under the bar into the jerk rack position and then stand to lift the bar off the pins. The lifter will hold the positions for 3-10 seconds, actively maintaining a strong rack position, before returning the bar to the pins.

Notes: It's important to keep the shoulders lifted slightly in a proper rack position to prevent compression of the carotid arteries and dizziness. For longer holds, lifters will need to release some of their air as well.

Purpose: The jerk rack support strengthens the jerk rack position, upper back and the trunk, and can help with confidence by getting the lifter accustomed to the feel of heavy weights in the rack position.

Programming: This exercise should be placed at or near the end of a workout. Use weights of 100% and above of the lifter's best jerk for holds of 3-10 seconds.

Jerk Recovery

The jerk recovery is a variation of the jerk support that begins in the split position. The lifter will set up a barbell in a power rack at a height 2-3 inches below where it would be if overhead in the split jerk receiving position. The lifter will take a jerk grip on the bar and step into the split position underneath it, lowering into a position with locked elbows. It's important the lifter is balanced directly under the bar—some lifters like to hang off the bar to get centered and then place their feet in the split. With the trunk and upper back locked tightly, the lifter will push with the legs straight up to lift the bar off the pins. Once supported securely, he or she will recover from the split position into a standing position by stepping back about a third of the distance with the front foot, and then bringing the back foot forward to meet the front foot. He or she will lower the bar back onto the rack by bending at the knees.

Notes: The most difficult part of the exercise is usually the initial break of the bar off the rack and ensuring it's balanced. Ensuring tension against the bar and pushing off the front leg somewhat more than the back will help move the bar vertically instead of forward.

Purpose: The jerk recovery is a way to strengthen the overhead position and the split position that allows the use of weights beyond what the lifter can jerk, or at least can or should jerk at that time. It can also be used to practice the footwork of the recovery from the split, and actively maintaining the balance and position of the bar overhead during the recovery. It will also help with confidence in the jerk.

Programming: The jerk recovery should generally be placed at or near the end of a workout. Single lifts or 2-3 repetitions are most common. Weights can range anywhere from 90% to over 100% of the lifter's best jerk. Often a lifter can just work up to the heaviest possible single on a given day.

Variations: Additional hold times overhead can be added in either the split position after the bar is lifted from the rack or once recovered. The jerk recovery can also be done as a power or squat jerk for lifters who use one of those styles.

Jerk Spring

The lifter will place the bar in the jerk rack position with the feet in the jerk drive position. He or she will bend at the knees only just as for the jerk and transition quickly in the bottom, aiming for a springy, elastic bounce in the bottom, and repeat this springy transition for the prescribed reps (usually 3-5) in a continuous series. It's not necessary to stand completely in each rep, and there is no active upward acceleration of the bar.

Notes: This exercise relies on finding a rhythm to synchronize the movement with the whip of the bar.

The heavier the weight, the easier this is to feel because the bar will bend more. Braking at the bottom of the dip must be abrupt—if it is slow, the weight must be reduced.

Purpose: The jerk spring helps train the elasticity of the transition between the dip and drive of the jerk. It can be helpful for improving the rhythm of the movement, especially for lifters who are not naturally quick and springy in the dip and drive of their jerks. It will also help improve the lifter's ability to brake quickly in the dip.

Programming: The jerk spring can be performed in isolation from a rack for 1-5 reps, or it can be done at the end of a set of cleans or front squats as some bonus work for the jerk. Weights can be very heavy and exceed the lifter's maximum jerk as long as the position and balance are correct and the movement remains quick and springy rather than slowing down into a grinding movement.

Variations: There are a few similar and related exercises to improve the jerk dip and/or drive (described in this chapter).

Jerk Support

The lifter will set up a barbell in a power rack at a height 2-3 inches below where it would be if overhead in a standing position with a jerk grip. The lifter will take a jerk grip on the bar and bend the knees slightly to position him- or herself under the bar with locked elbows in the proper overhead position. It's important the lifter is balanced directly under the bar—some lifters like to hang off the bar to get centered and then place their feet on the floor. With the trunk and upper back locked tightly, the athlete will push with the legs straight up to lift the bar off the pins and hold steady for the prescribed time—usually 3-5 seconds—then lower the bar back onto the rack by bending at the knees.

Notes: The most difficult part of the exercise is usually the initial break of the bar off the rack and ensuring it's balanced. It's important to ensure the upper back and trunk are locked in tightly and to squeeze the bar up off the pins rather than trying to lift it abruptly.

Purpose: The jerk support is a way to strengthen the overhead position for the jerk that allows the use of weights beyond what the lifter can jerk, or at least can or should jerk at that time. It can also help with confidence in the jerk.

Programming: The jerk recovery should generally be placed at or near the end of a workout. Single lifts or 2-3 repetitions are most common. Weights can range anywhere from 90% to over 100% of the lifter's best jerk. Often a lifter can just work up to the heaviest possible single on a given day.

Variations: The main variation of the jerk support is another exercise called the jerk recovery. The jerk support can also be performed in a split position without recovery to standing.

Jump to Split

The lifter will secure the barbell behind the neck as for a back squat, being sure to use a fairly narrow grip, and actively pulling the bar tightly against the body to ensure it doesn't shift during the exercise. The athlete will dip at the knees and drive upward slightly like a jerk with less upward power—just enough to create some time and space to split the feet. He or she will jump the feet out quickly into the jerk split position and absorb the weight tightly, making sure to land in the proper position with the weight balanced approximately evenly between the front and back foot, and keeping the trunk tight and upright. The lifter will recover by stepping back about a third of the way with the front foot, then stepping the back foot up to meet it.

Notes: This exercise can be very intimidating and may need to be introduced to a lifter with very light weights, although eventually heavy weights will be possible.

Purpose: The jump to split strengthens the split receiving position for the jerk, which can often be a weakness that limits an athlete's jerk. It also trains quick and accurate foot transition into the split position.

Programming: The jump to split should be done after the jerk and variants, but can be done before more strength-oriented work like squatting and pulling. Weights of up to 100% and more of the athlete's best jerk may be used for 1-5 reps, although 2-3 reps

will be most common. It can also be done with light weights before a jerk workout as a technique primer to practice footwork for 3-5 reps.

Variations: The jump to split can be done without any upward drive—that is, the athlete will just pick up and split the feet with no upward movement of the bar first. This will limit the weight that can be used somewhat, and the lift can then more accurately be called a drop to split.

Pause Jerk

The lifter will secure the bar in the jerk rack position with the feet in the jerk drive position, keeping the weight balanced toward the heels while maintaining full foot contact with the floor. He or she will dip and hold in the bottom position for 3 seconds, then drive aggressively with the legs against the floor with no preceding countermovement to accelerate the barbell upward and complete the jerk.

AKA: Jerk with pause.

Notes: Because the split jerk is the overwhelmingly dominant competitive jerk style, the term *jerk* implies split jerk except for athletes who use a different style as their primary jerk.

Purpose: Because the pause limits the power of the subsequent drive, it can be used as a way to force better power generation in the drive. It can be used to help train and reinforce the proper posture and balance in the dip for athletes who shift forward or collapse in the dip, or shift forward in the drive. It can also be used with light weights as a technique primer before jerk workouts for athletes with the aforementioned problems.

Programming: Sets of 1-3 reps are suggested with weights anywhere from 70% to the lifter's maximum jerk. Generally this exercise should be performed following any snatch variants and possibly before clean variants depending on what the intended emphasis of the workout is. As a technique primer before a jerk workout, weights should remain below 60%.

Variations: The pause jerk can be done with any style of jerk: power jerk, push jerk or squat jerk in addition to split jerk. Any of these pause jerk variations may also be performed from behind the neck.

Power Jerk

The power jerk is a jerk variation in which the feet land in the squat position rather than in the split, and the lifter does not squat below parallel depth. Its execution is described in detail in the Learning the Jerk chapter.

AKA: Push jerk.

Notes: Often the terms power jerk and push jerk are used synonymously, but they can be distinguished as two different exercises—the feet lift and move in the power jerk, and stay connected to the floor in the push jerk.

Purpose: The power jerk can be a lifter's chosen style of jerk in competition. As a training exercise, it serves weightlifters who split jerk as a way to train better and higher drive on the bar, balance in the dip and drive, a more precise vertical drive, a quicker transition between the drive and the movement down under the bar, and proper movement of the bar into position overhead for the split jerk.

Programming: Sets of 1-3 reps are suggested with weights anywhere from 70% to the lifter's maximum power jerk. Generally this exercise should be performed following any snatch variants and possibly before clean variants depending on what the intended emphasis of the workout is. With light weights, it can be used as a technique primer before split jerks to train a more vertical drive or higher drive. A common complex is power jerk + split jerk to improve the orientation of the dip and/or drive for the split jerk for lifters who tend to shift forward.

Variations: The power jerk can be performed without the feet leaving the floor, in which case it becomes a push jerk. It can also be performed from behind the neck, or with a snatch grip behind the neck as a snatch power jerk.

Power Jerk Behind the Neck

This is simply a power jerk in which the barbell begins behind the neck. It's important the lifter use the correct jerk grip, as there is a tendency for lifters to unintentionally widen their grips when lifting from behind the neck. Equally important, the lifter must

be cautious of leaning the chest forward and allowing the hips to move back in the dip.

AKA: Behind the neck power jerk, power jerk bnk, BTN power jerk.

Notes: Because the bar and the trunk begin in the same plane and orientation respectively that they should be in when the bar is overhead, the bar path should be perfectly vertical and the trunk should remain in the same orientation (inclined forward very slightly).

Purpose: The power jerk behind the neck can be used for the same basic reasons as the power jerk in training, but with the added element of reinforcing the proper position of the bar overhead and strengthening the upper back to support the overhead position.

Programming: Sets of 1-3 reps are suggested with weights anywhere from 70% to the lifter's maximum power jerk. Generally this exercise should be performed following any snatch variants and possibly before clean variants depending on what the intended emphasis of the workout is. With light weights, it can be used as a technique primer before split jerks or power jerks to reinforce the proper overhead position.

Variations: The power jerk behind the neck can be performed without the feet leaving the floor, in which case it becomes a push jerk behind the neck. It can also be performed with a snatch grip as a common way to secure the bar overhead for heavy overhead squats.

Press Behind the Neck

The lifter will simply perform a press with the bar starting behind the neck as it would for a back squat. It's important the lifter use the correct jerk grip, as the tendency will be to take a wider grip when lifting from behind the neck.

AKA: Behind the neck press, press bnk, BTN press.

Notes: If an athlete can't press from behind the neck without pain, this exercise shouldn't be used until mobility is improved—the push press behind the neck may be a possible alternative. When performing multiple rep sets of the press, reps after the first can be touch-and-go as long as they remain full range of motion (bar contacts the traps at the start of each rep). Because the bar and the trunk begin in the same plane and orientation respectively that they should be in when the bar is overhead, the bar path should be perfectly vertical and the trunk should remain in the same orientation (inclined forward very slightly).

Purpose: The press behind the neck serves like the press as basic upper body and overhead strength exercise, but emphasizes upper back strength and mobility more than the press. It can also be used to teach the proper overhead position for the jerk.

Programming: Sets of 1-10 reps can be used depending on the timing and the specific need. 6-10 reps will help more with hypertrophy and some strength; 3-5 reps will be generally the most effective for strength work and some hypertrophy; 1-2 reps will usually be used for testing maximum lifts but will also improve strength; however, this is generally inappropriate for this exercise. For teaching and reinforcing proper overhead position for the jerk, light weights and 3-5 reps should be used.

Variations: The press behind the neck can be performed with a snatch-width grip, known as a snatch press.

Press Behind the Neck in Split

The lifter will secure the bar behind the neck as for a back squat with a jerk grip while in a full jerk split position, making sure the weight is balanced equally between the front and back feet and the trunk is rigid and stabilized with air pressure and strong muscular tension. From this position, the athlete will press the bar straight up into the proper split jerk overhead position, being careful not to shift the balance or position in the split.

AKA: Split press behind the neck, split position press behind the neck, press bnk in split, BTN press in split.

Notes: If an athlete can't press from behind the neck without pain, this exercise shouldn't be used until mobility is improved. When performing multiple rep sets of the press, reps after the first can be touch-and-go as long as they remain full range of motion (bar contacts the traps at the start of each rep). Because the bar and the trunk begin in the same plane and orientation respectively that they should

be in when the bar is overhead, the bar path should be perfectly vertical and the trunk should remain in the same orientation (inclined forward very slightly).

Purpose: The press behind the neck in split can be used as an upper body strength exercise that improves the position, balance and strength of the split simultaneously just like the press in split, but can be more appropriate for lifters who don't have a consistently correct overhead position and will place more emphasis on upper back strength and mobility than the press from the front. It can also be used as a technique primer for lifters who tend to land in an improper or imbalanced split with a poor overhead position.

Programming: Sets of 3-5 reps can be used generally and can be performed with weights nearly as heavy as can be handled in the press. If used as a technique primer, light weights should be used.

Variations: The press in split can be performed from the front as a press in split, and pauses in the overhead position can be added.

Press in Split

The lifter will secure the bar in the jerk rack position while in a full jerk split position, making sure the weight is balanced equally between the front and back feet and the trunk is rigid and stabilized with air pressure and strong muscular tension. From this position, the athlete will perform a press, moving the bar up and back into the proper split jerk overhead position, being careful not to shift the balance or position in the split.

AKA: Split press, split position press.

Notes: When performing multiple rep sets of the press, the full jerk rack position does not need to be reset—the subsequent reps can be touch-and-go as long as they remain full range of motion (bar contacts the shoulders at the start of each rep).

Purpose: The press in split can be used as a basic overhead strength exercise just like the press, but with the added benefit of simultaneously practicing the position and balance in the split, and strengthening the proper split position for the jerk. It can also be used as a technique primer for lifters who tend to land in an improper or imbalanced split position.

Programming: Sets of 3-5 reps can be used generally and can be performed with weights nearly as heavy as can be handled in the press. If used as a technique primer, light weights should be used.

Variations: The press in split can be performed from behind the neck, and pauses in the overhead position can be added.

Press to Jerk

The lifter will begin a press, and as the bar reaches approximately halfway up, lift and transition the feet into the jerk split stance, aggressively punching the arms to move down into a locked-out split receiving position, attempting to lock the bar out in the overhead position at the same time the feet hit the floor. The athlete will secure and stabilize the bar overhead before recovering into a standing position with the bar still overhead by stepping about a third of the way back with the front foot, and then stepping the back foot up to meet it.

AKA: Press into jerk, slow jerk.

Notes: It's important to maintain proper balance in this exercise and not dive forward onto the front leg.

Purpose: The press to jerk can be used as an upper body strength exercise variation that also trains quick and precise foot movement into the split. It can also be used to train patience in the split jerk by simulating a higher drive on the bar prior to movement of the feet into the split position.

Programming: Sets of 3-5 reps are suggested. If trained with fairly heavy weights, it should be performed following jerk or jerk variant work of the day. With light weights, it can be used as a technique primer before split jerks to train the timing and aggressiveness of the split.

Variations: The press to jerk can also be performed from behind the neck, as a power jerk or push jerk, or by rising onto the toes during the press.

Press

The press is the most basic pressing and overhead strength exercise in weightlifting. It was formerly a contested lift (as the clean & press) and was dropped from competition after the 1972 Olympics. Its ex-

ecution is described in detail in the Learning the Jerk chapter.

AKA: Military press, overhead press, shoulder press.

Notes: When performing multiple rep sets of the press, the full jerk rack position does not need to be reset—the subsequent reps can be touch-and-go as long as they remain full range of motion (bar contacts the shoulders at the start of each rep).

Purpose: The press is a simple upper body strength exercise. It can also be used to teach and reinforce the proper mechanics of the upper body for the jerk.

Programming: Sets of 1-10 reps can be used depending on the timing and the specific need. 6-10 reps will help more with hypertrophy and some strength; 3-5 reps will be generally the most effective for strength work and some hypertrophy; 1-2 reps will usually be used for testing maximum lifts but will also improve strength. For use teaching and reinforcing proper upper body mechanics for the jerk, light weights should be used for 3-5 reps, each of which should begin from a dead stop and the full jerk rack position.

Variations: The press can be performed from behind the neck, and with pauses in the overhead position.

Push Jerk Behind the Neck in Split

The lifter will secure the bar behind the neck as for a back squat while in a jerk split position, ensuring the weight is balanced equally between the front and back feet and the trunk stabilized with air pressure and strong muscular tension. The athlete will dip straight down with the legs and drive straight back up to elevate and accelerate the bar. He or she will then push the bar off the back aggressively with the arms and into a fully locked overhead position behind the neck while sinking back down into the starting split depth. It's important to maintain the same posture and equal balance between the feet throughout the movement.

AKA: Split push jerk behind the neck, push press behind the neck in split, split push press behind the neck, push jerk bnk in split, BTN push jerk in split.

Notes: The push into the overhead position

should be aggressive and quick. Timing will improve if the athlete attempts to lock the elbows at the same time he or she returns to the starting split depth. It will help to keep the dip relatively slow and the drive only as hard as necessary so the focus can be speed back under the bar.

Purpose: The push jerk behind the neck in split is a helpful exercise for strengthening the split position and reinforcing the proper position and balance in the split, while also strengthening and reinforcing the proper overhead position for the jerk. It can also be used as a technique primer for lifters who tend to land in an improper or imbalanced split position.

Programming: Sets of 3-5 reps with moderate weights can be used. Some lifters will be able to move a lot of weight in this exercise, but should never be allowed to exceed what can be done properly, as it will defeat the purpose and simply reinforce the problems it's supposed to be correcting. If used as a technique primer, light weights should be used for 3-5 reps.

Variations: The push jerk behind the neck in split can be performed from the front as a push jerk in split.

Push Jerk in Split

The lifter will secure the bar in the jerk rack position while in a jerk split position, ensuring the weight is balanced equally between the front and back feet and the trunk stabilized with air pressure and strong muscular tension. The athlete will dip straight down with the legs and drive straight back up to elevate and accelerate the bar. He or she will then push the bar off the shoulders aggressively with the arms and into a fully locked overhead position behind the neck while sinking back down into the starting split depth. It's important to maintain the same posture and equal balance between the feet throughout the movement.

AKA: Split push jerk, push press in split, split push press.

Notes: The push into the overhead position should be aggressive and quick. Timing will improve if the athlete attempts to lock the elbows at the same time he or she returns to the starting split depth. It will help to keep the dip relatively slow and the drive only as hard as necessary so the focus can be speed

back under the bar.

Purpose: The push jerk in split is a helpful exercise for strengthening the split position and reinforcing the proper position and balance in the split, while also strengthening and reinforcing the proper overhead position for the jerk. It can also be used as a technique primer for lifters who tend to land in an improper or imbalanced split position.

Programming: Sets of 3-5 reps with moderate weights can be used. Some lifters will be able to move a lot of weight in this exercise, but should never be allowed to exceed what can be done properly, as it will defeat the purpose and simply reinforce the problems it's supposed to be correcting. If used as a technique primer, light weights should be used for 3-5 reps.

Variations: The push jerk in split can be performed from behind the neck as a push jerk behind the neck in split.

Push Jerk

The push jerk is simply a power jerk in which the feet remain in contact with the floor rather than being lifted and relocated. The heels may rise off the floor during the drive. Typically lifters will use a wider drive stance in this variation.

AKA: Power jerk.

Notes: Often the terms power jerk and push jerk are used synonymously, but they can be distinguished as two exercises—the feet lift and move in the power jerk, and stay connected to the floor in the push jerk.

Purpose: The push jerk can be a lifter's chosen style of jerk in competition. As a training exercise, it serves weightlifters as a way to train better and higher drive on the bar, balance in the dip and drive, a more precise vertical drive, a quicker transition between the drive and the movement down under the bar, and proper movement of the bar into position overhead, all of which will improve the split jerk. It can be used instead of the power jerk for lifters who have trouble properly timing the movement of the feet and cut off the upward drive prematurely, or move the feet improperly.

Programming: Sets of 1-3 reps are suggested with weights anywhere from 70% to maximum. Generally this exercise should be performed following any snatch variants and possibly before clean variants depending on what the intended emphasis of the workout is. With light weights, it can be used as a technique primer before split jerks to train a more vertical drive or higher drive.

Variations: The push jerk can be performed with the transition of the feet from the drive position to the squat position, in which case it becomes a power jerk. It can also be performed from behind the neck.

Push Press

The push press is a basic overhead strength exercise for the jerk, and also trains the position and timing of the dip and drive. Its execution is described in detail in the Learning the Jerk chapter.

AKA: Power press.

Notes: If the knees rebend at all after the initial dip and drive, the lift is no longer a push press, but a push jerk. If the feet remain totally flat during the drive of the legs, the drive is not hard or long enough—the heels will rise at least slightly if the leg drive is adequate. Each rep of multiple-rep sets should begin from a dead stop and the full jerk rack position.

Purpose: The push press is an effective upper body strength exercise for the jerk, used more commonly than the press because larger weights can be used. Additionally, it helps train the proper dip and drive for the jerk, as that part of the movement should be identical to that of the jerk.

Programming: Sets of 1-6 reps can be used depending on the timing and the specific need. 3-6 reps will help with hypertrophy and strength; 1-2 reps will usually be used for testing maximum lifts but will also improve strength.

Variations: The push press can be performed from behind the neck as a push press behind the neck.

Push Press Behind the Neck

The push press behind the neck is simply a push press with the bar started behind the neck in the same position it would be for a back squat. It's important lifters use the proper jerk grip, as the tendency will be to widen the grip when lifting from behind the neck.

AKA: Push press bnk, BTN push press, power press behind the neck.

Notes: If the knees rebend at all after the initial dip and drive, the lift is no longer a push press, but a push jerk. If the feet remain totally flat during the drive of the legs, the drive is not hard or long enough—the heels will rise at least slightly if the leg drive is adequate. Each rep of multiple-rep sets should begin from a dead stop to ensure proper positioning and balance, and to train the elasticity and timing of the dip and drive fully.

Purpose: The push press behind the neck is an effective upper body strength exercise for the jerk that can be used instead of the push press in cases of wrist or elbow injuries that prevent the lifter from lifting from the jerk rack position, to emphasize upper back mobility and strength, or to teach, train or reinforce the proper jerk overhead position.

Programming: Sets of 1-6 reps can be used depending on the timing and the specific need. 3-6 reps will help with hypertrophy and strength; 1-2 reps will usually be used for testing maximum lifts but will also improve strength.

Variations: The push press can also be performed from behind the neck with a snatch grip as a snatch push press.

Rebound Jerk

The rebound jerk is a variation of the jerk in which multiple reps are performed in series without resetting the initial tall position. The athlete will begin by performing a jerk as usual. After securing the bar overhead, he or she will bring the feet back into the drive position with the bar still overhead. The lifter will then lower the bar back to the shoulders, absorbing it by bending the knees exactly like a jerk dip, and use this knee bend as the dip for the dip and drive of the subsequent jerk rep without pausing.

Notes: This is a tricky exercise. If an athlete is not good at lowering jerks back to the shoulders, or has a bad habit of hinging at the hip and/or shifting forward in the dip and drive of the jerk, this is not an appropriate exercise.

Purpose: The rebound jerk helps train the elasticity of the legs for the dip and drive of the jerk.

Programming: Sets of 1-3 reps are suggested with weights anywhere from 70% to maximum attempts.

Variations: The rebound jerk can be done with any jerk variation such as power jerk, push jerk and squat jerk in addition to the split jerk. Behind the neck variations are not recommended because of the likelihood of hinging at the hips and performing an improper dip movement.

Squat Jerk

The squat jerk is a rare style of jerk infrequently used in competition, and even more rarely used in training by athletes who don't use it in competition. Its execution is described in detail in the Learning the Jerk chapter.

Notes: Because of the extremely low receiving position, the squat jerk requires less elevation of the bar for the athlete to get under it. However, it requires excellent mobility, precision, overhead stability and leg strength.

Purpose: The squat jerk can be a lifter's chosen style of jerk in competition. As a training exercise for athletes who don't use it in competition, it has fairly limited utility. It can be used to train overhead strength and stability for the jerk and even snatch to some degree, as a way to improve mobility in the bottom position (although there are better choices for this, such as clean-grip overhead squats), and as some variety in training to have fun or keep a lifter mentally fresh.

Programming: Sets of 1-3 reps are suggested with weights anywhere from 70% to maximum. Generally this exercise should be performed following any snatch variants and possibly before clean variants depending on what the intended emphasis of the workout is. With light weights, it can be used to work on overhead stability and mobility before a jerk workout.

Variations: The squat jerk can be performed without the feet leaving the floor. It can also be performed from behind the neck.

Step to Split

The lifter will secure the barbell behind the neck as for a back squat, being sure to use a fairly narrow grip. He or she will step out with one leg into the default split jerk receiving stance and tighten the position immediately—that is, rather than sinking into a deeper lunge, the lifter will lock out the split quickly at his or her default depth. It's important to maintain the upright posture and land with the weight balanced evenly between the front and back feet. After securing the split position solidly, the lifter will step the front foot back into the starting position; alternatively, the lifter can step the front foot back about a third of the distance first to practice the recovery from the split.

Notes: Depending on how strong the lifter is in the split position, this exercise can vary greatly in possible loading. Avoid overloading to the point that the lifter is unable to step into the proper split position or it defeats the purpose.

Purpose: The step to split strengthens the split receiving position for the jerk, which can often be a weakness that limits an athlete's jerk. To some extent, it will also train the proper movement of the front foot into the split position and the maintenance of the proper upright posture.

Programming: The step to split should be done after the classic lift and variants, but can be done before more strength-oriented work like squatting and pulling. Weights of up to 100% and more of the athlete's best jerk may be used for 3-5 reps.

Variations: The step to split can be done by alternating steps of each leg to "walk" forward, making it a walk to split.

Tall Jerk

There are four basic variations of the tall jerk—half-press with flat feet, half-press on toes, from the shoulders on flat feet, and from the shoulders on the toes. To do the lift from the shoulders, the lifter will secure the bar in the jerk rack position with the feet in the jerk drive position. Without any upward drive of the legs, the athlete will lift and transition the feet into the jerk split stance, aggressively punching the arms to move down into a locked out split receiving position, attempting to lock in the overhead position at the same time the feet hit the floor. The bar should be secured tightly overhead before the lifter recovers into a standing position with the bar still overhead by stepping about a third of the way back with the front foot, and then stepping the back foot up to meet it.

For the half-press variation, the lifter will press the bar about halfway up (approximately to the top of the head) and hold—this is the starting position for the lift. The athlete will then lift the feet and move into the split position as he or she punches under into a split jerk receiving position as described above. To go from a half-press on the toes, the lifter will press the bar into the half-press starting position, then rise on the toes and hold to begin from that position.

AKA: Jerk punch under, jerk push under.

Notes: In the starting position for the half-press variations, the head needs to be pulled back out of the way so the bar is vertically above the shoulders as it would be at this point of an actual press or jerk.

Purpose: The tall jerk is a technique exercise that helps with aggressiveness, timing and accuracy of the split and overhead position in the jerk.

Programming: Sets of 3-5 reps are suggested. The tall jerk is best used as a technique primer before jerks to train the timing and aggressiveness of the movement under the bar and the speed, timing and accuracy of the footwork.

Variations: The tall jerk can also be performed from behind the neck, or as a power jerk, push jerk or squat jerk.

Walk to Split

The lifter will begin by performing a step to split. Rather than bringing the front foot back into the starting position, the lifter will step the rear foot forward into a split position with that leg forward and repeat until he or she has performed the desired number of repetitions. Alternatively, the lifter can step the front foot back about a third of the distance to mimic the recovery from the split jerk and then step forward with the back leg. If needed, the lifter can step the back foot up to meet the front foot before stepping out into the next split. It's convenient to set up two squat racks facing each other to walk between on each set.

AKA: Walking split lunge.

Notes: Depending on how strong the lifter is in the split position, this exercise can vary greatly in possible loading. Avoid overloading to the point that the lifter is unable to step into the proper split position or it defeats the purpose.

Purpose: The walk to split strengthens the split receiving position for the jerk, which can often be a weakness that limits an athlete's jerk. To some extent, it will also train the proper movement of the front foot into the split position and the maintenance of the proper upright posture. The advantage over the step to split is training the non-dominant leg to help maintain a degree of strength balance between the two sides.

Programming: The walk to split should be done after the classic lift and variants, but can be done before more strength-oriented work like squatting and pulling. Weights of up to 100% and more of the athlete's best jerk may be used for 3-5 reps.

Variations: The walk to split can be done standing in place and simply stepping forward and then back into the starting position before the next rep, making it a step to split.

General Exercises

1¼ Squat

The 1¼ squat is a variation of either the back squat or front squat that focuses on the bottom of the movement. The lifter will perform the eccentric portion of the squat as usual, then recover only partially (about to parallel or slightly below), return to the bottom, then recover fully to standing, maintaining tension on the legs throughout the movement.

Purpose: The 1¼ squat is used to strengthen the bottommost part of the squat to aid in proper recovery posture in the squat, clean or snatch. It can also be used specifically to train VMO and glute activation and strength.

Programming: Typically the 1¼ squat will be performed at moderate to moderately heavy weights—it's not an appropriate exercise to take to maximal effort. If the positions are not correct, it's not effective. Sets of 2-5 reps are most common. Usually this would be done one day each week as a supplement to normal back and/or front squats other days of the week.

Variations: The 1¼ squat can be performed at a slow tempo throughout to maximize strength work, or it can be done with speed as a way to train the elasticity of the bounce in the squat or clean. Overhead squats can also be performed with the 1¼ movement.

Back Squat

The back squat is the most basic strength exercise in weightlifting, and one of the most commonly used exercises other than the competition lifts. The movement of the squat and proper bar placement are described in detail in the Squat chapter.

AKA: Squat.

Purpose: The back squat is the most effective exercise in weightlifting for building basic strength, particularly of the legs and trunk. It is used for general leg strength development primarily, although nearly always is used in combination with the front squat for weightlifting.

Programming: There are a huge number of possibilities when it comes to programming the back squat. Most commonly weightlifters will use sets of 1-6 reps, but it's not unheard of to use as many as 10 occasionally and far out from competition.

Variations: The back squat can be performed as a pause squat, parallel squat, with prescribed tempos (usually slow eccentric movement), and as a 1¼ squat.

Bent Row

The lifter will hold the bar with a clean grip, arch the back tightly, bend the knees, and hinge at the hips to bend forward until the trunk is nearing horizontal. Keeping the bar close to the legs, the lifter will pull the shoulder blades back and down and pull the elbows up to row the bar into the abdomen. The entire upper back should be squeezed tightly at the top of each rep, arching the length of the spine and pulling the shoulder blades back and down. The bar should be lowered under control to full elbow extension without losing the arched back position.

AKA: Bent-over row, bent forward row.

Notes: The bent row can be performed strictly with a controlled tempo, or with a little body English to put some speed on the bar and then reach the trunk into the bar at the top of the row.

Purpose: The bent row is a basic back strength exercise that helps develop the upper and middle back, and even the lower back through its role in holding the body in position throughout the movement. It will also strengthen the shoulders and arms. It can serve to help develop postural strength, shoulder stability, back arch strength, upper back arch strength in particular, and arm strength for the pull under the bar in the clean and snatch.

Programming: Sets of 5-10 reps are usually appropriate with weight that allows a full range of motion with proper posture.

Variations: The bent row can be done with a snatch grip, with hands supinated (palms facing forward), and with different trunk angles. It can also be done as a Pendlay row, in which each rep starts with the bar on the floor and the upper back rounded, and then the athlete extends the upper back during the rowing motion.

Bulgarian Split Squat

The Bulgarian split squat may be just a joke played on gullible Americans by a visiting Bulgarian coach, but it can still be a useful exercise in some cases. The exercise is simply a 1-legged squat with the rear foot elevated on a bench, box or similar. The lifter will hold the barbell behind the neck as for a back squat, and place what will be the front foot about 3 foot-lengths in front of a bench or box, and place the top of the rear foot on the top of the bench or box—this is the starting position. The distance of the front foot from the bench can be adjusted as needed to make sure the front shin is about vertical in the bottom of the squat. With a controlled speed, the athlete will bend at the knee with an upright trunk until the rear knee lightly contacts the floor, then stand again, pushing more through the heel than the balls of the foot. The position of the front knee should be maintained over the foot—it should be not allowed to collapse inward or be pushed outward.

AKA: RLE squat.

Notes: The length of the split can be adjusted to obtain somewhat different effects. The farther forward the front foot, the more the exercise will rely on the posterior chain and stretch the rear hip flexors; the farther back the front foot, the more the exercise will rely on the quads.

Purpose: The Bulgarian split squat can be used as a supplemental leg exercise to help balance weakness in one leg or hip, build better glute strength and hip stability, or as an exercise for hypertrophy at higher reps.

Programming: Sets of 5-10 reps are usually appropriate with weight that allows a smooth movement and no crashing into the bottom position.

Variations: The Bulgarian split squat can be loaded with any implement, from a barbell to single or double dumbbells or kettlebells held in any position. In the case of weightlifting, a barbell in the back squat position is most common.

Chin-up

The athlete will hang from a pull-up bar with the hands supinated (palms facing the athlete) and just outside shoulder width, allowing the shoulder to open completely. The athlete will squeeze the shoulder blades back and down and pull with the arms to bring the chin above the bar, trying to continue pulling the shoulders and arms back in the top position to finish with a strong arch in the upper back. The athlete will lower under control until the elbows are completely extended and shoulders are fully open again before beginning subsequent reps.

AKA: Chin, pull-up.

Notes: The natural tendency is to round the back at the top of the movement, but it's important to arch instead to fully engage all of the back musculature and maintain proper shoulder movement. It's equally important to ensure each rep starts from a genuinely open shoulder position—this will ensure proper shoulder mobility and health.

Purpose: The chin-up strengthens the back and arms in opposition to vertical pressing motions common in weightlifting training and helps keep the shoulders and upper back balanced and healthy. The chin-up emphasizes the biceps a little more than the pull-up and can also be used as an alternative to avoid pain in the pull-up and vice-versa.

Programming: Sets of 5-10 or more reps are usually appropriate, and often a good way to prescribe chin-ups is with a total number of reps to be completed as possible (i.e. as many reps per set as can be done until reaching the total). Resistance can be reduced for those unable to perform chin-ups with their full body weight by using elastic bands, or by standing on a box and using the legs to partially unload weight as necessary.

Variations: The chin-up can be done with wider or narrower grips, although usually the same grip width used for the jerk and press is ideal. The hands can be pronated (palms facing forward), in which case the exercise would then be called a pull-up.

Clean-Grip Overhead Squat

The clean-grip overhead squat is simply an overhead squat with a narrow grip. The overhead position should be established identically to the jerk, and the movement should be performed at a controlled tempo to maximize postural tension. The lifter can move the bar into the overhead position with his or her preferred style of push press or jerk (most commonly a push press or power jerk behind the neck).

AKA: Jerk-grip overhead squat, narrow-grip overhead squat, close-grip overhead squat.

Purpose: The clean-grip overhead squat can be used as a mobility exercise for the ankles, hips, shoulders and thoracic spine, and also a strength exercise for upper back extension, which will help posture in the snatch and clean, and stability overhead in the snatch and jerk.

Programming: Clean-grip overhead squats should typically be done for sets of 2-5 reps. If being used a strength exercise, they should be performed toward the end of a workout after more speed and technique dependent exercises. They can be performed before snatches or jerks with light weights as a way to activate the upper back, or to help warm-up and stretch for the snatch or jerk.

Variations: The most common variation of the clean-grip overhead squat includes a pause in the bottom position to further train stability, strength and balance. The clean-grip overhead squat is also very commonly combined into a complex with push presses behind the neck preceding it.

Front Squat

The front squat is a basic strength exercise in weightlifting, and one of the most commonly used exercises other than the competition lifts. Its execution is described in detail in the Squat and clean Receiving Position chapters.

Purpose: The front squat is a leg strength exercise very specific to the clean, but also will help the jerk by emphasizing quad strength, and improve the ability of lifters to pull from the floor with an upright posture. It is also an effective trunk and back (particularly mid and upper back) strengthening exercise. It is usually used in combination with the back squat for weightlifting.

Programming: There are a huge number of possibilities when it comes to programming the front squat. Most commonly weightlifters will use sets of 1-5 reps, but more often 1-3 reps. Weights can be very heavy to maximal for strength development, or more moderate for training speed, timing and position for the clean, or as a lighter squat day during preparation mesocycles.

Variations: The front squat can be performed as a pause squat, parallel squat, with prescribed tempos (usually slow eccentric movement), and as a 1¼ squat.

Good Morning

The lifter will place a barbell behind the neck as for a back squat, place the feet between the pulling position and squat position, and set the back tightly in a complete arch, locking it in position with tight abs. Allowing the knees to unlock and bend only very slightly, the lifter will hinge at the hip, maintaining the back arch aggressively, and bend forward as far as he or she can without losing the arch in the back. When the motion is reversed, the lifter needs to ensure the back arch is not allowed to soften or the knees allowed to bend more.

AKA: Bend over.

Notes: The good morning does not need to be loaded extremely heavily to be effective. The focus should be on an active and aggressive arch of the back and full range of motion. More bend in the knees will allow a better back arch and heavier loading, especially for lifters will relatively limited mobility; however, knee bend should be kept minimal. Belts should not be used.

Purpose: The good morning primarily strengthens the isometric position of the back arch used in the snatch, clean, squat and related exercises to improve the lifter's stability, power transfer and safety. Secondarily, it strengthens the glutes and hamstrings, and can improve hip mobility.

Programming: Sets of 3-6 reps are most common, but can be taken up as high as 10 reps. Weights can usually be 20-40% of the lifter's best back squat.

Variations: The good morning can be performed with a number of minor variations. It can be done with completely straight knees (more hamstring involvement), a wide stance (more hamstring and adductor), a narrow stance (more glute), with more bend in the knees (more weight and more focus on the back), and seated.

Lunge

The lifter will place a barbell behind the neck as for a back squat and pressurize and tighten the trunk, then step forward with one leg far enough that the front shin remains vertical into the bottom of the lunge, keeping the trunk as upright as possible and the weight balanced evenly between the two feet. He or she will sink to a depth at which the rear knee very lightly touches the floor, not allowing it to crash down or rest on the floor. The lifter will push off the front foot more through the heel to step back into the starting position. All reps on one leg can be performed before switching to the other leg, or legs can be alternated.

AKA: Barbell lunge.

Notes: Many athletes try to load lunges too heavily and lose the position in which the exercise will be most effective. If the athlete can't maintain a controlled descent into the bottom of the lunge, maintain an upright trunk, and maintain balance between the feet, the weight should be reduced.

Purpose: The lunge is the simplest unilateral leg exercise and can be used to improve strength and mobility balance in the hips, improve the strength of the split position for the jerk, or for hypertrophy in addition to squatting.

Programming: Sets of 3-10 reps per leg are usually appropriate with weight that allows a proper position, smooth movement and no crashing into the bottom position.

Variations: The lunge can be done with the bar

in the front squat (clean) rack position or using other implements to add weight. It can also be done as a walking lunge—rather than stepping back with the front foot after each rep, the athlete will step the back foot forward directly into the next lunge or to meet the front foot before stepping the other leg forward.

Overhead Split Squat

The overhead split squat is simply a split squat with the barbell locked out in the jerk overhead position. The lifter can secure the bar in place with a push press or jerk of his or her preference. The key to the exercise is maintaining strict stability of the bar, and maintaining the proper posture and balance in the split position.

Notes: The length of the split can be adjusted to obtain somewhat different effects. The farther forward the front foot, the more the exercise will rely on the posterior chain and stretch the rear hip flexors; the farther back the front foot, the more the exercise will rely on the quads. However, if using the exercise specifically to strengthen the receiving position of the split jerk, the stance should be identical to the lifter's split jerk receiving position.

Purpose: Like the split squat, the overhead split squat strengthens the legs, hips and trunk for the split receiving position of the split jerk, but it also adds some upper body strength and stability development.

Programming: Sets of 3-6 reps are usually appropriate with weight that allows a smooth movement and no crashing into the bottom position, as well as a fully locked overhead position throughout the set.

Variations: The overhead split squat can be performed to maximal depth (i.e. the rear knee as close to the floor as possible), or just to the lifter's normal split jerk receiving depth. In the latter case, heavier loading will be possible.

Parallel Squat

Any type of squat—back squat, front squat or overhead squat—can be performed as a parallel squat. The only difference from the standard squat is that the lifter will squat only to parallel depth—the thighs in a horizontal orientation. Otherwise all other elements of the squat's execution are identical. It's particularly important in the parallel squat to enforce proper posture and position, as the tendency will be for lifters to sit the hips farther back to shift more of the work to the hips.

Notes: Parallel squats can place a lot of additional strain on the knees and patellar tendons, and excessive use can produce tendonitis. Volume and frequency should be prescribed accordingly.

Purpose: Parallel squats help develop strength in the most mechanically disadvantaged position in the squat. This position is where the typical lifter will have the worst leverage and slow down when recovering from a squat. Parallel squats can help strengthen this position to help lifters move through it more quickly and with less effort during cleans and other squats.

Programming: Parallel squats should typically be used as only one squat variation among others during a training week. They can also be used in back-off sets following heavier standard squats. Sets of 3-6 reps are typically ideal—very heavy singles and doubles are more likely to force the lifter out of position.

Variations: The parallel squat can be performed with a pause in the parallel position.

Pause Squat

Any type of squat—back squat, front squat or overhead squat—can be performed as a pause squat. The lifter will perform the squat as usual, but hold in the bottom for 3 or more seconds before standing without any bouncing action—that is, the recovery must be initiated from a dead stop. The lifter should attempt to accelerate maximally and immediately.

AKA: Stop squat.

Notes: A pause of 3 seconds is adequate to eliminate the stretch-shortening reflex entirely. Longer holds can be done for additional posture strength work (i.e. trunk strength), but will not increase the effect on rate of force development. It's important the athlete not sneak in some subtle bouncing when initiating the recovery in order to stand more easily, as this will reduce the effectiveness of the exercise.

Purpose: The pause squat can serve a few purposes. First, it helps train rate of force development

in the squat by eliminating the stretch-shortening reflex that normally occurs. It will also improve trunk strength and postural strength, improve mobility and comfort in the bottom of the squat, and can help correct improper movement in the squat such as leading with the hips (as long as reps are performed with proper posture).

Programming: Pause squats can be programmed in the same way as their standard counterpart squats, although usually reps above 5 are not recommended. Weights of course will be limited relative to the standard squat, although by how much will vary depending on how much elasticity the lifter relies on when squatting normally.

Pulling-Stance Back Squat

The pulling-stance back squat is simply a back squat in which the lifter's feet are positioned in the same stance used to pull the snatch or clean.

AKA: Narrow-stance squat, close-stance squat.

Notes: This lift is sometimes done with the knees directed nearly forward, although if being used specifically to strengthen the snatch or clean pull, they should be oriented exactly how they are in that lifter's pull.

Purpose: The pulling-stance back squat can be used to strengthen a lifter's pull from the floor in the snatch and clean, or to emphasize quad strength.

Programming: The pulling-stance back squat would most often be used once weekly in addition to normal back squats and front squats. Generally sets of 3-5 reps are most effective at 70% of the lifter's best back and higher.

Variations: The pulling-stance back squat can be performed as a pause squat, with prescribed tempos (usually slow eccentric movement), and as a 1¼ squat. It can also be performed with an even narrower stance and the knees moving nearly straight forward.

Pull-up

The pull-up is a simple and effective upper body pulling strength exercise that also can help with shoulder mobility. The lifter will hang from a pull-up bar with the hands pronated (palms facing forward) and just outside shoulder width, allowing the shoulder to open completely. He or she will squeeze the shoulder blades back and down and pull with the arms to bring the chin above the bar, trying to continue pulling the shoulders and arms back in the top position to finish with a strong arch in the back. The athlete will lower under control until the elbows are completely extended and shoulders are fully open again.

AKA: Chin-up, chin.

Notes: The natural tendency is to round the back at the top of the movement, but it's important to arch instead to fully engage all of the back musculature. It's equally important to ensure each rep starts from a genuinely open shoulder position—this will ensure proper shoulder mobility and health.

Purpose: The pull-up strengthens the back and arms in opposition to vertical pressing motions common in weightlifting training and helps keep the shoulders and upper back balanced and healthy.

Programming: Sets of 5-10 reps or more are usually appropriate, and often a good way to prescribe pull-ups is with a total number of reps to be completed as possible (i.e. as many reps per set as can be done until reaching the total). Resistance can be reduced for those unable to perform chin-ups with their full body weight by using elastic bands, or by standing on a box and using the legs to partially unload weight as necessary.

Variations: The pull-up can be done with wider or narrower grips, although usually the same grip width used for the jerk and press is ideal. The hands can be supinated (palms facing toward the athlete), in which case the exercise would then be called a chin-up.

Romanian Deadlift

The Romanian deadlift's exact origins and original execution are points of contention. It certainly originated when Nicu Vlad of Romania and his coach, Dragomir Cioroslan, were in the US in 1990 for the Goodwill Games. Vlad was performing an exercise that hadn't been seen before, and someone (Jim Schmitz at the Sports Palace or one of the lifters at the Olympic Training center, possibly both at separate times) suggested the exercise be called the Romanian deadlift when Cioroslan said they didn't have

a name for it.

With the feet in the pulling position and holding the bar in a clean grip, the lifter will bend the knees slightly with the trunk vertical—this is the starting and ending position for each rep. Maintaining the same slight bend in the knees throughout the movement, the lifter will set the back in a tight arch and hinge at the hips as far as he or she can without losing any arch in the back. Once the lowest possible point is reached, the lifter will return to standing while maintaining the same slight bend in the knees. Straps should be used.

AKA: RDL, Stiff-Legged Deadlift (incorrectly).

Notes: The Romanian deadlift and stiff-legged deadlift are often considered the same exercise, but the two can be distinguished by the action of the knees. In the stiff-legged deadlift, the knees start fully extended and unlock slightly as part of the forward hinge rather than remaining bent throughout the entire movement.

Purpose: The Romanian deadlift strengthens the back arch along with the glutes and hamstrings, but places somewhat less emphasis on the hamstrings because the knees remain bent throughout. Because of this bend, it can also be used as a way to reinforce the knee movement under the bar as occurs in the snatch and clean pulls. It also strengthens the lats and shoulders because of the effort to keep the bar close to the legs with the shoulders in front of the bar.

Programming: Sets of 3-6 reps are most common. Weights usually start around 50% of the lifter's best back squat and often are very heavy, sometimes as much as 70-80% of the back squat.

Variations: The Romanian deadlift can be done with a snatch grip and with more bend in the knees to be able to handle more weight for increased back arch strengthening. It can also be done without straps for more grip strength work.

Seated Good Morning

The seated good morning is fairly uncommon variation of the good morning that requires very good hip mobility. The lifter will place a barbell behind the neck as for a back squat while sitting with the legs straddling a bench, knees bent and feet flat on the floor farther forward than the knees. The back will be arched completely and tightly, and the trunk position locked in with tight abs. The lifter will hinge at the hip, maintaining the back arch, and bend forward as far as he or she can without losing the arch in the back, then reverse the motion and return to the original upright position.

Notes: The seated good morning does not need to be loaded extremely heavily to be effective. Focus should be on an active and aggressive arch of the back and full range of motion and loading should not exceed what allows this perfect movement and position.

Purpose: The seated good morning primarily strengthens the isometric position of the back arch used in the snatch, clean, squat and related exercises to improve the lifter's stability, power transfer and safety. Secondarily, it strengthens the glutes and hamstrings, and can improve hip mobility. The seated good morning is somewhat more specific to the squat position and starting position of the snatch and clean as opposed to the pulling position than the conventional good morning. It can also be used as an alternative to the good morning in cases of lower leg injuries that prevent standing.

Programming: Sets of 3-6 reps are most common, but can be taken up as high as 10 reps. Weights can usually be 20-40% of the lifter's best back squat.

Split Squat

With a barbell behind the neck as for a back squat, the lifter will step into a lunge stance long enough that the front shin will remain approximately vertical when in the bottom of the movement, keeping the weight balanced evenly between the front and back feet. With a controlled speed, the athlete will lower him- or herself with an upright trunk until the rear knee lightly contacts the floor (without letting it crash down or rest on the floor), then stand again maintaining the balance between the feet. The position of the front knee over the foot must be maintained rather than allowing the knee to move inward or outward relative to the foot. The athlete will perform the total number of reps on one leg before switching to the other leg.

Notes: The length of the split can be adjusted to obtain somewhat different effects. The farther forward the front foot, the more the exercise will rely on the posterior chain and stretch the rear hip flexors; the farther back the front foot, the more the exercise will rely on the quads. However, if using the exercise specifically to strengthen the receiving position of the split jerk, the stance should be identical to that position.

Purpose: The split squat is primarily an exercise to strengthen the split receiving position of the split jerk, but it can also be used as a supplemental leg exercise to help balance weakness in one leg or hip, build better glute strength and hip stability, or as an exercise for hypertrophy at higher reps.

Programming: Sets of 5-10 reps are usually appropriate with weight that allows a smooth movement and no crashing into the bottom position.

Variations: The split squat can be loaded with any implement, from a barbell to single or double dumbbells or kettlebells held in any position. In the case of weightlifting, a barbell in the back squat position is most common.

Stiff-Legged Deadlift

The stiff-legged deadlift is a very effective back strength exercise often confused with or considered a synonym for the Romanian deadlift. With the feet in the pulling position and holding the bar in a clean grip, the lifter will set the back tightly in a complete arch. He or she will hinge at the hips as far as possible without losing any arch in the back, bending the knees as he or she hinges and allowing them to remain slightly bent until returning to standing vertically, straightening them as the hips are extended. Straps should be used.

AKA: Romanian deadlift (incorrectly).

Notes: The stiff-legged deadlift and Romanian deadlift are often considered the same exercise, but the two can be distinguished by the action of the knees. In the stiff-legged deadlift, the knees start fully extended, bend slightly as part of the forward hinge, then straighten again as the hips extend, rather than remaining bent throughout the entire movement as they do in the Romanian deadlift.

Purpose: The stiff-legged deadlift strengthens the back arch along with the glutes and hamstrings. It also strengthens the lats and shoulders because of the effort to keep the bar close to the legs with the shoulders in front of the bar.

Programming: Sets of 3-6 reps are most common. Weights usually start around 50% of the lifter's best back squat and often can be very heavy, sometimes as much as 70-80% of the back squat.

Variations: The stiff-legged deadlift can be done with a snatch grip and with more bend in the knees to be able to handle more weight for increased back arch strengthening. It can also be done without straps for more grip strength work.

Straight-Legged Deadlift

The straight-legged deadlift is one of the few exercises in weightlifting in which the back is actually flexed and extended rather than held in a static extended position. The lifter will stand on a box with the feet in the pulling position, holding the bar in a clean grip, and the legs tight to keep the knees straight. He or she will hinge at the hips and bend forward as far as possible by allowing the back to round forward, keeping the knees straight and the bar close to the legs, then return to standing by extending the hips and straightening the back again into a vertical position.

AKA: Stiff-legged deadlift (incorrectly).

Notes: The straight-legged deadlift is often avoided because of the fear of back injury. It should not be used by athletes with existing back problems, and used only by athletes with good hip mobility. The exercise should be introduced in very small doses and with very light weights.

Purpose: The straight-legged deadlift strengthens the back with dynamic work rather than the isometric work typically done in weightlifting. It can also be used for some variety and mobility.

Programming: Sets of 5-10 reps are most common. Weights should be relatively light and never heavy enough to force the athlete to noticeably strain. It should be stopped at the first indication of any lower back discomfort.

Variations: The straight-legged deadlift can be done with a snatch grip. It can also be done without lifting straps for more grip strength work.

Upper Back Extensions

The upper back extension is a simple, short range of motion exercise to strengthen thoracic spine extension. The athlete will lie prone (face down) on the floor with the feet anchored under a piece of equipment or with a partner holding the legs down. Holding a dumbbell or plate behind the neck, he or she will arch the upper back forcefully and maximally at a controlled tempo to maintain tension through the entire range, which will be short. The athlete will return to lying flat at a similarly controlled tempo to maintain tension. It's important the upper back is the focus of the extension effort rather than the lower back. It will help to keep the head lifted.

Purpose: The upper back extension is a good partner to thoracic spine mobility work to ensure that new range of motion is supported with strength and activation. It can help with stability in the overhead position for the snatch and jerk, and with postural strength in the clean and squats.

Programming: Extensions can be done for 3-4 sets of 8-20 reps with as much weight as will allow complete extension and a controlled tempo. They should be performed with other trunk strength and accessory exercises at the end of the workout.

Introduction to Nutrition

The fundamental goal of any athletic nutritional approach is to support continued performance gains. Depending on the sport in question, performance-oriented nutrition may or may not be optimally supportive of health; however, nutrition for weightlifting can generally be accomplished with high food quality and does not require excesses of any particular macronutrient to the point of potential health concerns. Super-heavyweights are an exception in most cases because the remarkably great demand for total calorie intake reaches beyond what can be achieved in an entirely healthy fashion; in addition to this is simply forcing, in most cases, the body to carry significantly more mass than it was intended to, which in and of itself is unhealthy to some degree.

There are three fundamental components of nutrition: quantity, quality, and macronutrient composition. None can be neglected in the pursuit of optimal performance, but as specific goals vary during different periods of training over the long term, the importance of one may temporarily eclipse the others. The additional two elements to consider are macronutrient timing and supplementation (the latter will be addressed it its own chapter).

Quantity

Quantity is the simplest value to understand. It refers to the total amount of food being eaten in a given period of time, measured in calories, or more accurately, kilocalories (kcal). This gives us a measure of the amount of energy being taken in, and can be considered a kind of gross adjustment tool, the manipulation of which can produce the most dramatic changes in the body such as large degrees of weight gain and weight loss.

Quality

Food quality is a more nebulous value than quantity, with widespread and occasionally vehement contention existing. The guiding principle in food quality is remarkably simple: natural foods are generally superior in terms of their support of basic health. This leaves meat, fish, eggs, vegetables, fruit, tubers, nuts and seeds, certain oils, and possibly certain dairy products as the types of foods that will ideally comprise the bulk of the athlete's intake.

A discussion of the depth required to fully explain the science behind this perspective is better left for more appropriate channels and those with greater expertise on the subject. The take-home point is that processed foods cannot compete with the nutritional density of natural foods, and often carry with them numerous potential health risks, even if performance and body composition metrics can be achieved with the lower quality foods. The quality of foods is what will supply required micronutrients, help prevent autoimmune disorders, and support long-term health.

To a great extent, food quality will also support athletic performance, but as health and performance diverge at times, so too will this relationship change occasionally to some degree. For example, a large serving of carbohydrates at a certain time (such as post-workout to replenish glycogen stores and aid in the recovery process) is far easier to achieve (and arguably more effective) with more processed foods (with a consequently higher glycemic index and rate of assimilation) that might normally be avoided for the sake of health.

Macronutrient Composition

The final fundamental element of nutrition is macronutrient composition: the relative quantities of protein, fat and carbohydrate that produce the total caloric intake. With the total quantity acting as our gross adjustment tool, macronutrient composition provides us a tool for generally more minor but potentially significant adjustments. We can consider macronutrient composition within a single meal or in terms of daily totals depending on the purpose.

Protein should be considered the first priority in terms of macronutrients, particularly for strength athletes. Recommendations for protein intake vary from extremely minimal to quite epic. The numbers on the lower end of the spectrum are put forth by most of the medical community and government organizations and are reflections of absolute minimal intakes to support life, not optimal intakes to support athletic performance, health or longevity.

The recommended baseline for protein intake is 1 gram per pound (or approximately 2 grams per kilogram) of bodyweight (Zatsiorksy 1995). This is an arbitrary number in a sense, but its efficacy has been well demonstrated for many years in the strength training world. From this starting point, adjustments can be made as needed for each individual. Many will find they operate better with intakes twice as high at times (and even more during periods of weight gain). Experimentation is recommended without dipping below the 1g/1b/day baseline.

The quality of protein varies with its source. Meat, fish, eggs and high-quality egg and whey supplements will provide protein of the greatest bioavailability and amino acid profiles. The protein content of nuts and seeds, grains, and legumes is negligible in terms of both quantity and quality and these foods should not be considered legitimate protein sources that would act as substitutes for the previously listed sources. Soy has been pushed for years as a source of quality protein, but the claims are largely unfounded, and more research on soy's effects on health are producing frightening results; soy in any considerable quantity does not belong in the diet, with the occasional exception of fermented products such as soy sauce (ideally tamari, which is made without wheat). Supplemental protein will be discussed in more detail

in the Supplements chapter.

Fat has been thoroughly demonized, but is not only not inherently a threat to health, but is absolutely necessary to support it. Mono-unsaturated fats should make up the bulk of fat intake. These will be supplied by foods such as nuts and seeds, avocado, and olive oil, and even by many meats (approximately half of the fat in beef is mono-unsaturated, for example). Poly-unsaturated fats such as vegetable oils should be used sparingly, particularly when using oil to cook at high heats, such as with fried foods. The poly-unsaturated fat is a very unstable molecule and is easily damaged, creating unhealthy substances such as trans-fats and lipid peroxides.

Saturated fat like that found in animal products should not necessarily be sought out in great quantities, but as a stable molecule among other features, it's preferable over poly-unsaturated fat. Saturated fat is widely associated with dietary cholesterol, which is widely associated with heart disease. No research to date has conclusively demonstrated any causative relationship between fat or dietary cholesterol and heart disease, and more recent work is demonstrating that the relationship between cholesterol levels and heart disease risk is far from straightforward. This again is well outside the scope of this book, but the reader is strongly encouraged to do some homework if concerns about consumption of saturated fat and cholesterol exist. Keep in mind when encumbered by the fear of saturated fat and cholesterol that's been instilled in most of us that cholesterol is a structural component of every single cell in the body, and, among many other things, required in the production of steroid hormones (e.g. testosterone). It is absolutely essential to life, and the majority of cholesterol in the body is produced by the liver. This is why efforts to lower cholesterol levels through the extreme reduction of dietary cholesterol invariably fail—the body simply manufactures what it needs to take up the slack, just as it reduces production in the presence of adequate dietary cholesterol.

Omega-3 fatty acids are an essential fatty acid largely absent from most individuals' diets with the rare consumption of organ meats and only somewhat more common consumption of O-3-rich fish, although in recent years awareness has increased considerably and we are seeing more and more products with Omega-3 fatty acids, from Omega-3 supplements to eggs with added Omega-3 content. Omega-6 fatty acids are also essential, but their consumption is typically sufficient and often excessive relative to O-3s due to their natural presence in common foods such as meat, eggs and nuts; they are also pro-inflammatory. Few are willing to add organ meats to their diets and increase fish consumption adequately, so other sources of Omega-3s are usually necessary. Eggs enriched with O-3s are a wise choice since this will help balance the naturally high levels of O-6 in eggs; grass-fed beef is also higher in O-3s than grain-fed. Reducing O-6s is a better idea than increasing O-3s dramatically to improve the ratio.

In addition to supporting optimal health, fat can be used, due to its far greater caloric density relative to carbohydrate and protein, to supply a large quantity of daily calories if energy requirements are extremely high. That said, most athletes find it much easier to consume large quantities of carbohydrate than fat, as the former tends to be more palatable and actually often increases appetite, while the latter tends to be more satiating.

The third and final macronutrient is carbohydrate, which continues to be promoted as the cornerstone of great health as much as fat is vilified. This again is a subject demanding a venue other than this book for its due; suffice it to say claims of carbohydrates' role in health are often exaggerated. In fact, carbohydrates are technically the one of the three macronutrients not actually required to keep humans alive. This doesn't mean they are inherently bad or unhealthy, but that they, like the other two macronutrients, should be understood and used properly for each athlete's needs.

Carbohydrate requirements vary considerably among athletes and among periods of training. Low-repetition, high-intensity lifting is not demanding on glycolytic metabolism like somewhat more sustained, relatively intense activity is. With such training, carbohydrate intake can usually be kept relatively low with no negative effect on performance (note that this does not mean extremely low carbohydrate intake). However, with higher training volume or efforts at weight gain, carbohydrate intake will need to be increased. How much will vary, and experimentation will be important for each athlete. In any case, weightlifters will not have the carbohydrate requirements of endurance athletes or even those who engage in extended sprint-type efforts like football. Superheavyweights will generally require higher carbohydrate intakes simply to sustain their bodyweight.

Vegetables and some fruit should be the foundation of carbohydrate intake because of the micronutrient density. More energy-dense carbohydrate sources like tubers, corn products and rice can be added to fill out total carbohydrate need as determined by each athlete. Wheat products, if tolerated by the athlete, can also be added to fill out carbohydrate needs.

Macronutrient Timing

The timing of macronutrient consumption will have the least significant effect on performance, body composition and health relative to quantity, quality and macronutrient composition, but certain practices around training can be helpful. As with nearly all subjects in the realm of nutrition, much of the more detailed practices are largely speculative and certainly subject to individual experimentation—any such experimentation should be clearly documented to allow accurate evaluation.

Pre-Workout: The pre-workout period will most often involve nothing more than the athlete's normal eating habits—a balanced meal of protein, fat and carbohydrate. Timing of the last meal before training will vary among athletes depending on what the meal is comprised of and how the athlete tolerates such foods with training, but typically 1-2 hours prior to training is optimal as this provides enough time for at least partial digestion and assimilation so that the athlete has energy for training but does not feel bloated or otherwise uncomfortable from eating.

For athletes attempting to gain weight, 20-40 grams of easily-digested protein (supplemental whey protein) 10-20 minutes prior to training may create a more anabolic environment and encourage greater muscle growth. Instead of or in addition to this, athletes may find similar results from a high dose of a branched-chain amino acid supplement, although this will often create GI discomfort.

Pre-workout energy supplements are also used commonly. Most contain at least some amount of caffeine and usually a collection of amino acids and other substances that may (or may not) help provide the athlete more energy or a feeling of alertness. This could be something as simple as black coffee to expensive pre-workout powders or drinks with incredible claims. Each athlete will respond differently to every pre-workout supplement, so experimentation is encouraged. However, as with all supplements, competitive lifters need to be very cautious about what they use as many stimulants or similar compounds are banned by WADA/USADA.

Athletes should also ensure they're adequately hydrated in preparation for training. An easy method is simply making a habit of drinking 8-16 oz of water on the way to the gym or during the warm-up. This may be accomplished with a pre-workout energy drink.

Peri-Workout: During the training session itself, nutrition should not be an issue in most cases. For particularly lengthy training sessions, the same quality food eaten throughout the day can be eaten during breaks in the session—deli meat, nuts and fruit are convenient. Carbohydrate-based drinks work well for some individuals, but are usually unnecessary except for cases of unusually large training volumes or people whose blood glucose levels tend to drop dramatically.

Maintaining hydration will be the primary concern, particularly during the hotter months of the year during which athletes can lose significant quantities of water. In such circumstances, athletes may be well served by adding some kind of electrolyte mixture to their water (electrolytes are addressed in the Supplements chapter). For those attempting to gain weight, another dose of BCAAs in water or protein supplement can be sipped during the training session, provided the athlete has determined that neither causes gastrointestinal discomfort during training.

Post-Workout: Post-workout nutrition should aim to replace what has been used during training and assist the body in recuperating maximally. A common practice is to use a 3:1 carbohydrate to protein mixture. This ratio can be altered according to each athlete's needs with regard to carbohydrates and the volume of training: lower volume will require fewer carbohydrates. Fat intake in this meal should be minimal (as close to zero as possible) to prevent the slowing of digestion.

This post-workout meal can consist of whole foods such as a combination of grilled chicken and sweet potatoes, or it can be comprised of supplements like a combined protein and carbohydrate powder, or protein powder and a carbohydrate drink. The supplemental method is typically preferable, as it is digested and assimilated much more quickly, and athletes typically will not have much of an appetite immediately after training. In either case, this meal should be consumed immediately after the workout.

The post-workout meal can help encourage the anabolic processes in response to training. More recent research is suggesting that pre-workout protein might be more effective, but in most cases, both are advisable. A complete balanced meal should follow within 1-2 hours.

Planning Nutrition

To assemble this into practical application, first we need to know that protein and carbohydrate provide approximately 4 kcals per gram and fat 9 kcals. Next we need to determine the athlete's approximate daily caloric needs. To do this, we can use any number of formulas, none of which are ever remarkably accurate, or we can use a food journal to track food consumption and bodyweight for at least a week. Using online or other resources, calorie content can be determined for the food in the journal and daily totals can be calculated, from which a daily average over the period of the food journal can then be calculated. This average will be the starting point for daily calorie consumption (This assumes bodyweight is presently static—weight loss, gain, and maintenance are covered in the next chapter).

Since we've made protein the first priority and defined a clear quantitative guide for its consumption, we can determine the baseline daily protein requirements of the athlete: 1 gram of protein per pound of bodyweight per day. So with an 85kg athlete, we would end up with a starting point of 187 grams of protein per day (748 kcal).

Next, we can calculate a baseline carbohydrate intake level. This should be done in consideration of both bodyweight and activity quantity and na-

Day/Training	Carbohydrate Intake
Rest Days	< 1.1g/kg/day (0.5g/lb/day)
Low Volume Workouts	2.2g/kg/day (1.0g/lb/day)
Moderate Volume Workouts	3.3g/kg/day (1.5g/lb/day)
High Volume Workouts	4.4g/kg/day (2.0g/lb/day)

TABLE 48.1 Optimal carbohydrate intake guidelines. (Adapted from Israetel, Case, Hoffman, 2014)

ture. The higher the activity level, and the higher the average repetitions per set, the higher the carbohydrate intake should be; for example, during periods of high volume training such as during preparation mesocycles, lifters will typically need higher levels of carbohydrates to support muscle and liver glycogen replenishment as well as the actual carbohydrate needs for fueling the workouts themselves. We can also modulate carbohydrate intake day to day to suit that day's training workload (Table 48.1). In this way, we can be sure to consume optimal amounts on average without excessive intake when unnecessary, maximizing the performance results and minimizing any potential negative effect on body composition (and even health).

For our 85kg lifter, this would look like:

Day	Carbohydrate Intake
Rest Day	< 96g/day (384 kcal)
Low Volume Workouts	187g/day (748 kcal)
Moderate Volume Workouts	281g/day (1124 kcal)
High Volume Workouts	374g/day (1496 kcal)

Next, we simply need to fill the rest of the total daily caloric needs with fat. By tracking intake with the food journal for 2 weeks during a period of constant bodyweight, we can find an average number of daily calories for the athlete by adding each day's total calories and then dividing the sum by the number of days. We then know this is the caloric intake that will preserve the lifter's current bodyweight, and can make adjustments for weight loss or gain from this baseline.

We want to adjust daily caloric intake according to daily activity level in the same manner carbohydrate levels were adjusted, however, so we need to do a little math.

First, we add the protein and carbohydrate calories for each type of training day we have planned in a week. For example:

Day	Training	Protein/Carb
Monday	Heavy	2244 kcal
Tuesday	Moderate	1872 kcal
Wednesday	Heavy	2244 kcal
Thursday	Moderate	1872 kcal
Friday	Rest	1132 kcal
Saturday	Heavy	2244 kcal
Sunday	Rest	1132 kcal

This gives us a weekly total of 12,710 kcals, and a daily average of 1820 kcal (weekly total divided by 7 days). Next we use this average and our determined daily average from the food journal to create a multiplier by dividing the determined total by the combined protein/carbohydrate total. If we've determined through the food journal that our 85kg lifter needs about 2500 kcals/day to maintain his weight, we would divide 2500 by 1820, which gives us a multiplier of 1.37.

We can then use this multiplier with the combined daily protein/carbohydrate calorie number to get a total daily calorie number that is proportional to the carbohydrate intake, which we will likely then alter a bit to get rid of extreme fluctuations.

Day	Training	Protein/Carb	Total
Monday	Heavy	2244 kcal	3074 kcal
Tuesday	Moderate	1872 kcal	2565 kcal
Wednesday	Heavy	2244 kcal	3074 kcal
Thursday	Moderate	1872 kcal	2565 kcal
Friday	Rest	1132 kcal	1551 kcal
Saturday	Heavy	2244 kcal	3074 kcal
Sunday	Rest	1132 kcal	1551 kcal

This gives us an average for the week of 2493 kcal/day, which closely matches our desired total. If we want (or need) to reduce the range of extremes, we can simply move some of the calories from the heavy days to the light or rest days. For example, we can knock 200 kcal off each heavy day, which gives us 600 total calories, which we can then split between our two rest days (300 kcal each), giving us 2874 kcal on the heavy days and 1851 kcal on the rest days. This will usually be preferred by athletes because it makes meal planning a little easier and tends to help with recovery on off days.

Finally, we can determine our daily fat intake by simply finding the daily difference between the total calories and the combined protein/carbohydrate calories and dividing by the 9 calories per gram that fat contains. For example, a moderate training day has a total of 2562 kcal and a combined protein/carbohydrate total of 1872 kcal, leaving a difference of 690 kcal, which, divided by 9, gives us 77 grams of fat.

Again, these figures are loose starting points and will more than likely need to be adjusted based on how the lifter feels and performs. For example, some lifters may want to increase their daily protein intake, which means they can simply remove the additional calories from their fat intake. Or an athlete who finds he or she feels better with a somewhat lower carb intake can make up the caloric difference by increasing protein and/or fat.

Depending on the nature and volume of training, and the athlete's individual recovery capacity, recovery may be better if rest day carbohydrates are not reduced as dramatically. This is more likely the higher the training volume is, and if the athlete trains late in the day and consequently consumes fewer carbohydrates after the workout to replenish glycogen before a low-carbohydrate rest day. In these cases, the carbohydrate intake can be balanced more or completely across all days of the week while maintaining the same totals.

Alternatively, if the food journal method of determining average daily calorie needs is not possible, such as in the case of changing bodyweight, we can get an estimate of average daily caloric needs using a rough BMR (basal metabolic rate) estimate and a multiplier based on activity level. This can be done with several online sources quickly and easily. Bear in mind this is very much an approximation, as it involves multiple steps of estimation and assumption, and not as accurate as the food journal method, which reflects the individual's actual metabolic activity—it is merely a starting point and adjustments will need to be made in response to weight and performance changes. Using the food journal to track bodyweight and performance for 2 weeks at the daily calorie intake determined with this method will let the athlete know if this number is too high or low, and it can be adjusted accordingly.

This takes care of the quantity and macronutrient composition elements—these must simply now be fulfilled with food of the appropriate quality. It's easy these days to determine macronutrient and calorie quantities of any imaginable food with online sources, and to track daily consumption. Keep in mind that any supplements that contain calories (such as fish oil and pre-workouts) need to be considered in the daily macronutrient and calorie figures.

Water Intake

There should be no need to make a case for the importance of adequate hydration here—make it happen. Intake recommendations vary dramatically, and recently some have begun to lean toward lower quantities. A reasonable starting point is:

Bodyweight (kg) X 0.026 = L/day
or
Bodyweight (lbs) X 0.4 = oz/day

For our 85 kg (187 lb) athlete, we would end up with about 2.2 L (75 oz) per day. This is a baseline intake and doesn't take into account water loss during physical activity. Before, during and after any activity, water should be consumed according to the intensity and duration of the activity and obvious loss through sweat. For more accurate re-hydration, replace every kilogram of bodyweight lost during activity with 1 liter of water (or every pound of bodyweight with 16 ounces of water).

Bodyweight

Managing bodyweight is primarily a concern of competitive weightlifters, although most athletes will certainly have reason to control their weight within at least general ranges in order to optimize performance and body composition. There are three basic bodyweight scenarios: maintaining weight, losing weight and gaining weight. All three have the implicit goal of maximizing functional muscle mass at a given weight, which means achieving relatively low body fat levels. However, this does not necessarily mean weightlifters need or want to reach extremely low body fat percentages, and, in fact, extreme leanness arguably does not allow for maximal performance unless an athlete is naturally very lean.

Bodyweight can be controlled by both training and nutrition. However, training should be focused as much as possible on achieving specific athletic and functional objectives—that is, the training program should remain designed to elicit adaptations for improved weightlifting ability, and not diverge to any significant degree from this to achieve bodyweight changes. A minor exception to this would be in cases of bodyweight gain in which training may temporarily increase in volume and number of repetitions per set for certain exercises to encourage greater hypertrophy, supported by appropriate nutritional changes. Additionally, while training influences the nature of weight gain or loss to some extent (i.e. relative fat and lean mass levels), nutrition is what ultimately allows the most significant gains or losses.

A fundamental principle of bodyweight is the First Law of Thermodynamics: Neither matter nor energy can be created or destroyed. The two can be converted, but there is never any net change in the total quantity. What this means in terms of bodyweight manipulation is that weight cannot be reduced without a deficit of energy, and weight cannot be increased without a surplus of energy. No amount of heavy back squatting will make a skinny kid huge if said skinny kid fails to eat more energy and material than his body is using simply to survive—as remarkable as the human body is, it cannot create tissue from thin air. This would be akin to building an addition to a house without using any new materials or performing any work: impossible.

Likewise, no amount of physical activity will cause a reduction in bodyweight if the individual is consuming more food energy than is being used in a given period of time. When evaluating a bodyweight plan, always return to and rely on this fundamental principle to guide your decisions.

The above said, it's unfortunately not such a simple equation—human metabolism manages to be remarkably complex and remains incompletely understood in the context of bodyweight and body composition even by experts in the field. The first complication is the second law of thermodynamics—entropy. Entropy is the transfer of a percentage of the energy during a chemical reaction to the realm outside the reaction—commonly this transfer is referred to as a "loss", but because, according to the first law, energy cannot be lost, it is simply being relocated, usually in the form of heat. Macronutrients ultimately provide different net calories because of the variation the efficiency of their metabolism. For example, protein has fewer usable calories per gram than carbohydrate because the greater number of chemical reactions required to use protein as energy result in a lower net amount of energy with the increased entropy (although this is a very small difference) (Eades M.R., Eades M.D., 2001). This of course does not alter the fact that a calorie is a calorie—it only forces us to consider calories in terms of net instead of gross. And it certainly does not change the fact that an individual cannot gain weight without a net calorie surplus, or lose weight without a net calorie deficit.

To complicate things further, it turns out that the basic energy balance equation that's relied on for most bodyweight recommendations is widely misinterpreted (Taubes, 2007):

Change in energy stores = Energy intake – Energy expenditure

This is commonly understood to mean that the change in bodyweight is entirely and exclusively a product of the relationship between calories consumed and calories expended. In other words, it's assumed that any increase in energy intake will cause an increase in bodyweight, and any reduction in energy intake will cause a reduction in bodyweight, because the equation has to remain balanced or the universe will fall apart.

However, real-world evidence demonstrates that the response to changes in caloric intake is not rigid and perfectly predictable. That is, a given reduction in calories does not necessarily produce the exact reduction in bodyweight predicted by the relevant mathematics in all individuals.

Instead, the body apparently has a fairly well-established set point in terms of bodyweight and composition that it attempts to maintain—changes in energy intake will cause the body to make changes in its energy expenditure in order to maintain that set point. For example, if an individual increases his calorie consumption, the body will find ways to expend more energy through generally unnoticed processes that convert the excess energy to heat. This is why dieting of the basic calorie-reduction form fails so much—the dieter's body simply reduces its energy expenditure to match intake as much as possible (Taubes, 2007).

All this said, pursuit of bodyweight changes is not hopeless, just more complicated, and requires a bit more finesse. In the case of weight gain, it appears that the body can only increase its energy expenditure so much—this simply means that calorie surpluses will often need to be even greater than expected to exceed the body's ability to compensate. After an athlete lives at a greater bodyweight for a period of time, the set point seems to be adjusted upwards, making maintenance and further gains easier.

With regard to weight loss, the issue appears to be one largely of macronutrient composition and its effect on metabolic status. That is, management of proper hormonal levels, gut health and systemic inflammation coupled with a series of incremental calorie reductions rather than a single dramatic one, seems to be far more productive than extreme calorie restriction. Again, with time at a new bodyweight, the set point seems to be readjusted. In all cases, slower changes seem to be more effective than attempts at rapid ones.

Of course, each athlete will respond differently to any given change in caloric intake or macronutrient ratios, and each will need to be adjusted accordingly. Additionally, just as each athlete has a ceiling for certain performance characteristics determined by genetic factors, each athlete's genetics will largely control the rate of weight and body composition changes, as well as the ultimate states of each. No matter how precise an athlete's nutrition is, he or she may never achieve the level of leanness, for example, of another athlete. Again, just like training, nutrition can be used to reach each athlete's ultimate genetic potential, but never actually alter it. The actual alteration of genetic potential is the exclusive realm of pharmaceuticals.

Maintaining Weight

Bodyweight maintenance can range from requiring no work at all to being extremely troublesome. For those who maintain their weights without any thought, the only remaining issue is that of body composition.

The maintenance of bodyweight is simply a matter of balancing energy consumed as food and energy expended through metabolism. For those whose bodyweights fluctuate continually, the goal is developing consistency in eating and activity—to establish the body's set point at the desired weight and body composition and then support its maintenance.

The first step is to assess the current situation. A detailed food journal should be kept for at least a week and ideally two, describing accurate quantities of all food and any beverages, including water—daily weight fluctuations are often simply the result of varying levels of hydration. Online programs can be used to then calculate calories and macronutrients for each day. In this journal, records of bodyweight can be kept as well. Weight should be taken at the same time and under the same conditions every time. The typical recommendation is to weigh first thing in the morning on an empty stomach; however, we're concerned with bodyweight two hours prior to competition. This being the case, for the most accuracy, weight should also be checked at the same time every afternoon so both measurements can be tracked. The food and weight journal should be paired with the athlete's training records to provide a complete picture.

The first thing to look at is water consumption—1 lifter of water weighs 1 kg (and 16 ounces of water weighs 1 pound). Much bodyweight fluctuation can be attributed to inconsistent hydration, particularly considering most individuals are not extraordinarily disciplined with their water intake. If the food log shows large changes in water consumption that correspond with bodyweight changes—that is, lower water intake is associated with lower bodyweight and vice versa—the first step should be equalizing daily water consumption for a period of time and evaluating its effect on bodyweight.

If during a period of consistent hydration bodyweight does not stabilize satisfactorily, it will be necessary to make additional adjustments. Start by averaging the daily calorie totals from the food log to arrive at a baseline. From this, determine a daily calorie intake: if the weight fluctuation tends to be heavy, start with 5-10% fewer calories than the average; if the weight fluctuation tends to be light, start with 5-10% more calories than the average. Attempt to hit this calorie number every day for a week and assess its effect on bodyweight. Continue making minor calorie intake adjustments accordingly until the desired bodyweight is reached and maintained. Be patient and give each intake level at least a week before adjusting. Again, this more deliberate approach is more effective than attempting dramatic changes, which will be resisted by the body through adjustments in energy expenditure and will not provide reliable responses.

Once the correct bodyweight has been achieved, more focus can be directed to improving body composition through macronutrient ratios and food timing. If the desired bodyweight requires unusually difficult food intake, whether too little or too much, the athlete should consider changing weight classes to allow living closer to a natural bodyweight if it will not negatively impact performance. That said, patience is important—over time, the body will adjust more to a given weight and maintenance will become less of a struggle.

Losing Weight

Losing weight is achieved by creating a calorie deficit while supporting healthy metabolic activity, largely through the management of relevant hormone levels, intestinal health and systemic inflammation. This is done primarily through incremental reductions in calorie intake, improvement of food quality, and lifestyle components like adequate sleep and stress reduction. Because of the body's natural reaction of metabolic adjustment, the more gradual the weight loss, the less of a negative effect on performance it will have. Sudden large calorie deficits will produce systemic fatigue and decreases in strength and stamina, will be psychologically taxing, and will typically result in less weight loss than expected.

Plan weight loss as far out from a competition as possible to allow continued successful training during the drop. Too often weightlifters are content to remain overweight most of the year and then struggle to lose significant amounts in very little time for competition, often unsuccessfully or with considerable detriment to performance. This stress, performance reduction and potential failure can be avoided easily through better planning and weight management.

Our weight loss plan begins in the same way as our maintenance plan—we first need to record and find our average daily calorie intake over a week. From here, we'll drop this figure and consume the calculated number of calories consistently for 1-2 weeks, evaluate the progress, and readjust if necessary.

How much we drop the calorie level will depend on two things. First, is bodyweight constant, increasing or decreasing at present? Second, how quickly does the weight need to come off?

If bodyweight is constant and we have no time constraints, we may drop the calories by 10-15% or so for 1-2 weeks and monitor weight and performance. If the weight is dropping at a reasonable rate—probably around 0.25 – 1% of bodyweight per week—and performance has not been negatively affected to any degree beyond what is acceptable, this calorie level can be maintained until weight loss begins to slow. At that point, the calorie intake will have to be again dropped to account for the lower bodyweight. In this fashion, a gradual but steady rate of weight loss can usually be maintained with minimal disruption to performance.

If bodyweight is already dropping, the goal is either to maintain the current rate of decrease or accelerate it if and when necessary. In the same manner, calculate current average daily calorie intake and continue adhering to this level until progress slows, at which time calorie intake can be decreased another 10% or so.

If bodyweight is currently increasing, the initial calorie decrease will simply need to be greater. Depending on how quickly weight is increasing, this initial cut may be as much as 20%. Unusually large drops are not advisable because of their potential to cause counterproductive metabolic shifts and impact on performance.

If time for weight loss is limited, more aggressive calorie deficits can be created; however, it's important to keep in mind that the greater the deficit, the greater its impact on performance will be, and that there's no guarantee it will be successful because of the body's attempt to readjust. As much as possible, this situation should be avoided.

Last minute weight loss in order to make weight for competition (weight cutting) is covered in the Competition section.

Gaining Weight

While in theory gaining weight is no more complex than either maintaining or losing it, in practice it invariably proves difficult for a variety of reasons. Foremost of those reasons is that the discipline required by the pursuit of functional mass often surpasses that of even aggressive weight loss.

The fundamental principle of weight gain is merely the opposite of weight loss: create a surplus of energy and material while attempting to prevent compensatory metabolic adjustment by the body to maintain its set point bodyweight and encourage the accumulation of muscle mass over body fat. In cases of aggressive weight gain, simply consuming the necessary quantity of food is uncomfortable at best and seemingly impossible at worst. Contributing to the difficulty is the great importance of food quality and macronutrient composition. A great enough calorie surplus of any composition will produce at least some weight gain—but the role of additional weight is to provide additional functional capacity. The difficulty lies in encouraging the body not to simply increase its mass, but to do so through functional muscular hypertrophy—this demands the control of food quality and macronutrient composition, as well as factors like sleep quantity and quality, and creating a hormonal state that encourages lean tissue growth.

As is the case with weight loss, the longer the period of time over which weight is gained, the more the quality of the added mass can be controlled. There are limits to the rate at which the body's lean mass can grow, and reaching beyond these limits will unavoidably result in greater gains in body fat relative to muscle mass.

That said, weightlifting is a sport with broad weight classes and essentially no off-season, and often weight must be gained rapidly in order for an ascending lifter to remain competitive. In these cases, quality will take a back seat to quantity with the presumption that efforts will be made to improve quality once the lifter has settled into the higher weight.

For gradual weight gain, the process is in essence no different than gradual weight loss, the difference being only that the daily calories will be incrementally increased instead of decreased. Accurate record keeping is equally important—the same ease of self-delusion during weight loss applies to weight gain. Protein intake can be adjusted up to as much as 2-3 grams per pound of bodyweight per day. How well this higher protein intake accelerates muscle gain seems to vary among individuals, but it has certainly never hurt. Carbohydrate intake should be increased as well as an easy, palatable way to increase total caloric intake, but also to support the increased training volume the athlete is likely undertaking in order to stimulate muscular hypertrophy. Fat intake can then be increased as needed to achieve the determined total daily caloric needs.

For more aggressive weight gain, the rules must be changed somewhat. The rule standing high above all is *eat more*. More than you ate before, more than what you want to eat, more than what you think you can eat. Quality and macronutrient composition are irrelevant until quantity has been taken care of. This is by no means intended to dissuade attempts to maintain quality and composition, but to more forcefully underscore the importance of a large and consistent calorie surplus. In other words, if the only options are eating fast food and eating little or nothing, the choice must be fast food, and more than is appealing. Always remember—if you're not uncomfortable, you're not eating enough, and if you're hungry, you're failing miserably.

With gradual weight gain, the body is allowed time to adjust to progressively larger quantities of food; with rapid weight gain, there is no such luxury. In order to mitigate this problem, foods with the greatest possible caloric density will become necessities. Fats will be instrumental considering that a given quantity has over twice the calorie content of the same quantity of either protein or carbohydrate. Nut butters, olive oil, and coconut milk are relatively easily stomached but extraordinarily calorie-dense. For those who can tolerate dairy, whole milk should replace its reduced-fat counterparts (and those who are lactose intolerant can still include whole milk along with lactase supplements). In the same vein is supplemental protein, which will provide an extremely helpful service considering the physical difficulty of eating enormous quantities of meat. This will be discussed more in the Supplements chapter.

Fitting in another meal in the middle of the night has been a successful tactic for many. Typically this meal is in the form of a shake consisting of supplemental protein, milk, nut butter, coconut milk, and possibly fruit. This can obviously increase the number of quality calories in a 24-hour period significantly, and will consequently be successful if eating the rest of the day is in order. However, the quality and quantity of sleep, particularly during times of weight gain, is of great importance. Because of this, the recommendation is to prepare a shake and place it in the refrigerator. If the athlete wakes naturally during the night, he or she can drink the shake. If not, he or she can drink it the next morning. Intentionally disrupting sleep is potentially more detrimental than night feedings are beneficial. If an athlete is the kind of individual who can be awakened, drink a shake, and fall immediately back to sleep, this may not be an issue. But for some, a five-minute task can result in multiple hours of lost sleep.

Just as with weight loss, individuals will respond very differently during weight gain. That is, with a given calorie surplus, athletes will gain different amounts of weight of different qualities, according to genetic predisposition. Again—if no weight is being gained, not enough is being eaten.

Milk

Milk is commonly endorsed among old school strength coaches and athletes as the ultimate weight gaining food. There is no question that milk offers a generally easily consumed and inexpensive source of potentially enormous amounts of protein and calories, and consequently can help encourage rapid weight gain. Whether or not milk actually produces gains in muscle mass any better than the equivalent totals of quality protein, fat and carbohydrate is not as clear, but anecdotal evidence seems to suggest it may. In any case, its convenience and affordability is hard to beat.

Lactose intolerance can be managed with inexpensive lactase supplements. Raw milk is another option that will itself supply some of the needed lactase enzymes, as well as some colostrum, both of which will reduce the cost of supplementation for these two items. Whole milk with 100% of the lactose removed is also available.

The Superheavyweight

As has been alluded to previously, the super-heavyweight lifter is somewhat of a special case in terms of nutrition. In essence he or she is eternally attempting to gain weight, and doing so at an already very large body mass. This extreme demand on the body often necessitates more extreme measures.

Ideally the superheavyweight follows the same basic nutritional prescription as any other lifter; that is, a foundation of quality animal-source proteins, vegetables and fruits, and quality fats, but supplemented to increase caloric level with additional food of all macronutrient content, and likely a greater proportion of dense carbohydrate sources.

Carbohydrate is only slightly more energy-dense than protein in terms of net calories, and is less than half as dense than fat, by the gram, but it's invariably much easier to consume in great quantities, and its elicitation of insulin secretion appears to help with weight gain both by encouraging nutrient storage and promoting hunger. Because of this, for many superheavies, carbohydrate intake will typically need to be much greater (both in absolute and relative terms) than what would normally be considered necessary or healthy. However, being a superheavyweight is not an excuse to entirely abandon quality nutrition. The same foundation of quality food should remain in place, not be replaced.

Genetic Predisposition

As with all morphological changes in the body, genetic factors will affect an individual's ability to both gain muscular weight and to lose body fat. As a consequence, a great deal of variation among athletes will be seen even with identical protocols. Athletes must simply work with what they have and maximize gains underneath their genetic ceilings. With this in mind, expectations for gaining or losing weight or shifting body composition must be considered realistically, and nutrition must be altered to best suit each athlete.

Supplements

Nutritional supplementation is an enormous industry populated overwhelmingly with overpriced and ineffective gimmicks supported by inaccurate, cleverly manipulated, misunderstood, or occasionally non-existent science. There are, however, a few supplements that deserve discussion, experimentation, or recommendation. The following supplements are considered effective and useful to a degree that warrants at least educated experimentation.

Competitive weightlifters are encouraged to verify with the US Anti-Doping Agency (USADA), World Anti-Doping Agency (WADA), or the appropriate national organization the legality of supplements in and out of competition before beginning use. Ignorance of the rules is not grounds for immunity or leniency.

Additionally, competitive weightlifters need to be cautious about what they use as supplements are often manufactured in facilities and with equipment used for other supplements. This means that even a supplement that does not contain any banned substances in its listed ingredients may still produce a positive drug test result due to being contaminated by residue from other supplements. A few companies guarantee their products to be free of banned substances, and these products should be relied on primarily.

Protein

With the importance of quality protein and the difficulty of consuming large amounts of it in whole foods, as well as the need for rapidly digesting and assimilating protein post-workout, supplemental protein is commonplace in weightlifters' diets. The abundant use of supplemental protein means the availability of a wide range of type and quality. There are only three types of supplemental protein that should even be considered: whey, egg and casein. Each can be used in different situations primarily depending on the need for absorption rate. For example, whey is very rapidly absorbing and consequently ideal post-workout, whereas casein is more slowly digested, making it better (often in combination with whey) for other times of day.

Supplemental protein should contain precisely what the name implies: protein. There will typically be trace amounts of fat and carbohydrate in any protein supplement, but it should be minimal because any added fat or carbohydrate will generally be of poor quality and better supplied by whole foods (An exception to this would be a combination protein and carbohydrate supplement intended for use post-workout as long as it's in the correct ratio for the athlete). Also look for supplements with no or minimal amounts of artificial sweeteners and unnecessary additives.

For athletes needing to consume unusually large amounts of protein, a hydrolyzed supplement will be a wise choice if not entirely necessary. Hydrolyzation breaks down the proteins into smaller peptides, making the supplement easier to digest. If hydrolyzation proves inadequate to prevent digestive trouble, additional digestive enzymes can help.

And don't forget to chew your protein shakes as you would solid food—you may feel silly, but this action helps fully stimulate the digestive process and improves the ultimate assimilation of the protein.

Vitamin D

Vitamin D supplementation is becoming more and more popular as increasingly individuals are being found deficient. Many of us spend the vast majority of our time indoors and as a consequence are exposed to very little sunlight. Vitamin D levels can be tested easily with routine blood work and supplementation can be based on the level of deficiency. Typically it will be recommended in cases of deficiency to start with a higher dose and step down to a lower maintenance dose after a month or so. Supplemental Vitamin D in cases of deficiency can have dramatic effects on energy, mood and recuperation.

Creatine

The effectiveness of creatine probably varies among individuals more than any other supplement. For 20-25% of the population, response is immediate and measurable. For many, there may be marginal results, but nothing remarkably convincing and possibly not worth the cost and hassle of taking it. And for a final group, there will be no apparent response at all, although bodyweight may increase slightly from water retention with no accompanying performance gains.

Creatine is inexpensive and certainly merits experimentation. While some athletes may not noticeably respond in terms of performance, creatine may decrease cortisol levels and oxidative damage, and taken at bedtime may increase growth hormone secretion during sleep. Because of this, even non-responders may consider supplementation.

There is no need for a loading period—simply start with the normal dose of 5-10 grams/day in water or protein shakes. For larger athletes taking higher doses, the total can be split and taken at different times—typically pre- and post-workout, or post-workout and bedtime.

It appears the body may have a saturation point, after which it will reduce its own production of creatine to return quantities to below its natural level. Cycling 2-6 weeks on and 1 week off should help counteract this to keep the average level over time above normal. A simple and effective way to cycle creatine is to simply time it with training cycles; that is, during weeks of reduced intensity and/or volume, creatine use can be stopped, and then resumed with normal training. In any case, it's important to ensure use is timed appropriately for competitions, and should not be used pre-competition without previous experience.

Fish Oil

Available as either liquid or in capsules, fish oil provides the Omega-3 fatty acids that are essential to health, performance, and life itself, but are often largely absent in the typical diet. Fish oil has a number of beneficial effects with regard to performance, including increasing protein synthesis, reducing cortisol levels, increasing testosterone levels, and reducing inflammation.

The compounds in which we're interested are EPA and DHA, and how much is contained in the total amount of fish oil is the number with which to be concerned. For example, some fish oil supplements will have a combined total of 300 mg of EPA and DHA per 1000 mg serving, while others will have 600 mg of EPA and DHA in a 1000 mg serving. The former will often appear less expensive, but with a direct comparison of EPA and DHA content with the latter, the price gap will typically disappear.

A starting dose should be 1-2 grams of total EPA/DHA per day, ideally taken with fat-containing meals to improve digestion and absorption. After 1-2 weeks, the dose can be increased 500 mg – 1 g. This can be repeated until no further benefits are noticed or digestive discomfort appears. It's advisable to reduce excessive Omega-6 intake and other pro-inflammatory foods more than increase Omega-3 intake to counteract it; a top-end dose would be 4-6 grams daily. If any amount of fish oil produces digestive problems, it can be accompanied by ox bile, which will help with the fat's digestion. Make sure to keep fish oil in the refrigerator or freezer to prevent untimely oxidation.

Multi-Vitamin/Mineral

Depending on the quality of food being consumed consistently by an athlete, it may or may not be necessary or beneficial for an athlete to take a multi-nutrient supplement. Generally a wise approach for athletes who eat well consistently is taking a multi-nutrient every other day or even less frequently. Athletes for whom food quality is inconsistent may take one more frequently. Keep in mind that repeatedly it has been shown that vitamin and mineral supplementation does not have beneficial effects beyond eliminating deficiencies. More recent research actually suggests that excessive intake can have negative effects on health.

Digestive Enzymes

For the rapid weight gain crowd, digestive enzymes can be the difference between success and failure. Typically in cases of quick weight gain, the sheer volume of food being consumed will exceed the body's ability to digest it adequately, resulting in anything from discomfort to serious GI distress. Enzymes are relatively inexpensive and will greatly improve the usability of the food being eaten. Take with meals.

Ox bile is an inexpensive supplement that will aid in the emulsification of fats and reduce fat-related digestive discomfort. It can be taken with high-fat meals and with fish oil as needed to improve digestion.

Branched-Chain Amino Acids

The branched-chain amino acids are luecine, isoleucine, and valine. Use of BCAAs appears to assist in muscle growth, although many claims of effectiveness are greatly exaggerated. Supplementation with large dose BCAAs is worth experimenting with during periods of mass gain. Some will find these large doses to cause GI discomfort and will need to reduce the dosage, although if the necessary reduction is dramatic, it's likely not worth continuing use. Some BCAA supplements are combined wisely with glutamine to improve muscle protein sparing and muscle growth response. Be sure to purchase as powder instead of capsules for better cost per dose. Often protein supplements will have additional BCAAs and/or glutamine included, which is a convenient way to increase intake, although it limits the possible timing of ingestion.

Vitamin C

Vitamin C is an inexpensive supplement that can be helpful in a number of ways. As an immune function supporter, it can obviously help keep athletes healthy and training at full speed. It can also help lower cortisol levels, and for this purpose can be taken post workout and at bedtime. Supplements that contain bioflavanoids rather than only ascorbic acid are more effective in general, and in particular for adrenal function support. As mentioned with regard to multi-vitamin and mineral supplements, excessive consumption is not recommended. It may be a good idea to only add vitamin C during periods of extremely strenuous training when immune function will be the most susceptible to compromise, when around other people who are sick, or leading into a competition to help prevent becoming sick at that critical time.

Probiotics

Probiotic supplements encourage the proliferation and maintenance of the natural microorganisms that inhabit the human gut. This is a commonly underappreciated element of general health, and consequently athletic performance. Probiotics come in a multitude of forms, from pills to powder, or can be ingested as part of fermented foods if preferred.

Glutamine

Glutamine is an amino acid often used in large quantities, and often added to branched-chain amino acid supplements. Research has suggested it can increase growth hormone levels, improve protein synthesis, and improve immune system function. Like creatine and BCAAs, individuals seem to respond to glutamine supplementation very differently, some feeling significant improvement in recovery from training and others experiencing no noticeable benefit. Glutamine should be purchased in bulk powder form as beneficial doses will be multiple grams. Generally, it should simply be added to the lifter's post-workout protein & carbohydrate drink.

Glucosamine / Chondroiton / MSM

Glucosamine, chondroiton and MSM have all been demonstrated widely to improve connective tissue repair and joint health, and are most commonly taken in combination with each other. Considering the abuse the joints will take when exposed to weightlifting over any extended period of time, this is a wise addition to the nutrition program.

Colostrum

Bovine colostrum is typically sold as an immune function supporter, but its effects at high doses on muscle growth have been demonstrated in at least a few studies and in much real world experience. The dosage required to elicit measurable lean mass gain makes colostrum an expensive supplement, but for those having trouble gaining weight, it's worth evaluating. Dosage in pertinent studies has been 20 grams daily; athletes can adjust for their bodyweights by using about 10% of bodyweight in pounds per day in grams, e.g. a 230-lb athlete would use 23 grams daily.

Caffeine

Caffeine is a substance that attracts as wide an array of opinions as any other. There is little argument regarding its ability to improve athletic performance in the short-term; the more contentious issue is its effects on long-term health, particularly its potential impact on adrenal function. As long as adrenal problems don't exist presently, dosing is appropriate, and caffeine is not relied on as a substitute for adequate quantity and quality of sleep, there is little concern.

Because caffeine's effects vary among individuals, it's important for lifters to have experience training while caffeinated before bringing it into a competitive situation. Keep doses reasonable—there will be a point at which more caffeine will fail to improve performance and instead begin disrupting it. Further, excessive caffeine use and the resulting high level of arousal during training can increase systemic fatigue and lead more easily to overtraining.

A wise approach to caffeine intake might be cycling. After a period of normal caffeine use, a significant reduction or elimination of intake for a week or two may provide time for the body to recover from any accumulated systemic fatigue that has developed from the greater degree of physical excitement experienced with caffeine use and reset caffeine sensitivity to a lower baseline. This back-off period may be particularly beneficial in the 1-2 weeks prior to a competition, with the reintroduction of caffeine just prior to the event, and then in the 1-2 weeks following a competition when training will be less demanding and the body will need to recover. Experiment with this outside of competition first to gauge response, as it may be dramatically different than expected.

Electrolytes

During intense training in the summer months, athletes can lose considerable amounts of water, along with which will come electrolytes—sodium, potassium and chloride. Electrolyte replacement drinks or powders can be purchased, typically combined with sugar, which is fine if it's determined the athlete will benefit from this during or after training. To make an effective electrolyte solution without sugar if needed or wanted, add about a half-teaspoon of salt and half-teaspoon of potassium chloride (sold commonly as a salt substitute) to each liter of water.

Pre-Workouts

Pre-workout energy drinks are extremely popular for obvious reasons. The first concern with these supplements is the possible presence of banned substances—both as legitimate ingredients and due to contamination from other products. The second concern regards excessive nervous system fatigue due to frequent over-stimulation. Long term frequent use of stimulants results in much a greater systemic fatiguing effect from training that can create serious problems for a lifter, essentially accelerating the process of overtraining and even creating a state of overtraining from training that would otherwise not cause it. This is an instance in which the concept of minimal effective dose is important to keep in mind—use of stimulants for training should be judicious and prevented from becoming excessive. Additionally, it's a good idea to cease use periodically for a week, such as during periods of light training in a cycle, to give the body a chance to recover; this will also make the supplement more effective and lower doses when used again.

Introduction to Mobility & Flexibility

Weightlifting demands a high degree of mobility relative to many other sports, and certainly to any other strength sport. The hips, shoulders, wrists and ankles primarily must be able to move unimpeded through the necessary ranges of motions in order to allow the proper performance of the lifts and avoid unnecessary stress and potential injury; additionally, above average mobility of the thoracic spine is required for optimal structure.

When athletes begin training for weightlifting at the ideal young age, typically mobility is naturally adequate or nearly so and will require relatively little work to develop to the optimal degree. In these cases, the preservation of the natural youthful mobility and achieving any additional mobility not naturally present is the goal, along with the development of the necessary strength and stability to support the range of motion. This can usually be accomplished indirectly without any specific mobility work through the typical training program, which at this early stage should include a wide array of general physical activities including large amplitude and gymnastics-type bodyweight movements.

More often than not, athletes who begin weightlifting later in life will initially possess inadequate mobility for the movements and positions, and will need to improve their mobility in order to train effectively and safely. While barbell training itself will contribute to improving mobility to some extent for these athletes, specific and direct mobility work will need to be included in the training program to both maximize and accelerate improvements.

While the terms *flexibility* and *mobility* are often used interchangeably, and arguably the precise definitions are unimportant in a practical sense, we can specify for the sake of thoroughness. *Flexibility* typically refers to the extensibility of a specific muscle, while *mobility* refers to the potential range of motion of a specific joint (which is affected in part by the flexibility of the related muscles).

In addition to this is the element of *stability*, which is the ability of the athlete to securely support all positions within the possible range of motion—this is an issue of strength and motor control. A lack of stability in a certain position or range of motion can present as immobility, as the body will naturally protect itself by avoiding entering unsupportable positions and movements. This is the primary reason why strength and technique training must play a role in mobility improvements—these things allow the body to develop increasing ranges of motion in concert with the motor abilities to control the related positions and movements effectively and safely. A limitation based on instability rather than flexibility or mobility can usually be discovered through identifying a disparity between the range of motion in a passive movement (e.g. a static stretch in a supported position that does not require any stabilization) and the range of motion of the same joint(s) in the same basic position in which there is a stability and strength component (e.g. a squat). However, a great enough degree of mobility will eclipse the limitations of instability in the absence of significant resistance—this does not mean we necessarily want athletes to possess extreme mobility, but that flexibility and mobility themselves cannot be neglected.

Optimal Mobility

The field of athletic training is abounding with conflicting information regarding mobility and stretching. The reigning popular notion of mobility and stretching is that their relationships to both athletic performance and injury protection are positive and linear; that is, as stretching and mobility increase, so do athletic performance and injury protection. The actual research and experience of coaches and athletes, however, have failed to demonstrate this relationship, and the evidence in concert with a dose of reason suggests a different association.

It's more likely that the relationship of mobility to both injury and performance describes a modified bell curve; that is, both hypomobility and hypermobility increase the risk of injury and may limit performance. However, in close proximity to the apex representing optimal mobility—the degree of mobility associated with the least risk of injury and the greatest performance—hypomobility is associated with greater injury risk and greater performance inhibition than is hypermobility (Figure 51.1). In other words, excessive mobility is only slightly more desirable than inadequate mobility.

It's important to understand the difference between reducing or eliminating a performance-limiting factor and actually improving performance. It's also important to visualize this trend on the bell curve described in Figure 51.1 and note that past the apex, the increasing mobility that initially improved performance may begin to harm it instead. In terms of athletic performance, optimal mobility will not improve strength, power, speed or any other physiological capacity. It will simply eliminate hypomobility-related performance limitations. If those limitations in a particular athlete are extraordinarily great, however, the improvement in performance gained from increased mobility may be dramatic.

Accordingly, optimal mobility is not technically a performance enhancer, but an impediment reducer. This is important to keep in mind when considering the mobility-injury-performance curve: increasing mobility will increase performance and decrease risk of injury if an athlete is presently hypomobile, but that trend will not continue indefinitely. Beyond the apex of the curve representing optimal mobility, the trend prior will invert, and it's likely that increasing mobility will increase the risk of injury and decrease performance.

This can be seen, for example, with limited thoracic spine and shoulder mobility in the jerk. The poor rack position may prevent a solid connection between the bar and torso, limiting the athlete's ability to accelerate the bar upward; it may place the bar

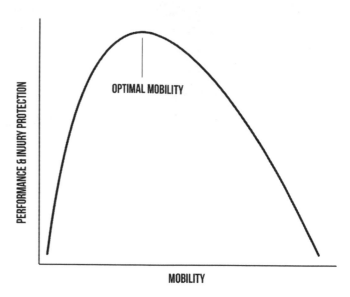

FIGURE 51.1 The relationship of injury protection and performance to mobility describes a modified bell curve. The apex represents optimal mobility—the degree of mobility that allows the greatest performance and provides the greatest protection from injury. Note that the curve is steeper on the hypomobility side of the apex—in proximity to optimal mobility, a given degree of hypomobility impedes performance and increases the risk of injury to a greater extent than that same degree of hypermobility.

too far forward of the spine and create an excessive moment on the back, encouraging forward collapse during the dip and a subsequent forward bar path; and it may place the arms in a very disadvantageous position for pushing under the bar; and restrictions in range of motion may prevent a structurally sound overhead position. These things will all undoubtedly limit the athlete's maximal jerk. As the immobility that prevents proper positioning is reduced, the athlete's ability to jerk will increase accordingly within his or her strength, explosiveness and technical capacity. Once the athlete has achieved as much mobility as is required for perfect jerk positions and motions, further increases in mobility will have no more positive effect on jerk performance, and in fact are likely to begin reducing stability.

Supported & Unsupported Range of Motion

The issue of stability brings into consideration the idea of supported and unsupported ranges of motion. The supported range of motion is the portion of the movement in which the athlete is able to maintain stability through the effort of the muscles and nervous system feedback and responses; the unsupported range of motion is the portion of the movement through which the athlete is still able to move, but in which he or she is unable to create adequate stability.

The goal of mobility work for the weightlifter is to minimize and eventually eliminate any unsupported range of motion to reduce the potential for instability and injury. The process can involve both increasing stability and actually reducing mobility; how much of each is required depends on the athlete's present levels of stability and mobility relative to what is optimal.

For example, an immobile new lifter will not have any unsupported range of motion because his or her range of motion has not even reached the minimal requirement. This athlete will require specific flexibility and mobility work to increase range of motion; the weightlifting training will help maintain the balance between mobility and stability as the range of motion increases, as the body will be continually learning to control the incrementally greater amplitude of movement.

A hypermobile athlete, on the other hand, may have range of motion that exceeds what is necessary for weightlifting, and in the range beyond necessary is likely to be unstable, as his or her training will not address such positions and that portion of motion. This athlete may be stable within the range of motion used in lifting, but the additional range beyond this creates potential for unwanted movement, and its reduction can further improve stability. Finally, an athlete with optimal mobility for weightlifting may have a lack of stability, in which case only stability work is necessary. In the latter two cases, strength work will play a critical role, and specific flexibility and mobility work should be eliminated for all joints with excessive range of motion.

Determining Mobility Demands

As should be clear with any consideration, the demands of mobility will vary, sometimes greatly, among sports. The first step of developing any mo-

bility protocol is determining the needs of the athlete. There are two categories of mobility requirements—universal and sport-specific. That is, there is a range of motion for each joint and a degree of collective mobility that can be considered necessary to support orthopedic health and functional capacity for any human being irrespective of any chosen physical activities with which they occupy themselves; and there is a range of motion for each joint and a degree of collective mobility required by the demands of the chosen sport.

Universal mobility requirements include the ability to squat with the thighs past a horizontal position while maintaining a neutral spine, properly aligned knees and flat feet; the ability to achieve 90 degrees of bilateral hip flexion while maintaining a neutral spine; and the ability to completely open the shoulder joint while maintaining a neutral spine.

The degree to which sport-specific requirements differ from the universal requirements is wholly dependent on the unique demands of the sport. In most cases, sport-specific mobility requirements will involve greater ranges of motion than the universal requirements, but this is not a rule without exception. Distance runners, for example, have relatively little demand for mobility; the sport requires a very limited range of motion of all joints. On the other end of the spectrum is gymnastics, which demands movement and the control of great resistance through ranges of motion far beyond those found in universal requirements. Weightlifting certainly falls much nearer to gymnastics on this spectrum.

Weightlifting Specific Mobility Requirements

Specific mobility requirements are simply the positions and ranges of motion demanded by the athlete's sport. Any experienced athlete or coach will be able to quickly and easily identify these with little effort. For weightlifting, the necessary positions have been described in great detail throughout this book. Weightlifters are required to be capable of achieving the following positions according to the criteria discussed in the relevant chapters:

- Front Squat
- Overhead Squat
- Clean Rack Position
- Jerk Rack Position
- Jerk Overhead Position
- Jerk Split Position
- Snatch & Clean Starting Positions

Generalizations can certainly be made with respect to the mobility limitations of new adult weightlifters. Problems tend to exist with thoracic spine and shoulder mobility in the overhead position for both the snatch and jerk; with the hips at the bottom of the squat and the starting position of the snatch and clean; with the ankles in the bottom of the squat; and with the shoulders and wrists in the clean and jerk rack positions. Each athlete will present somewhat differently in terms of the nature and degree of immobility, so mobility training, like all training, will need to be addressed individually to maximize its effectiveness and efficiency.

Expectations

Extremely mobile athletes have preserved and improved upon the natural mobility of youth, and in many cases, are predisposed anatomically to allow maximal range of motion. There is unquestionably a limit to how much mobility can be improved in an adult athlete; however, it can be improved with consistent long-term hard work. An adult who has allowed his or her natural juvenile mobility to be reduced through a lack of adequate movement will never be able to achieve the same degree of mobility as an athlete who has worked continuously since youth to preserve and improve that level of mobility. Expectations should be adjusted accordingly, but the pursuit of improved mobility by adults should not be abandoned.

Mobility Training Protocols

In order to effectively improve mobility, we need to understand the available methods and determine which are most appropriate—this considers not only the effectiveness, but also the efficiency and accessibility. The most effective stretch in the world is only effective if it can be and is done by the athlete with adequate frequency and regularity.

It is unnecessary to identify the actual muscles in need of stretching; attempts at naming such muscles are typically inaccurate and incomplete anyway. There are approximately 640 skeletal muscles in the human body—it's extremely uncommon to find a coach or athlete who can name more than 10% of them, and even less common for those coaches and athletes to be able to accurately identify that 10% with respect to the source of immobility. Additionally, the mobility of a joint involves more than just the extensibility of the muscles that control it; consequently, joint mobility is much easier to improve if it is approached collectively rather than by individual elements.

Just as we approach training from the perspective of movement and position rather than the use of specific muscles, so too should we primarily concern ourselves with positions and motions rather than specific muscles or structures with respect to mobility. In other words, we need to determine in which positions an athlete is immobile, and then find or create exercises that improve these inadequate ranges of motion.

The two broadest categories of stretching are static and dynamic. Generally speaking, static stretching should be used primarily for remediation of immobility, and dynamic stretching for both remediation and maintenance. Dynamic stretching should also play a role in training preparation and warm-up.

In addition to stretching protocols, soft tissue work with implements like foam rollers, balls and the like can play a role in improving mobility though the release of trigger points, clearing of adhesions in the muscle, fascia, and joint connective tissue, and general improvement of the fluidity of the muscles. This is discussed in more detail in the following chapter.

Static Stretching

Static-Passive Stretching The most common type of mobility training is static-passive stretching—entering a stretched position and maintaining it for a given period of time, using anything but the antagonists of the stretched muscles to achieve and hold the position. For example, leaning forward over an extended leg to stretch the hamstrings, using gravity and/or pulling against the leg with the hands to pull the muscles into a stretched position, and holding the stretched position without movement.

Static stretching offers the most potential for dramatic increases in mobility, and is the easiest, most accessible method, but should be primarily considered a remediation tool. That is, aggressive static stretching should be employed to bring an athlete's mobility up to optimal as quickly as possible, but once that optimal mobility has been achieved, static stretching can become gentler and less frequent to simply help maintain mobility as needed (or to help with recovery between workouts).

Research has demonstrated that static stretching may temporarily disrupt nerve function, resulting in diminished force production capacity and delayed reaction to proprioceptive input. This means the possibility of slightly less strength and speed and greater injury risk if static stretching is performed immediately prior to activity. For this reason, in addition to the fact that static stretching prior to activity that has warmed the muscles and maximized their pliability is not particularly effective, static stretching of significant duration and intensity should generally not be done prior to training or competition.

However, the potential functional reductions resulting from pre-activity static stretching are extremely minor. Further, any athlete whose mobility is limited to such a degree that static stretching is even a consideration pre-training is not performing at a high enough level for this issue to matter. Athletes at this stage will arguably benefit orders of magnitude more from the additional mobility work than their strength and power will be compromised by it.

There are situations in which pre-activity static stretching is advisable. This practice will be limited to athletes with extreme immobility that prevents their ability to achieve necessary positions within a safe range. For example, an athlete with extraordinarily tight hips may be unable to squat to full depth with the maintenance of proper lumbar extension. In such a case, time spent stretching prior to a squat workout (after a more dynamic warm-up and in between sets) may loosen the muscles enough to allow a safer position, and this improvement outweighs any potential force-production problems. In addition to the previous exceptions are the ankles, wrists and shoulder girdle in particular. This pre-activity static stretching should be preceded with a thorough warm-up to ensure safety and effectiveness, and was discussed in the Warming-up chapter in more detail.

On training days, static stretching should be performed immediately following the training session when the muscles will be the most pliable and receptive to adaptation (if foam rolling or similar soft tissue work is also being performed, stretching should follow it). On rest days, static stretching should ideally be preceded by a hot shower or hot bath, or at least performed later in the day following some kind of physical activity. Static stretching should generally not be performed in the early part of the day, as mobility will be most limited and stretching will produce less of an effect.

Static stretches should be entered gradually until reaching the ultimate range to be held. If holding the stretch for an extended duration, this range can be incrementally increased as the muscle(s) relax. Contraction of the antagonistic muscles can improve relaxation of the muscles being stretched through reciprocal inhibition. For example, contracting the quads can allow a more effective stretch of the hamstrings.

Recommendations for durations of static stretches range from 2-120 seconds. A solid guideline for static stretches is 30-90-second durations. Athletes may find stretching more effective—or possibly more tolerable—by holding each stretch for 20-30 seconds and performing 2-3 circuits of the selected stretches in series.

The simple reason for such a wide array of duration recommendations among sources, arguably, is that nearly any stretching protocol can improve mobility—the true deciding factor in effectiveness is consistency at the right frequency over a long enough period of time, not the actual stretching protocol used (assuming the protocol is reasonably sound).

PNF Stretching PNF (Proprioceptive Neuromuscular Facilitation) stretching is a more aggressive type of static stretching that can deliver improved mobility in less time. It can be employed in essentially any stretch, although some may prove more difficult—generally working with a partner is ideal. The athlete will first assume a normal static stretch and hold for approximately 30 seconds. The athlete will then isometrically activate the muscle being stretched against resistance (his or her own or a partner's) for 5 seconds. At the end of that 5 seconds, the athlete will shut off the activation immediately and pull the stretch slightly farther (or the partner will increase the stretch) to hold for 5 seconds.

This contract-relax cycle should be repeated 5 times, increasing the degree of the stretch each time, then followed by a final 30-second static stretch in the final position. The athlete should hold his or her breath during the contraction phase, and release it abruptly along with the contraction as he or she moves into the increased stretch. Contractions should not be of maximal intensity; 20-50% effort has been shown to be as effective and poses less of a risk of injury.

Pulse Stretching A variation of static-passive stretching is to use a series of brief (2 second) pulses rather than a longer duration continuous stretch. This is not an abrupt, aggressive movement like a ballistic stretch, but simply a very brief hold in the stretched position. Each subsequent stretch should increase the range slightly relative to the previous. This variation can be used as an alternative to static-passive stretching to give the athlete some variety day to day and reduce the monotony of the mobility program.

Static-Active Stretching Static-active stretching is a form of static stretching that uses the control of antagonist muscles to pull the agonists into an extended position. The contraction of the antagonist(s) also creates a reciprocal inhibition response to help relax the agonist(s). A simple example would be, from a standing position, lifting a straight leg to the front with the hip flexors to extend and stretch the hip extensors. Isolated active stretches like this have limited utility, at least for weightlifting.

However, active stretches are continually performed naturally during weightlifting training. For instance, sitting in the bottom of a squat or setting the proper starting position for the snatch or clean involves active stretching of multiple muscle groups. Active stretching will be performed unavoidably by all weightlifters in the course of normal daily training and does not need to be employed in addition to this unless desired by a lifter.

Dynamic Stretching

Dynamic Range of Motion Drills (DROMs) The type of stretches that will remain an indefinitely valuable tool irrespective of the athlete's present level of mobility are dynamic range of motion drills (DROMs). These are drills like those discussed in the Warming Up chapter of the book.

Training itself may be considered a form of dynamic mobility work because the movements—assuming they're being performed correctly through the full range of motion—will preserve that range of motion quite well, and even help improve it to some extent. Additional dynamic mobility work serves more as a bridge between inactivity and activity in the context of a warm-up or to ensure more balanced mobility for athletic specialists.

DROMs upon rising in the morning can help improve mobility throughout the day by essentially helping to neurologically reset muscle length that diminishes due to the limited movement during sleep. The morning is not the time to go for extensive ranges of motion—this should be gentle, incrementally increasing movement comfortably below the ranges of motion possible later in the day when warm. This practice takes little time and can make significant improvements in mobility and joint comfort. A series of arm circles forward and backward, torso rotations, and leg swings forward and backward is adequate. Some light calisthenics can also be helpful.

Lifting Interestingly enough, working on the actual exercises or positions we're trying to improve—performing the lifts themselves—is itself effective mobility training. The benefit of this approach is that both mobility and specific stability are being trained simultaneously, helping to prevent the creation of any unsupported range of motion. However, this should not be misinterpreted to mean that additional mobility work is never necessary.

Creating a Mobility Program

The process of developing an individual mobility program includes several steps. First, we must define and understand the program's goal: achieving optimal mobility to reduce performance impediments and the risk of injury as much as possible. Next, we must determine the requirements to define the individual's optimal mobility: this will simply be a comparison of the athlete's present mobility to the mobility requirements of weightlifting. Once we know the requirements, we can develop the actual training methods to satisfy them, including specific stretches and protocols. Very importantly, we must actually ensure the program is being implemented properly by the athlete, which means not only the correct execution of stretches, but the consistent, regular performance of the program at the necessary frequency. And finally, we must continue re-evaluating the athlete's mobility and adjusting the training accordingly.

Improving Effectiveness

Any mobility program is only effective if it's actually executed correctly with the necessary frequency and regularity. This is possibly the most common impediment to improving mobility—often the program is unable to succeed because the athlete simply fails to implement it.

With little exception, stretching is not an activity athletes enjoy, particularly after taxing training sessions and when time is limited. If the coach can create a mobility program that both minimizes the necessary time and effort of the athlete while delivering measurable gains in performance, athletes will be much more likely to remain consistent and reap the potential benefits. Encouraging an athlete to stretch more than necessary or in inappropriate manners has the potential to be counterproductive and to discourage adherence to the program.

The coach actually assisting the athlete with partner stretches when possible is an easy way to ensure stretching is being undertaken as well. Similarly, encouraging a team of athletes to stretch together is often much more effective than athletes stretching individually due to the elements of accountability and social interaction. In addition, the more specific a stretching program is, the more likely an athlete will be to perform it; vague programs or suggestions by the coach with the expectation that the athlete will take the initiative and choose stretches, methods, durations, and times often results in the athlete doing very little at all. The consequent lack of progress often then encourages a poor opinion of mobility work generally, further impeding the ability of the athlete to make progress.

The following chapter contains a collection of stretches effective for addressing the common mobility limitations specific to weightlifting.

Stretches

The following selection of stretches addresses the most common mobility problems of new weightlifters. Stretches can be selected to address specific areas in need of improved mobility, or the collection in its entirety can be used as a basic starting routine.

Stretches are in general quite intuitive and easy to create—if an athlete has a mobility issue not satisfactorily addressed by any of the following stretches, he or she is encouraged to experiment with positions that reach the areas in need of stretching. Caution should be exercised to not place stress on joint structures directly by ensuring tension is felt in the appropriate muscles only.

As was discussed in the previous chapter, these stretches should be used frequently and aggressively to bring the immobile athlete to a state of optimal mobility as quickly as possible. After this has been accomplished, static stretching can be reduced dramatically to only the minimum necessary to, along with lifting and dynamic mobility work, maintain mobility.

It should be understood clearly that aggressive stretching implies discomfort, not pain. At no time should a stretch feel injurious, and soreness following a bout of stretching is indicative of excessive intensity.

Wrist Stretches

Addresses: Clean and jerk rack positions, snatch and jerk overhead positions

The positional demands on the wrists by weightlifting are great, and immobility will limit performance and expose the athlete to pain and injury. Wrist mobility can be a constant struggle because of the large volume of flexor work from gripping a barbell. Over time, athletes will likely find themselves habitually performing wrists stretches throughout the day to relieve the residual tension. For improving mobili-

ty, they should be done at minimum before and after training.

The primary issue will be the finger and wrist flexors—these will potentially be, in part, what limit the athlete's ability to assume the clean and jerk rack positions or hold a bar properly overhead. The remaining stretching is more for balanced mobility than direct effect on positions.

The wrist is comprised of a large number of small bones and deals regularly with high degrees of compression. This compression can become residual and leave the wrist in a condition of reduced mobility. In order to stretch the wrists effectively, they should be first decompressed—this will allow a fuller stretch and prevent unnecessary stress on the carpals from compression. When initiating a stretch, the hand should simply be pulled straight out from the forearm before it's extended. This pulling action should continue during the stretch, directed toward the tips of the fingers. Simply shaking the hands out as well is effective for loosening up the structures of the wrist before and after stretches.

There are many ways to stretch the wrist flexor and extensor muscle groups; which variations are used is largely a matter of personal preference based on what each athlete feels is both most effective and convenient. Basic and effective variations are described and illustrated below.

Flexor Stretch Flexor stretches can be performed to emphasize either the finger or wrist flexors. Finger flexor flexibility will always be accompanied by the need for wrist flexor flexibility—in the clean rack position, for example, when both are in an extended position—but wrist flexibility can be necessary without accompanying need for finger flexor flexibility, such as is the case with the jerk rack position in which the wrists may be extended to a great degree while the fingers remain flexed.

In order to emphasize the wrist flexors, the stretch should be performed by pressing against the palm of the hand rather than the fingers—this will ensure the fullest possible extension of the wrist (Figure 52.1a). To stretch the finger flexors as well, the fingers will be pressed, bringing them and the wrist into extension (Figure 52.1b). This will be the default stretch because it will hit both flexor groups, but often the fingers will limit the range of motion of the wrist somewhat, so more direct wrist flexor stretching may be necessary.

Flexor stretches can be performed with one hand pressing against the other, but are often easier when pressing the hand against the floor while kneeling or against a wall while standing. Different degrees of internal/external rotation of the arms (fingers pointing up, to the side, or down) can be used to change the stretch somewhat. These flexor stretches can also be done against a barbell in a squat rack (usually one hand will need to hold the bar and provide resistance while the other hand is pushed against the bar to be stretched).

Extensor Stretch In order to promote full mobility and balance, the extensor groups should be stretched as well. This is done simply with the reverse action as the flexor stretches—pressing against the back of the hand to flex the wrist (Figure 52.2). As with flexor stretches, the extensors of the wrist and fingers can be emphasized by changing the location of pressure application from the hand to the fingers, respectively.

Hook Grip Stretch A final useful stretch will address the thumb and related structures, and can often be helpful for new lifters experiencing discomfort or pain. Make a fist with the thumb held inside the fingers, as if hook-gripping a bar, then ulnar deviate the hand—tilt it the opposite direction of the thumb and hold this position (Figure 52.3).

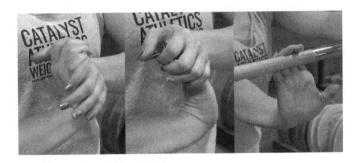

FIGURE 52.1 Wrist flexor stretches

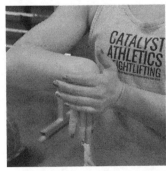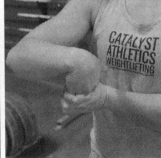

FIGURE 52.2 Wrist extensor stretches

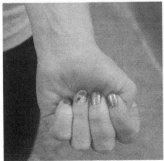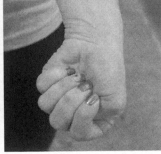

FIGURE 52.3 Hook grip stretch

Leaning Bar Hang
Addresses: Snatch and jerk overhead positions

The leaning bar hang is a simple, general stretch for the shoulder girdle and arm adductors—all of the muscles that can restrict complete opening of the shoulders in the overhead position. The athlete will hold a pull-up bar with a jerk-width grip and place the toes on the floor 1-2 feet behind the bar. If the bar is too high, the feet can be placed on a plyo box or bench. Keeping the toes on the floor, the athlete will hang from the arms and lean forward, letting gravity pull the body down and adding a forward push of the chest through the arms. Keeping the feet on the floor behind the bar will allow the forward lean that improves the stretch of the shoulder girdle, as well as allowing the muscles to relax more. The width of the grip can be changed for somewhat different effects. (Figure 52.4)

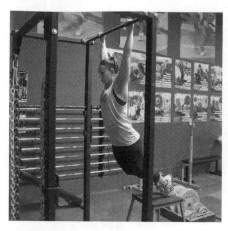

FIGURE 52.4 Leaning bar hang

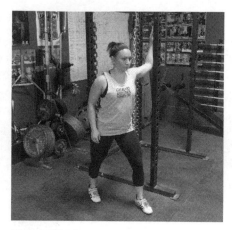

FIGURE 52.5 Doorjamb shoulder girdle stretch

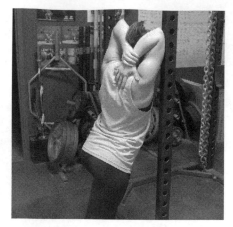

FIGURE 52.6 Underarm rack stretch

Doorjamb Shoulder Girdle Stretch
Addresses: Snatch and jerk overhead positions

This is another simple but effective stretch to help open up the shoulder girdle for better overhead positioning in the snatch and jerk. The athlete will place the forearm vertically against a doorjamb, the upright of a power rack, or a similar solid structure, keeping the elbow higher than the shoulder, and push the chest forward. The height of the elbow relative to the shoulder can be changed along with the inclination of the chest (i.e. adding a forward lean rather than remaining vertical) to achieve a somewhat different stretch. (Figure 52.5)

Underarm Rack Stretch
Addresses: Snatch and jerk overhead positions, jerk and clean rack positions

The underarm rack stretch directly addresses muscles such as the lats and triceps that limit the opening of the shoulder when attempting to achieve the overhead position. The athlete will bend one arm at the elbow completely, then lift the elbow above the shoulder and place the back of the upper arm near the elbow against the upright of a power rack or similar structure, keeping the trunk squared off facing the rack. If possible, the lifter should grip the wrist of the arm being stretched with the free arm and push it out to the side slightly. From this position, the athlete will simply lean into the rack to push the elbow back. (Figure 52.6)

Back Squat Push Through
Addresses: Clean and jerk rack positions, snatch and jerk overhead positions

The back squat push through is a unique stretch for the shoulders and elbows that will for some lifters be both helpful and enjoyable, and for others totally unnecessary—it should be quickly obvious based on feel along which it is for a given lifter. It will stretch the shoulder girdle somewhat, but also the internal rotators of the upper arm.

Gripping a barbell in a squat rack with a jerk-width grip, the lifter will reach the head under the bar as if getting into position to back squat, but will instead simply keeping pushing the chest forward through the arms, keeping the trunk and forearms approximately parallel with each other. The width of the grip can be changed to move the emphasis of the stretch somewhat. (Figure 52.7)

Apley Push
Addresses: Clean and jerk rack positions

This stretch is named the Apley push because of the resemblance of the position to the common physical therapy assessment, the Apley scratch test. The athlete will place the back of one hand against the lower back so that the elbow is bent approximately 90 degrees and protruding straight out from the side of the body. The lifter will then use the upright of a power rack or similar structure to push the arm forward by rotating the body. (Figure 52.8)

Greg Everett

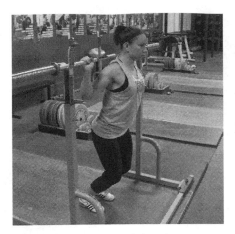

FIGURE 52.7 Back squat push through

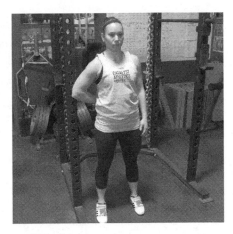

FIGURE 52.8 Apley push

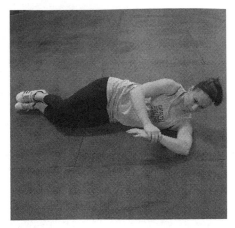

FIGURE 52.9 Sleeper internal rotation stretch

Sleeper Internal Rotation
Addresses: Snatch and clean third pull

This stretch is a simple way to improve internal rotation of the arm, which will allow a better elbow path in the initial phase of the third pull of the snatch and clean, allowing the elbows to move higher with the bar in closer proximity to the body.

Lying on his or her side, the lifter will rest the upper arm against the floor at a 90 degree angle from the body with the elbow bent to 90 degrees to orient the forearm vertically. Keeping the upper arm in the same position, the athlete will use the opposite hand to push the palm down toward the floor. (Figure 52.9)

PVC External Rotation
Addresses: Clean and jerk rack positions

This stretch works to improve the lifter's ability to establish secure and comfortable clean and jerk rack positions by helping the upper arm externally rotate farther and allow a greater range of possible grip widths.

Standing, the athlete will hold up one arm with the elbow bent and pointed straight forward, the upper arm horizontal, and a PVC pipe hanging down from the hand outside the upper arm. With the other hand, the athlete will pull the PVC pipe across the body away from the stretching arm to externally rotate the upper arm. (Figure 52.10)

Burgener Bar Stretch
Addresses: Clean and jerk rack positions

This stretch comes from coach Mike Burgener and is an easy way to work on shoulder and elbow mobility for both the clean and jerk rack positions. The athlete will take a jerk-width grip on a barbell and place it behind the neck as if preparing for a back squat. Keeping a full grip on the bar, the athlete will bring the elbows forward and up, reaching them as high and as far forward as possible (protracting the scapulae). The width of the grip can be changed to shift the emphasis of the stretch to different locations in the shoulders and elbows. (Figure 52.11)

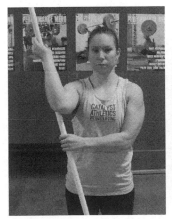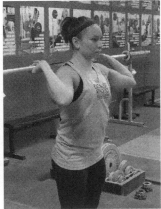

FIGURE 52.10 PVC external rotation stretch (left)

FIGURE 52.11 Burgener bar stretch (right)

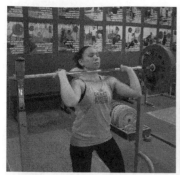
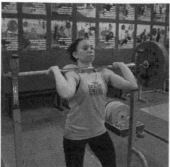
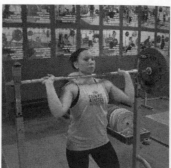
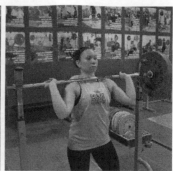

FIGURE 52.12 Rack elevators: clean (left) and jerk (right)

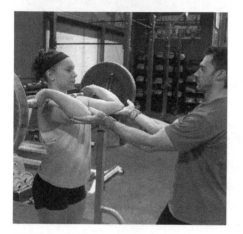

FIGURE 52.13 Partner clean rack stretch

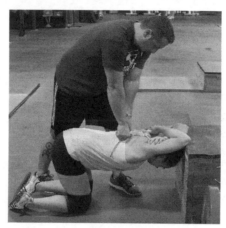

FIGURE 52.14 Partner T-spine mobilization

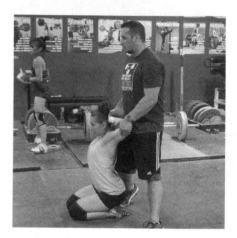

FIGURE 52.15 Partner shoulder girdle stretch

Rack Elevator

Addresses: Clean or jerk rack position

The rack elevator stretch can be used for both the clean and jerk rack positions. With a loaded barbell in a squat rack, the athlete will step the feet directly under the bar and set the clean or jerk rack position with some space between the bar and the shoulders—enough to allow the best possible hand and elbow positions for the athlete's present mobility. The athlete will then stand, pushing the shoulders up into the bar, using the legs to stretch into the correct rack position. The position can then be held for the chosen duration. (Figure 52.12)

Partner Clean Rack Stretch

Addresses: Clean rack position

If the athlete is unable to elevate the elbows adequately in the clean rack position due to immobil-

ity (not because of proportions, inappropriate grip width, or the like), the clean rack position can be taken on a loaded barbell in a squat rack and a partner can gradually push the athlete's elbows up to achieve a stretch. This can also be used for lifters who want to transition from an open-hand to full grip in the clean rack position and need additional mobility to do so. (Figure 52.13)

Partner T-Spine Mobilization

Addresses: Overhead positions and starting positions

Thoracic spine mobility is both critical for proper overhead structure, and commonly limited in athletes beginning weightlifting past the optimal age. As part of a warm-up, following a workout, or both, a training partner or coach can help mobilize the T-spine. The athlete will kneel on the floor and place the elbows overhead and on a bench or box to open the shoulders and orient the trunk horizontally. The partner will place the thumbs or knuckles on the spinal erectors on either side of the thoracic spine and push down momentarily before moving the hands along the spine slightly, working gradually up and down the length of the T-spine 2-5 times. Pressure can be increased each pass as long as it does not become painful. (Figure 52.14)

Partner Shoulder Girdle Stretch
Addresses: Snatch and jerk overhead position

An effective bilateral variation of the doorjamb shoulder girdle stretch will require a partner. The athlete will kneel on the floor and place the hands behind the head. The partner or coach will place one knee behind the athlete's upper back to support it, and then pull the athlete's elbows back to stretch the shoulder girdle. The athlete needs to keep the abs tight to prevent the back from arching excessively. The stretch should be gradually increased for the duration of the hold, which can be 20-60 seconds. Contract-relax PNF stretching can also be easily incorporated. (Figure 52.15)

Russian Baby Maker
Addresses: Squat

The Russian baby maker (The reader may be assured that the backstory behind this name is hilarious) is a good stretch for opening the hips to improve the bottom position of the squat. With the feet wider than the normal squat stance, the athlete will place the hands on the tops of the feet and wedge the elbows inside the thighs as deep as possible (back to-

ward the groin). He or she will then sit the hips down into a squatting position while pushing the elbows out, trying to spread the legs apart at the proximal ends (i.e. pushing the legs apart where they meet the hips, not at the knees). The back does not need to be arched and the athlete does not need to be in an upright squat position, and in fact the trunk will be close to horizontal. In the lowest position, at least some of the athlete's bodyweight will be supported on the elbows. (Figure 52.16)

Squat with Knees Out
Addresses: Squat

Pushing the knees out to the sides while sitting in a squat is a simple way to stretch the adductors to improve the squat position for lifters who are unable to keep the knees out enough to maintain alignment of their knees. The stretch should be performed in a close to a proper squat position as possible, i.e. with a properly extended spine, full depth and balance over the feet. (Figure 52.17)

Lying Hamstring
Addresses: Squat, snatch and clean starting position

The hamstrings are notoriously resistant to stretching and consequently notoriously tight. For weightlifters, this means an inability to maintain correct spinal extension in the squat and possibly in the early stages of the snatch or clean pull from the floor. This is not only detrimental to performance, but unsafe.

A contributor to the hamstrings' seeming resistance to flexibility is the simple yet overlooked

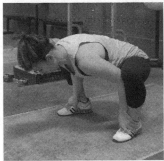
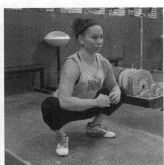

FIGURE 52.16 Russian baby maker   **FIGURE 52.17** Squat with knees out

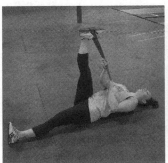
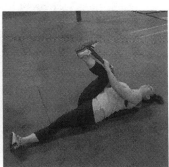

FIGURE 52.18 Lying hamstring stretch

fact that the vast majority of hamstring stretching is performed incorrectly or in manners that inherently prevent adequate stretching. These practices limit the extension of the hamstrings by relying on lumbar flexion to give the appearance of increased range of motion—this flexion allows the pelvis to rotate posteriorly and consequently the insertions of the hamstrings don't travel far enough from their origins to cause an adequate stretch. This also develops excessive mobility of the lumbar spine, exposing it to greater injury risk, particularly in concert with tight hamstrings.

The key to all hamstring stretching is that the hamstrings originate on the pelvis—they have nothing to do with the spine beyond the fact that the spine is also attached to the pelvis. That means in order to stretch the hamstrings, the thigh must move relative to the pelvis, not the spine.

The ideal position to ensure the hamstrings are being stretched while the curve of the lumbar spine and its integrity are preserved is lying on the back. A towel roll or similar can be placed under the lower back to support a normal arch and further isolate hip flexion. Leaving one leg straight and flat on the floor to help prevent the pelvis from rotating posteriorly and reducing hamstring tension, the athlete will bring the other leg up by flexing at the hip and hold it in a stretched position. This stretch should be performed both with a straight knee and with a partially flexed knee. To stretch straight-legged, the knee should be locked and the hip gradually flexed; to stretch bent-legged, the hip should be fully flexed (bringing the knee to the chest), and the knee gradually extended

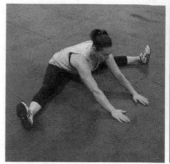
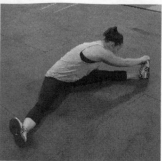

FIGURE 52.19 Straddle

while maintaining the hip flexion. In both straight and bent knee stretches, the leg can be moved laterally to emphasize the stretch on the inner or outer hamstrings as needed.

Athletes should avoid holding the toes during the straight knee stretch—this can place undue stress on nerve structures in the leg. A length of nylon webbing or similar can be hooked over the middle of the foot to provide the athlete a convenient handle with which to draw the leg toward the chest. This is a perfect stretch with which to use the PNF protocol. (Figure 52.18)

Straddle

Addresses: Squat, snatch and clean starting position

The seated straddle is performed by simply sitting upright and extending the legs into the widest angle relative to each other possible. Some forward pelvic tilt will introduce an additional stretch—but this

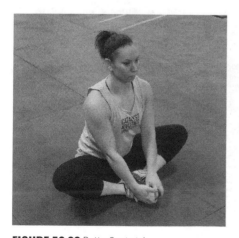

FIGURE 52.20 Butterfly stretch

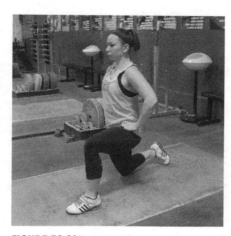

FIGURE 52.21 Lunge stretch

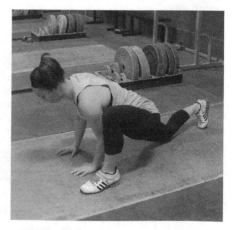

FIGURE 52.22 Spiderman lunge

Greg Everett

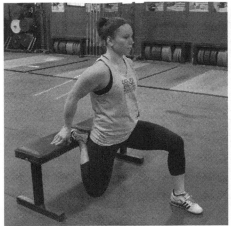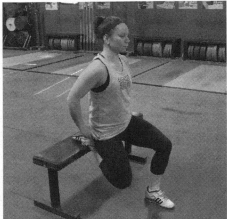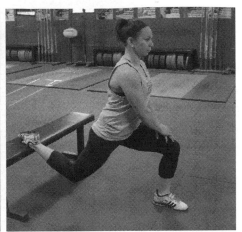

FIGURE 52.23 Death stretch

should not be confused as flexing the lower back, which will accomplish nothing. The athlete simply needs to attempt to sit erect with lumbar extension and as flexibility allows, lean forward while maintaining the pelvis-spine relationship. Along with a direct forward reach, the athlete can turn toward one leg and reach both hands to that foot. (Figure 52.19)

Butterfly
Addresses: Squat, snatch and clean starting position

The butterfly stretch is performed in a seated position with the knees bent to bring the soles of the feet in contact with each other as close to the body as possible. The knees can be pushed toward the floor by the elbows with the hands grasping the feet as an anchor. Like in the straddle, the athlete should attempt to sit upright with normal lumbar extension, and eventually to tilt the pelvis forward. (Figure 52.20)

Lunge
Addresses: Jerk split position, squat, snatch and clean starting position

The hip flexors can be stretched with the lunge and its variations. Further stretching of the hip flexor can be achieved in the lunge position by rotating the vertical torso to the side of the front leg. In all cases of hip flexor stretching, the glute on the side being stretched should be contracted to help relax the hip flexor and prevent hyperextension of the lower

back (which will allow the hip flexor to be stretched more in addition to being safer for the spine). (Figure 52.21)

Spiderman Lunge
Addresses: Squat, snatch and clean starting position

The spiderman lunge is simply a very long lunge in which the athlete tries to lower the trunk to the floor inside the forward knee and drop the hips as low as possible—bringing the elbow to the inside of the front foot is a good target, but the primary focus is lowering the hips. This is an excellent stretch for all of the hip extensors and adductors that tend to interfere with deep squatting, and will generally improve movement in the hip capsule. The athlete should attempt to rotate the pelvis forward as the torso drops rather than simply bending the back. (Figure 52.22)

Death Stretch
Addresses: Jerk split position, squat

Tight quads and hip flexors are extremely common sources of knee pain among weightlifters. It can be remarkable to witness the speed at which knee discomfort abates with a short period of flexibility and SMR work (covered in the following chapter). Likewise, lower back tightness and pain can often be traced to tight hip flexors. With the exception of the back leg in the split jerk, the rectus femoris (midline quad muscle that crosses both the knee and the hip) is always in a relatively shortened position, and is often encouraged to shorten further by ab work that includes large volumes of hip flexion without commensurate stretching. Bringing the hip flexors and quads to a point of optimal flexibility can result in dramatic improvements.

With a single position, we can stretch both the quads and hip flexors extremely well, and with slight modifications, emphasize one over the other. The athlete will place the top of his or her foot on a chair, box or similar object approximately knee height behind him or her. Entering into a lunge position, the athlete will attempt to flex the back knee completely while simultaneously extending the hip completely. This will be the most advanced position and will cover both the quads and hip flexors equally. To reduce the stretch on the hip flexors while continuing to stretch the quads, the hip can be flexed partially and the knee kept flexed completely. To reduce the stretch on the quad and emphasize the stretch of the hip flexors, the front leg can be stepped farther forward, the knee opened somewhat, and the hip extended fully. In any variation, the trunk can be rotated toward the front leg to increase the stretch on the hip flexors. (Figure 52.23)

Pigeon
Addresses: Squat, snatch and clean starting position

The pigeon stretch addresses the lateral glutes and hip, which often become tight in weightlifters as they are nearly always in a shortened position. With the front shin perpendicular to the body and lying flat on the floor and the back leg extended straight back, the athlete will lean forward over the front leg. It's important the lower leg remain flat on the floor—the athlete can press the knee and ankle down with the hands or elbows.

In addition to leaning straight forward, the stretch can be modified by reaching the arm opposite the front leg across the body toward the side of the front leg and creating some rotation at the hips. (Figure 52.24)

Seated Glute Crossover
Addresses: Squat, snatch and clean starting position

Seated with one leg extended forward and flat on the floor, the athlete will bend the other knee and bring that foot outside of the straight leg. Reaching the

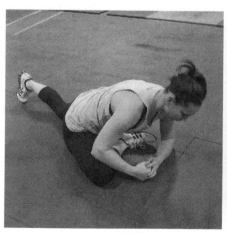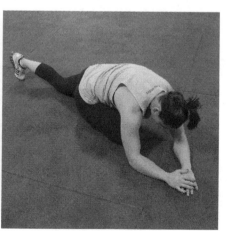

FIGURE 52.24 Pigeon stretch

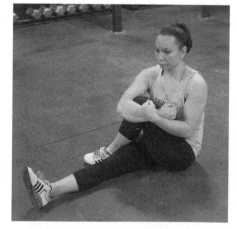

FIGURE 52.25 Seated glute crossover

arm around the knee (it's easiest to hook the crook of the elbow around it), the athlete will pull the knee across the body toward the opposite shoulder. (Figure 52.25)

Calf Stretches
Addresses: Squat, jerk split position

The calves are comprised of the gastrocnemius, which crosses both the ankle and the knee, and the soleus, which crosses only the ankle (and the plantaris, which is generally not a concern). The soleus is the source of most problems related to weightlifting since the ankles are at their greatest flexion in the bottom of the squat and tension on the gastrocnemius is minimal due to knee flexion.

For the preferred soleus stretch, the athlete will assume the bottom position of a squat, and by leaning his or her elbows onto one knee, will attempt to flex the ankle as much as possible. It's important the foot remain flat on the floor to ensure the mid-foot isn't stretched along with the calf; lifting shoes should also be worn to make sure the arch of the foot remains intact. A similar stretch is often performed by sitting in the bottom of a squat and pressing down on a barbell lying across the thighs near the knees—this is a decent stretch, but makes aggressive focus on one ankle more difficult. If an athlete is not mobile enough to sit in a squat position for this ankle stretch, it can be modified and done in a lunge position.

If the gastrocnemius does require attention, stretching must be done with a straight knee. The athlete can place the toes against a wall with the heel on the floor and lean the body forward to flex the ankle. The heel being supported on the floor is important—hanging off an edge on the balls of the feet means the calf being stretched must help support the weight of the body and cannot relax into a legitimate stretch. Better than a wall is the upright of a power rack. This will provide the surface needed for the foot, but will also give the athlete something to hold onto and pull against as needed. (Figure 52.26)

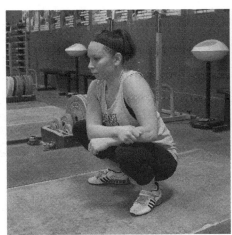
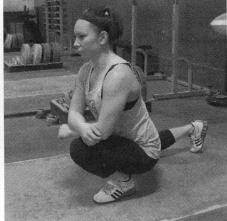
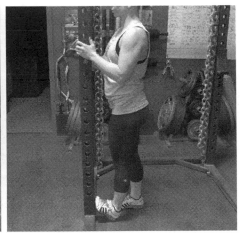

FIGURE 52.26 Calf stretches

Self-Myofascial Release

Self-Myofascial Release (SMR), commonly referred to as foam-rolling, although other implements are often used, can benefit athletes dramatically in both remediation and maintenance capacities. Its value lies primarily in economics and convenience—a $30 cylinder of foam can routinely provide much of the results of soft tissue work by a manual therapist and can be done with a frequency that would be financially impossible for actual therapy.

The science behind SMR is not settled and there exists some contention among sources regarding the actual mechanisms behind the observable results, as well as some disagreement on exact protocols, but little if any argument regarding its effectiveness and benefits. Like with many elements of training, understanding the science is not entirely necessary if the protocol has proven effective in practice.

SMR has two basic functions: to help break up adhesions in fascial tissue, and to release excessive muscle tension through autogenic inhibition.

Muscles are sheathed in connective tissue called fascia that encases the entire muscle belly continuously with the tendons, and layers within the belly surrounding both fascicles and individual muscle fibers. These fascial sheets can develop scar tissue and other irregularities that disrupt the smooth movement of the muscle internally and in relation to surrounding structures. This disruption can produce anything from chronic pain to dysfunctional movement to reduced range of motion to injury. Like deep-tissue massage, foam-rolling and similar myofascial release techniques can break up the adhesions within the connective tissue and promote improved fluidity in the muscles (Robertson 2008), improving function, increasing joint range of motion, and reducing injury risk.

Autogenic inhibition refers to the releasing of muscle tension by the golgi tendon organs (GTOs). GTOs are mechanoreceptors in the tendons of muscles that sense tension and shut down or reduce muscular contraction when tension becomes excessive, presumably to try to prevent injury to the muscles and tendons. By creating additional tension with the pressure of a foam roller or other implement on an area of excessive residual muscular tension (a knot or trigger point), we can cause the GTO to signal the body to relax the muscle. This release requires the maintenance pressure for 20 seconds or longer (Alexander 2011).

SMR Protocol

For most athletes, foam-rolling will be painful, occasionally excruciatingly so in certain locations. However, the pain produced by the practice will abate to some degree with regular performance, although it's unlikely any weightlifter will ever achieve complete clearance of painful areas.

Foam rolls should be selected according to density and size. A 6-inch roll of the densest foam is generally appropriate (usually black in color), and will conveniently be durable. Soft rolls (white) fail to produce adequate pressure on the muscles, especially for heavier athletes. That said, certain athletes may need to start with softer rolls until a reasonable degree of improvement is attained and harder rolls can be tolerated.

The basic self-myofascial release protocol is extremely simple. With the foam roller on the floor, the athlete will place the body part to be treated on top of it. He or she will begin with gentle rolls across the foam, possibly with reduced pressure from support of partial bodyweight by the arms and/or legs, making alternating passes across the length of the muscle or targeted area for around 15-30 seconds.

The athlete will then stop with the roller under each particularly painful point, giving the pressure time to help release any trigger points (20 or more seconds). Once all the hotspots have been covered individually, the athlete can finish the body part with another series of complete passes.

For some locations, a foam roller may prove unsuitable because of its size. In cases of small, less accessible points needing to be reached, alternatives such as lacrosse balls or softballs can be used (tools made specifically for this use are also available). With these implements, smaller points can be reached more effectively, such as areas of the scapular musculature or points under the arm.

This aggressive and focused SMR should be performed after training along with, and preceding, any static stretching. It can and should also be performed on rest days along with any necessary static stretching, but like static stretching, is best preceded by a hot bath or shower, or at least some physical activity, to improve the compliance of the muscles. As discussed in the Warming Up chapter, foam rolling with lighter passes and little or no aggressive focus work on specific points is an effective element of training preparation.

The most helpful rolling locations and positions are described in the Warming Up chapter. These can also be used as the foundation (or entirety) of the post-workout SMR routine.

Thoracic Spine Mobility

Although not actually myofascial release, weightlifters will find foam-rolling helpful for improving thoracic spine mobility, both before and after training. The upper back is often very immobile and locked into a limited range of motion with exaggerated kyphosis. This prevents the establishment of a proper overhead position in the snatch and jerk, and a proper rack position in the clean, reducing structural integrity and consequently both performance and safety.

The athlete will lie supine on the roller with the spine perpendicular to it. Crossing the arms over the chest and loosely holding the upper back straight, the athlete will roll back and forth along the length of the thoracic spine, allowing the vertebrae to release and shift slightly around the curve of the roll, and attempting to allow the back to curve progressively more around the roll with subsequent passes. The athlete will typically be met initially by audible cracking, but this will invariably be both temporary and extremely satisfying. With regular rolling, cracking will decrease and may stop entirely.

In addition to this basic rolling, the athlete can also perform rolls with the arms stretched overhead to simultaneously stretch the shoulder girdle and encourage more thoracic extension, and can pause at points along the thoracic spine and try to relax over the roller for 10-30 seconds.

Competition

Weightlifting competition is remarkably simple in theory—the athlete snatches three times and clean & jerks three times, attempting to total as much weight as possible with the best of each lift—but the details governing how this actually occurs can be overwhelming. As with anything, knowledge will provide the athlete and coach the basic tools for the job, but only experience will allow the comfort and confidence necessary for the highest levels of success.

Weightlifting competition rules in the USA comply with the rules set forth by the International Weightlifting Federation (IWF). Free copies of the rules manuals for both the IWF and USA Weightlifting can be obtained from the organizations' websites. Each country will have at least one federation with a relationship with the Olympic committee and IWF who will observe the same rules.

Age Categories

There are a number of age categories in weightlifting to allow more appropriately matched competition. To determine eligibility for an age category, subtract the athlete's birth year from the year of the competition, e.g. an athlete born in 1998 would be eligible for

Category	Age
Youth	13-17
Junior	15-20
Senior	15 & older
Master	35 & older

TABLE 54.1 IWF Age Categories

the 2015 Junior National Championships (2015-1998 = 17). The month of birth is not relevant.

The senior class is open to all athletes 15 and older who are able to make any required qualifying totals for particular competitions. For example, athletes under the age of 21 or over the age of 35 may compete in the senior category if their lifts qualify them for a given meet. The youth category is typically broken up in national competitions into 13 & Under, 14-15 and 16-17 categories.

The minimum age for participation in the senior, junior and university world championships is 15, and the minimum age for participation in the Olympics is 16.

Bodyweight Categories

As of July 2018, there are 10 all new weight classes each for senior and junior men and women for all IWF competition, and another 10 classes for each gender in the youth category. For the 2020 Olympics, only 7 of these 10 classes will be used. This may change in future Olympic quads, as this is the first time the sport has used such a system and will likely require refinement.

The weight of each class indicates the top-end limit, e.g. a 94 kg lifter may weigh between 85.01-94.00 kg. The superheavyweight class (109+ for men and 87+ for women) has no upper-end limit.

Athletes are best served by training and competing at the heaviest bodyweights allowed by their classes. In the case of tying lifts or totals, the lighter athlete is given the win; however, this is not a wise strategy for competition unless useable by chance in a particular situation. Instead, the athlete should take advantage as much as possible of the allowable weight.

Senior & Junior Men	
kg	lbs
55*	121
61	134
67	148
73	161
81	179
89*	196
96	212
102*	225
109	240
109+	240+

TABLE 54.2 Senior & Junior weight categories. * Not Olympic classes.

Senior & Junior Women	
kg	lbs
45*	99
49	108
55	121
59	130
64	141
71*	157
76	168
81*	179
87	192
87+	192+

Youth 14-15 Boys	
kg	lbs
39	86
44	97
49	108
55	121
61	134
67	148
73	161
81	179
89	196
89+	196+

TABLE 54.4 Youth 14-15 weight categories

Youth 14-15 Girls	
kg	lbs
36	79
40	88
45	99
49	108
55	121
59	130
64	141
71	157
76	168
76+	168+

Youth Men	
kg	lbs
49	108
55	121
61	134
67	148
73	161
81	179
89	196
96	212
102	225
102+	225+

TABLE 54.3 Youth weight categories

Youth Women	
kg	lbs
40	88
45	99
49	108
55	121
59	130
64	141
71	157
76	168
81	179
81+	179+

Youth 13 & Under Boys	
kg	lbs
32	65
36	79
39	86
44	97
49	108
55	121
61	134
67	148
73	161
73+	161+

TABLE 54.5 Youth 13 & Under weight categories

Youth 13 & Under Girls	
kg	lbs
30	66
33	73
36	79
40	88
45	99
49	108
55	121
59	130
64	141
64+	141+

When registering for competition, athletes declare their weight class. The weight class can be changed (assuming the athlete has made any necessary qualifying totals at the new weight or is otherwise already qualified) up to the verification of entries meeting that is typically held the day before the event begins.

In national and international competition, if an athlete fails to make weight at the weigh-in, he or she is disqualified from competition. Typically in local meets, a lifter will be allowed to lift in the next category up.

Greg Everett

Qualifying Totals

Certain competitions (regional and national) require athletes to achieve certain totals in sanctioned competition within the qualifying period to be eligible. Qualifying periods are typically from one year prior (or the competition's last occurrence) to about one month prior to the competition in question. The actual qualifying period and totals will be posted for each competition by the sanctioning organization. The qualifying total must be made at the correct bodyweight category or lighter (it's assumed, naturally, that an athlete who increases a weight category will be able to lift that same total or more, but not necessarily if they drop a weight class).

In other cases, such as international competition, the qualification procedure will involve an athlete ranking system based on certain competitions that essentially predict how each athlete will place in the competition in question. The higher an athlete will place theoretically, the higher the ranking. The lifters will be selected based on this ranking list to fill the available team spots, with the caveat that there may not be more than 2 lifters per weight class—that is, the third highest-ranked lifter in a given weight class will not make an international team even if ranked higher than the next highest-ranked lifter in another weight class. The selection process varies among countries and can change periodically within a given federation. Each federation will publish qualifying information each year.

Clothing & Personal Gear

Competitors' attire must conform to a number of rules. Athletes will be required to wear a tight-fitting one-piece singlet that covers neither the knees nor the elbows and has no collar. Additional garments such as T-shirts and tight shorts can be worn underneath, but none of these may cover the elbows or knees. Singlets can be purchased through a number of weightlifting equipment suppliers.

Recently a new rule has been added to allow lifters for religious reasons to wear a single, tight-fitting unitard under the singlet that covers the arms and legs, but it must be a single solid color with no patterns on it.

While the actual rules regarding footwear are quite vague, athletes should be wearing weightlifting shoes, just as they should in training. These shoes may not be taller than 130 mm from the top of the sole to the top of the shoe; there is no limit on heel elevation; no restrictions on materials; the sole may not extend horizontally from the rest of the shoe more than 5 mm at any point. Socks may be of any length, but may not cover the knees, may not touch knee sleeves or wraps, and may not cover any illegal wraps or bandaging.

Belts of any type may be worn outside of the singlet, and cannot be more than 120 mm tall. One-piece sleeves or wraps without any reinforcement can be worn on the knees and must be less than 300 mm tall.

Wraps or tape under 100 mm wide can be worn on the wrists. Tape or plasters may be worn on the hands and fingers. These can be attached to the wrist, but may not protrude past the tips of the fingers.

Tape or bandages cannot be worn on the elbows, thighs, shins or arms, with the exception of bandages placed by meet staff to cover bleeding. Only one type of wrap is allowed per bodypart, e.g. an athlete cannot tape the wrists and wear wraps over the tape.

It's common for athletes to wear a short-sleeved T-shirt or similar garment under the singlet to provide a more secure surface for the bar during clean & jerks. Sweat on bare shoulders can cause problems with cleans that are not racked deeply enough.

No personal electronic equipment like iPods may be worn on the competition platform. If a hat is worn (strongly discouraged), it is considered part of the athlete's head, and the barbell may not touch it at any point of the lift.

Nutrition

Nutrition prior to and during competition should vary as little as possible from the athlete's customary routine. The athlete's daily nutrition should already be optimal to support recovery and performance, and no last-minute changes prior to competition will produce any considerable improvements. Absolutely the worst possible idea is to experiment with un-familiar practices during competition. Any desired protocols should be tested thoroughly long before competition to evaluate the athlete's response. The key to successful competition is maintaining as much consistency with training as possible—to minimize variables and allow the athlete to focus on nothing more than the lifts themselves.

Generally athletes will want to eat something between snatch and clean & jerk sessions. Small protein shakes and bars, deli meat, nuts and fruit are easy options, and quantities should be limited to what is necessary to prevent GI discomfort during competition. The classic weightlifter's meal between snatches and clean & jerks is a Snickers bar—this should only be used by lifters who are not overly sensitive to sugar and know exactly how they will respond to it.

Athletes should be conscious of water intake during a meet to ensure adequate hydration is maintained. A combination of fatigue and dehydration can make the athlete's clean & jerks remarkably difficult.

Travel

For national meets in which travel is required, a few things need to be kept in mind. Time zone changes will affect the lifter's sleep and energy, and considerable climate differences can also negatively influence the lifter. Because if this, and the generally stressful and fatiguing nature of travel, it's important to schedule travel at least a full day prior to the date of competition to allow for rest and acclimation. For example, if a lifter competes on Saturday, travel should be no later than Thursday. This is even more important if the lifter is scheduled for an early session.

All personal gear necessary for the competition should be kept in carry-on baggage, never in checked baggage. If a checked bag is lost, the lifter will still be able to compete.

Finally, lifters should expect a loss of bodyweight with air travel—approximately as much as they typically lose overnight. This can be a product of dehydration to some extent, which is easily enough remedied, but can also be a result of stress.

Making Weight

Most athletes train close to the upper limit of their weight classes. For some, it's matter of trying to keep weight on, while others must be cautious of gaining too much weight unintentionally. Another group of athletes intentionally train heavier than their competition weight, generally as a way to handle heavier loads in training. As long as an athlete does not have unusual difficulty dropping weight for competition, this is acceptable. Weight surpluses should be kept reasonable to prevent unnecessarily draining weight loss for competition and to ensure better predictability of competition performance; depending on the weight class, generally 1-3% of bodyweight.

Typically athletes will lose some amount of weight simply as a result of increased nervous energy in the final days before the contest—sometimes as much as 3 kg—but with experience, athletes will be able to predict this weight loss accurately enough to plan for it. If an athlete expects such a weight loss, he or she should plan to approach the contest with the according excess of weight. It's also particularly important for such athletes to ensure quality sleep and adequate nutrition as a competition nears. Additionally, athletes will typically lose a consistent amount of weight overnight (usually up to about 1% of bodyweight), and this must be factored into weight cutting plans. For example, if a lifter weighs in early in the morning and is 0.5 kg heavy the night before, last-minute weight cutting should not be necessary, as that weight will come off overnight and any additional weight cutting will just be unnecessarily draining. Of course, lifters should monitor their bedtime and waking bodyweights periodically to become familiar with how much they can rely on losing.

In the final days leading into the contest, the athlete's bodyweight can be closely monitored and eating and drinking can be managed accordingly. It's important the athlete approach the final days before competition near enough to the competition weight that a severe weight cut that damages performance will not be necessary.

Whatever the reason for an excess of bodyweight, athletes will occasionally have to drop sometimes considerable weight immediately prior to competition in order to successfully weigh in. While some athletes intentionally drop weight in such a manner in the belief that it gives them a competitive advantage, nearly all the evidence suggests this belief is unfounded in the case of weightlifting because of the proximity of the weigh-in to the contest; this differs dramatically from other sports such as boxing in which weigh-ins are commonly held as much as 24-hours prior to the event, providing the athletes adequate time to rehydrate completely and consequently to dehydrate to extreme degrees in order to make weight without detriment to performance. Relatively small weight cuts should have little or no detriment as long as they are done properly and the lifter is accustomed to the practice.

It's likely a lifter will encounter a situation in which he or she will need to drop weight at the last minute at least once in his or her competitive career. Whatever the reason may be, there are a number of strategies to consider, many of which may be implemented together, and all of which rely on dehydration. Note that any water-reducing protocol is not particularly healthy, although for presently healthy individuals, it should create no problems. Athletes with health problems should avoid it, or at least consult with a physician prior to experimenting.

Some basic rules, which may be obvious, but are violated surprisingly frequently because athletes simply aren't thinking include not showering prior to the weigh-in after a weight cut to ensure water is not absorbed by dehydrated skin to add to bodyweight; all fluids count, not just water; and be ready to begin rehydrating immediately after weighing-in.

Sauna Probably the most traditional method of dehydration weight loss is the use of a sauna to accelerate sweating. The effect of the heat can be accentuated by wearing warm clothing and/or non-breathable clothing such as plastic sweat suits that prevent the evaporation and cooling effect of sweat and consequently encourage even greater sweating. Aside from being remarkably uncomfortable, this approach to rapid weight loss can be extremely draining on the athlete both physically and psychologically. It's common for combat athletes to perform some kind of activity such as jumping rope or calisthenics while in the sauna to increase sweating even further, but this is well beyond what most weightlifters will be able to manage. In consideration of the brief time between

weigh-in and competition, this method of weight loss should be limited to relatively small increments of weight that weren't able to be lost in time through less taxing methods.

Boiling Boiling is essentially a method of mimicking the effect of the sauna when one isn't available but a bathtub is, such as in the athlete's hotel room at the competition venue. The athlete will sit in a bath of the hottest water he or she can stand, ideally wearing a towel or other warm item on the head to further increase body temperature. Once the athlete is as warm as the water will get him or her, the athlete will wrap him- or herself in towels or put on a sweat suit or similar to force as much sweating as possible as a result of the heat from the bath. This process can be repeated, re-entering a freshly-warmed bath as soon as the rate of sweating seems to start slowing. Similarly, an athlete can dress in warm clothing and run a hot shower in a closed bathroom to simulate a steam room. Typically the athlete should spend about 8-10 minutes in the bath and 8-10 minutes out.

Heater Another option in the absence of either a sauna, bathtub or shower is using the heater of a home, hotel room or car in concert with warm clothing to produce sweating. Be sure to periodically dry your sweat and change into dry clothing so you minimize the cooling effect of the sweat.

Spitting Spitting is as simple and accessible a weight-cutting tool as exists. You need nothing at all to do it, although a cup to spit in is usually appreciated by the people around you. Additionally, chewing gum or sucking on sour hard candies can increase the amount of saliva produced that can then be spit out. One L of water equals 1 kg, so whatever fraction of a liter the lifter is able to spit will be the same fraction of a kilogram he or she has lost; e.g. if an athlete spits out 0.1 L, he or she has lost 0.1 kg.

Hyperhydration Although hyperhydration is not actually a last-minute weight loss protocol, it warrants mention here because of its ability to help athletes lose water weight in a less physically taxing manner, which means better performance at any given weight. By initially over-hydrating and then systematically reducing water intake, we can encourage the body to

Away From Meet	Water Intake
5 days	5 liters
4 days	4 liters
3 days	3 liters
2 days	2 liters
1 day	No water
Day of meet	Rehydrate after weigh-in

TABLE 54.6 The basic hyperhydration protocol

shed water weight without the use of forced sweating and its draining effects on energy and confidence. The water intake protocol is simple and can be adjusted slightly for the size of the athlete, but the basic protocol is outlined in Table 54.6.

The following rehydration can be accomplished fairly quickly. It will be more effective with electrolytes and an isotonic solution (same salt content as body's cells) such as Gatorade, Pedialyte or a homemade recipe of about a half-teaspoon of salt and half-teaspoon of potassium chloride (sold commonly as a salt substitute) per liter of water in addition to plain water. If the lifter has had to cut down carbohydrate intake in the weight-cutting effort, Gatorade is a good choice to quickly get some simple carbohydrates back into the system.

This rehydration needs to begin immediately following the weigh-in because of the brevity of the timeframe. The quantity of liquid needing to be replaced can be estimated according to the weight loss—again, 1 kg of lost bodyweight will need to be replaced by approximately 1 L of water; however, more than this will be necessary because some will be lost through urination as the lifter is rehydrating.

This protocol should be tested at least once well prior to any competition to evaluate the athlete's response in terms of weight loss, rate of rehydration, and performance following the process. Notes should be taken each day of the process that the athlete can refer to later when preparing for an actual competition to ensure he or she is on track and the predictions that have been made can be relied upon. Hyperhydration can be used to help drop the bulk of necessary weight and supplemented with one or more of the last-minute methods above as needed.

Examples Tables 54.7 and 54.8 are actual bodyweights and water intakes for two different athletes to provide an idea of what can be expected from the hyperhydration protocol. How much weight loss occurs will depend on a few factors, such as how much water the athlete drinks regularly, reduction or lack thereof of sodium and/or carbohydrate during the course of the week, alterations of caloric intake, etc. A common mistake is for lifters to panic during the week when they don't see their weight dropping—it needs to be understood that weight will not drop significantly, if at all, until the last 1-2 days. This again is a reason to test the protocol and document daily bodyweights to reassure the athlete that the protocol will work.

Monday	2 gal	54.7 kg
Tuesday	2 gal	54.5 kg
Wednesday	2 gal	53.7 kg
Thursday	1 gal	53.8 kg
Friday	1 gal	53.7 kg
Saturday	1/2 gal	52.8 kg
Sunday (meet)	0	52.66 kg (weigh-in)

TABLE 54.7 Example daily bodyweight and water intake for a 53kg female during a hyperhydration protocol.

Monday	6 L	105.9
Tuesday	5 L	106.1
Wednesday	4 L	106.5
Thursday	3 L	105.8
Friday	1 L	105.5
Saturday	0	104.5 (weigh-in)

TABLE 54.8 Example daily bodyweight and water intake for a 105kg male during a hyperhydration protocol.

Greg Everett

Competition Preparation Training

Weightlifting competition is about as stressful as it gets due to the circumstances—an athlete has spent months and years training for a grand total of six lifts that matter. There are countless factors that contribute to performance, and many are beyond the athlete's control, such as stress unrelated to training and problems with the venue or travel.

However, there are a lot of factors the athlete and coach can control, and a lot of little ones that may never even occur to them. Following are some of those little considerations that together can make a big difference. Athletes can make competition a lot more controlled and a lot less intimidating and overwhelming by paying attention to the details, and always remembering that experience will be the best teacher.

Use Collars Weightlifters commonly train without ever using collars in the gym. They're not only a hassle to use, but often gyms aren't equipped with enough competition-style collars for everyone to use. However, a bar feels and sounds significantly different with collars on it, and this change can throw a lifter off in competition if he or she not accustomed to it. Athletes should use collars on all heavy snatches and clean & jerks as they approach a competition so they don't even have to think about it.

Load the Right Way Another issue for a lot of athletes is seeing plates on the bar they're not used to seeing—like those red ones. Often women especially will never use red plates, and over time, a subconscious belief takes form that red plates are much heavier than a blue and a five. The lifter sees a bar loaded with red plates awaiting them on the platform and believes it to be heavier than it really is. This rule goes right along with the above rule about using collars—load the bar exactly how it would be loaded in competition. That means once a female is at 65 kg or a male at 70 kg, red plates should be on the bar.

Control Your Rest Periods Typically weightlifters rest according to feel in training. Unfortunately, for some athletes, this means excessive rest, and often times warm-ups and competition lifts in a meet have

to be done at a much faster pace. In the last few weeks leading into a meet rest periods should be kept to about 2 minutes. This will help condition the lifter both physically and mentally if and when it's needed.

Use Waves Wave loading is good training protocol generally, but it can be very helpful to prepare for competition specifically. In a competitive weight class, several lifters may be taking the same or similar attempt weights, which can create extremely long waits between a given lifter's first, second and third attempts. In some cases, a lifter may have to drop down to a lighter weight and warm back up to the next attempt because there will be so much time. If a lifter has never done this in the gym, it will not only be tough physically, but can be devastating mentally.

Practice Your Warm-up Progressions A lifter should never get to a meet and not know exactly what warm-up lifts he or she will be taking. Not only should that be planned ahead, it should be something the lifter is largely accustomed to. Again, changes between training and competition should be minimal—using a totally different weight progression in competition than the lifter uses in the gym every day is an enormous mental issue. If a lifter's warm-ups feel routine, their competition lifts are much more likely to feel routine. Leading up to competition, lifters should follow the same warm-up progressions for the snatch and clean & jerk that they plan to use in competition. This is also a chance to find out if something doesn't work well in time to make an adjustment.

Snatch and Clean & Jerk on the Same Day Often in training, athletes will perform snatch and clean & jerk related lifts on different days. This is generally good practice for motor learning and reinforcement reasons, but if a lifter never trains the snatch and clean & jerk together, competition can be extremely difficult physically and mentally.

Rest between Snatch and Clean & Jerk Because in competition, there will be a short break between the end of the snatches and start of the clean & jerks, depending on where an athlete finishes with the snatch and starts with the clean & jerk, the rest can be significant. By practicing at least some days resting about

10 minutes between snatches and clean & jerks, the athlete can simulate the meet environment somewhat and learn how to stay warm during that period and also stay calm without losing control of the focus and psychological arousal needed for clean & jerks.

Change Your Lifting Environment Competition lifting can be intimidating simply because of the different location with different things to look at. Many a lifter has missed a lift for no reason other than that they didn't find a good focal point. A lifter doesn't necessarily even need to leave his or her own gym for this one, although that is an option. Athletes should practice lifting on different platforms, and even facing the opposite direction on a given platform. Lifters should also train on different bars—even from set to set occasionally, just like a lifter will change to a different bar between the last warm-up and the first competition lift.

Embrace Chaos A lot of weightlifting spectators are weightlifters themselves or are well-versed in weightlifting etiquette… and many are not. There will always be noise and distractions in a competition venue, sometimes of a nature and magnitude that's unexpected. If an athlete controls the training environment completely to the point that one little unexpected distraction throws him or her off, that athlete is going to have a lot of trouble in a meet. Athletes should let people walk in front of them, stare at them, talk loudly around them, have their phones make noise, and the like periodically. It doesn't need to always be like this (and shouldn't), but athletes need to be exposed to it and toughen up so they will be better prepared for imperfect situations in competition.

Practice Your Caffeine If an athlete uses pre-training and competition caffeine, he or she should do it the same way every max day in the gym as it will be done in competition. That means type, timing, and amount. If an athlete normally drinks a cup of coffee an hour before training, drinking two Redbulls before he snatches in competition is a potential disaster. The opposite is true as well—if an athlete is accustomed to training under the influence of caffeine, that athlete needs to have the same ready to go for the meet. Caffeine intake leading into a competition can be tapered down to help with restoration

and re-sensitize the body to it, but this should be practiced outside of competition first.

Practice the Time of Day If the meet schedule has the athlete lifting at a time of day significantly different than what he or she is accustomed to, he or she should try to get at least some training in around that time. The athlete will better know what changes if any need to make to the warm-up—afternoon lifters who have to lift early may find they need considerably more time to get loose, for example—and better know what to expect to feel like. For some lifters, there isn't much of a difference, but for others, this is a real game-changer. Don't just wonder—find out.

Train Hot If an athlete is fortunate enough to train in a gym with air conditioning and/or fans, that athlete should train without them sometimes. More often than not, the warm-up rooms at meets are crowded, hot and stifling, and doing a big clean & jerk in that environment is considerably different than in a comfortable one.

Weigh In Frequently Bodyweight is a touchy subject for a lot of lifters, and many like to ignore it until they absolutely have to pay attention. This can cause a lot of problems, both physically and psychologically. Lifters should weigh in frequently—even daily. Not only does this help them control their weight and hydration like they need to, it makes the weigh-in routine instead of some monumental event they spend months dreading. As an aside, noting bodyweight in the training logs is a great piece of data to consider later down the road.

Pre-Competition Preparation

The athlete's activity prior to competition can have a considerable effect on performance. Essentially, we want to minimize fatigue, both physical and psychological, and maximize confidence.

Smaller local competitions can last many hours, and national and international competitions are typically spread over three or more days. Depending on the athlete's weight class, this can mean a lot of waiting either at the venue itself or in the case of longer distance travel, in a hotel. The natural desire for most will be to watch other lifting sessions, particularly if friends and teammates are competing. This should be avoided as much as possible—it's very psychologically tiring and distracts the athlete from his or her own upcoming performance. Whenever possible, the athlete should remain in his or her hotel room or in a part of the venue in which he or she can relax and focus.

Ideally the athlete is relaxed and resting, but not entirely sedentary. Some light movement throughout the day such as the dynamic range of motion exercises used to warm-up will better prepare the body for performance.

Additionally, visualization of the upcoming performance can be helpful. Such visualization should of course consist of successful lifting. The athlete should attempt to perform such visualization without getting excited—psychological arousal at this point can be tiring and detract from the athlete's performance when it matters. Visualization should be an exercise in composure, focus and confidence. The more extensive and accurate the visualization, the more effective it will be. The common practice for weightlifting is to visualize the entire competition from the first warm-up lift until the last competition lift. The idea is to create realistic imagery that includes every sense: what the athlete sees, hears, smells, etc. In essence, the athlete is experiencing the entire competition mentally, seeing and feeling the successful outcome before it happens.

Competition Procedure

Local weightlifting meets can vary considerably in how they're run in terms of formality. Generally they will be more casually administered, although the same basic procedure will be followed. National level meets will involve more complicated administrative elements, but also tend to be better organized.

Athlete & Coach Check-in The first step is for the athlete and coach to check in at the meet. At a local meet, this may not be necessary; at a national meet, both the athlete and coach will need to obtain their credentials to get access to the warm-up room.

Technical & Verification Meetings The technical meeting and verification of entries are usually held the night before the first day of competition. The meet organizers will discuss any technical changes or possible issues so that all coaches may be informed. The verification of entries meeting is the last chance to make changes to athletes' weight classes. Coaches and athletes are not required to attend either, but it's recommended they do when possible to gain the experience.

Early Preparation Before the weigh-in, the athlete needs to ensure he or she is prepared in every way for the upcoming meet, as time between the weigh-in and start of competition will be limited and stress needs to be minimized. This means having all water, energy drinks, Gatorade, food for during the meet, and all personal gear packed and ready to go. The lifter also needs to have a clear plan for eating and rehydrating immediately after the weigh-in. The initial post-weigh-in rehydration fluid of choice should be brought to the weigh-in so the lifter can begin drinking immediately. The lifter should eat as soon as possible after the weigh-in also to ensure the food has enough time to digest adequately both so that it can actually contribute energy to performance and not create GI distress.

Additionally, it's advisable to run through a quick series of DROMs immediately prior to the weigh-in to begin the warm-up process. This activity doesn't replace any of the warm-up activity that will be done immediately before the session begins. It's a way to loosen up the lifter, who has likely been largely sedentary for 1-3 days, and begin the initial warming of the body and neurological resetting of muscle length and tension. This will make the actual warm-up more effective and ensure the lifter feels as good as possible during the session.

Lifters should also check their bodyweights periodically leading into the competition to properly control food and water intake and plan any necessary cutting procedures. Venues will provide check scales for this purpose in addition to the official scale used for weigh-in. Occasionally the check scales will not be perfectly accurate, but any inaccuracies are typically noted for lifters to determine their weight better—for example, a scale may be 0.1 heavy at 40kg.

Weighing In The earliest stage of competition is the weigh-in. Weigh-ins begin two hours prior to the beginning of the lifter's session. In national meets, weigh-ins will typically be of a single weight class, but occasionally may be two combined classes. In local meets, a single session may have several weight classes. In either case, all athletes for the given session weigh in together. Athletes will be called to weigh in according to the order of assigned lot numbers; in local meets, it may be a first-come, first-served order.

Athletes need to make sure to have the proper credentials and ID. This usually means a driver license or equivalent and the meet-issued credential. It's important to find out exactly what is needed before the weigh-in to ensure no time is wasted.

Weigh-ins must be done in undergarments or nude—no additional clothing may be worn. An official will verify the lifter's weight and enter it in the system and/or on the attempt card. The lifter will have an opportunity to review and verify the weight. The athlete will also provide the official his or her intended opening lift weights for the snatch and clean & jerk. These may be changed later, but these numbers will be used to create the initial order of lifting. The lifter will then sign the card to verify the numbers are correct. The lifter will be assigned a lot number, which will be used during the competition to determine lifting order in some cases, and should be what the coach references to the marshals, rather than the lifter's name, when declaring weights for the lifter.

Competition

Minor details will differ among local, national and international competition, but the basic structure will always be the same.

In a national or international meet, the athletes will be introduced on stage to begin the session. Once completed, a 10-minute clock will begin; at the end of this clock, the first lifter will be called for the session. Generally local meets will not involve introductions, and the first lifter will be called at the listed session start time.

The snatch is performed first by all athletes and the clean & jerk second. Athletes are allowed three attempts with each lift. To begin each lift's session, the barbell is loaded to the lowest opening weight for the session stated on the weigh-in cards, and the weight on the bar will be progressively increased according to the lifters' declared attempt weights until all attempts in the session have been made.

Each lifter's best snatch and best clean & jerk are added to make a total, and the lifters are ranked in order of total, with the highest total winning the weight class. In cases in which two or more lifters make the same total, the lifter who completed the total first wins—as of 2016, it is no longer possible to win with an identical total by weighing less. In addition to the total, which wins the competition, some events will also award medals for the top 3 snatches and clean & jerks.

Lifting Order The lifters in the session are ordered according to four figures, listed in order of priority: the attempt weight; current attempt number; increase in weight from last attempt; lot number.

The lifters are ordered primarily by the weight of their attempts—that is, the bar moves continually from lowest to highest weight and the athletes make their attempts as those attempts meet with the weight on the bar.

If two lifters have declared the same weight, the lifter with fewer completed attempts goes first—for example, if two lifters are attempting 120kg, the lifter for whom it will be a first attempt goes before the lifter for whom it will be a second or third attempt.

If there are two lifters on the same attempt number with the same weight, the lifter taking the largest weight increase will lift first. If Lifter A's first attempt was 110kg and Lifter B's first attempt was 115kg, Lifter A would take 120kg for a second attempt before Lifter B.

If the weight, attempt number and increase are all the same among two or more lifters, the lifter with the lowest lot number will lift first.

Time & Weight Changes The first lifter's name is announced and he or she then has 1 minute to begin the lift (separate the barbell from the platform). Until the lifter has 30 seconds or less remaining on the clock, the weight of the attempt may be changed. There are two allowable changes to each declared attempt weight—if the declared weight is 120kg, the lifter may first change to 122kg, and then change again to 123kg. These changes must be made with at least 30 seconds remaining on the lift clock. The clock is paused during the changing of weights and resumed when the loaders are again off the platform.

However, if this new weight is no longer the lowest one in the cards, this lifter will no longer be up. The lifter with the new lowest weight will then be called and a new 1-minute clock started for him or her after the barbell is loaded to that weight (or it may remain if another lifter is taking the original weight).

After completing the attempt on the platform, the athlete (or coach) will declare to the officials his or her next attempt if there is one. A successful lift is not required to increase the weight of the next attempt—the athlete can declare any weight greater than his or her last attempt , and can declare a repeat of a missed weight.

If no declared attempts exist between the lift just taken and that lifter's next declared attempt, that lifter will follow him- or herself. In this case, he or she will be given a 2-minute clock following the loading of the barbell within which the lift must be started.

Caution should be taken in certain cases regarding the 2-minute clock. If the lifting order is Lifter A, Lifter B, then Lifter A, and lifter B declares a change *after being announced* to a weight greater than Lifter A's second attempt, lifter A will in a practical sense be following him- or herself. However, there will be no 2-minute clock because Lifter B was announced prior to the weight change, which means that technically Lifter A is not following him- or herself. This rule is occasionally used to try to create a disadvantage to Lifter A, but often it happens inadvertently—in either case, the lifter and coach need to be prepared.

Weight changes are often used as a strategy to increase the rest time for the athlete to prepare for a heavier lift because the clock is stopped during the change. For example, if an athlete will be following him- or herself after a lift at 120kg with 125kg next, he or she may declare 122kg (declaration) immediately following completion of 120kg. Shortly after 122kg is loaded, the athlete may change the attempt to 124kg (change 1). Again waiting until shortly after 124kg is loaded, the athlete may finally declare his 125kg (change 2) with his last weight change. Depending on the proficiency of the loaders at the meet, this can buy significant additional rest time for the lifter, and in any case, more than none.

Athletes can reduce the weight of their next attempts only if the desired weight is still equal to or greater than what's currently on the bar—that is, the weight on the competition bar can never be lowered. Practically speaking, this means the athlete can only lower a declared attempt weight well prior to being called for that attempt. Attempts can be declined and athletes can withdraw from competition. Neither decision can be reversed once the official announcement has been made.

Break and Clean & Jerk This process of progressive loading and lifting will continue until all athletes have made their three snatch attempts (unless any athletes decline to take any attempts or withdraw from the competition in case of injury, for example).

When all snatching is complete, a 10-minute break is taken before the clean & jerk attempts begin (occasionally if the meet is running behind, this break is shortened or eliminated at the discretion of the officials). This allows lifters who will be near the beginning of the order adequate time to warm-up. These lifters will often need to begin warming up for their clean & jerks while the snatch session is still underway.

During the break, the barbell will be loaded to the first clean & jerk attempt weight. The process used for the snatch is then repeated identically for the clean & jerk. Once all attempts have been completed, each lifter's best snatch and best clean & jerk are added to produce his or her total. In national and international competition, medals are awarded for best snatch, best clean & jerk, and best total within each weight class. Generally in local meets, only the totals are considered, and physical awards may or may not be given.

Drug Testing In national and international meets (or any other that is being drug tested), following the final lift of an athlete who will be tested (usually the medalists and possibly one or more random athletes from each session), a representative from the testing agency (WADA, USADA or other national equivalent) will meet the lifter and let him or her know he or she will be tested. The representative will then stay with the lifter until testing is completed. It's generally a good idea for athletes to remain in the warm-up area for 10 minutes following the completion of the competition to ensure they are not being tested before leaving.

Technical Rules & Procedures Prior to competition, athletes and coaches should be familiar with the technical rules of weightlifting with respect to the performance of the lifts, familiar with the etiquette of weightlifting competition, and should have an idea of what to expect on the competition platform. Obviously understanding will increase with experience, but having a baseline of knowledge is important. Equally important for the beginner athlete or coach is to be respectful of the other lifters, coaches and officials at the meet, and of the system and procedures themselves; defer to the more senior participants when appropriate. The overwhelming majority of coaches and lifters are more than happy to help new lifters and coaches, but their willingness to do so will evaporate instantaneously, and justifiably, in response to displays of arrogance, disrespectfulness and the like by new coaches and lifters. Consider the early stages of your lifting or coaching career to be the time to listen, watch and learn, not try to gain attention for yourself.

The competition platform is 4x4 meters—considerably larger than the typical training platform. The lifter must start each lift facing forward, but may, due to the need to make adjustments during the lift, complete a successful lift facing any direction and in any area of the platform.

If an electronic timing system is being used, there will be a clock visible to the lifter from the platform so that the remaining time to start the lift can be monitored. Chalk and possibly rosin for the shoes will be at some place near the competition platform.

There will be three officials judging each session—one directly in front of the platform and one to either side at an oblique angle. At local meets, it's common for the competition platform to be on the floor, placing the center judge directly in front of the lifter; lifters will need to find a focal point just over the official's head or even on the chest to minimize distraction. Platforms at national and international meets are typically raised on a stage, placing the referees at a lower lever and eliminating this problem.

Following each lift, these officials will provide their decisions—either passing or not—based on whether the lift was executed legally. With light systems, a white light indicates the judge has declared a good lift, and red indicates a no-lift. At smaller local meets, the judges may have red and white flags or similar, or may even simply use a thumbs-up/thumbs-down system. For a lift to count, it must be passed by at least 2 of the 3 judges.

With electronic scoring systems, after all three officials have declared their decisions, some kind of light and sound will signal the lifter that the weight can be dropped. Otherwise, or in case the system is malfunctioning or the lifter does not respond to the signals, the center judge will give a down signal manually and audibly.

The down signal will not be given until the lifter has returned to the final standing position with the feet in line with each other and has the weight under control overhead. If the weight is dropped before the officials give the down signal, even if the athlete appears to have had the weight under control, the lift will not count.

The bar must be dropped in a clearly intentional manner in front of the athlete, the athlete must keep the hands on the bar until it passes the shoulders, and the bar must land on the platform. USAW provides the director of any sanctioned meet the discretion to impose and enforce a rule that prevents intentionally slamming the bar down onto the platform following a lift. This should never be an issue, as doing so is generally considered disrespectful, and athletes should have the presence of mind to avoid behaving this way in competition. In no way does this imply that athletes are not allowed to celebrate successful lifts; it should just be done in a way that is respectful to the officials, athletes and coaches.

In national and international competition, there will be a jury of 3 or 5 officials in addition to the referees. This jury may overturn the referees' decision if they agree unanimously to do so.

While the bar must simply leave the platform before the lifter's time runs out, the lift officially begins when the bar reaches the knee with regard to the movement being considered an attempt. That is, as long as time remains on the clock, a lifter may lift the bar slightly off the floor, return it to the floor, and then perform the lift legally; the bar must start from a dead stop on the floor, however (i.e. it cannot be lifted first and then bounced off of the platform to begin the actual attempt). Only one attempt at the lift can be made each time the lifter is on the platform, regardless of the time on the clock.

The snatch and clean & jerk are considered complete when the athlete is standing erect with both feet next to each other in an orientation parallel with the bar—that is, they cannot be staggered—but may be at any width, and the barbell is held overhead with straight elbows.

No part of the body other than the feet may touch the platform at any time, such as knees during a split or the glutes during a squat. The arms may not touch the legs during the receipt of the clean. The barbell may not touch the head, including the hair or any hat being worn.

In the clean, the bar cannot be moved from the initial receiving position—that is, if the lifter receives the bar low on the chest, it cannot be subsequently lifted up onto the shoulders.

The athlete must be motionless before beginning the jerk following the clean. There may be only one drive attempt for the jerk—the athlete can bend the knees and bounce the bar in order to adjust the hands and arms, but once he or she begins to dip for a jerk attempt, it cannot be aborted and repeated.

With the snatch and jerk, the bar must be received with the elbows locked, and they must remain locked until the lift is completed. A pressout is defined as continued extension of the elbows after the athlete's body has reached its lowest position.

For athletes who have anatomical conditions preventing the full lockout of the elbows, this condition must be demonstrated to the officials prior to the athlete lifting, usually by pointing to the elbow of the raised arm before beginning the lift.

Judges are not perfect and their decisions may not be consistent from lifter to lifter and session to session. At times mistakes may be in the lifter's favor, and at other times, they won't be. Athletes and coaches should avoid arguing with officials except in cases of grievous and obvious mistakes or failures.

Knowing that judges are capable of missing technical mistakes, the athlete should never indicate that he or she is aware an error has been made and complete the lift as if it is successful until told otherwise. For example, an athlete may feel a slight pressout with the elbow, but this may not be seen by the judges (and often what feels like a failing pressout is actually minimal enough movement to be passable). If the athlete in some manner indicates knowledge of the error, it's more likely the judges will notice it and call a no-lift. In short, the athlete should assume the lift is good until the officials indicate otherwise.

Timing Warm-Up Lifts

Warming up properly in preparation for competition attempts is considerably more complicated than warming up in the gym because of the need to time the athlete's warm-up lifts to properly coincide with the time he or she will be called to the platform. This unfortunately means the process is neither simple nor perfect, but with experience, coaches will be able to achieve very high accuracy.

The method to time warm-up lifts relies on maintaining a running count of how many competition attempts remain to be taken prior to the lifter's opener. Counting attempts is not an exact practice—there is some degree of unpredictability involved. This unpredictability is a result primarily of the uncertainty of the amount of weight each lifter will increase after each attempt. The coach must estimate the count number and continually monitor the progress to maintain an accurate count.

Determining Warm-up Lifts First, the lifter and coach need to determine the warm-up sequence for the snatch and clean & jerk based on the selected opening weights. This will provide the coach with the number of lifts that need to be taken prior to the opening attempt so that the warm-up can be properly timed.

The goal with the warm-ups is to ensure the athlete is fully prepared while minimizing unnecessary fatigue. This will usually mean approximately 6-9 sets; it is typically advisable to perform fewer sets in the clean & jerk than in the snatch, as the movement is more fatiguing, but the somewhat lower precision allows fewer lifts and larger weight increases between lifts.

Ideally, any additional sets are done at the athlete's starting weight; this will allow more extensive warming of the lifter with insignificant additional fatigue. For example, if a lifter's first warm-up weight for the snatch is 50kg, he may elect to do 2-3 sets with the weight before moving to his next.

The newer the lifter, the closer the last warm-up weight will be to the opener. In fact, in some cases with new lifters, the opening weight can even be taken as the last warm-up. This is a good way to build confidence for new competitors; at the early stage, their weights will not be very physically taxing, so such a practice will have little or no noticeable negative effect.

An example snatch warm-up sequence for a 140kg snatch opener may look like the following:

Bar
50
50
50
70
90
110
120
130
135

An example clean & jerk warm-up sequence for a 175 kg opener may look like the following:

Bar
70
70
70
110
140
155
165

Initial Count Prior to the start of the session, the coach must obtain an initial count. In a national or international meet, there will be a scoreboard that shows all of the lifters and their declared attempts—at the start of the session, this means only the opening attempts. In a local meet, there will typically only be the attempt cards arranged on the marshal's table. The cards will usually be ordered on the table according to the sequence of lifting and therefore constantly changing position, but in some meets the cards may be attached in static positions to the table.

The coach will use either the cards or the scoreboard to make an initial count of attempts. This is done by predicting how many attempts each lifter will make before our lifter's opening attempt. Generally speaking, the farther the previous attempts are from our lifter's opener, the more reliable the count; the closer, the more educated guesswork is required.

If our lifter is opening in the snatch at 120kg and another lifter is opening at 100kg, we can reliably predict that the first lifter will take all 3 attempts before our lifter, as there is a 20kg spread. If another lifter is opening at 119kg, we will plan for only 1 attempt from that lifter. This can change, of course, if that lifter misses and repeats, but that is a detail that has to be dealt with during the course of the warm-up. If a lifter is opening at 115kg, we have to make a decision.

Generally lifters will not make more than a 5kg jump in the snatch. If this lifter takes 115 and then 120, that will be 1 attempt because our lifter will take 120 first, as it's his first attempt and the other lifter's second. However, that lifter may take only 117-119, in which case it's 2 attempts.

	LOT	NAME	Y-O-B	TEAM	BDWT	NEXT	SNATCH					CLEAN & JERK					TOTAL		Sinclair Formula
							1	2	3	Res	Pl	1	2	3	Res	Pl	Res	Pl	
On the Clock	1	BARARI Mohammadreza	1988	IRI	104.56	221	170	-175	175	170	11	211			211	10	381	10	416.183057
On Deck	4	BONK Bartlomiej	1984	POL	104.25	221	185	-189	-190	185	4	215			215	5	400	4	437.389333
In the Hole	6	KLOKOV Dmitry	1983	RUS	104.60	221	187	192	196	196	2	220			220	2	416	1	454.354811
	8	KIM Chul-Min	1986	KOR	104.62	221	172	-178	-178	172	10	213			213	8	385	9	420.468770
	10	TOROKHTIY Oleksiy	1986	UKR	104.27	221	176	181	-185	181	5	220			220	1	401	3	438.453455
	11	EFREMOV Ivan	1986	UZB	103.35	221	175	-180	-185	175	9	215			215	4	390	8	427.758100
	5	ISTOMIN Sergey	1986	KAZ	104.41	221	178	-182	-182	178	8	210	215		215	6	393	6	429.505400
	3	AKKAEV Khadzhimurat	1985	RUS	104.44	222	190	195	198	198	1				0	11	0	11	0.000000
	9	MACHAVARIANI Gia	1985	GEO	104.00	222	180	184	187	187	3	212	218		218	3	405	2	443.228846
	2	NASIRSHELAL Navab	1989	IRI	103.91	223	175	180	-185	180	6	211	211		211	9	391	7	428.037395
	7	AUDZEYEU Mikhail	1982	BLR	104.71	215	175	-180	180	180	7	-210	210	215	215	7	395	5	431.261588

FIGURE 54.1 In a national or international meet, there will be a scoreboard that shows all of the lifters and their declared attempts.

Greg Everett

The coach can assume that lifters will typically increase 2-5 kg between snatch attempts and 3-8 kg between clean & jerk attempts and use this to make the initial count (women generally more toward the lower end of the range and men more toward the higher end). Additional information can be used when available for a more reliable count. For example, if the coach is familiar with any of the other lifters, he or she may know what those lifters are capable of lifting and what kind of weight increases they typically take.

Another consideration are potential 2-minute clocks, as these will extend the duration considerably. If there are lifters before ours who will likely follow themselves—for example, if a lifter is opening at 90kg and the next lowest opener is 105kg—we need to count each 2-minute clock as 2 attempts.

This will give the coach the initial count of attempts until his or her athlete takes the first lift. The lifter's warm-up lifts can then be timed accordingly (explained below).

An exception to this process would be when an athlete is the first to lift in the session or is early enough in the session that his or her warm-up attempts must begin before the first lifter is on the platform. In these cases, the clock must be used instead of or along with the attempt count by having the lifter take a warm-up lift every 3 minutes. With clean & jerks, this is a little more complicated because there will likely not be enough time between the snatch and clean & jerk sessions for the athlete's entire warm-up, so it must be started while the snatch session is still in progress. In this case, the coach can count the remaining snatch attempts, the time of the break, and/or any attempts in the clean & jerk that will come before his or her lifter's opener.

Timing Warm-up Attempts Once the coach has the initial attempt count, the athlete's warm-up attempts can be planned. Generally lifters will take a warm-up lift every 3 attempts on the competition platform, which results in an approximately 3-minute rest between sets.

Prior to the start of the session, the coach should have determined the warm-up lifts the lifter will take. Each lift can now be assigned to a "time"—a number of attempts remaining (or as described above, it may be a literal time on the clock). Using the every-3-attempt protocol, each successive warm-up lift will be taken with 3 fewer remaining attempts. That is, the lifter's last warm-up will be taken when there are 3 attempts remaining; the second to last warm-up with 6 attempts remaining; the third to last with 9 attempts; etc.

The lifter will then take his or her first warm-up when the remaining lifts equals the number of lifts planned for that warm-up. For example, if the lifter is 36 attempts out from the start of the session and his or her first warm-up needs to be taken with 30 attempts remaining, the first warm-up will be taken after 6 attempts have occurred on the competition platform.

Using our previous snatch warm-up sequence, we would assign a count for each set as follows:

NAME		LOT #	
BODYWEIGHT		DOB	
USAW #		AGE CLASS	
TEAM		WEIGHT CLASS	

LIFT	1	2	3	BEST
SNATCH				
CLEAN & JERK				
			TOTAL	

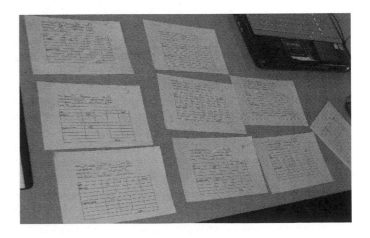

FIGURE 54.2 Attempt cards will be used by the marshals to control the meet. In a local meet, these will usually be the only part of the system; in a national or international meet, these will be used in conjunction with a scoreboard.

Bar - 30
50 - 27
50 - 24
50 - 21
70 - 18
90 - 15
110 - 12
120 - 9
130 - 6
135 - 3

With this sequence, the lifter would need to begin warming up with the empty barbell when 30 attempts remain before his opener, and be lifting 110kg when 12 attempts remain.

As mentioned above, in some cases, a lifter will be too early in a session to have time to take all warm-up attempts during the session itself. Using our same example, if our lifter is only 15 attempts out from the start of the session, he would need to begin warming up before the first lift of the session is taken. The coach can then use a combination of attempt counts and a number of minutes prior to the session start time as follows:

Bar - 15 min
50 - 12 min
50 - 9 min
50 - 6 min
70 - 3 min
90 – 15 (start of session)
110 - 12
120 - 9
130 - 6
135 - 3

The coach can track warm-ups and attempts by making a simple notecard for the session. This warm-up card should list the athlete's warm-up lifts in sequence as well as other procedures to be planned (such as pre-barbell warm-ups that need to be accounted time), and alongside each, note how many attempts out it should be performed (Figure 54.3).

Other notes can be made as the session progresses to help the coach keep track, as the process can get confusing with all of the possible distractions, particularly if managing more than one athlete in a session.

For example, the coach may decide to make hash marks to log completed competition attempts to help remain on schedule—this can reduce the number of times the coach has to return to the attempt cards to recount. Of course, the coach should still recount periodically to ensure no unexpected changes have occurred for which he or she hasn't accounted. This also allows more opportunities to recognize previous mistakes and adjust accordingly.

When instructing the athlete to take a warm-up attempt, the coach should take into consideration any additional demands on time. For example, if an athlete is sharing a bar with another, the weight may need to be changed; the athlete may have to cross a large warm-up room to get chalk; and nervous athletes may find themselves needing to visit the restroom frequently during their warm-ups.

Bars should be loaded for the athlete's next warm-up immediately following the previous lift, or immediately following another athlete's warm-up if necessary. Whenever possible, the coach or another assistant should load the bar to allow the athlete to continue resting. The coach may instruct the athlete

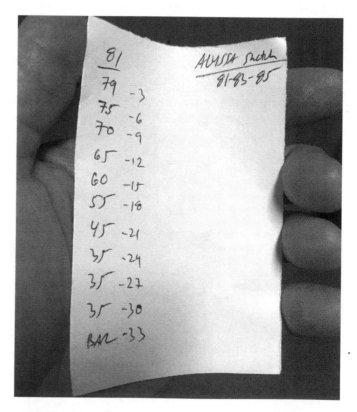

FIGURE 54.3 A warm-up card to help the coach keep track of the athlete's warm-ups and the competition attempts.

Greg Everett

to get chalk one attempt before the intended attempt for the athlete's warm-up to ensure he or she can make the lift at the correct time. Restroom breaks should always be taken immediately after the bar is dropped following a warm-up attempt to make the best use of the limited time.

In some cases, whether due to unpredictable weight changes, missed lifts and repeats, or a mistake on the coach's part, there may be more or less time before the athlete's first attempt than expected and the warm-ups must be altered. The coach needs to continually update the attempt count so that the pacing of the warm-ups can be adjusted appropriately. If a significant change occurs, a warm-up lift may need to be omitted entirely or additional warm-up attempts added—ideally this is done as early as possible so it's one of the lighter weights.

If the mistake is realized early on in the warm-up process and the time will be longer than expected, the athlete should remain at the current warm-up weight until the time gap is closed. That is, if the athlete has just taken 60kg and the coach realizes there will be 6 more attempts than expected, that athlete may take 60kg for 2 more warm-up lifts before proceeding to the next planned weight to get the warm-up progression back on schedule.

If the weight is already beyond what the athlete can reasonably take more than once, the weight may need to be dropped and then the athlete will work back up. Obviously this is not ideal, but this should underscore the importance of making and keeping an accurate count right from the start.

In the opposite situation—the coach miscounting, a lifter withdrawing, or unexpectedly large weight increases, and there being fewer attempts than expected—the warm-up process will need to be shortened. How this is done may vary among athletes depending on what they're comfortable with. For example, some athletes may prefer to omit a warm-up completely and alter the next warm-up weights a little to account for it. If there is enough time, the athlete may be able to take the planned warm-up lifts but at shorter intervals, such as every 2 attempts instead of 3, if preferred.

Continuing the Count

As the session progresses and the lifter nears his or her opener, more accurate counts can be continually made due to a decreasing total number of lifters and the consequent reduction in uncertainty, other lifters declaring second attempt weights so subsequent weight increases can be more accurately predicted, and the ability to account for misses and 2-minute clocks. It should also be kept in mind that lifters commonly take smaller jumps between their second and third attempts than between their first and second attempts.

In addition to the cards and scoreboard, coaches should pay attention to what's happening in the warm-up room as much as possible, as it can be a source of helpful information with regard to predicting other lifter's upcoming attempt weights. For example, overhearing a lifter and coach discussing withdrawing because the lifter is hurt, the coach can expect to lose whatever attempts that lifter has before his or her lifter and not be surprised when the withdrawal is announced, which could be at the very last moment with respect the lifter's last warm-up. Another example is watching the competitors' current warm-up weights in relation to their openers and the timing. If a lifter has declared a 100kg opener but is snatching 100kg in the warm-up room, there's a nearly 100% chance that lifter will increase the opening weight. Similarly, if a lifter seems to be behind on the timing of the warm-ups, this suggests he or she is going to increase the opening weight. On the other hand, if a lifter looks terrible or is missing warm-ups, the opener may be lowered. Any other information gleaned during or before the competition about the other competitors can become useful during the warm-up.

Competition Attempts

After each competition attempt, an automatic 1kg increase will be entered for the athlete's next lift. The next attempt must be declared with the first 30 seconds by the athlete or coach, this 1kg increase will become the declared attempt, and no changes will be allowed. To avoid any possible confusion or problems, it is best practice to always declare the next attempt as quickly as possible, even if it is only a 1kg increase. This not only ensures that there will be 2 changes available, but it helps the marshals and other coaches do their jobs more easily.

Choosing Weights Decisions will need to be made by the athlete and coach regarding the weights the athlete will take for each attempt. Opening weights can be chosen well prior to a meet, and adjusted if necessary during the warm-up process. Generally, openers should be lifts with which the athlete is wholly confident—a successful opening attempt will ensure the lifter makes a total, and will provide confidence for the subsequent attempts; missed openers can be devastating psychologically and often prevent athletes from successfully making subsequent lifts even well within their physical abilities.

The second and third attempt weights will be determined according to the athlete's performance on the preceding lifts and competition strategy. Generally, of course, the goal is to increase as much as is believed possible in order to make the heaviest lift possible; how easily the athlete made the previous lift will be the best indicator of what weight can be expected to be made next.

However, at times the athlete and coach may decide to take smaller jumps to ensure a win over a competitor. For example, in a situation in which an athlete is 1kg behind a competitor who has no further attempts, that athlete may decide to increase only 2kg even if he or she feels more is possible to make a successful lift and consequently a win more likely. This is particularly important in team competition—athletes should generally make attempts based on earning necessary team points rather than individual goals.

Strategies for competition lifts vary among coaches and athletes. One approach is to use competitions as an opportunity to make personal records, as this is generally the most appropriate time—the athlete is recovered and prepared specifically for lifting maximal weights, and will be under the influence of the greatest possible levels of physiological and psychological arousal. Exceptions, of course, are athletes who are not particularly good at dealing with pressure and tend to actually perform worse in meets, those who cut significant weight for competition, or those who train in a more Bulgarian fashion, in which case competition lifts may never exceed gym lifts. In such cases, the goal should be to continually improve on the competition PRs rather than the overall PRs in competition.

The other approach is to make records in the gym, and make lifts in competition. That is, the competition is viewed as a time to make as many successful lifts as possible; in order to ensure high success rates, competition attempts do not exceed the athlete's best lifts in the gym. While this certainly improves the number of successful attempts a lifter is likely to have in competition, it also limits the potential maximal weights. This is also necessary for athletes who cut significant weight.

Ultimately, an athlete only needs to make one snatch and one clean & jerk to win; this is certainly a riskier strategy, but has the potential to pay off more. Typically a balance between the two strategies should be taken, especially with regard to mindset—that is, lifters and coaches should be attempting to lift the heaviest possible weights in competition, but should also be attempting to make as many of the competition attempts as possible.

Of course, not all competitions need to be approached the same way. For lifters at the national and international level, occasional lower level competitions may be used simply for practice, and the weights will not be pushed like they would be in more meaningful meets. Using such competitions as a chance to work on preparation, consistency, and making all 6 lifts, rather that hitting absolute maximal attempts, is an effective approach.

Making Changes & Buying Time As was mentioned previously, changes can be made to declared attempt weights. When declaring opening attempts during the weigh-in, it's wise to declare weights slightly lower than intended if an athlete has been inconsistent or unexpectedly fatigued leading up to the meet. These can be increased later if determined appropriate, but will allow the athlete some security in case the warm-ups indicate he or she is not performing as well as hoped. This can also be done if necessary for a strategic advantage, but otherwise should be avoided, as it only complicates the warm-up procedure for everyone else unnecessarily—if a lifter is going to place 15th in a local meet, there is no need to try to fool opponents with a low opening declaration that will be increased later.

In cases in which the coach or athlete wants to allow more time for the athlete to recover between attempts, a lower weight than actually wanted can be declared. Once the athlete is called for the attempt, two changes to the weight can be made before the final 30 seconds. Because the clock is stopped while the loaders change the weight on the bar, this can increase the rest time between lifts significantly, especially if a declared change requires new bumper plates and not just change plates.

Warm-ups for Subsequent Attempts Generally, most of the stress of the warm-up is over once the lifter takes the first attempt. In some meets, however, the stress will continue because the durations between each lifter's three attempts can sometimes become unexpectedly long.

In a very large session (more common in local meets), there may be several lifters calling the same or similar weights; in very competitive sessions, many lifters may be attempting the same or similar weights. The result of each is the same—even a relatively small weight increase will require a long wait because of the unusually large number of attempts by other lifters at weights in between the previous and next attempt.

Additionally, a series of missed lifts can create unexpected additional attempts and 2-minute clocks. For example, if our lifter snatches 120, then declares 125 for his second attempt, and there is a lifter at 122 and 124, that would in ideal circumstances be two attempts before our lifter was called again. If the first lifter misses and repeats, he will have a 2-minute clock, and if he misses again, he'll have another 2-minute clock; this means that the wait has increased from 2 lifts to the equivalent of 5 lifts. Multiply that potential by more lifters, and it's obvious how wait times can unexpectedly increase dramatically.

In any case, a lifter cannot wait idly for too long between attempts, and the coach and lifter need to have a protocol for managing waits. There are multiple methods, and which is used will depend on both the duration of the wait and what works best for each lifter. The purpose of all methods is to keep the athlete warm and prepared while minimizing fatigue.

First, the time between lifts can be extended beyond what was used in the initial warm-up; in fact, athletes will typically not mind getting a little more rest between their competition attempts. Beyond 5-6 minutes, however, and most athletes will begin to stiffen up and lose focus and aggression. Consequently, some kind of lift should be taken during waits to prevent resting more than 5-6 minutes at a time. For example, if there is a wait of about 10 minutes or 10 attempts, a single lift can be taken around the midpoint; or, a lifter may prefer to split that 10 minutes with 2 lifts. Again, the coach and athlete need to have discussed a strategy beforehand so decisions can be made quickly. The more experience the coach and lifter have in such situations, the better the decisions and strategies for each will become.

The first method is to perform a full lift (snatch or clean & jerk) at a lighter weight. For example, our lifter waiting for a 125kg second attempt may take an 80-90kg snatch in the warm-up room during the wait. The benefit to this is that the lifter is performing the complete movement and the light weight will not be taxing; the drawback is that returning to a significantly heavier weight on the platform may be mentally tough.

The next method is to perform a power snatch or power clean & jerk, also at a reduced weight. This is essentially the same as the previous in terms of benefits, with the addition of even less work for the legs, and drawbacks, with the addition of the lifter having to readjust to a full lift again.

Next is to take a snatch pull or clean pull rather than a full lift. This may be the most common method, but it has its own drawbacks. Primarily, pulls usually feel very heavy even relative to full lifts at the same weights, especially without straps, and consequently this can be very mentally problematic. The additional drawback is a more extensive variation of the power strategy: the athlete has to readjust mentally and physically from a pull to a full lift, and in the clean & jerk, the jerk is left out altogether.

Finally, for extremely long waits, the best approach is to perform waves, sometimes called segments. Using our same example, the lifter waiting for the 125kg second attempt who needs to take 3 lifts in the warm-up room may snatch 110-115-120 and then take his competition attempt at 125. Essentially, the athlete is performing an abbreviated warm-up to the next attempt like he did for his opener. While this is arguably the best approach for such a situation, it will still be exhausting physically and difficult mentally. It's helpful when athletes train with waves periodically in the gym to be prepared for such circumstances in competition.

While waiting between lifts, athletes need to stay warm, covering with a towel or blanket, or draping warm-ups over themselves. After a fairly long wait between lifts in which the athlete has been sitting still, it's helpful to perform 1-2 squat jumps right before heading to the competition platform to help wake the body up.

Warm-Up Room Etiquette

While much warm-up room etiquette is no different than in any other area of life, there are a few issues specific to weightlifting, and an apparent need to reiterate even things that may seem obvious.

First and foremost, be polite and respectful. Whether you're a first time competitor or a veteran, there is no better way to establish a bad reputation that will follow you forever in the sport than by being rude and disrespectful to other lifters, coaches or officials. Showing some basic courtesy is not difficult—say your pleases and thank yous and don't act like anyone knows who you are, should know who you are, or owes you anything.

Warm-up rooms can get very crowded and hectic. No one likes this situation any more than you do, so don't act like you're the only one put out by it. It's traditional to reserve a warm-up platform by placing a chair on it—if you see this, respect it. Someone was there before you. If you're not sure if someone is using a particular platform, ask.

On the other hand, if you reserve a platform with a chair or training bag and disappear, don't be surprised if someone is using the platform when you return. Explain to them the convention and then be gracious about either sharing with them or moving to a different platform. The best course of action with regard to reserving a platform is to post a coach or someone else on it who can be there when someone else wanders over and wants the platform.

Another issue with crowded warm-up rooms is that there will very likely be a shortage of equipment—most commonly change plates. You will possibly have to share certain plates with other lifters from other platforms. Never steal weights from another platform—ask. Other lifters and coaches will be more than willing to let you use them as long as you're polite about it. They'll also tell you when you can use them without interfering with a lifter's warm-up timing. Always return borrowed plates as soon as you're done with them.

On the subject of sharing, it's inevitable at meets that you'll have to share a platform with another lifter, and possibly more than one. This is not ideal and can make warming up complicated, but keep in mind that you're not the only one who doesn't like it—the other lifters and coaches don't want to share a platform with you any more than you want to share one with them. Make the best of an unavoidable situation and cooperate to keep everyone's warm-ups as smooth and timely as possible. Communicate with the other coaches and lifters with regard to timing—if you need to take your next lift before the other lifter, speak up.

As in any other training situation, do your best not to walk or stand in front of an athlete who is taking a lift. If it's obviously a very light weight, don't worry too much about it, but otherwise, either stop and wait for the lift, or walk behind the platform if you can. Also be sure you're not standing in the way of a lifter trying to lift, and as much as possible, walk around platforms instead of over them.

Similarly, be respectful of the lifters and coaches with regard to noise and general distraction. You or your lifter may not currently be in need of focusing for a lift, but chances are someone else is. Keep your noise to a reasonable level and be aware of what's going on around you.

Don't bring an entourage into the warm-up room. There is very likely limited space already—your five friends don't need to be back there with you taking up space and making noise. They can go sit out with the crowd and cheer you on from there.

Always leave chairs and sitting space for the lifters. If you're not lifting, stand up and get out of the way. Don't steal chairs from other platforms either—just like with equipment, ask first.

Take care of the equipment. More often than not,

the equipment at a meet is being loaned by coaches and gyms for the event, and these people get nothing in return. The least you can do is be respectful of the gear and not go out of your way to destroy it.

Once you or your lifter begins, be aware of how you act with the officials and other coaches. Again, most of this is common courtesy and simply being polite. Say please and thank you when making changes with the marshals. Don't chew out a marshal or official for being slow to respond or making a mistake—they're juggling a million things and doing their best. If they've made a mistake, point it out and help them correct it.

Declare your or your lifter's next attempt promptly. Technically you have 30 seconds to do so, but dragging it out unnecessarily just makes everyone else's life more difficult and slows the competition. Unless it's necessary for a specific strategic move, just get it done.

On the subject of strategy, use it wisely and reasonably. This largely means that jockeying and tricks with attempt declarations and changes should be reserved for lifters who are genuinely in the mix for medals, records, or similar and for whom such things are legitimately helpful. If you or your lifter are duking it out for 18th place, be reasonable and don't mess with other lifters' warm-ups by misleading people with low opening attempts or unnecessary weight changes. Along these same lines, if another coach asks you what you or your lifter is going to declare next so they can better time their own warm-ups, tell them if it's not going to hurt your own lifter—if it's a lifter competing directly with your own for placing, obviously you shouldn't share your plan and you can politely decline to provide the information.

Pay attention to where you're standing during the meet. If you're not actively looking at the cards or scoreboard, move out of the way so other coaches can get a view. Likewise, don't block walkways coaches and lifters need to be moving through to get to the competition platform.

At national level meets, there will be athlete introductions on the competition platform at the start of each session. Be prepared for this with your warm-ups, but also so you don't hold up the process for everyone else because you're not paying attention or ready to line up.

Platform Etiquette

Competition platform etiquette, like warm-up room etiquette, is largely just common sense and basic sportsmanship on the part of both athletes and coaches. Show the other participants respect and behave respectably, and you'll receive respect in return. As was mentioned earlier, a single display of disrespect or poor sportsmanship can and will follow you for an entire career.

Whether you're the best or the worst, behave in a way that represents yourself, your coach, your team and the sport well. Don't make excessive displays on the platform—let your lifts speak for you. Great lifting can quickly and easily be forgotten if accompanied by juvenile, disrespectful behavior.

Remember that you are one of many lifters in a given meet—don't linger on the platform after your lift and delay the competition.

Step onto the stage or platform only after being called by the announcer and wait for the previous lifter to get off—make sure you give that lifter space to do so as well.

Respect the judges' and/or jury's decisions. Arguing or throwing a tantrum like a whiny child has never once resulted in a change of call, and never will. The only thing it can accomplish is creating a reputation for yourself as a lifter or coach no one respects regardless of the actual lifts you perform.

Never speak ill about other competitors or coaches at the meet. You can prove your superiority with the performances on the platform if that's your goal. If you have a problem with given lifters or coaches, bring it to their attention at the appropriate time.

Coaches need to observe the same basic rules as their athletes. Aside from damaging your own reputation in the sport, you're damaging all of your athletes' reputations with poor behavior. Along the same lines, as a coach it's your responsibility to teach your athletes how to behave properly in competition and to enforce that behavior.

As a coach, mind your business, which is your own athletes and their performances. Don't interfere with other lifters unless they come to you and expressly ask for help. If an athlete obviously is without a coach, feel free to offer to help warm him or her up if you're able, but stay out of other coaches' ways. It doesn't matter whether or not you agree with how they're doing things—it's their responsibility.

While it doesn't fall into the category of etiquette, a final word on coaching is warranted here. Avoid over-coaching your lifters in competition. It's far too late to teach them anything with regard to lift technique by the time you arrive at a meet. All you can do is remind your lifters of things you've already taught them with judiciously-metered and properly-timed cues. Just like you can't overwhelm a lifter with information in the gym, the lifter can only handle so much in competition, and arguably far less than in the gym. Competition is the time for a lifter to demonstrate what he or she knows and has practiced, not to learn how to lift. Save the lessons for after the competition is completed.

Appendix

Progression Summaries

Breathing & Trunk Stabilization

Relax the abdominal muscles.

Initiate the breath through the nose and fill the trunk with air from the bottom up.

Tighten the trunk musculature circumferentially without drawing the abs in excessively.

The Squat

Place the heels slightly outside hip-width with toes turned out comfortably.

Sit the hips down and relax in the bottom position, adjusting the foot position until the thighs are parallel with the feet and the hips comfortable.

Stand, arch the entire back and pressurize the trunk, and squat slowly to maximal depth with the back remaining arched and the torso upright.

Keep the feet flat and the weight balanced over the front edge of the heels.

Foot Transition

Start with the feet approximately under the hips and turned out comfortably

Weight slightly more on the heels than the balls of the feet

Rise to the balls of the feet and then quickly lift and move the feet to the squat position, landing flat-footed.

Initially land in quarter-squat depth

On each subsequent transition, land in a deeper squat until finally transitioning into a full squat as quickly as possible.

Snatch Grip

Take a wide grip on the bar using the hook grip.

Stand tall and adjust the hands until the bar contacts the crease of the hips just above the pubic bone.

Adjust from this starting point to accommodate unusual proportions as needed.

Snatch Overhead Position

Squeeze the upper inside edges of the shoulder blades together forcefully.

Squeeze the elbows forcefully in full extension.

Orient the bony points of the elbows approximately halfway between down and back.

Allow the hand and wrist to settle in with a relatively loose grip, keeping the bar in the palm slightly behind the middle of the forearm.

Keep the head up and pushed forward slightly through the arms.

Keep the barbell vertically above the base of the neck.

Overhead Squat

Lock the barbell into the proper snatch overhead position.

Place the feet into the proper squat stance.

Pressurize and stabilize the trunk.

Squat by bending at the knees and hips together to maintain an upright posture.

To recover, push up on the bar and follow it with the body, maintaining the upright posture.

Pressing Snatch Balance

Start with the feet in the receiving position and the bar behind the neck.

Hold the bar with a snatch grip and squeeze the upper inside edges of the shoulder blades together.

Pressurize and stabilize the trunk.

Slowly press against the bar as you squat straight down.

Lock the elbows into the final overhead position as you reach the bottom of the squat.

Recover to the standing position with the bar locked tightly overhead.

Drop Snatch

Start with the feet in the pulling position and the bar behind the neck.

Hold the bar with a snatch grip and squeeze the upper inside edges of the shoulder blades together.

Pressurize and stabilize the trunk.

Lift the feet and punch against the bar to push yourself down into a squat.

Lock the elbows into the final overhead position at the same time your feet reconnect flat with the floor.

Recover to the standing position with the bar locked tightly overhead.

Heaving Snatch Balance

Start with the feet in the receiving position and the bar behind the neck.

Hold the bar with a snatch grip and squeeze the upper inside edges of the shoulder blades together.

Pressurize and stabilize the trunk.

Bend at the knees smoothly and drive with the legs up against the bar enough to unweight it without elevating it significantly.

As the bar moves up, punch against the bar to push yourself down into a squat, keeping your feet flat on the floor.

Lock the elbows into the final overhead position and sit into the bottom of the squat as quickly as possible.

Recover to the standing position with the bar locked tightly overhead.

Snatch Balance

Start with the feet in the pulling position and the bar behind the neck.

Hold the bar with a snatch grip and squeeze the upper inside edges of the shoulder blades together.

Pressurize and stabilize the trunk.

Bend at the knees smoothly and drive with the legs up against the bar enough to unweight it without elevating it significantly.

As the bar moves up, lift and transition your feet into the receiving position, landing flat.

As the feet move, punch against the bar to push yourself down into a squat, trying to lock the bar out overhead at the same time the feet reconnect with the floor.

Recover to the standing position with the bar locked tightly overhead.

Snatch Mid-Hang Position

The feet are in the pulling position with the weight balanced over the front edge of the heel.

The shins are approximately vertical.

The knees are bent slightly, and the back is set tightly in continuous extension with the trunk pressurized.

The shoulders are slightly in front of the bar and knees.

The bar is held in light contact at the mid-thigh.

The arms are long and loose with the elbows turned to point to the sides.

The head and eyes are directed forward.

Mid-Hang Snatch Jump

Start in the mid-hang position with the weight properly balance over the front edge of the heel.

With no countermovement, jump vertically as high as possible.

Keep the bar in light contact with the body throughout the movement.

Mid-Hang Snatch Pull

Start in the mid-hang position with the bar hook-gripped at snatch-width.

Push against the ground aggressively with the legs, using the lats and shoulders to keep the bar in immediate proximity to the thighs.

Reach the final extended position with the legs vertical and the shoulders slightly behind the hips.

Actively push the bar back into light contact with the hips.

Shrug the shoulders up to allow the bar to continue traveling momentarily without swinging forward.

Do not prolong this extended position.

Tall Muscle Snatch

Stand tall with the bar at arms' length, the elbows turned out, and the weight balanced over the front edge of the heel.

Pull the elbows as high as possible and to the sides and squeeze the shoulder blades back, shrugging naturally with this movement and keeping the bar as close to the body as possible.

As the elbows reach maximal height, rotate the arms to bring the bar overhead, keeping the bar close to the face.

As the bar is turned over, release the hook grip quickly and let the hands and wrists settle into the correct overhead position.

Punch up vertically against the bar and secure the overhead position aggressively.

Scarecrow Snatch

Begin standing tall with a snatch-width grip on the bar, the elbows elevated as high as possible and out to the sides, and the bar in light contact with the body.

Simultaneously lift and move the feet into the receiving position and turn the bar over into the overhead position to move down into a squat.

Lock the bar out overhead at the same time the feet reconnect flat with the floor.

Recover to standing with the bar held securely overhead.

Tall Snatch

Begin standing tall with a snatch-width grip on the bar, and the bar hanging at arms' length in light contact with the body.

Simultaneously lift and move the feet into the receiving position and pull the elbows up and out, then turn the bar over into the overhead position to move down into a squat.

Lock the bar out overhead at the same time the feet reconnect flat with the floor.

Recover to standing with the bar held securely overhead.

Mid-Hang Snatch

Begin in the mid-hang position with a snatch-width grip.

Initiate the movement by pushing with the legs against the floor.

Maintain the bar's proximity to the body with the lats and shoulders.

Snap the hips open and continue to drive with the legs to achieve complete extension with the legs vertical, shoulders slightly behind the hips and bar against the hips, naturally moving up onto the balls of the feet.

Lift the feet and pull the elbows as high as possible and to the sides to move down, maintaining the bar's proximity to the body.

Turn the bar over and lock it in the overhead position at the same time the feet reconnect flat with the floor.

Recover to a standing position with the bar secured aggressively overhead.

Snatch Starting Position

Place the barbell over approximately the balls of the foot.

Turn the feet out slightly and balance the weight evenly across them.

Hold the bar with the hook grip at snatch-width.

Assume an upright posture that orients the arms approximately vertically when viewed from the side.

Pressurize the trunk and fix the back securely in a continuous arch.

Keep the head up with a focal point straight ahead or slightly above.

Push the knees outward inside the arms and over the bar.

Internally rotate the arms and keep them passively extended.

Snatch Segment Deadlift

Set the starting position tightly and hold momentarily.

Push with the legs to separate the bar from the floor 1 inch and pause for 3 seconds.

Push with the legs and shift the weight back to the front edge of the heel to bring the bar to the kneecap, maintaining a similar back angle, and hold for 3 seconds.

Push with the legs to move into the mid-hang position and hold for 3 seconds, maintaining balance over the front edge of the heel.

Return the bar to the floor at a controlled speed, trying to move through the same correct positions on the way down.

Halting Snatch Deadlift

Set the starting position tightly and hold momentarily.

Push with the legs to separate the bar from the floor smoothly.

Maintain approximately the same back angle and shift the weight to the front edge of the heels as the bar moves toward the knees.

Continue pushing with the legs, maintaining the balance over the front edge of the heel, and allow the shoulders to move forward slightly to reach the mid-hang position.

Hold the mid-hang position for 3 seconds.

Return the bar to the floor at a controlled speed, trying to move through the same correct positions on the way down.

Segment Snatch + Snatch

Set the starting position tightly and hold momentarily.

Perform a halting snatch deadlift to the mid-hang position and hold for 3 seconds.

Directly from this pause position, perform a mid-hang snatch.

Return the bar from the floor and reset the starting position.

Perform a snatch with no pause, but keep the lift from the floor

to mid-thigh slow to ensure correct positions, balance & timing.

Snatch

Set the starting position tightly and hold momentarily.

Initiate the lift by pushing with the legs against the floor.

Shift the weight back to the front edge of the heel by the time the bar reaches knee height.

Continue pushing with the legs until reaching the mid-hang position, maintaining the balance over the front edge of the heel.

Execute the final upward explosion by pushing with the legs against the ground and extending the hips aggressively, actively maintaining the proximity of the bar to the body.

As you reach the final extended position with the legs vertical, bar against the hips, and shoulders slightly behind the hips, lift the feet and pull the elbows high and out.

Keep the bar as close to the body as possible, turn the arms over and bring the bar into the overhead position, locking it out at the same time the feet land flat on the floor in the receiving position.

Continue sitting into the bottom of the squat fluidly with the bar secured tightly overhead.

Recover to a standing position by pushing straight up against the bar and following it with your body.

Clean Grip

Hold the bar half a fist-width outside the shoulders or slightly more with the hook grip.

Adjust from this starting point to accommodate unusual proportions as needed.

Clean Rack Position

Hold the bar in a clean-width grip.

Extend the upper back.

Push the shoulders forward as much as possible and up slightly.

Place the bar in the channel between the throat and the highest point of the shoulders.

Keep as full of a grip around the bar as possible without squeezing tightly.

Elevate the elbows as much as possible without compromising the position of the shoulders or bar.

Front Squat

Secure the bar in the clean rack position.

Place the feet into the proper squat stance.

Pressurize and stabilize the trunk.

Squat by bending at the knees and hips together to maintain an upright posture.

Use the elastic bounce in the bottom to transition and accelerate up.

Push up the shoulders and elbows, maintaining your upright posture as you stand.

Clean Mid-Hang Position

The feet are in the pulling position with the weight balanced over the front edge of the heel.

The shins are approximately vertical.

The knees are bent slightly, and the back is set tightly in complete extension with the trunk pressurized.

The shoulders are slightly in front of the bar and knees.

The bar is held in light contact at the mid-thigh.

The arms are long and loose with the elbows turned to point to the sides.

The head and eyes are directed forward.

Mid-Hang Clean Jump

Start in the mid-hang position with the weight properly balance over the front edge of the heel.

With no countermovement, jump vertically as high as possible.

Keep the bar in light contact with the body throughout the movement.

Mid-Hang Clean Pull

Start in the mid-hang position with the bar hook-gripped at clean-width.

Push against the ground aggressively with the legs, using the lats and shoulders to keep the bar in immediate proximity to the thighs.

Reach the final extended position with the legs vertical and the shoulders slightly behind the hips.

Actively push the bar back into light contact with the hips.

Shrug the shoulders up to allow the bar to continue traveling momentarily without swinging forward.

Do not prolong this extended position.

Clean Segment Deadlift

Set the starting position tightly and hold momentarily.

Push with the legs to separate the bar from the floor 1 inch and pause for 3 seconds.

Push with the legs and shift the weight back to the front edge of the heel to bring the bar to the kneecap, maintaining a similar back angle, and hold for 3 seconds.

Push with the legs to move into the mid-hang position and hold for 3 seconds, maintaining balance over the front edge of the heel.

Return the bar to the floor at a controlled speed, trying to move through the same correct positions on the way down.

Halting Clean Deadlift

Set the starting position tightly and hold momentarily.

Push with the legs to separate the bar from the floor smoothly.

Maintain approximately the same back angle and shift the weight to the front edge of the heel as the bar moves toward the knees.

Continue pushing with the legs, maintaining the balance over the front edge of the heel, and allow the shoulders to move forward slightly to reach the mid-hang position.

Hold the mid-hang position for 3 seconds.

Return the bar to the floor at a controlled speed, trying to move through the same correct positions on the way down.

Segment Clean + Clean

Set the starting position tightly and hold momentarily.

Perform a halting clean deadlift to the mid-hang position and hold for 3 seconds.

Directly from this pause position, perform a mid-hang clean.

Return the bar from the floor and reset the starting position.

Perform a clean with no pause, but keep the lift from the floor to mid-thigh slow to ensure correct positions, balance and timing.

Clean

Set the starting position tightly and hold momentarily.

Initiate the lift by pushing with the legs against the floor.

Shift the weight back to the front edge of the heel by the time the bar reaches knee height.

Continue pushing with the legs until reaching the mid-hang position, maintaining the balance over the front edge of the heel.

Execute the final upward explosion by pushing with the legs against the ground and extending the hips aggressively, actively maintaining the proximity of the bar to the body.

When complete extension is reached with the legs vertical, bar against the upper thigh, and shoulders slightly behind the hips, lift the feet and pull the elbows high and out.

Keep the bar as close to the body as possible, turn the arms over and secure the bar in the rack position at the same time the feet land flat on the floor in the receiving position.

Continue sitting into the squat fluidly and rebound immediately from the bottom.

Recover to a standing position by leading with the head, shoulders and elbows to maintain bar security and upright posture.

38 Progression Summary / Page 200
Jerk Grip

Hold the bar half a fist-width outside the shoulders or slightly more with no hook grip.

Adjust from this starting point to accommodate unusual proportions as needed.

39 Progression Summary / Page 200
Jerk Overhead Position

Squeeze the top inside edges of the shoulder blades together forcefully.

Squeeze the elbows forcefully in full extension.

Allow the hand and wrist to settle in with a relatively loose grip, keeping the bar in the palm slightly behind the middle of the forearm.

Keep the head up and pushed forward slightly through the arms.

Keep the barbell vertically above the base of the neck.

40 Progression Summary / Page 202
Jerk Split Position

Stand in a partial lunge position with the weight balanced between the feet.

The front foot should be straight forward or turned in slightly and flat on the floor.

The rear foot should be turned in slightly to align it with the lower leg, the heel elevated, and the pressure on the balls of the foot.

The width of the feet should be similar to the squat or slightly wider.

The lead shin should be vertical and the thigh at about a 20-40 degree angle relative to the floor.

The trunk should be pressurized and tight and approximately vertical.

41 Progression Summary / Page 205
Jump to Split

Stand tall with the feet under the hips.

Bend slightly at the knees only and drive up in a slight jump.

Keeping your trunk upright, move quickly into the split position to land with equal balance between the feet.

Adjust the position and balance if needed and hold for 3 seconds.

Step a third of the split length back with the front foot, then bring the back foot up to meet it.

42 Progression Summary / Page 206
Jerk Rack Position

Hold the bar in a jerk-width grip.

Extend the upper back.

Push the shoulders forward as much as possible and up slightly.

Place the bar in the channel between the throat and the highest point of the shoulders.

Keep as full of a grip around the bar as possible without squeezing tightly.

Bring the elbows down until slightly in front of the bar and spread them to the sides without changing the shoulder or bar positions.

43 Progression Summary / Page 209
Jerk Dip

The feet are slightly wider than hip width and turned out 10-20 degrees, with the weight primarily on the heels but with full foot contact.

The knees are bent to lower the athlete 8-10% of his or her height.

The knees are pushed out to remain aligned with the feet.

The trunk is vertical with the barbell, hips and ankles remaining in the same vertical plane when viewed from the side.

Press

Stand with the feet in the drive position, the bar secured in the jerk rack position, and the trunk pressurized and tight.

Push the bar slightly back as it leaves the shoulders, spreading the elbows out and under the bar as it rises.

Pull the face back to clear a path for the bar, moving it back through the arms after the bar has passed.

Secure the bar actively in the overhead position.

Push Press

Stand with the feet in the drive position, the bar secured in the jerk rack position, and the trunk pressurized and tight.

Keep the weight balanced primarily on the heels with full foot contact on the floor and the quads tight.

Dip smoothly at the knees to about 8-10% of height and drive back up immediately and aggressively.

As the legs finish extending, keep the knees straight and quickly push the bar up and back off the shoulders with the arms.

Move the head back out of the way of the bar and spread the elbows out and under the bar as it rises.

Bring the head back through the arms and secure the bar tightly

in the correct overhead position.

Tall Power Jerk

Begin standing tall in the drive position, the hands in a jerk-width grip, and the bar pressed to the top of the forehead with the head back out of the way.

Lift and plant the feet quickly into the power receiving position.

As the feet are transitioning, punch against the bar with the arms to push down into quarter-squat depth.

Move the head back through the arms and fix the bar in the proper overhead position forcefully.

Attempt to lock the bar in the overhead position at the same time the feet reconnect with the platform.

Hold the receiving position 3 seconds before recovering to standing with the bar still overhead.

Power Jerk

Begin with the feet in the drive position and the bar secured in the jerk rack position.

Pressurize and stabilize the trunk, settle the balance over the heels with full foot contact with the floor, and keep the knees straight but unlocked.

Dip at the knees only while maintaining connection with the bar, brake quickly, and drive straight up aggressively.

As the legs near complete extension, push against the bar with the arms to begin moving it into the overhead position, moving the head back out of the way.

As the arms push against the bar, lift and move the feet to plant them flat in the power jerk receiving position.

Lock the bar forcefully in the overhead position at a quarter squat depth at the same time the feet reconnect with the platform.

Hold the receiving position aggressively for 3 seconds before standing with the bar still locked tightly overhead.

Split Jerk Behind the Neck

Begin with the feet in the drive position and the bar secured behind the neck with the elbows down.

Pressurize and stabilize the trunk, settle the balance over the heels with full foot contact with the floor, and keep the knees straight but unlocked.

Dip at the knees only while maintaining connection with the bar, brake quickly, and drive straight up aggressively.

As the legs near complete extension, push against the bar with the arms to begin moving it into the overhcad position, moving the head back out of the way.

As the arms push against the bar, lift and move the feet into the split receiving position quickly and aggressively, moving the hips and trunk straight down under the bar.

Lock the bar forcefully in the overhead position at the same time the feet reconnect with the platform.

Hold the receiving position aggressively for 3 seconds before recovering by stepping a third of the way back with the front foot, and then bringing the back foot forward to meet it, with the bar still locked tightly overhead.

Jerk Balance

Begin with the feet in a partial split position approximately two-thirds the length of the full split position and the bar secured in the jerk rack position.

Dip straight down and drive straight back up to accelerate the bar upward.

As the bar leaves the shoulders, keep the back foot planted and lift the front foot to step out into the full split length.

Keep the trunk upright and land in the full split length with equal balance between the two feet.

Punch the bar up into the overhead position and lock it as the front foot reconnects with the floor.

Split Jerk

Begin with the feet in the drive position and the bar secured in the jerk rack position.

Pressurize and stabilize the trunk, settle the balance over the heels with full foot contact with the floor, and keep the knees straight but unlocked.

Dip at the knees only while maintaining connection with the bar, brake quickly, and drive straight up aggressively.

As the legs near complete extension, push against the bar with the arms to begin moving it into the overhead position, moving the head back out of the way.

As the arms push against the bar, lift and move the feet into the split receiving position quickly and aggressively, moving the hips and trunk straight down under the bar.

Lock the bar forcefully in the overhead position at a quarter squat depth at the same time the feet reconnect with the platform.

Hold the receiving position aggressively for 3 seconds before recovering by stepping a third of the way back with the front foot, and then bringing the back foot forward to meet it, with the bar still locked tightly overhead.

Glossary

Absolute Intensity: An objective measure of the difficulty of a lift measured in terms of actual weight (e.g kilograms).

Anthropometry: Also anthropometrics. The proportions of the human body. See brachiomorph, dolichomorph and mesomorph.

Bounce: The bounce is the use of the elastic rebound at the bottom of the squat or clean to recover from the bottom position more easily and with more speed. It is the combination of three elements: the literal bounce of the upper leg off the lower leg, the stretch-shortening reflex in the muscles of the legs and hips, and the elastic whip of the barbell. The bounce should generally be used in training with the clean and front squat to train the reflex and timing.

Brachiomorph: An athlete with a relatively long trunk and short limbs.

Center of Gravity (COG): For the purposes of weightlifting, *center of gravity* may be used interchangeably with *center of mass*. They diverge only when gravity does not act uniformly on an object—in the context of weightlifting, they refer to the same point.

Center of Mass (COM): The point around which an athlete's total mass is equally distributed in all directions. An object will be balanced with the base of support vertically under the center of mass. For the purposes of weightlifting, *center of mass* may be used interchangeably with *center of gravity*.

Center of Pressure (COP): The location of an object's base of support at which the pressure of the object's weight is centered.

Complex: A complex is the combination of two or more distinct exercises into a series. Complexes can be used for technical reasons or for training elements such as speed, explosiveness or strength.

Concentric: The concentric phase of a lift is that during which the acting muscles are contracting. As an example, the concentric phase of the squat is the phase of returning to a standing position from the bottom position.

Consistent Minimum: The minimum weight an athlete is capable of lifting in a given lift in a given period of time when making appropriately heavy or maximal attempts. This is a baseline of ability that measures preparedness.

Dolichomorph: An athlete with relatively short trunk and long limbs.

Double Knee Bend: AKA Scoop, transition. The double knee bend is the temporary cessation of extension and forward movement of the knees during the final explosive extension of the snatch or clean. This is a natural reaction if the position is correct upon initiating the second pull and does not need to be performed intentionally.

Drive Position: The drive position is the position of the feet (stance) during the drive of the jerk.

Dynamic Start: A dynamic start is a method of beginning a pull from the floor (such as in the snatch or clean) in which the athlete moves continuously into the position in which the bar is first separated from the floor; that is, the athlete never sets and holds a starting position before beginning the lift as they would in a static start. This allows the lifter to move the bar from the floor with more speed and less fatigue.

Eccentric: The eccentric phase of a lift is that during which the acting muscles are extending. It is sometimes referred to as the "negative" phase of the lift. As an example, the eccentric phase of the squat is the movement down from the standing position into the bottom position.

First Pull: The first pull of the snatch or clean is the movement of the bar from its starting point on the floor until it reaches approximately mid-thigh, the point at which the final upward explosive effort is initiated.

Floating: *Floating* indicates that the barbell is not allowed to touch the floor between the reps of a set. For example, in a *floating clean pull*, the lifter lowers the bar as close to the floor as possible without allowing the plates to touch in between reps.

Frequency: How often a weightlifter trains, usually expressed in training sessions per week.

Halting: *Halting* refers to pulling exercise variations in which the athlete stops at a point before full extension. For example, in the *halting snatch deadlift*, the lifter will deadlift the bar typically to mid-thigh and hold this position for 2-3 seconds before returning to the floor without ever standing completely.

Hang: Hang refers to a starting position for a lift with the bar above floor level, e.g. hang clean. At what height a hang lift is started needs to specified, such as mid-thigh, knee or below the knee.

Hook Grip: The hook grip is used in the pull of the snatch and clean to ensure a secure grip during the aggressive acceleration of the bar. The lifter first wraps the thumb around the bar, then grips the thumb with usually the first and second fingers and pulls it tightly around the bar.

Intensity: A measure of the difficulty of a lift, measured either in absolute terms (actual weight in kilograms) or relative terms (the percentage that weight represents of the lifter's maximum). May also be expressed subjectively at times as a measure of perceived effort.

Line of Gravity: An imaginary vertical line that passes through the base indicating the balance point of the center of mass; this indicates where over the foot a lifter's weight is balanced as well as where (in terms of fore-aft position usually) the center of mass is located.

Mesomorph: A lifter with balanced proportions, i.e. relative trunk and limb lengths. (Also may refer to a balanced body type in terms of muscular development and leanness).

Power Position: The position during the pull of the snatch or clean when the knees have moved forward under the bar during the double knee bend, the bar is in contact with the body, and the trunk is approximately vertical.

Power: (1) The term power refers to a receiving position of the snatch, clean or jerk in a partial squat. Most commonly the cut-off point is a parallel squat—if the lifter receives and stops the bar before squatting below parallel, the lift qualifies as power snatch, power clean or power jerk. It is also sometimes defined as no more than a 90-degree bend in the knees. (2) The combination of strength and speed. Technically defined as force over time; in other words, the movement of heavy weights quickly.

Preparatory Position: The position a lifter assumes once at the barbell, prior to actively setting the starting position. This is a relaxed or semi-relaxed position the lifter habitually holds at least momentarily while focusing and finalizing any pre-lift mental rituals.

Pulling Position: Pulling position refers to the position of the feet (stance) during the pull of the snatch or clean.

Receiving Position: Receiving position refers to the position of the feet (stance) when receiving the snatch, clean or power jerk. It is most often the same as the lifter's squat stance.

Relative Intensity: A measure of the difficulty of a lift measured in terms of the weight's relation to the athlete's maximum, usually single repetition, in that lift, listed as a percentage.

Scoop: AKA transition, double knee bend. The forward movement of the partially-bent knees under the bar during the double knee bend of the snatch or clean.

Second Pull: The second pull of the snatch or clean is the final upward explosive effort of the lift, beginning when the bar reaches approximately mid-thigh and ending with the complete extension of the hips and knees.

Split: The split is the receiving position for the split jerk, which is a partial-depth lunge. Also used in the split snatch and split clean.

Starting Position: The position or posture from which the lifter begins the separation of the barbell from the floor in the snatch or clean.

Static Start: A static start is a method of beginning a pull from the floor (such as in the snatch or clean) in which the athlete sets and holds the starting position at least momentarily before actually lifting the bar from the floor.

Straps: AKA lifting straps. Straps are fabric or leather strips that wrap around the lifter's hands and bar to secure the grip on the bar. Most often used for snatch or clean pulls or deadlifts and snatches from the hang position.

Technical Consistency Threshold: This is the weight (expressed as absolute or relative intensity) of a given lift at which the lifter remains consistent in his/her technical performance—the last point after which technique begins to break down and diverge from ideal. The goal of training is to continually elevate this threshold, both relatively and absolutely.

Technique Primer: This is an exercise performed before a primary exercise to practice and reinforce certain technique points of the primary exercise.

Third Pull: The third pull of the snatch or clean is the movement of the lifter under the bar after the final upward extension.

Warm-up Couplet: Term that describes the use of a technique-reinforcing exercise with a primary exercise in a complex during the warm-up for that primary exercise. Examples would be muscle snatch + snatch, snatch + snatch balance, push press + jerk, etc. This complex would be repeated with progressively increasing weights as the athlete warmed up the primary lift, and then the technique exercise removed once heavier weights were reached.

Index

References

Alexander, J. (2011) *The Alexander Method: The Fundamentals*. Costa Mesa, CA: Network Fitness.

Bompa, Tudor O. (1999) *Periodization: Theory & Methodology of Training*. Champaign, IL: Human Kinetics.

Dvorkin, L.S. (1992) *The Junior Weightlifter*. (A. Charniga, Trans.) Moscow, Russia: Fizkultura i Sport. (Original work published 1982)

Eades, M.R. & Eades M.D. (2001) *The Protein Power Lifeplan*. New York, NY: Grand Central Publishing.

Glyadkovsky, V.S. & Rodionov, V.I. (1992) *Variations of the Dynamic Start for the Snatch*. (A. Charniga, Trans.) Tyazhelaya Atletika. Sbornik Statei. Fizkultura i Sport, Moscow, Russia. (Original work published 1971)

Hatfield, F.C. (1989). *Power: A Scientific Approach*. New York, NY: Contemporary Books.

Israetel, M, Case, J., Hoffmann, J. (2014) *The Renaissance Diet*. Charlotte, NC: Renaissance Periodization.

Kanyevsky, V.B. (1992) *Teaching the Starting Position of the Snatch and the Clean & Jerk to Novice Weightlifters*. (A. Charniga, Trans.) Moscow, Russia: Lenin State Institute of Physical Culture. (Original work published 1982)

Laputin, N.P., Oleshko V.G. (2007) *Managing the Training of Weightlifters*. (A. Charniga, Trans.) Kiev, Russia: Zdorov'ya. (Original work published 1982)

Lorenz, D. (2011) *Postactivation Potentiation: An Introduction*. International Journal of Sports Physical Therapy. 2011 Sep; 6(3): 234–240.

Medvedyev, A.S. (1995) *A Program of Multi-Year Training in Weightlifting*. (A. Charniga, Trans.) Moscow, Russia: Fitzkultura i Sport. (Original work published 1986)

Medvedyev, A.S. (1989) *A System of Multi-Year Training in Weightlifting*. (A. Charniga, Trans.) Moscow, Russia: Fitzkultura i Sport. (Original work published 1986)

Robertson, M. (2008) *Self-Myofascial Release: Purpose, Methods and Techniques*. Indianapolis, IN: Robertson Training Systems.

Takano, B. (2012) *Weightlifting Programming: A Winning Coach's Guide*. Sunnyvale, CA: Catalyst Athletics.

Taubes, G. (2007) *Good Calories, Bad Calories*. New York, NY: Alfred A. Knopf.

Vector Forces. (2011, August 12). Retrieved from http://www.ropebook.com/information/vector-forces

Zatsiorsky, V. (1995) *Science and Practice of Strength Training*. Champaign, IL: Human Kinetics.

Zhekov, I.P. (1992) *Biomechanics of the Weightlifting Exercises*. (A. Charniga, Trans.) Moscow, Russia: Fitzkultura i Sport. (Original work published 1976)

Zhongshan Camry Electronic Co. Ltd (2015) *Camry Hand Dynamometer EH101-17: User Manual*. Guangdong, China: Zhongshan Camry Electronic Co. Ltd.